Bone Disorders

Reiner Bartl • Christoph Bartl

Bone Disorders

Biology, Diagnosis, Prevention, Therapy

With a contribution by
Andrea Baur-Melnyk and Tobias Geith

Springer

Prof. Dr. med. Reiner Bartl
Osteoporosis Center Munich
Kaufingerstr. 15
Munich
Germany

PD Dr. med. Christoph Bartl
ZOOOM (Center of Orthopaedics, Osteoporosis and Sports Medicine, Munich)
Rosa-Bavaresestr. 1
Munich
Germany

With a contribution by

Prof. Dr. med. Andrea Baur-Melnyk and Dr. med. Tobias Geith
Department of Clinical Radiology
University of Munich-Grosshadern
Marchioninistrasse 15
Munich, Germany

All coloured illustrations from Harald Konopatzki, Heidelberg.
All two-coloured and blackline illustrations from Reinhold Henkel†, Heidelberg.

ISBN 978-3-319-29180-2 ISBN 978-3-319-29182-6 (eBook)
DOI 10.1007/978-3-319-29182-6

Library of Congress Control Number: 2016944148

Printed on acid-free paper

This Springer imprint is published by Springer Nature
The registered company is Springer International Publishing AG Switzerland

Preface

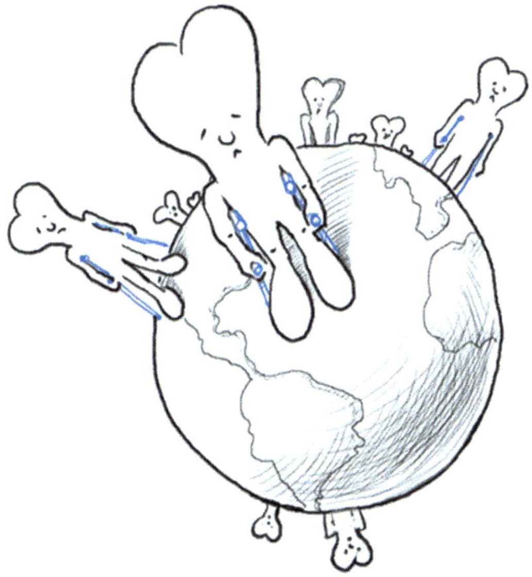

Fig. 1 Bone disorders: a worldwide challenge!

With the dawn of the twenty-first century has come the realisation that bone and joint diseases are the major cause of pain and physical disability worldwide. Moreover, according to the WHO Scientific Group, there are more than 150 diseases and syndromes of musculoskeletal conditions, usually associated with pain and loss of function. It is undoubtedly these insights that prompted the WHO to declare the first 10 years of the new century as "The Bone and Joint Decade 2000–2010". This declaration obviously made a highly significant impact on international, national and medical authorities, as well as on physicians, scientists and citizens worldwide as evidenced by an overwhelming flood (a regular tsunami) of articles, studies and books on the subject in the last few years alone! Not to mention the coverage in newspapers and journals, on the radio and television, and of course all the up-to-date information freely available on the Internet. The number of people suffering from these diseases – already many millions in the developed and underdeveloped countries in the world – is expected to double within the next 20 years. In many countries, this increase will be even greater due to the longer survival and consequently larger numbers of older people in the population. It is therefore inevitable that the

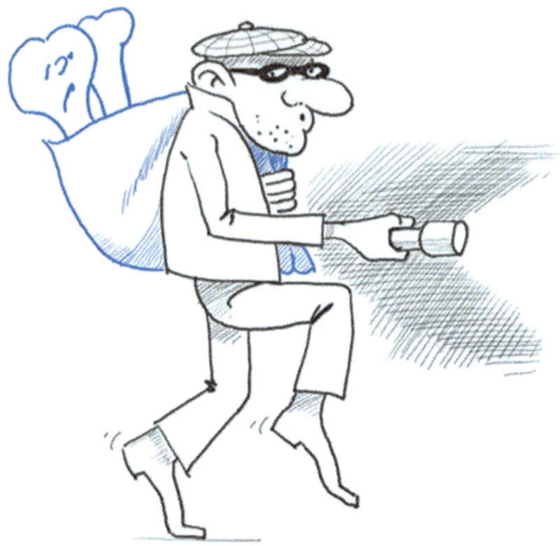

Fig. 2 Osteoporosis: a silent thief!

already astronomical costs of health care will rise proportionally. According to the International Osteoporosis Foundation (NOF), the worldwide incidence of hip fracture is projected to increase by 240 % in women and 310 % in men by 2050, unless appropriate preventive measures will be taken on sufficiently large national and international scales, for which, hopefully, this book will provide a stimulus!

On the positive side, the enormous amount of work, research and study of disorders of bone over the past 10–20 years or so has contributed greatly to our understanding of the causes, treatment and prevention of osteoporosis and other disorders. Most importantly, perhaps, the skeleton is now regarded in a new light, as a dynamic organ undergoing constant renewal throughout life from start to finish, from the cradle to the grave. And what is more: it is now abundantly clear that the skeleton participates, usually not to its advantage, in almost every condition that may affect the organs and tissues in the body! This applies especially to *osteoporosis*, which is now under control!

How did this come about?

- Because of the elucidation of many of the factors involved in osseous remodelling.
- Because of the development of simple, fast, reliable and non-invasive methods for measurement of bone density, and for testing other factors such as mineralisation, trabecular architecture, cortical thickness, and the bone cells themselves.
- Because of the identification of general and individual risk factors, so that appropriate measures can be taken to prevent development of osteoporosis and/or its progression, if and when fractures have already occurred.
- And finally, because effective medication for prevention and therapy is now readily available worldwide.

The efficacy of the classes of compounds known as "bisphosphonates" as well as of the "selective oestrogen receptor modulators" (SERMs) and more

Fig. 3 Be active and be happy!

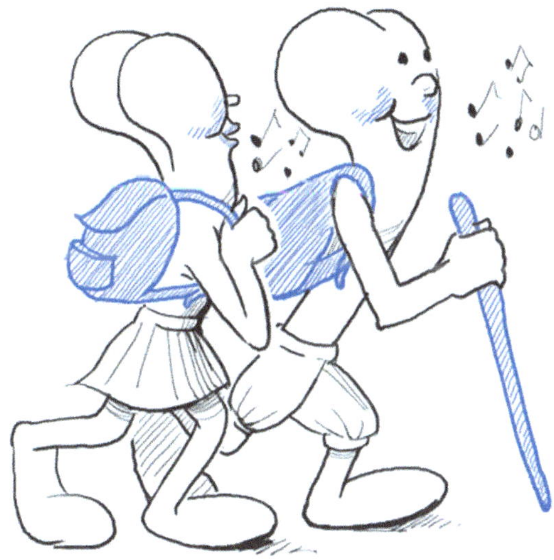

recently of the anabolic parathyroid hormones and denosumab has now been unequivocally established by numerous large multicentre trials involving literally millions of patients. In addition, simple methods such as a healthy lifestyle, adequate nutrition, sufficient physical activity, vitamin D and calcium supplements, as required, can be recommended and adopted on a large scale, beginning with the responsible authorities and reaching to the individual citizens.

Introduction and acceptance of these methods require public awareness and support and the realisation that every individual is the guardian and caretaker of his/her own bones and responsible for their structural and functional integrity. Fortunately, some progress has been made, as shown by the numerous articles recently published from the "four corners of the globe" which unequivocally establish the epidemic proportions of the problem. Well-founded diagnostic techniques and effective therapies – both antiresorptive and osteoanabolic – are now available for prevention, diagnosis and treatment of bone disorders. It should be emphasised that the treatments recommended in this text are all founded on "evidence-based medicine" (unless otherwise stated) for which the appropriate references are given at the end of the text.

The aim of this book is to demonstrate that "Bone is EveryBody's Business" and especially every patient's and doctor's, and to provide guidelines for the diagnosis, therapy and prevention of bone disorders – from paediatrics to geriatrics. It is hoped and anticipated that this book will raise awareness and provide information to anyone seeking it, and especially to doctors across all disciplines concerned with various "bone problems". Clinical osteology is now an independent specialty which nevertheless encompasses all branches of medicine and affects each and every one of us.

Consequently we have adhered stringently to simplicity, comprehensiveness, and to practicality of approach to examinations, methods and implementation of up-to-date testing, to strategies for prevention, to criteria for

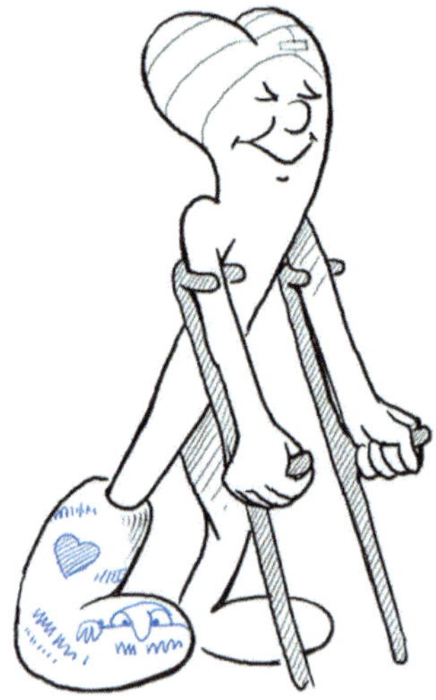

Fig. 4 Fragility fractures: focussing not only on prevention and treatment but also on ways to deal with the personal and social consequences of the disease such as pain, depression, loss of self-esteem and social isolation!

diagnosis, and to presentation of therapeutic possibilities, as well as to our own particular goal which is to keep this text as "user-friendly" as possible, so that any doctor seeking information on a particular topic in bone disorders has uncomplicated and time-saving access to it.

We wish all our readers success in their endeavours to help patients and to reduce suffering in this strife-ridden, beautiful planet of ours!

Munich, Germany

Reiner Bartl
Christoph Bartl

Contents

Part I

Evolution and Biology of Bone

1 Evolution of the Skeleton

1.1 From the Primeval Sea to the Precambrian Period

The earth had existed for about 4500 million years. This corresponds to about a third of the time since the creation. The oldest animal fossils (multicelled) come from the time 500–1000 million years before the evolution of mankind. A dive through the primeval sea about 600 million years ago would be very colourless and unspectacular. Ten million years earlier, the earth had emerged from an ice age which had lasted for many million years with glaciers at the equator. The earth had over many million years the same appearance of the Jupiter moon Europa today, whose whole surface is covered by a very thick layer of ice. Sunlight and therefore photosynthesis was blocked and totally absent. Living organisms had a difficult time, so only the simplest organisms could exist in the oceans. The seafloor was covered by a solid mat of bacteria and along the coasts grew, by the photosynthesis of blue algae, huge chalk towers, "stromatolites". There was no trace of higher, differentiated animals.

On the floor of the ocean along the tectonic plates between the smoking chimneys of the "black smokers" swarmed bizarre life forms. Experts estimate the biomass in these deep sea oases to be many kilogrammes per square metre. The photosynthesis of the vegetation in the coastal areas could not be the basis of the ecosystem in this underworld but was a chemical synthesis of microbes: sulphur-containing bacteria oxidised there in the chimneys giving rise to hydrogen sulphide.

Multicelled organisms first developed in the closing Precambrian period: sponges and Cnidarians, primitive precursors of all modern animal stems. Considerably more complex, mirror invert constructed life forms (bilateralia) developed slowly: these animals had for the first time different tissues, a nervous system, a blood circulation, internal organs, as well as mouth and intestinal openings. In stone, which is more than 550 million years old, hardly any traces of the existence of these animal species can be found. The animals were apparently too small and too soft and did not have a skeleton and thus did not leave any recognisable fossils behind in the rock.

1.2 The "Cambrian Explosion"

Fifty million years later, the picture basically changed: the whole sea swarmed with life forms of many types. At the beginning of the earth epoch Cambrian, 550 million years ago, an unexpected sediment was deposited full of small shells, small teeth and spines. Considering the sheer endless period of more than 3 billion years, in which only the primitive single-cell organisms populated the oceans, an event must now have occurred which was the decisive ignition of this

R. Bartl, C. Bartl, *Bone Disorders*, DOI 10.1007/978-3-319-29182-6_1

"origin of life". This "Cambrian explosion" probably had both internal and external causes:

- *Warming and circulation of the ocean and an increasing oxygen concentration in the atmosphere:* Nourishment-rich deep water flowing to the top and flooding the continental shelf areas with nourishment.
- *Enrichment of the ocean with calcium:* Following the erosion of the primeval continents, huge amounts of calcium and other minerals were spewed into the sea. Calcium in too high concentration is in fact a cell poison; however, the life forms made a virtue out of a danger: they process the calcium into shells and armour – the birth of the outer skeleton (exoskeleton) (Fig. 1.1). At the beginning, the hard shell served as protection against high waves and the movement of currents and marked the start of the "Cambrian radiation (family tree)" with the development of ever more refined skeletons, which guaranteed survival.
- *Development of meat eaters:* The occurrence of the first predators was a considerable catalyst for evolution and it began a continuous armament race between the hunter and the hunted with manifold possibilities through new genealogy: tentacles, spines, fins and eyes. With that came a new order in the evolution of the world: eat or be eaten. Naturally under these conditions, those which could protect themselves with armour had an advantage.
- *Development of armours and shells:* The great amount of calcium and other minerals in the water accelerated the development of a variety of hard parts for protection from the "hunters". Skeletons proved to be the breakthrough in the point of evolution. The storage of calcium carbonate in organic tissue matrix created protective armour: shells and thorns for the "hunted" (Fig. 1.2a, b), but also new types of hunting tools like teeth and claws for the "hunters" (Fig. 1.3). The hard parts of the animals from the time of the "Cambrian explosion", a geological short period of only 10–20 million years, are found in the basins of the former seas as metre-thick sediment layers.

The Cambrian ocean proved to be the "playground of evolution" with the development of remarkable creatures. The earliest life form, which used the high concentration of minerals in the ocean, is *Cloudina*, a 1.5 cm small, elongated creature, which successfully protected itself against enemies by the production of tubes in which it lived. The predominant part of these creatures died out, but some of them which could win through, were the predecessors of all animals which populate the earth today. Biologically successful models of them like the *Monoplacophora*, a primitive predecessor of the snail have survived almost unchanged for 450 million years. For example, *Neopilina* can be found as a living fossil at a depth of 3000 m in the Pacific. Also today there are still creatures with a suitable outer skeleton, which are encased with a shell or armour, for instance, mussels, insects or spiders.

1.3 Development of the External Skeleton

Only a few creatures like the jelly fish (Cnidarians) exist completely without body support; however, with the deployment of strong poisons, they have developed other strategies for defence. A great disadvantage for animals with armour or shells lies in the lesser movement and in the lesser

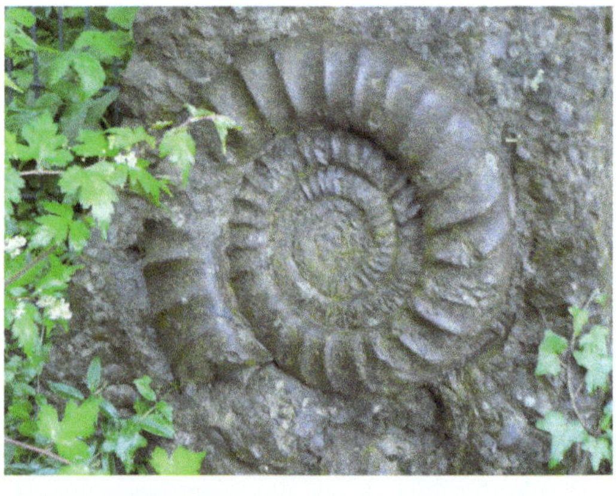

Fig. 1.1 Fossilisation of a huge ammonite, a cuttlefish fossil which died out at the end of the chalk age with 4–12 turns of rolled chalk housing. Ammonites had a diameter from 2 to 200 cm with many separating walls and gas-filled chambers

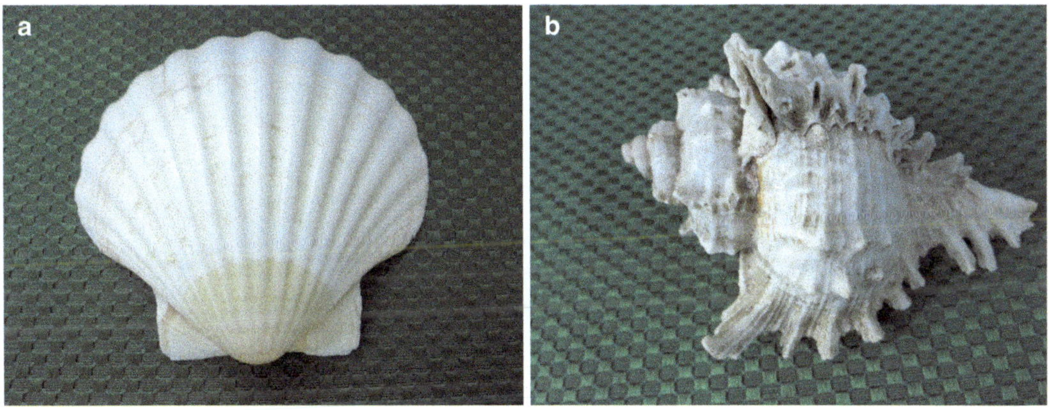

Fig. 1.2 (**a**, **b**) Two variants of exoskeletons: examples of effective shells, beautiful in their shapes

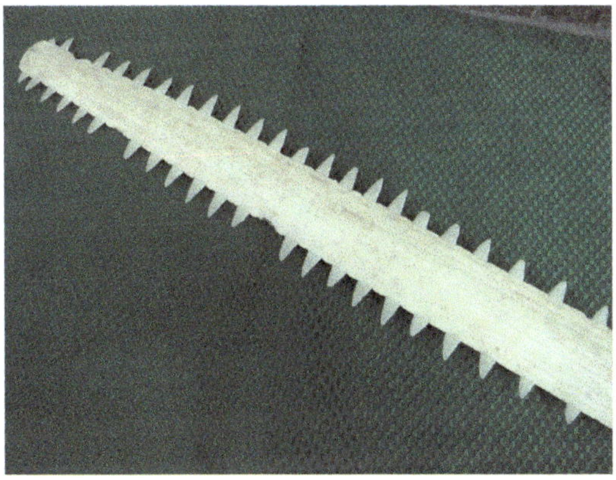

Fig. 1.3 Variant of a hunting tool, with numerous teeth

potential for escape against the increasingly faster emergent hunters. An important development produced powerful muscles, which joined the body of snails with the shells. At time of danger, they were able to retreat into the protective chamber. The hinged connection between shell and muscle enabled a rearward movement and further mobility. One animal group surpassed all others on diversity with the help of an ingenious muscular-skeletal system and its segmentation: the arthropod. All insects, crustaceans, spiders and millipedes descend from them. The ingenious mixture of calcium, protein and carbohydrate, known as chitin, allowed the construction of different organs such as tentacles, claws, pincers and masticatory organs. But the exterior skeleton of the arthropod had one great disadvantage: it constricted the animal in a stiff corset and did not allow any further growth. The act of "skinning" meant a deadly failure in development in the dangerous underwater world.

1.4 Development of the Internal Skeleton

Animals with an inner skeleton, a structure of cartilage, bones or a combination of both, are fishes, amphibians, birds and mammals. The successor of the chordate, today's vertebrates, moved the supporting exterior skeleton (*exoskeleton*) to inside (*endoskeleton*), developed an ingenious muscle system and gained thereby a considerably higher movement capability. The act of switching from an external to an internal skeleton brought a decisive advantage for the development of the movement apparatus and enlarged the radius of action. The speed of movement was decisive for survival and thereby the driver for further evolution. The growth of the life forms was also no longer limited.

1.5 Calcium Phosphate: The New Building Material

A further step in the development of a stable but light internal skeleton (Endoskeleton) and for movement lies in the chemical situation: the hard parts built of calcium carbonate were replaced by crystalline calcium phosphate. In the seawater and on the land, huge quantities of the mineral calcium complex with pyrophosphate were deposited. Pyrophosphates were split by enzymes into phosphates. This highly insoluble calcium phosphate, in the form of *hydroxylapatite* $Ca_{10}(PO_4)_6\,(OH)_2$, was stored in the newly developed bone matrix (Fig. 1.4). This building material consisted of collagen and, a few nanometres larger, calcium phosphate crystals. In comparison to the nonelastic, brittle and readily soluble calcium carbonate of the shelled creatures, it was firmer, more elastic and more acid resistant – the ideal building material for the demands of lightweight construction.

1.6 Development of the Backbone

About 500 million years ago, a small, inconspicuous and primeval fish appeared, which in the survival struggle no longer had an armour, but had built a simple pliable support rod out of connective tissue in the interior of the body. This made it an especially fast and nimble swimmer. From this rod gradually developed the jointed backbone, at the start out of cartilage, later of bone (*Chondrichthyes* and *Osteichthyes*). On the vertebrae followed bones, e.g. ribs, which protected the body and offered further muscle support. Alongside the optimisation of movement, a bony jaw emerged in the area of gill, with which the fish could grip and crush their prey. A few species became the largest predators of the oceans: the great sharks weighing several tons.

1.7 Invasion of the Dry Land

After the divide of the Silurian/Devonian periods, the plants increasingly inhabited the dry land, and in their wake, animal organisms also followed. Towards the end of the Devonian period

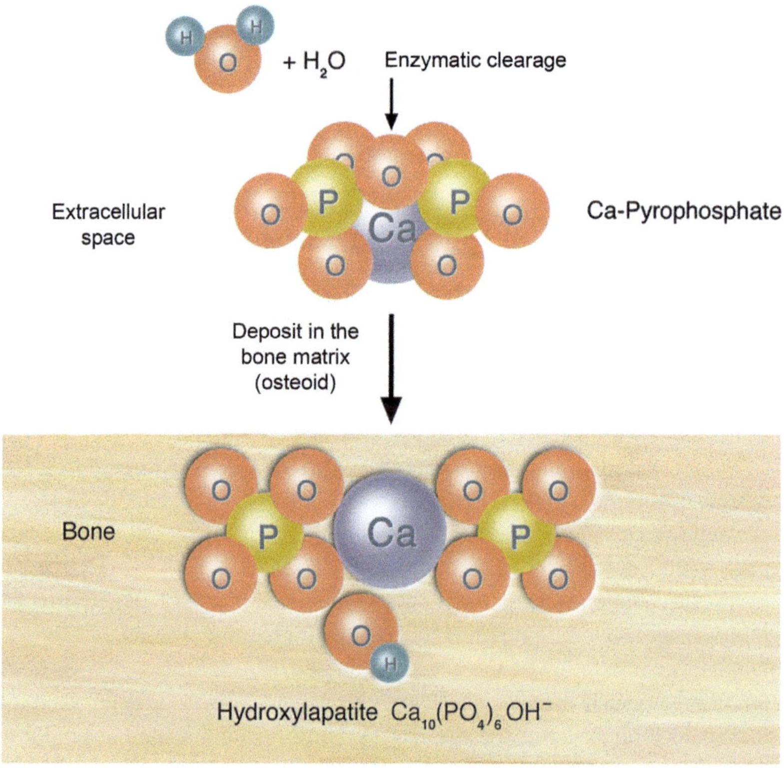

Fig. 1.4 Enzymatic splitting of calcium pyrophosphate in the extracellular space and formation of crystalline calcium phosphate in the form of hydroxylapatite in the bone matrix

(about 350 million years ago), the amphibians separated from the bony fish group and began to move to the dry land (Fig. 1.5). The reptiles which developed from them became the main type of vertebrate from the carboniferous period. The loading on the bones, caused by the gravity on land, placed particular demands on their capacity, but was overcome by diverse innovations relating to lightweight construction: the "spongification and lamination" of the bone construction. Additionally the development of core cavities provided space for blood formation, for the marrow.

The next development period, the dinosaurs were the lords of the earth, until the end of the chalk age (about 60 million years ago). The *Ankylosaurus* protected itself with thick bone plates on its skin (the principle of the impregnable castle against meat eaters). This armament developed in the first year of life and utilised enormous quantities of calcium and phosphate. Palaeontologists from Bonn (Germany) could recently show that the armoured dinosaurs used their long skeletal bones as a mineral source and probably in their youth suffered periodically from strong bone shrinkage. As soon as the armour was complete, the bones at the extremities were again strengthened.

Before the abrupt extinction of the dinosaurs, a bird developed on the model of especially lightweight bones (the principle of elastic, load-bearing spongy bones). The triumphant march of the predatory animals, which remains to today, began with the extinction of the dinosaur about 60 million year ago.

1.8 Bone and Blood Formation

Further progress in the evolution of the skeleton produced the combination of blood formation and bones. The bone marrow finds protection in

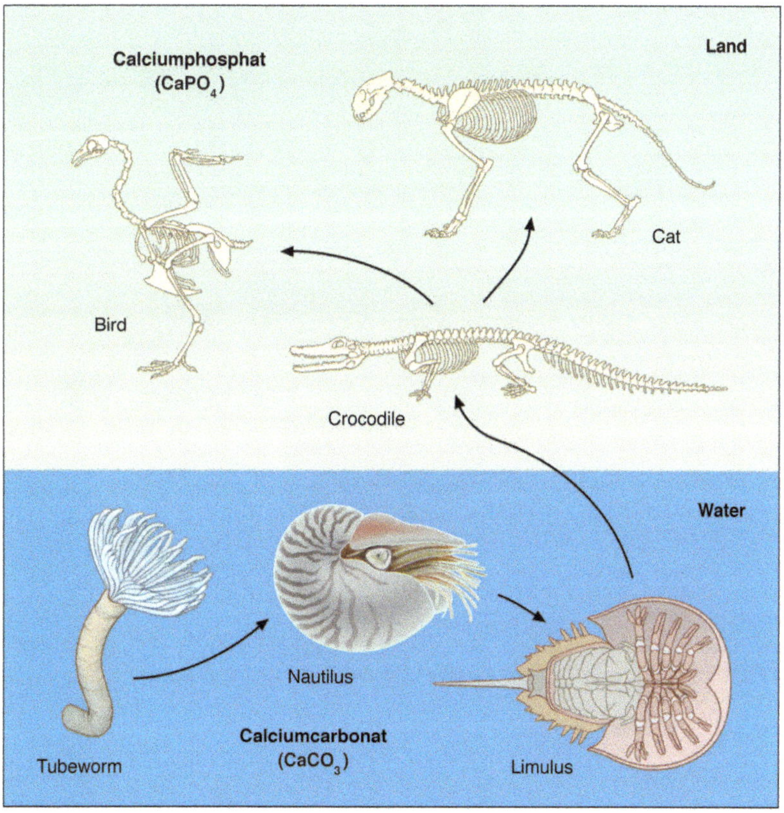

Fig. 1.5 Evolution of the skeleton, from tubeworms to mammals

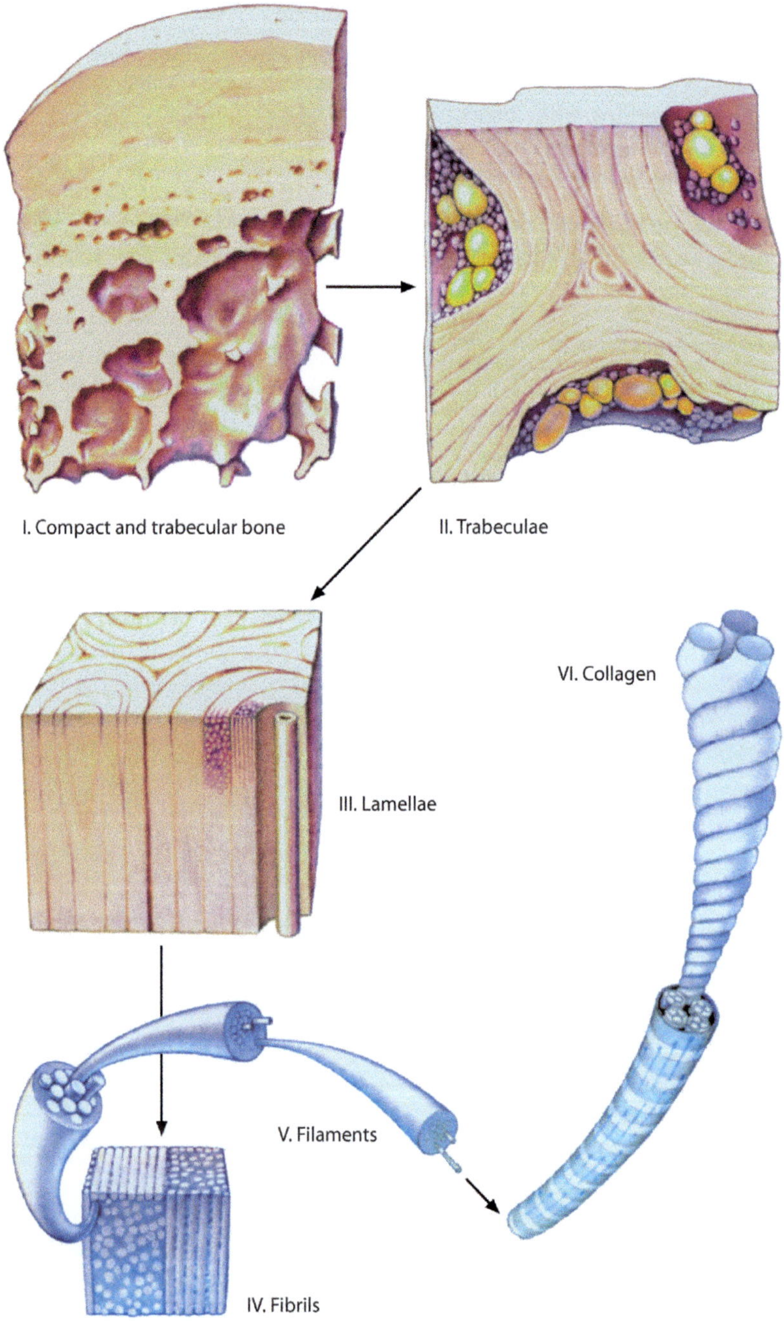

Fig. 1.6 Organisational levels of bone structure, which ensure both flexibility and rigidity of the skeleton: from macroscopic via microscopic to molecular levels

many spongy cavities of the skeleton; on the other hand, important bone cells are recruited direct from the bone marrow (osteoclasts from the haematopoietic stem cells and osteoblasts from the stroma cells), so that one correctly speaks about a functional anatomical unit, the "bone-bone marrow system". The continually running bone rebuilding ("modelling and remodelling") and the fracture healing would not be thinkable without recruitment of haematopoietic cells and without blood supply from the neighbouring bone marrow.

1.9 The Human Skeleton

These stages of the development of life in water and on the earth are substantiated by fossil finds. Thereby the impressive chronology of the development of the intelligent inner skeleton from simple exterior shells and armour can be understood in the fossilisation. The current modern skeleton of the predatory animals combines on one side through its strength and flexibility (resistance against the omnipresent gravity), on the other side through its low weight (advantage for movement and fast locomotion). This occurs in particular in the skeleton of a bird, through the refinement of its light construction, which first enabled flight.

The current modern human skeleton, in all structure orders – from molecular via microscopic and to the macroscopic levels – which took place over more than 500 million years of continual development, is a masterpiece of bio-architecture (Figs. 1.6 and 1.7).

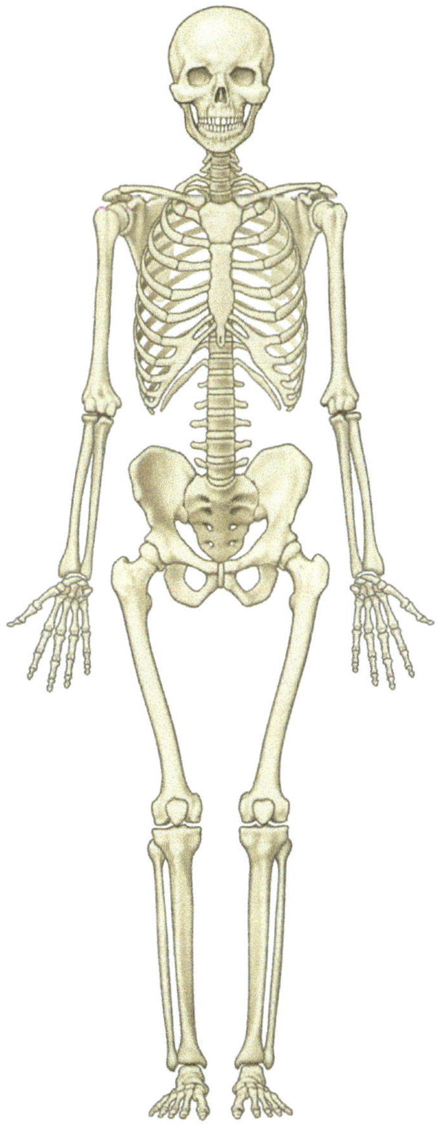

Fig. 1.7 The adult human skeleton – a masterpiece of architecture. It comprises about 210 individual bones, each of which is sculpted by the process of "modelling" and constantly renewed by the process of "remodelling". It has a total weight of about 10 kg (minerals 50–70 %, organic matrix 20–40 %, water 5–10 % and fats 3 %) and contains 15 % of the body weight

2 Structure and Architecture of Bone

The human skeleton has 204–214 individual bones; it weighs about 10 kg and accounts for about 15 % of the body weight. A rough breakdown differentiates the skeleton of the trunk (trunk or axial skeleton) from the skeleton of the extremities (peripheral skeleton). The skeleton includes the following bones:

- 29 cranial bones (including 6 in the auditory canal)
- 28–32 bones in the vertebral column
- 25 in the ribcage
- 4 in the shoulder girdle
- 2 hip bones
- 60–62 in the upper and
- 60 in the lower extremity

2.1 Function of the Skeleton

Bone has five main tasks to fulfil:

- *Support and locomotion:* of the body as a whole and of its individual components, e.g. from the smallest, the toes, to the largest, the legs and the spine.
- *Protection:* the skeleton protects internal organs from possible harmful outside effects. For example, the ribs shelter the heart and lungs; the cranial bones protect the brain.
- *Storehouse for minerals:* the skeleton is the largest depot for minerals in the body. 99 % of the calcium, 85 % of the phosphate and 50 % of magnesium are stored in the bones. Approximately 1–1.5 kg of calcium is built into the skeleton in the form of hydroxyapatite.
- *Storehouse for bone matrix proteins:* the mineralised bone substance consists of about 50 % organic material – 25 % matrix (ground substance) and 25 % water. The matrix contains 90 % collagen type I and 10 % other proteins such as glycoprotein, osteocalcin, osteonectin, bone sialoprotein, osteopontin, fibronectin as well as various proteoglycans. All these proteins are synthesised and secreted by osteoblasts and have a variety of functions, such as seeding crystal formation, binding calcium crystals and serving as sites for attachment of bone cells. Collagen also has direct effects on important bone cell functions including apoptosis, cell proliferation and differentiation, which are under complex control from the cell surface to the nucleus. Although collagen may have less effect on bone strength and stiffness than mineral does, it may still have a profound effect on bone fragility. Collagen changes that occur with age and reduce bone toughness or stiffness may be an important factor in the risk of fracture. Bone matrix also contains proteins such as bone morphogenetic proteins (BMPs), thrombospondin-2 and metalloproteinases that stimulate or inhibit the actions of bone cells. Some studies have

R. Bartl, C. Bartl, *Bone Disorders*, DOI 10.1007/978-3-319-29182-6_2

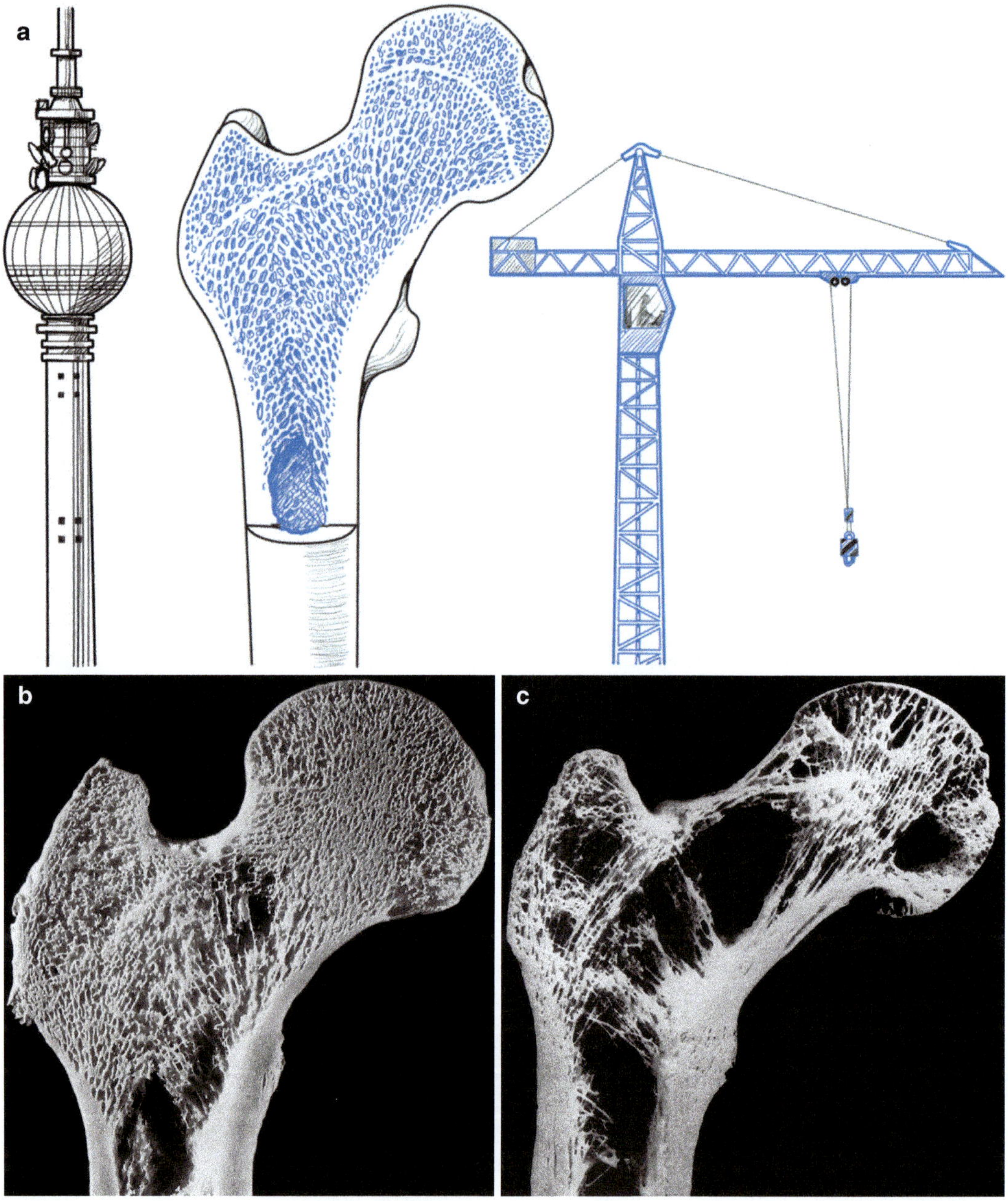

Fig. 2.1 (**a**) Architectural organisation of femoral head, neck and shaft, combining the two principles of construction for maximal weight-bearing: tubular structure illustrated by the television tower and trabecular structure by the crane. (**b**) Normal cortical and trabecular structure of the proximal femur (With kind permission of Springer, from [28]). (**c**) Proximal femur of a patient with severe osteoporosis. Note destruction of the trabecular (trajectorial) network indicating a high fracture risk (With kind permission of Springer, from [28])

shown that bone also contains growth factors and cytokines, such as TGF β1.

- *Endocrine regulation of energy* by means of mechanisms involving leptin and osteocalcin, by which glucose levels in the serum as well as adiposity are both affected: in this context, it is clear that the processes involved in energy balance influence many organs and tissues,

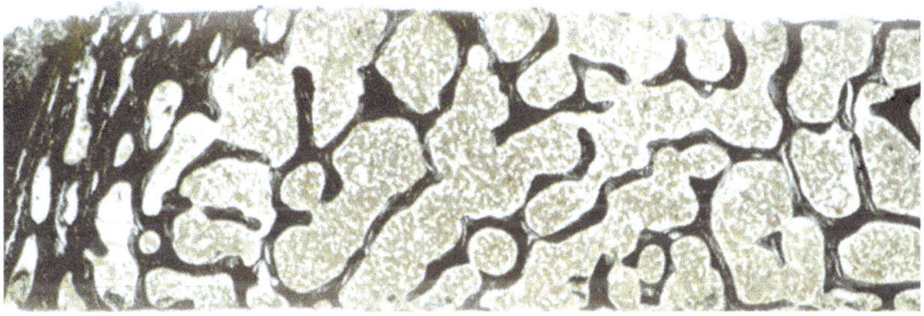

Fig. 2.2 Overview of section of normal bone biopsy of middle-aged man showing wide cortex and uniform, connected trabeculae. Gomori staining

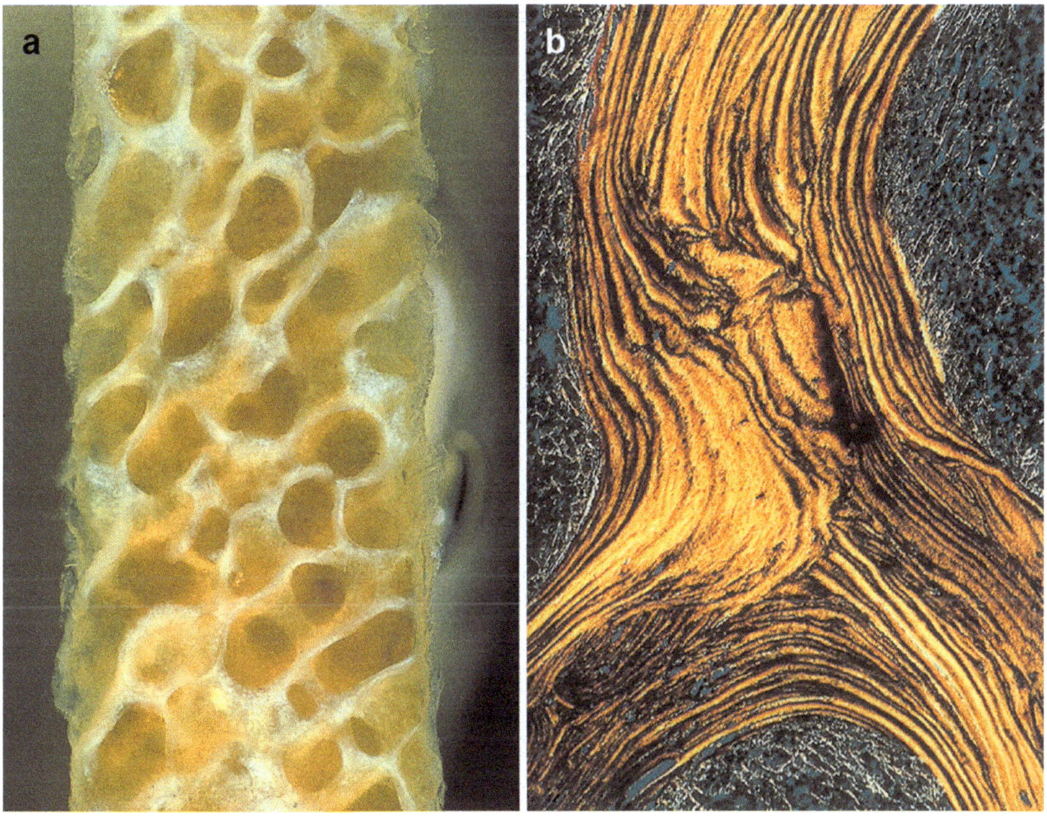

Fig. 2.3 (**a**, **b**) Normal trabecular bone. (**a**) Cut surface of a bone biopsy showing trabecular network and intertrabecular spaces. Note the honeycomb-like arrangement of the interconnected horizontal and vertical trabeculae and the nodes connecting them. The density of these "nodes" ensures mechanical strength. (**b**) Trabecula consisting of parallel layers of collagen fibrils. These lamellae ensure flexibility of bone. Gomori staining, polarisation

while imbalance induces adverse effects in the liver, in the pancreas and in skeletal muscle, which in turn affect the bones.

Bone has two mechanical functions to fulfil: weight-bearing and flexibility (Fig. 2.1a–c). Specific *structural organisations*, from the macroscopic through the microscopic to the molecular, enable bone to perform these functions:

- Configuration and size of bones
- Proportion of compact (cortical) to cancellous (trabecular) bone; adapted to weight-bearing (Fig. 2.2)
- Lamellar organisation of osseous tissue
- Trabecular bone structure with "nodes" to support weight (a "node" comprises the nodular junction of three or more trabeculae) (Figs. 2.3a, b and 2.4)

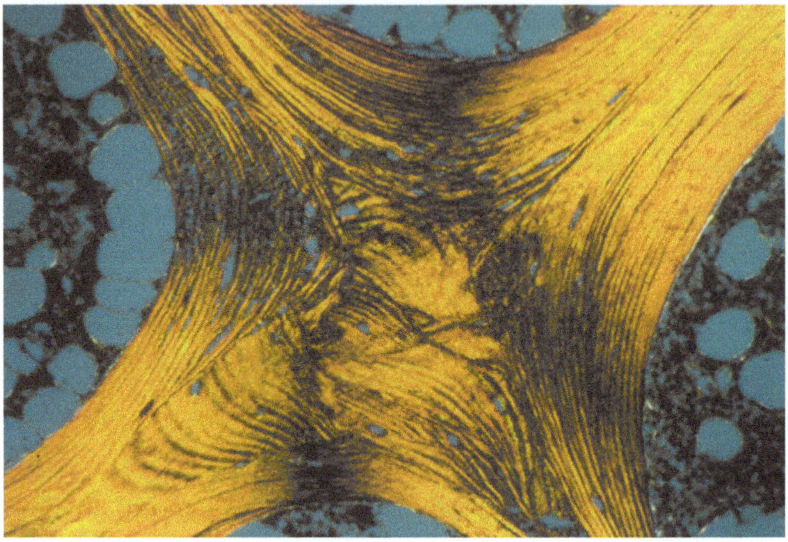

Fig. 2.4 "Node" at the intersection of four trabeculae with concentric lamellae. Gomori staining, polarisation

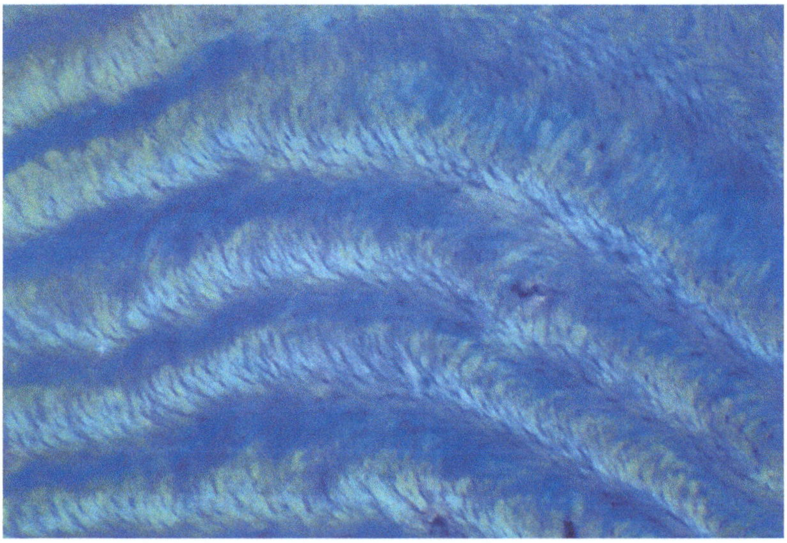

Fig. 2.5 Alternating light and dark "undulating" lamellae due to arrangement of collagen fibres. Giemsa staining, polarisation

- Degree of mineralisation of osseous tissue
- Arrangement of collagen fibres and filaments, together with non-collagenous matrix proteins (NCPs)
- Cable-like organisation of collagen molecules and their "cross-linking"

The elasticity of bone is achieved mainly by a special mixture of its component parts, known as "two-phase component" in the building industry. Bone consists of the matrix (the material laid down by the osteoblasts) made up of layers of collagen molecules between which crystalline calcium and phosphate are deposited (Fig. 2.5). This "passive gradual mineralisation" increases density as the bone gets older. The new matrix begins to mineralise after about 5–10 days from the time of deposition (*primary mineralisation*) (Fig. 2.6). On completion of the bone remodelling cycle, a phase of *secondary mineralisation* begins. This process consists of a gradual maturation of the mineral component, including an increase in the amount of crystals and/or an augmentation of crystal size towards its maximum dimension. This secondary mineralisation progressively increases the mineral content in bone

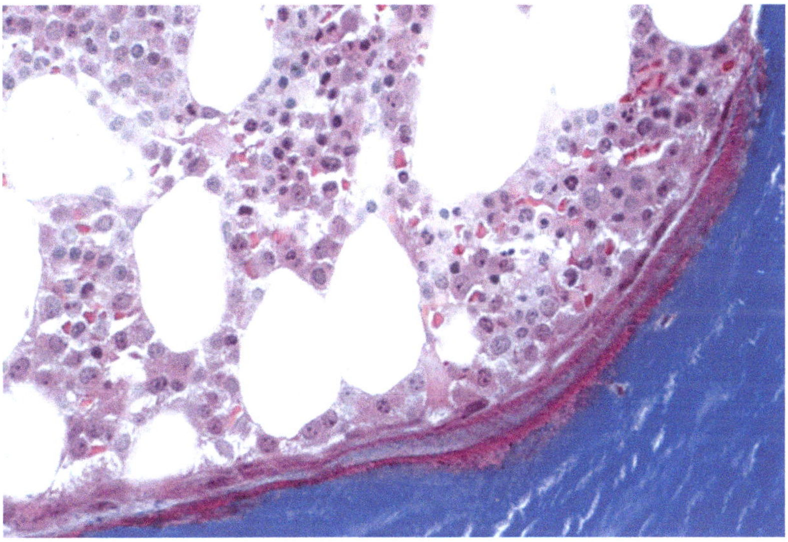

Fig. 2.6 Flat osteoblasts and layers of newly formed osteoid (*various shades of red*) on mineralised bone (*blue*). Ladewig staining

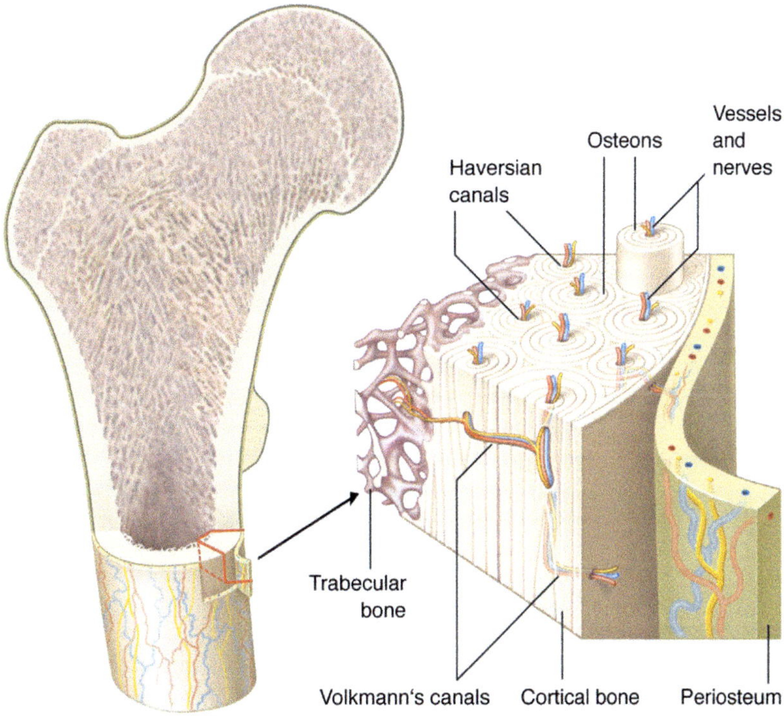

Fig. 2.7 Structure of bone: periosteum and cortical bone together with their vascular and nervous system surround the trabecular network

matrix. At the end of the primary mineralisation, mineral content represents only about 50 % of the maximum degree of mineralisation obtained at the end of the secondary mineralisation phase. Various trace elements, water and mucopolysaccharides serve as binding material ("glue") which binds the proteins and minerals firmly together. Collagen is responsible for the elasticity, the flexibility of bone, while the minerals provide strength and rigidity. The bundles of collagen fibres are arranged parallel to the layers of matrix and are connected by cement lines. In adult bone, the degree of mineralisation depends on the rate of remodelling. That means that the biologic

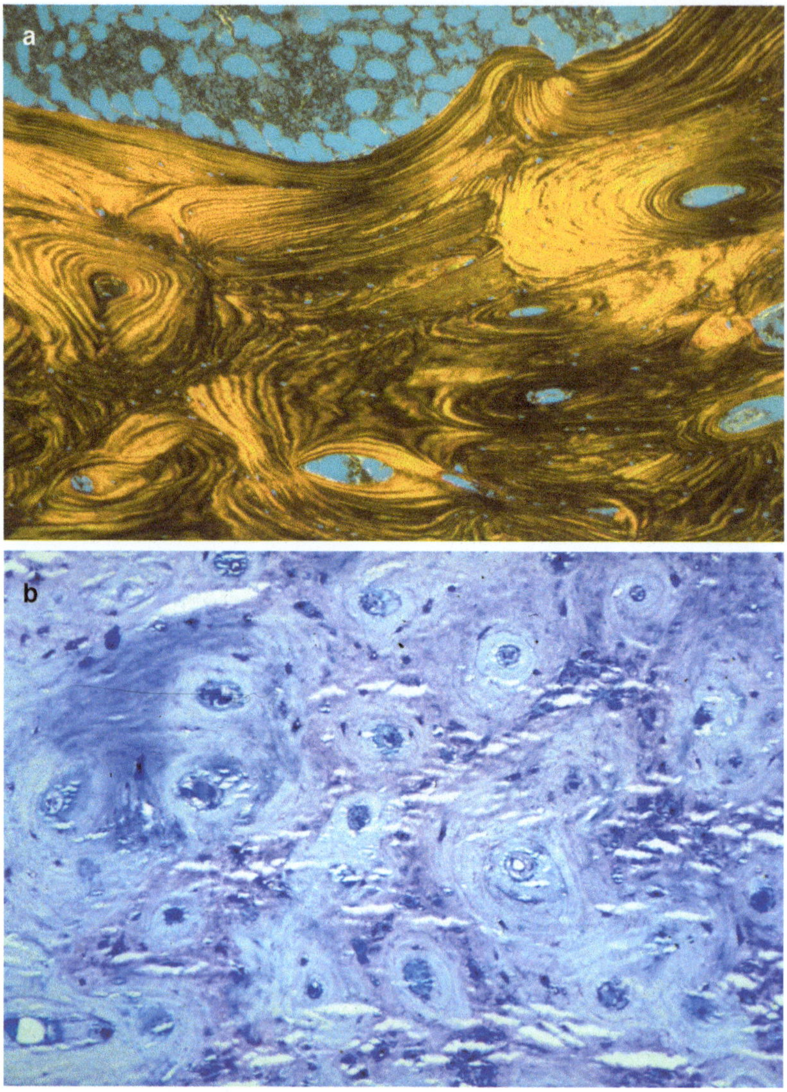

Fig. 2.8 (**a**) Cortical bone with multiple osteons and adjacent bone marrow (*upper half*). Gomori staining, polarisation. (**b**) Cross sections of multiple osteons in the cortical bone. Giemsa staining

determinant of mineralisation is the rate of bone turnover. These correlations also demonstrate that "bone mass" and "bone mineral density" (BMD), though often used synonymously, are two different entities. Indeed, the term "bone mineral density" has been introduced in the interpretation of the positive effects of the bisphosphonates on fracture risk.

2.2 Architecture of Bone

The external aspect of bone conceals its inner architecture (Fig. 2.7). The two main supporting *structures of bone* are only recognised in X-ray films or bone biopsy sections:

- *Compact, cortical bone*: It forms the outer layer of the long bones, is very densely packed and hard and has a slow metabolic rate. Therefore, cortical bone is resorbed and replaced at a much slower rate than trabecular bone. The layer of cortical bone of the long tubular bones (femur, humerus) consists of osteons also called Haversian systems, which are longitudinally oriented cylinders about 5 mm long and made up of 5–20 "rings" (Fig. 2.8a, b).

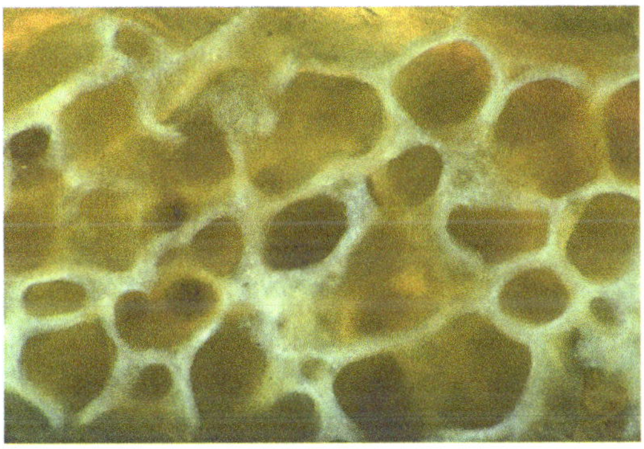

Fig. 2.9 Surface of a trimmed plastic block showing a fairly uniform trabecular network

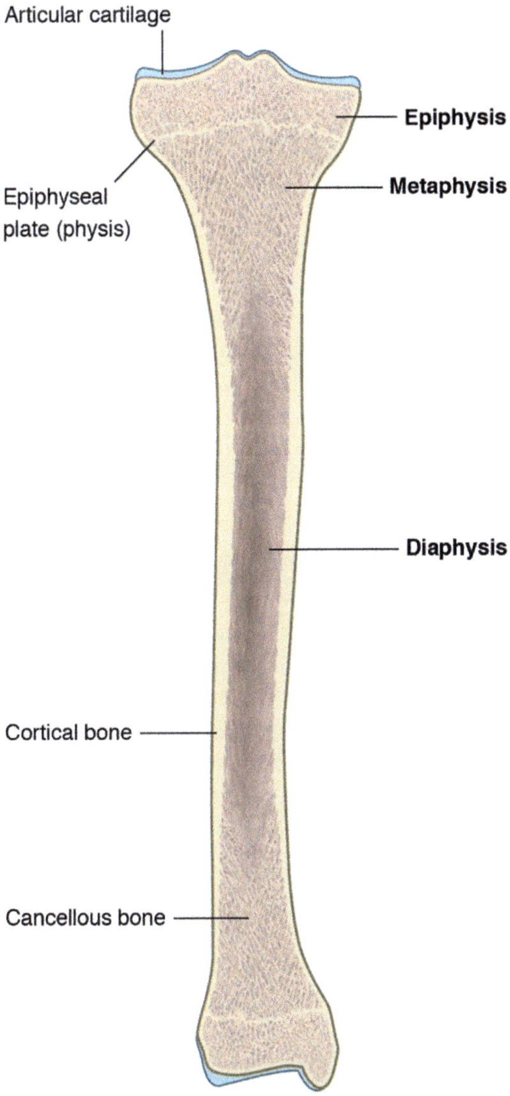

Fig. 2.10 Three main topographic parts of long bones

- *Spongy, cancellous, trabecular bone,* sometimes also known as ossicles: The axial skeleton (cranium, vertebral column, thorax and pelvis) has a specialised construction. At first glance, the trabeculae appear to be randomly distributed, but closer inspection reveals that they are oriented precisely along the lines of stress and weight-bearing ("trajection lines"), producing sponge-like and lattice-like structures (Fig. 2.9). The more closely the trabecular "nodes" are spaced, the greater the stability and strength of the bone, while the trabecular plates dominate the elastic properties of the trabecular bone.

Cortical bone has three surfaces and each has different anatomic features:

- The endosteal envelope faces the marrow cavity and comprises a high surface area and therefore supports a high bone turnover.
- The periosteal envelope, the outer surface of the bone to which the tendons, ligaments and muscles are attached, is capable of remodelling as is the intracortical surface.
- The intracortical envelope, with bone surfaces inside the Haversian system, i.e. the osteons.

The skeleton can be divided into two main compartments:

- *Axial skeleton*: This refers to the spine and proximal femur. The bone in this area is primarily trabecular with a high turnover.
- *Appendicular skeleton*: This refers to the long bones of the legs and arms. The bone in these areas is primarily cortical with a low turnover.

Approximately 80 % of bone is cortical and only 20 % is trabecular, and they undergo different rates of remodelling:

- Cortical bone is dense, is 90 % calcified, has a low surface/volume ratio and therefore has a slow remodelling rate.
- In contrast, cancellous bone has a porous structure and a large surface area. About 25 % of cancellous bone is remodelled annually compared to only 2.5 % of cortical bone. It therefore follows that any decrease in bone is

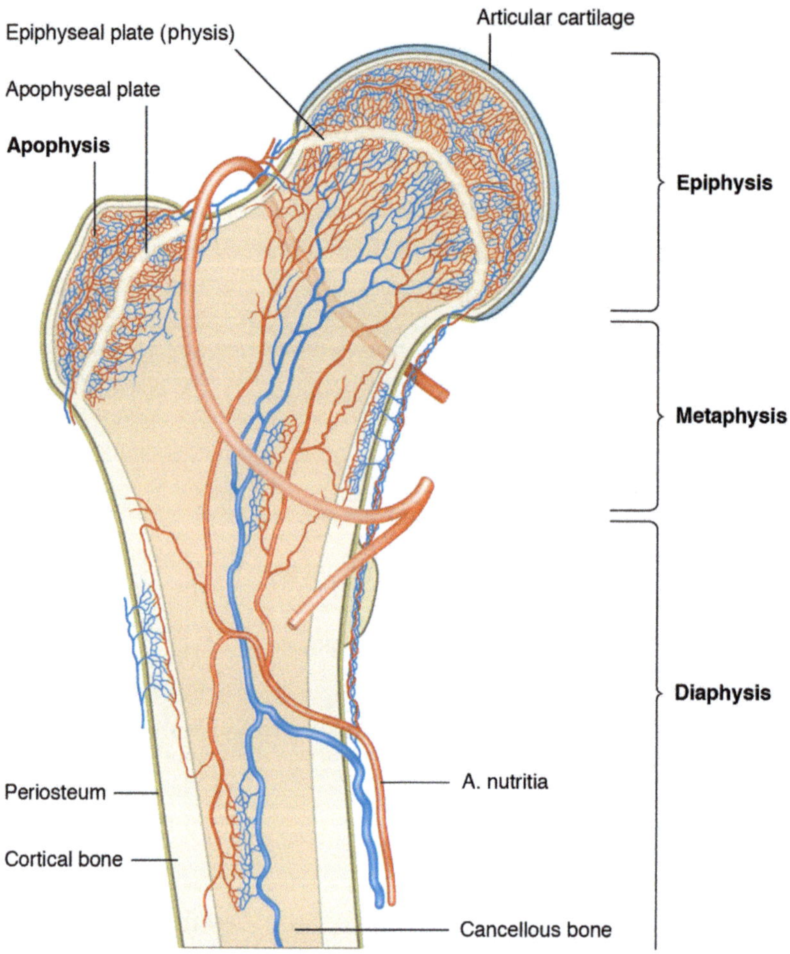

Fig. 2.11 Arterial and venous blood supply of long bones

first manifest in bones with a large proportion of trabeculae and therefore with a higher surface area.

The *proportion of trabecular bone* varies in different skeletal regions:

- Lumbar vertebrae 75 %
- Heels 70 %
- Proximal femur 50–75 %
- Distal radius 25 %
- Middle of the radius <5 %

Long bones consist of four main topographic parts (Fig. 2.10):

- Epiphysis, the end of a tubular bone, lying between the growth plate and the articular cartilage
- Growth plate (physis), the region of bone elongation in children
- Metaphysis, the widened part of bone occupying the region between the cylindrical diaphysis and the physis
- Diaphysis (shaft), the middle cylindrical part of the long bone, with a thick cortex and a central marrow space

2.3 Blood Vessels and Nerves of Bone and Marrow

Bone and marrow are highly vascularised organs which account for about 10–20 % of cardiac output. Diaphyseal nutrient arteries, the principal source of blood for bones, penetrate the cortex through the nutrient canal (Fig. 2.11). There are also metaphyseal and epiphyseal arteries

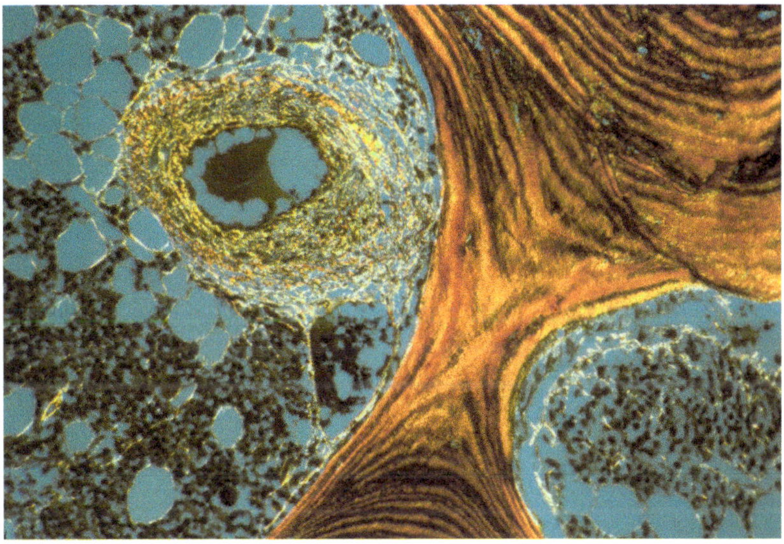

Fig. 2.12 Cross section of an artery in the bone marrow close to the trabecular network. Gomori staining, polarisation

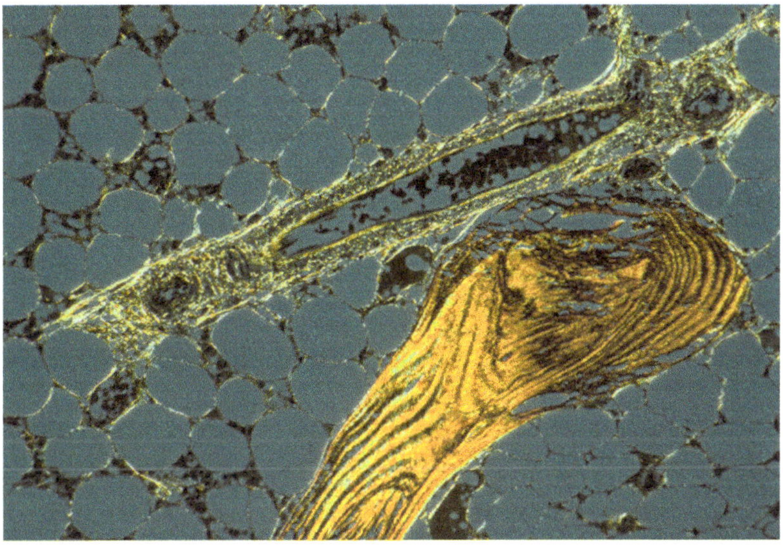

Fig. 2.13 Longitudinal section of an arteriole in the bone marrow adjacent to a trabecula. Gomori staining, polarisation

supplying the ends of long bones and the adjacent joints. Periosteal vessels supply the outer layer of the cortical bone. Each nutrient artery is accompanied by nerve fibres, and it branches within the marrow cavities. In long bones, it bifurcates into ascending and descending branches from which radial arteries arise, but this does not occur in flat bones like the pelvis. The smaller branches divide into arterioles and capillaries which either enter the cortex via Volkmann's canals to become cortical capillaries or lead to a highly branching network of medullary and endosteal sinusoids. These form a spongy network of channels of variable width and length, physiologically characterised by a very low rate of blood flow. A retrograde venous blood flow caused by muscle contractions has been observed in the endosteal sinusoids, and this may play an important role in the process of osseous metastases (Batson's vertebral venous plexus). At any particular time, portions of the sinusoidal channels may be collapsed and therefore difficult to identify even in semithin sections. The microvascular system is in a state of constant dynamic change, and its expansion and contraction are probably controlled by locally

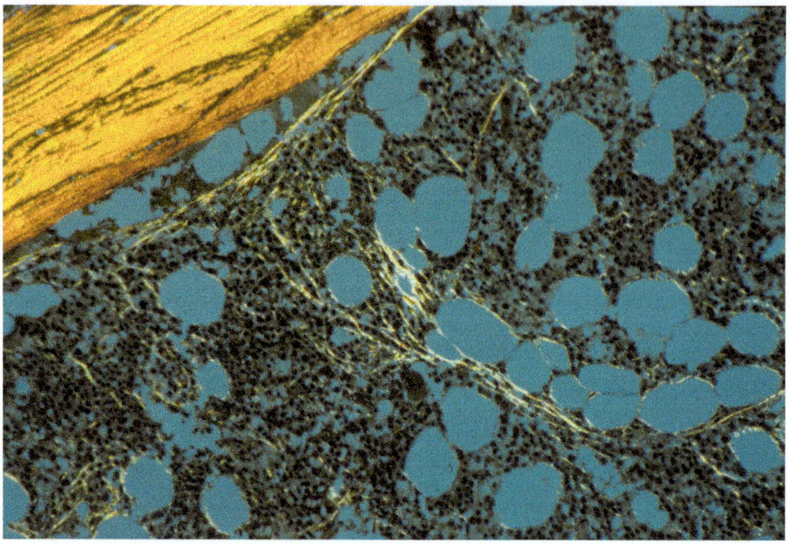

Fig. 2.14 Endosteal sinusoid close to the trabecular surface. Gomori staining, polarisation

produced factors and by the accompanying nerve fibres, which innervate the sphincter mechanisms and specialised thickened endothelial cells present at the bifurcation of smaller arteries. These regulate the blood flow in the different regions of bone and marrow (Figs. 2.12 and 2.13). Within the intertrabecular space, central sinusoids are associated with erythrons and megakaryocytes, while endosteal sinusoids (Fig. 2.14) of variable number and width accompany the trabeculae and supply the osteoblasts and osteoid seams. The medullary sinusoids drain into the periosteal venules and veins, which accompany the arteries and leave through foramina near the articular ends of the long bones. Lymph vessels are present in the periosteum. Traction of attached muscles may also assist venous drainage. There are close vascular relationships between bone and marrow. For example, changes in haematopoietic activity modify the dynamics of the regional circulation and set up a new equilibrium between bone cells and their environment, resulting in alterations in remodelling and possibly structure, while interference with the blood supply may lead to avascular necrosis of bone.

Nerve fibres accompany the blood vessels to the bone marrow and to the periosteum.

Nerve fibres of bone and marrow may be categorised into:

- Sensory (pain) nerves in the periosteum
- Vasomotoric nerves inside the bone controlling blood supply of the different regions
- Sympathetic nerves controlling bone remodelling and maturation of haematopoiesis

Modelling and Remodelling of Bone

3

Bone is a dynamic organ, highly vascularised and very active metabolically (Fig. 3.1). As the bones are not completely developed at birth, they continue to be formed slowly out of cartilage or connective tissue, which are converted into the hard, lamellar components of the bone. Growth of the bones (*modelling*) comes to an end at puberty with ossification of the "growth plates". Modelling is of particular interest as the bone is much more capable of reacting to external loads during growth than at any other time. About 90 % of adult bone is formed by the end of adolescence, and subsequent gains during adulthood are very small.

During adulthood, there is a continuous process of remodelling which maintains the bones and the bones adapts to the changing external circumstances (Fig. 3.2). Nevertheless, as the body ages, the bone loses some of its strength and elasticity and therefore breaks more easily. This is due to loss of mineral and changes in the bone matrix. Bones undergo a constant process of removal and replacement so that the components of the bone are exchanged at regular intervals. This process is called remodelling and serves the following purposes (Table 3.1):

- Mobilisation of calcium in the framework of calcium homeostasis
- Replacement of old osseous tissue
- Overall skeletal and individual local adaptation to different loads, weight-bearing and stress
- Repair of damaged bone, both microscopic and macroscopic

The last refers not only to repair or healing of fractures of whole bones but also to the countless perforations, breaks or cracks of the trabeculae, the "microfractures", "microdamage" or "fatigue damage" which occur constantly and which together with the thickness of the bones determine the fracture risk. As these tiny breaks, cracks or fractures accumulate, they weaken older bones and contribute to fracture risk if not quickly and adequately repaired. This, in addition to a slightly negative bone balance over time, eventually leads to reduction in structural continuity of the trabecular network and thereby loss of strength. In cortical bone, microcrack density is greater in older individuals, and on average, the microcracks are shorter in areas of the cortex with more resorption spaces, indicating a relationship with the rate of bone remodelling.

R. Bartl, C. Bartl, *Bone Disorders*, DOI 10.1007/978-3-319-29182-6_3

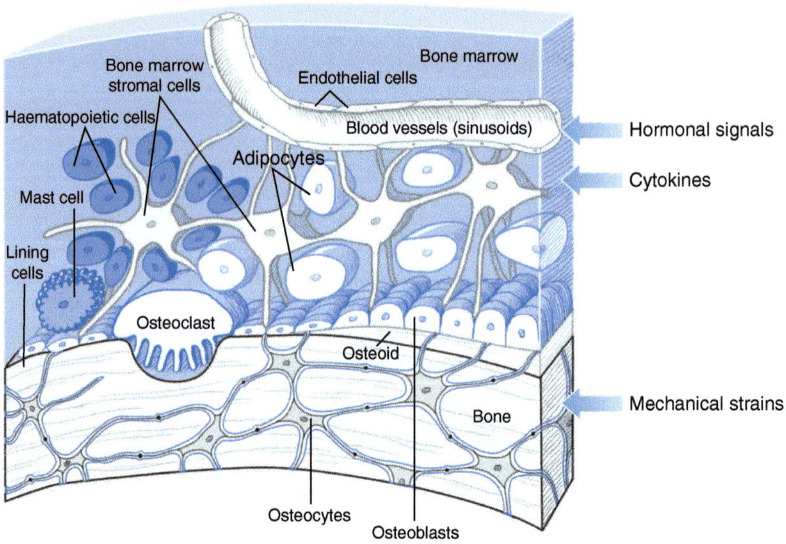

Fig. 3.1 Interdependence of the bone and marrow: together they form a single structural and functional entity: the "bone and marrow" system

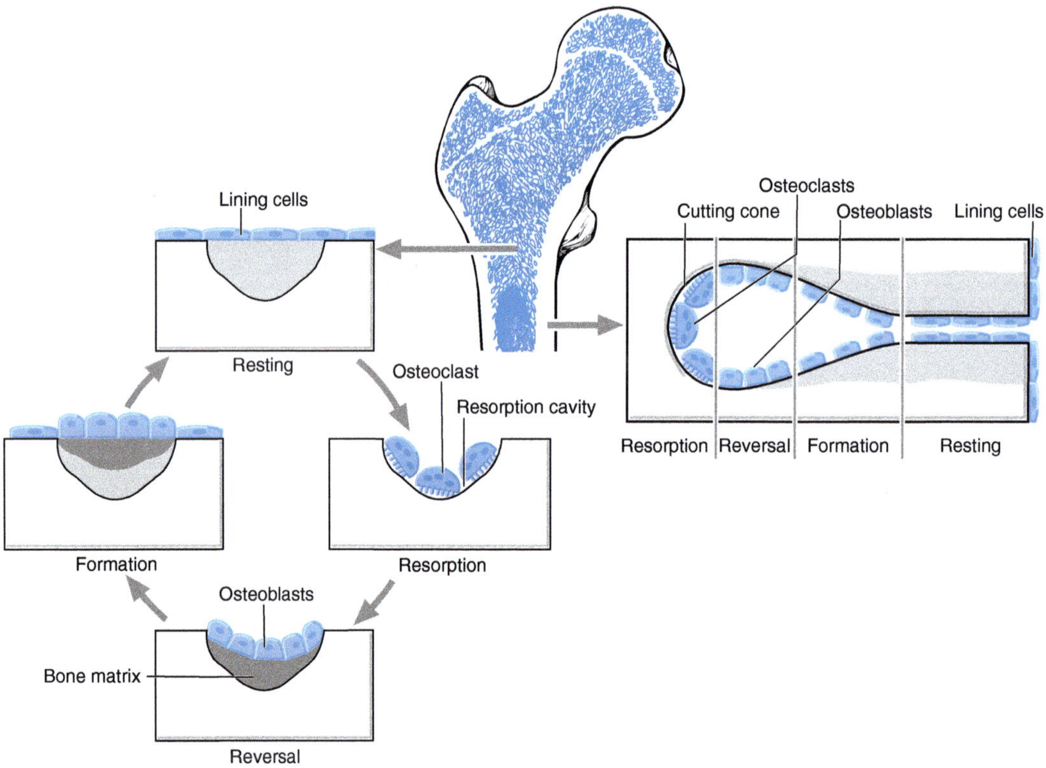

Fig. 3.2 Different bone remodelling in cancellous (*left*) and cortical (*right*) bone

Table 3.1 Quantitative parameters of bone remodelling in normal adults

Trabecular bone surface covered with	
Lining cells	90 %
Osteoblasts	2–7 %
Osteoclasts	1 %
Life span	
BMU[a]	6–9 months
Osteoclast	3 weeks
Osteoblasts	3 months
Number of active BMUs at any time	1 million
BMUs initiated per year	3–4 million/year
BMU size	1–2 mm long and 0.2–0.4 mm wide
Mean time for renewal of the bones	10 years
Renewal per day	0.027 % (1 BMU/7 s)

[a]BMU, bone multicellular unit

3.1 Bone Cells

The bone cells constitute a specialised osseous cell system responsible for the repair, maintenance and adaptation of the bone:

- *Osteoclasts* ("bone resorbers", "bone breakers", "bone carvers") can resorb old, weak bone in a short period of time (Fig. 3.3). These multinucleated giant cells are derived from monocytes of the bone marrow that is from a haematopoietic cell line and have a life span of up to 7 weeks. The cell membrane consists of numerous "folds" – the "ruffled border" which faces the surface of the bone (Figs. 3.4 and 3.5). The major function of osteoclasts is to destroy the surface of old and fractured bone. The osteoclasts release quantities of proteolytic and other enzymes into the space between the ruffled membrane and the bone. These substances dissolve the minerals and some of the bone matrix; the rest is phagocytosed and metabolised in the cytoplasm of the osteoclasts (Fig. 3.6). The osteoclasts also release protons directly via H^+-ATPase located in the ruffled border. The resulting acidification causes dissolution of bone mineral. If the trabecula is thin enough, active osteoclasts may perforate and transsect it, thereby disconnecting it from the trabecular network which irreversibly weakens that area of the bone (Fig. 3.7a, b). Recruitment, differentiation and activation of osteoclasts are accomplished by numerous systemic hormones (such as parathyroid hormones, oestrogens, androgens, leptin and thyroid hormones) as well as cytokines. Various growth factors are also involved. Recent investigations of the RANK/RANKL signalling pathway in the osteoclast have clarified mechanisms of stimulation and activation of resorption. Osteoclasts possess oestrogen receptors, by means of which oestrogen inhibits their recruitment. Androgens also act on osteoclasts. The actions of sex steroids on bone cells are discussed below.
- *Osteoblasts* ("bone builders") are derived from the mesenchyme in the bone marrow. Osteoblasts are cuboid cells that form a continuous layer (seam) on the bone surface. The life span of osteoblasts ranges from months to about a year. They produce new bone slowly, over several weeks to replace that resorbed by the osteoclasts (Fig. 3.8). Their main function is the synthesis of bone matrix especially collagen type I but also osteocalcin, osteonectin and bone morphogenetic proteins (BMP). Osteoblasts also possess receptors for oestrogen.
- *Osteocytes* ("bone maintainers", "bone controllers"): The osteocytes are the most numerous of all the bone cells (Fig. 3.9). They develop from osteoblasts. Approximately every tenth osteoblast situated on the surface of the bone is entrapped by the newly formed bone matrix and thus becomes an osteocyte. Osteocytes lose their ability to secrete bone matrix. It possesses receptors for various hormones including PTH and sex hormones. The osteocytes occupy spaces in the bone called "lacunae" and are connected to each other and to the endosteal cells on the surface of the bone by thin channels called "canaliculi" within which long cytoplasmic processes join osteocytes to each other and thus form a cir-

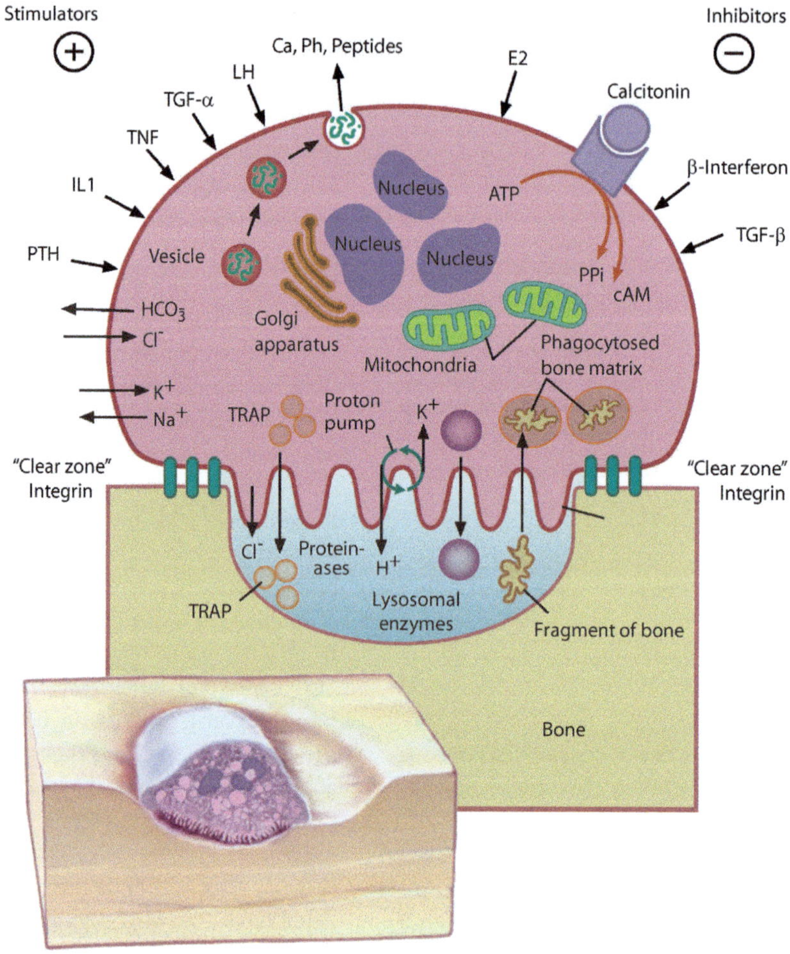

Fig. 3.3 Schematic drawing of structure and function of an osteoclast indicating stimulators and inhibitors of osteoclastic activity. The main targets of pharmacologic interventions are multiple signalling pathways, various enzymes produced, apoptosis, sealing zone, ruffled border and resorption pH

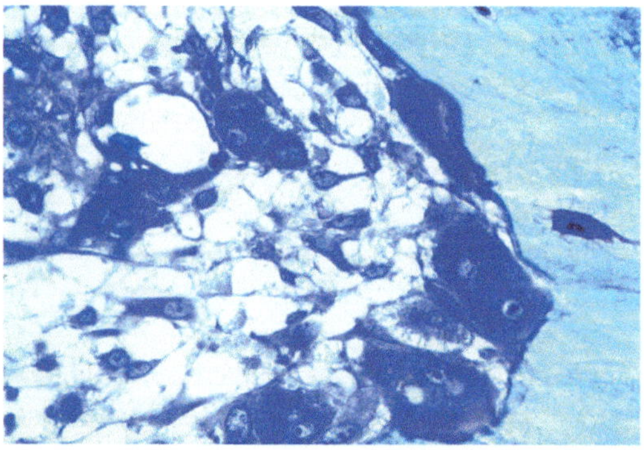

Fig. 3.4 Active osteoclasts in deep resorption bay. Giemsa staining

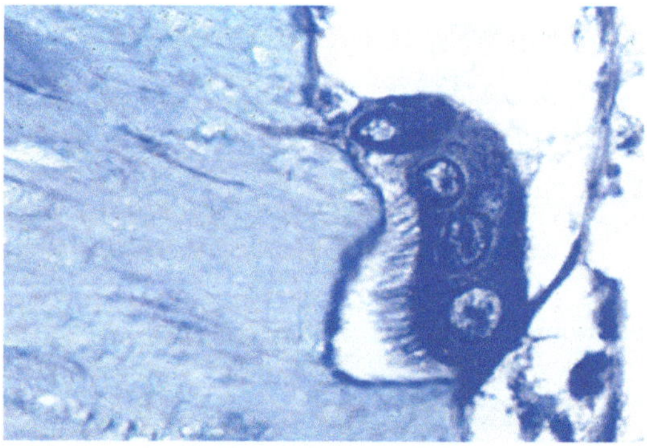

Fig. 3.5 Active osteoclast with ruffled border in lacuna with paratrabecular sinusoid. Giemsa staining

culatory system (Figs. 3.10 and 3.11). Osteocytes possess functional gap junctions enabling them to communicate with one another (like neurons) as well as with the surface lining cells – the endosteal cells. Therefore, osteocytes are in a position to transmit the load-induced signals to pre-osteoblasts which then differentiate and secrete osteoid. The total surface of combined lacunae and canaliculi has been estimated at 1200 sqm. The function of osteocytes has not yet been fully elucidated, but they are known to play an important part in the transport of organic and inorganic materials within the bones. Furthermore, their strategic location enables them to function as mechano-sensory cells and thus to detect the need for bone increase or decrease during functional adaptation of the bone as well as the need for repair of microfractures. Osteocytes detect changes in flow of the fluid in the canaliculi and in the levels of circulating hormones such as oestrogen, glucocorticoids and raloxifene, which influence their activities and their survival. Recent data suggest that mechanical loading decreases the osteocyte´s potential to regulate local osteoclastogenesis by direct cell-cell contact and/or via soluble signals. Quite possibly they also receive impulses from the muscles which they relay to the cells of the remodelling units at the surface of the bone. They also register the age of the bone and initiate its remodelling. Osteocytes also produce various factors, notably sclerostin, a molecule that regulates osteoblast activity as well as DMP 1 and FGF 3, a factor also involved in the regulation of renal phosphate uptake. To summarise the function of the osteocytes, osteocytes are actively involved in remodelling and in its control mechanisms. Osteocytes actively participate in ion exchange. Osteocytes are mechano-sensory cells with a major part in the functional adaptation of the bone. The number (density) of

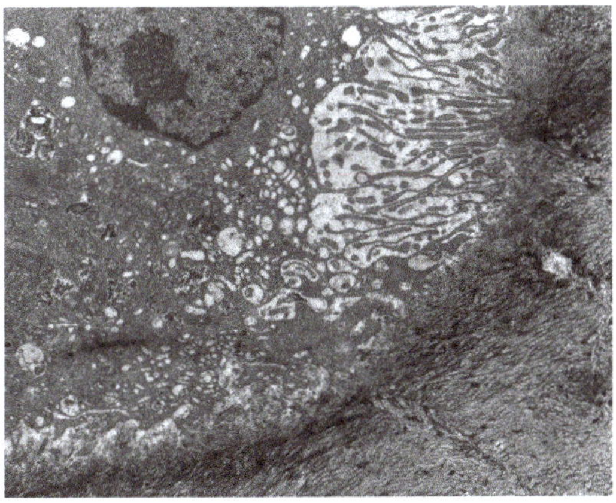

Fig. 3.6 EM of an osteoclast (*upper left*) attacking mineralised bone matrix (*lower right*). Note cross- and longitudinal sectioned villi of ruffled membrane as well as fragments of matrix in osteoclastic vacuoles (*left*)

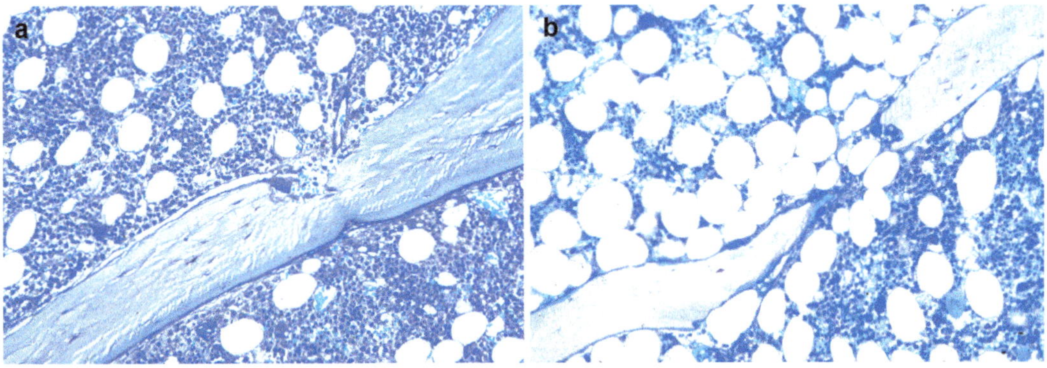

Fig. 3.7 (**a**, **b**) Osteoclasts perforate a trabecula (**a**) and transsect it (**b**) thereby disconnecting it from the trabecular network which irreversibly and mechanically weakens that area of the bone. Giemsa staining

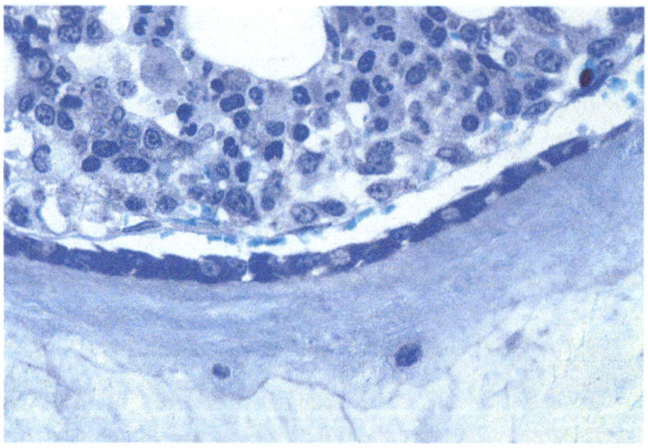

Fig. 3.8 Active cuboidal osteoblasts on osteoid seam of variable width. Giemsa staining

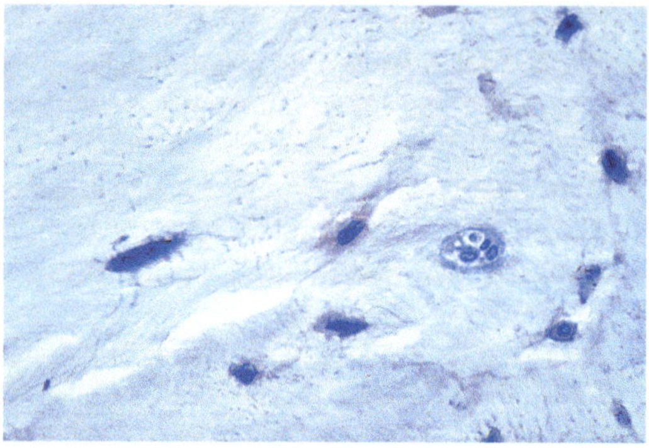

Fig. 3.9 Osteocytes cut at different angles in trabecular bone. Note a narrow trabecular canal containing a blood vessel. Giemsa staining

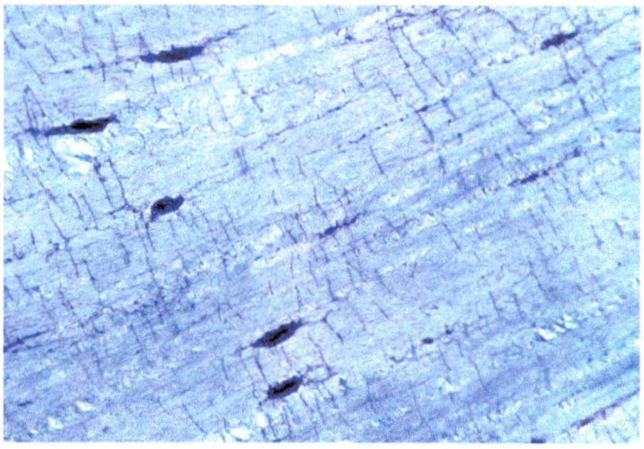

Fig. 3.10 Osteocytes connected by numerous channels ("canaliculi"). Giemsa staining

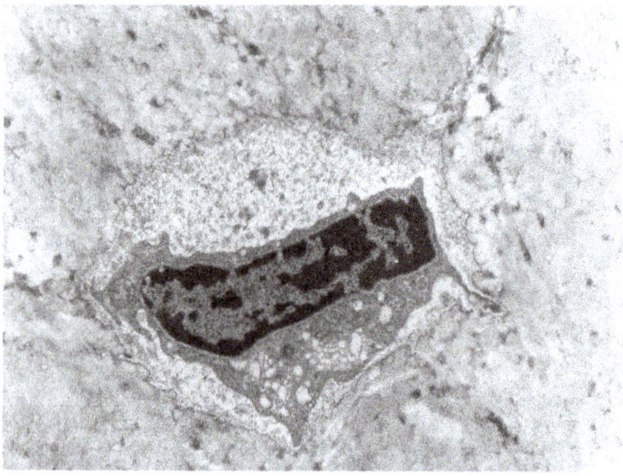

Fig. 3.11 Osteocyte nucleus with clumped heterochromatin and numerous cytoplasmic organelles including a centriole. EM

osteocytes determines bone mass both for cortical and trabecular bone. Disruption of the osteocyte network and decrease in osteocyte number with age is inevitably accompanied by a decrease in bone mass as well as by a decrease in bone quality by impairment of repair of microfractures. Though regulated by all the control mechanisms outlined above, in the final analysis, it is the highly complex intercellular signalling between the osteoprogenitor cells and the mature osteoclasts, osteoblasts and osteocytes which balance their activities in growth and remodelling.

- *Endosteal lining cells* (bone "housekeepers"): These are flat cells that cover 80–95 % of the internal surface of the bones. They are presumed to develop from inactive osteoblasts. They form a protective layer and constitute a surveillance system for the bones (Fig. 3.12). They are connected to a thin collagenous membrane covering the mineralised bone surface, the osteocytic lacunae and their canaliculi (Fig. 3.13). Recently, it has been shown that the endosteal lining cells may participate in the activation of osteoclasts. Certain surface molecules expressed on lining cells and on osteoclast progenitors react with the receptor RANK (also found on osteoclast

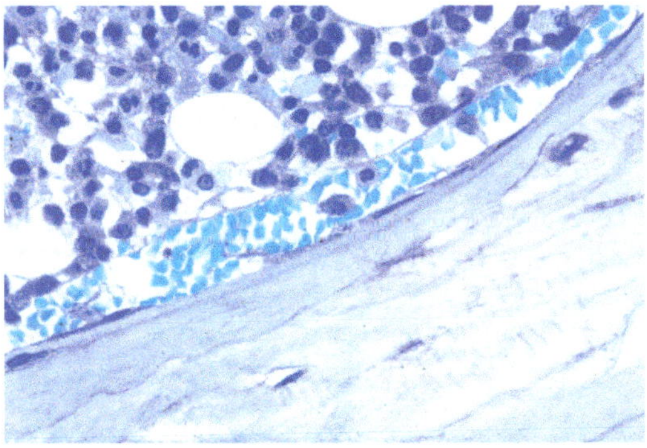

Fig. 3.12 Flat endosteal lining cells and paratrabecular sinusoid. Giemsa staining

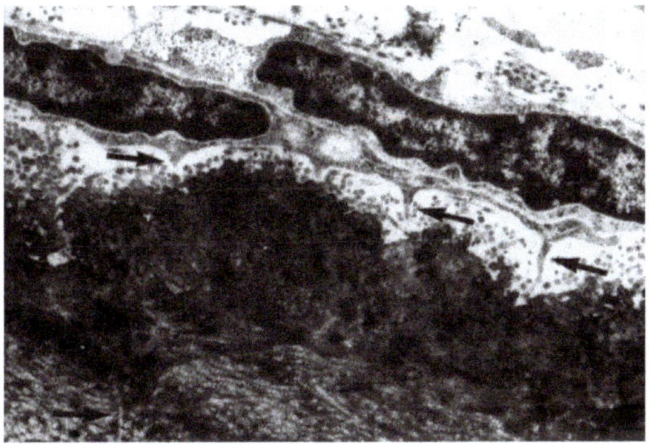

Fig. 3.13 At higher magnification, collagen in transverse section (thin collagenous membrane) under the flat endosteal lining cells and in longitudinal section (mineralised bone) in lower part of micrograph. Note processes of endosteal lining cells (at *arrows*) extending between collagen fibres, presumably to connect with processes of osteocytes within the canaliculi. EM

progenitors) and thereby set in motion a cycle of remodelling. Other important factors which participate in the remodelling cycle have also been analysed and these are ODF (osteoclast differentiation factor), OPGL (osteoprotegerin ligand), TRANCE and RANKL (RANK ligand). PTH, PGE_2, IL1 and 1,25 (OH) vitamin D exercise a negative influence on osteoprotegerin production and thereby stimulate resorption. Osteoblast precursors produce M-CSF which can activate osteoclasts. The endosteal lining cells also participate in bone remodelling. They remove fragments of bone collagen left by osteoclasts thereby cleaning up resorption pits and initiating formation of new bone.

3.2 Bone Remodelling Units

There are 2–5 million *bone remodelling units* (BRU) of the skeletal system (Fig. 3.14). These units, required for the maintenance and integrity of the bones, are of crucial importance for the development of osteoporosis (Table 3.2). The total quantity of the bone decreases if more bone is resorbed than is produced over the years. It has been estimated that osteoporosis develops when for every 30 units of bone resorbed, only 29 are produced. This negative "bone balance" has three possible causes:

- Increased osteoclastic activity without increased osteoblastic activity ("high turnover")
- Normal osteoclastic but decreased osteoblastic activity ("low turnover")
- Decreased osteoclastic and osteoblastic activity ("atrophic" or "adynamic" bone)

Consequently an overall decrease in the bone correlates primarily with the number of BRU and with the lack of coordination between the cells of the BRU. The level of excretion of calcium and collagen metabolites in the urine reflects the degree of resorption of the bone. The process of bone remodelling is as yet incompletely understood. One *remodelling cycle* takes approximately 120 days, and it has been divided into 6 *phases* (Fig. 3.15):

- Phase of quiescence: a layer of flat lining cells over a thin collagenous membrane covers the surface of the bone.
- Phase of activation: the quiescent bone surface is prepared for resorption. This involves retraction of the endosteal lining cells and removal of the thin collagenous membrane

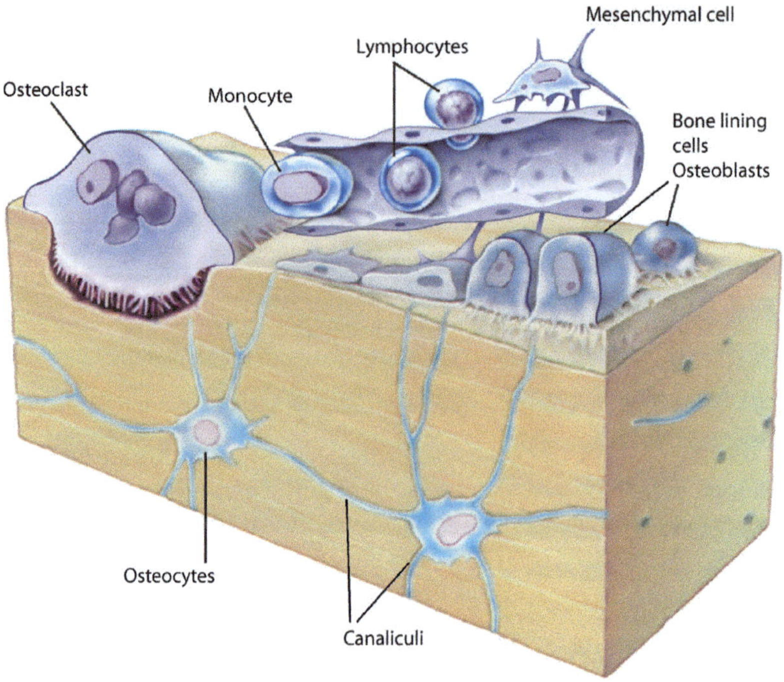

Fig. 3.14 Bone remodelling unit (BRU), consisting of bone resorbing cells (osteoclasts), bone matrix synthesising cells (osteoblasts) and bone protecting cells (osteocytes and endosteal lining cells) as well as various progenitor cells

Table 3.2 Bone remodelling and its clinical correlations

Phase of remodelling	Quiescence	Bone resorption by osteoclasts	Reversal	Bone formation by osteoblasts	Quiescence
Stimulating factors		Parathormone Vitamin D Thyroxine		Growth hormone Parathormone Oestrogen Testosterone Cytokines Prostaglandins Vitamin D	
Inhibiting factors		Oestrogen Calcitonin Testosterone Bisphosphonates Raloxifene		Corticosteroids Smoking Alcohol	
Bone markers		Pyridinoline, NTX, CTX		Bone specific Alk. phosph. Osteocalcin	

covering the bone surface. There is evidence that matrix metalloproteinases produced by osteoblasts are involved in this process. The site-specific activation may be achieved by mechanical stresses transmitted to the endosteal lining cells via the osteocytic-canalicular network.

- Phase of resorption: recruitment and fusion of osteoclastic precursors, preparation of osteoclasts for resorption and development of the ruffled membrane; osteoclasts resorb the bone, which leads to formation of lacunae or pits; osteoclasts migrate slowly or undergo apoptosis (Fig. 3.16).

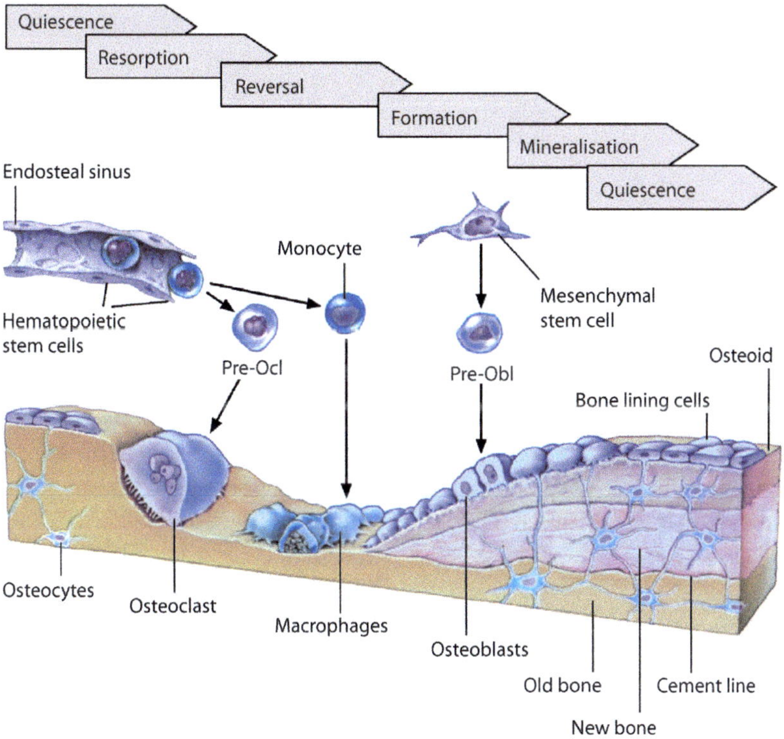

Fig. 3.15 Steps of bone remodelling in adult trabecular bone

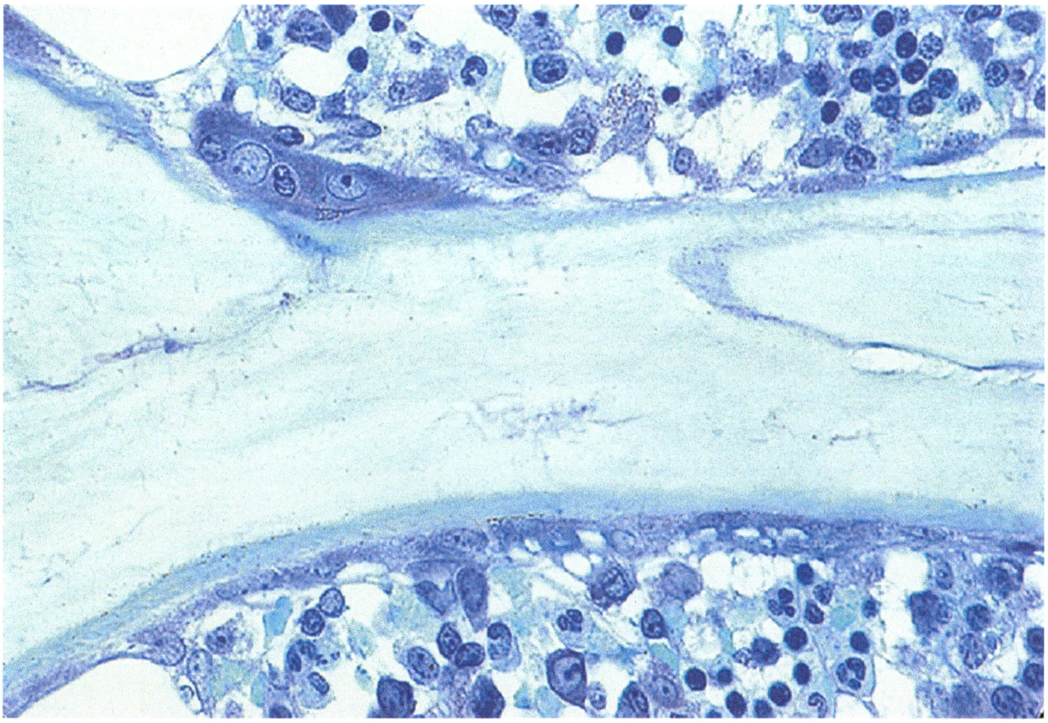

Fig. 3.16 Trabecula showing osteoclastic resorption (note osteoclast, left) on the upper surface and bone formation with layer of osteoblasts and osteoid seam (*darker blue*) on the lower surface. Example of normal, balanced remodelling of the bone. Giemsa staining

- Phase of reversal: osteoblast progenitors are attracted to the resorption pit, while monocytes and endosteal lining cells prepare the surface of the resorption pit for new bone production by removal of the debris left by the osteoclasts.
- Phase of early formation: production of osteoid by active osteoblasts.
- Phase of late formation: mineralisation of osteoid.
- Phase of quiescence: the osteoblasts turn into the flat endosteal lining cells or into osteocytes if trapped in the newly formed bone.

The phase of resorption is completed within 2 weeks, while that of mineralisation may take months and depends on the presence of active metabolites of vitamin D. On completion of a remodelling cycle, a *structural bone unit* is formed; about 35 million are present in the whole human skeleton. 8 % of the bone is replaced annually by the activity of the bone remodelling units (BRU).

The following four *stages of osteoclast activity* are involved:

- Formation and differentiation of osteoclasts from their precursors (RANKL)
- Migration and attachment of osteoclasts to the osseous surface (β3 integrins)
- Osteoclastic secretion of factors for acidification and solution of minerals (V-H+-ATPase, chloride channels)
- Dissolution of matrix (cathepsin K)

Currently, the majority of the treatments for osteoporosis tested so far target inhibition of bone resorption.

The resorption stage has a duration of about 30–40 days and is followed by a bone formation period of about 150 days. The surface of the spongiosa is totally remodelled every 2 years.

4 Control and Regulation of Bone Remodelling

During the first few years of the twenty first century, the complex mechanisms which characterise the control of bone remodelling were just beginning to be recognised and starting to be investigated. Results of the overwhelming amount of research subsequently published have illuminated the extreme complexity of the cellular and molecular interactions as well as the network of interwoven highways and byways representing the numerous pathways that transport factors to stimulate or to inhibit specific cellular activities. A highly significant aspect of the results of these investigations is the unequivocal demonstration of the participation of many of these pathways not only in the control of bone remodelling but also in numerous processes – both physiological and pathological – involving other organs and tissues and as such are examples of systems biology.

One striking demonstration of this is *osteoimmunology* in which the participation of lymphocytes and various immunological cytokines (among other factors) in the processes of bone remodelling has now been unequivocally established. Inflammatory reactions, acute and especially long-lasting chronic reactions, are major causes of local and even systemic bone loss. One such cause, for example, is the tumour necrosis factor (TNF) in inflammatory arthritis. Another example is the induction of bone destruction by the activation of T-cells by means of RANKL. In complete contrast, CD44 acts as an inhibitor of the deleterious consequences of TNF on bones and joints, similar to the effect of selectin-9 (a growth hormone) which stimulates the production of regulatory T-cells. Moreover, additional studies have pointed out that various signalling molecules, transcription factors and membrane receptors are also shared by the immune and skeletal systems. For example, NF-κ B is a vital component in inflammatory responses and also in osteoclast differentiation and osteolysis. Unhealthy life styles, including poor nutrition as well as overweight and morbid obesity, result in imbalances in the oxidation/redox systems, leading to inflammatory reactions and disorders of many organs including the bones and joints.

On the other hand, the localisation of the osteoclastic resorption may affect *haematopoiesis*, such as the mobilisation of haematopoietic progenitors when osteoclasts resorb an endosteal region of bone, with secretion and release of proteolytic enzymes, adjacent to stem cell niches. It has been speculated that this constitutes a link between bone remodelling and regulation of haematopoiesis.

Towards the end of the nineteenth century (in the1890s), researchers developed the hypothesis that mechanical loads affect the architecture of bone in living organisms. However, the processes by which this occurs were only investigated much later in the twentieth century when the weight-bearing and the load-bearing bones (not always the same) as well as various systems, including "feedback systems", were identified and subsequently

R. Bartl, C. Bartl, *Bone Disorders*, DOI 10.1007/978-3-319-29182-6_4

termed the *mechanostat* and which was held responsible for the strength of the bones.

The mechanostat hypothesis was then also applied in order to provide functional definitions of bone competence and of bone quality, in normal physiological conditions, as well as in pathological states, such as osteopenias and osteoporoses. Evidence was provided:

- That muscle strength largely determines the strength of the load-bearing bones
- That this in turn has implications for numerous aspects of bone physiology such as in modelling and remodelling and in interventions such as bone grafts, osteotomies and arthrodeses and possibly also in the actions of pharmaceutical agents

Additional discoveries during the first half of the twentieth century led to the formulation of the *Utah paradigm of skeletal physiology*, according to which the skeletal effector cells (osteoblasts, osteoclasts, chondroblasts, etc.) themselves determine the structure and function of bones, together with the fascia, ligaments and tendons. However, with the passage of time and a great deal of additional work, the results of studies on tissue-level mechanisms were added to the Utah paradigm, which by then also encompassed determinants of skeletal architecture and strength. Moreover, with the accumulating information on skeletal physiology, the Utah paradigm also came to include and integrate scientific evidence on anatomy and biochemistry – from histology to cellular and molecular biology – to pathologies of skeletal disorders and their clinical aspects.

The most significant for everyday medicine worldwide was and is the bottom line conclusion, which, simply expressed, states that strong muscles make and maintain strong bones throughout life!

The highly significant implications of this for diagnosis, for institution of preventive measures and for therapeutic interventions, are discussed later. Many studies have now been published on mechano-biology, that is, the relationship between mechanical forces and biological processes, including the specific pathways involved in the transmission of signals elicited by mechanical loading and stress, also known as *mechano-transduction* which is regulated by two structural combinations:

- Focal adhesions, linking cells to the extracellular matrix
- Junctional adhesions, linking adjacent cells to each other by means of adherins, and these, through the cellular circuits, coordinate tissue responses to mechanical loading or, in simple terms, enable cells to translate the signals produced by mechanical loading into biochemical responses.

But these biomechanical stimuli are only a few of the numerous signals, essential for an integrated osseous physiology, which are transported by the intra-osseous circulation formed by the dendritic extensions and gap junctions of the osteocytes and possibly also the hemichannels which contain connexin 43 (CX 43). Immunoreactive sites for CX43 have already been identified in mature osteoclasts, as well as in marrow stromal cells.

It should also be remembered that the osteocytes, among their other responsibilities, function as sensors for mechanical stimuli and as regulators of mineralisation in bone, which is part of their participation in overall mineral metabolism, particularly that of calcium. It is the gap junctions which enable adjacent cells to exchange second messengers, ions and cellular metabolites. The junctions also participate in development of bone cells, for example, providing signalling pathways downstream of RANKL, for osteoclast differentiation

4.1 Mechanisms Regulating Bone Mass

The bone possesses an efficient feedback-controlled system that continuously integrates both the signals and the responses which together

Table 4.1 Hormonal and local regulators of bone remodelling

Hormones
Polypeptide hormones
Parathyroid hormone (PTH)
Calcitonin
Insulin
Growth hormone
Steroid hormones
1,25-dihydroxyvitamin D_3
Glucocorticoids
Sex steroids
Thyroid hormones
Local factors
Synthesised by bone cells
IGF-1 and IGF-2
Beta-2-microglobulin
TGF-beta
BMPs
FGFs
PDGF
Synthesised by bone-related tissue
Cartilage-derived
IGF-1
FGFs
TGF-beta
Blood cell derived
G-CSF
GM-CSF
IL1
TNF
Other factors
Prostaglandins
Binding proteins

maintain its function of delivering calcium into the circulation while preserving its own strength. The question arises: How do mesenchymal and haematopoietic cells as well as the osteoclasts, osteoblasts and osteocytes cooperate to achieve such a perfect balance between resorption and formation of bone? This complex system is just starting to be unravelled (Table 4.1). There appear to be five groups of mechanisms regulating bone mass (Fig. 4.1):

- *Systemic hormones*: The most important hormones are parathyroid hormone (PTH), calcitonin, thyroid hormone T 3, insulin, growth hormone (GH) and insulin-like growth factor-1 (IGF-1) which mediates many of the effects of GH on longitudinal growth and on bone mass: cortisone, and sex hormones, and of these oestrogens regulate mainly osteoclastic activity and thus bone resorption. PTH together with vitamin D is the principal regulator of calcium homeostasis (Fig. 4.2). PTH exerts its effects by way of actions on the bone cells as well as on other organs such as the kidney and the gut. On bone, PTH exerts its influence mainly by participation in the mechanisms controlling bone turnover. Androgens are also important in bone formation. Osteoblasts and osteocytes as well as mononuclear and endothelial cells in the bone marrow possess receptors for androgen; the pattern and expression of the receptors is similar in men and women. Fat cells, the adipocytes, also have receptors for sex hormones which they are able to metabolise by means of the enzymes called aromatases. Sex steroids also influence lipid metabolism in pre-adipocytes. Significant levels of both oestrogens and androgens are present in the blood in men and in women, and both hormones play important, but not necessarily identical, roles in bone metabolism. For example, androgens may act on osteoblasts during mineralisation while oestrogens more likely affect osteoblasts at an earlier stage during matrix formation. Moreover, the sex hormones may also act at different sites of the bones – for example, androgens are important in the control of periosteal bone formation which contributes to the greater width of the cortex in men. There are receptors for oestrogen and for testosterone on osteoblasts, osteoclasts and osteocytes, but one or another of the sex hormones may dominate at different stages of the remodelling cycle. Androgens in particular exercise a strong influence on bone formation and resorption by way of local enzymes, cytokines, adhesion molecules and growth factors. Androgens increase BMD in women as well

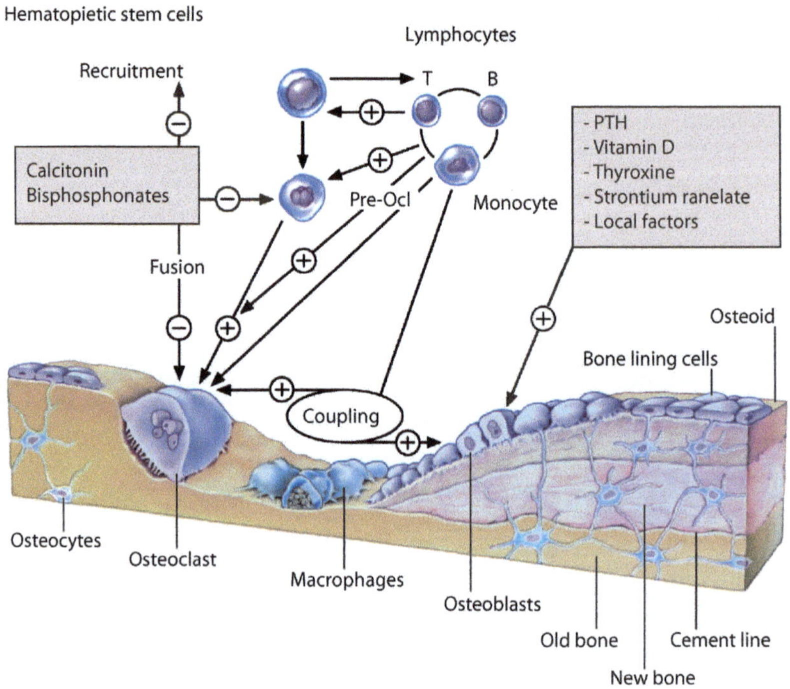

Fig. 4.1 Regulation of bone remodelling involves hormones, cytokines, drugs, mechanical stimuli and cellular interactions ("coupling" of bone resorption and formation)

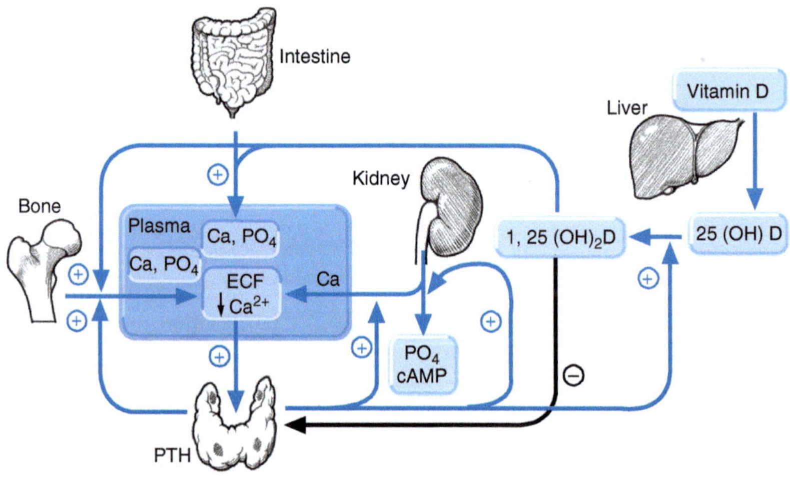

Fig. 4.2 PTH and vitamin D: control of calcium homeostasis (Modified from Brown et al. *Endocrinologist* 1994;4:419–426)

as in men, in normal as well as in some pathologic conditions. Moreover, when given together therapeutically, the two hormones increase BMD more than oestrogen given alone. Other influences such as muscular mass, strength, activity and mechanical strain may stimulate osteoanabolic activity – that is, bone formation while inhibiting bone resorption. Put briefly, during growth the processes of modelling and of remodelling optimise strength by deposition of bone where it is needed and by decrease in bone mass where it is not. It is essential to stress that the highly complicated mechanisms controlling bone remodelling are only briefly outlined here, and the elucidation of their pathways has already led to the disclosure of additional points of possible therapeutic intervention and undoubtedly will continue to do so in the future.

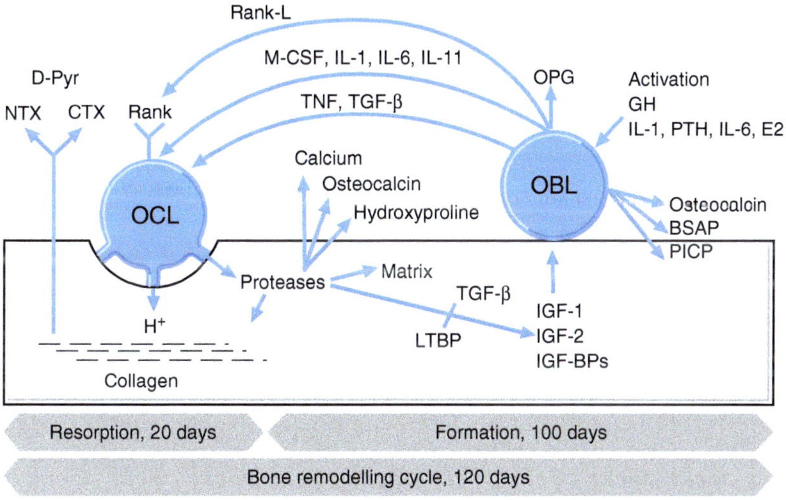

Fig. 4.3 Schematic illustration of factors controlling bone resorption and formation. Abbreviations: *OCL* osteoclast, *OBL* osteoblast. The osteoblast synthesises cytokines and growth factors that activate osteoclasts. The two major ones essential for osteoclastogenesis are macrophage colony-stimulating factor (*M-CSF*) and osteoprotegerin ligand (OPGL), also called RANKL. RANKL activates its receptor RANK on the osteoclast. Osteoprotegerin (*OPG*) is a dummy receptor for RANKL and can suppress osteoclastogenesis if it binds enough OPG (Modified from Rosen and Bilezikian 2001)

- *Local cytokines and signals*: Also significant are local cytokines, electromagnetic potentials and, most importantly, signals transmitted over intercellular networks. Bone cells synthesise whole families of cytokines: for example, IGF-1, IGF-2, beta-2-microglobulin, IL-1, IL-6, TGF-beta, BMPs, FGFs and PDGF (Fig. 4.3). Prostaglandins play a significant part in resorption of bone during immobilisation. Osteoprotegerin (OPG), a member of the tumour necrosis factor receptor family produced by osteoblasts, blocks differentiation of osteoclasts from precursor cells and thereby prevents resorption. In fact, OPG could represent the long sought-after molecular link between arterial calcification and bone resorption. This link underlies the clinical coincidence of vascular disease and osteoporosis, an association most frequent in postmenopausal women and in elderly people. OPG could represent a novel pathway for possible therapeutic manipulation of bone remodelling. Specific aspects of remodelling involve specific factors, as for example, the impact of VEGF (vascular endothelial growth factor) in angiogenesis and endochondral bone formation, in ossification of mandibular condyles and in the growth of the long bones.
- *Vitamins and minerals*: The bone cells as well as the surrounding cell systems are also influenced by various vitamins, minerals and other factors. Vitamins D, K, C, B_6 and A are all required for the normal metabolism of collagen and for mineralisation of osteoid.
- *Mechanical loading*: Exercise may improve bone mass and bone strength in children and adolescents. However, the osteogenic potential diminishes at the end of puberty and longitudinal growth of the bones. The adult bone is only moderately responsive to mechanical loading. A new way which might be useful to manipulate bone tissue is high-frequency, low-amplitude "vibration" exercise, combined with rest periods between loading events. Bone tissue cells must transduce an extracellular mechanical signal into an intracellular response. A mechanoreceptor is known to be a structure made up of extracellular and intracellular proteins linked to transmembrane channels. Touch sensation, proprioception and blood pressure regulation are mediated by ion channels. It has been

proposed that osteocyte processes are tethered to the extracellular matrix and that these tethers amplify cell membrane strains. Presumably the extracellular fluid flow creates tension on the tethers; this in turn stretches the cell membrane.

- *Transcriptional regulation and genes:* There exist a number of transcriptional factors that control osteogenesis and differentiation of osteoblasts. These include runt-related transcription factor 2 (Runx2), Osterix (Osx) and sex determining region Y-box 9 (Sox9), "master" regulators of osteogenesis. Also new genes responsible for hereditary skeletal disorders could provide new therapeutic opportunities. For example, the identification of LRP5 as a key molecule in bone regulation was shown recently to promote osteoblastic differentiation. Finally, it should be noted that research is still ongoing concerning the cells involved; their origin and differentiation; the control mechanisms of remodelling, particularly at different sites, for example, endosteal and periosteal, adjacent to haematopoietic (red) marrow or to adipocytic (yellow) marrow; as well as the activities (if any) of the endothelial cells of the blood vessels connected to the active remodelling units. Results of these studies may reveal additional aspects of remodelling.

4.2 Osteoimmunology

It is important to emphasise that elucidation of the mechanisms underlying metabolism of bone has revealed that these mechanisms include elements of the immune system. This in turn has led to the establishment of the new interdisciplinary field. *Osteoimmunology*, originally triggered by the observation that the increased bone resorption in inflammatory disorders such as rheumatoid arthritis, is caused by increased expression of RANKL (receptor activator of nuclear factor kappa B ligand), which induced accelerated osteoclastic differentiation and activity. Moreover, such interplay/crosstalk also provides bridges for many factors – cytokines, signalling molecules, transduction factors, receptors, etc., which implement bone remodelling, are involved in the homeostasis of bone and are essential participants in the regulation of other organs and systems such as cardiology, nephrology, hepatology, gastroenterology as well as in cardiovascular, hormonal and endocrinological disorders. This multisystem participation provides a well-nigh irrefutable explanation for the fact that the bone is affected one way or another by disorders of practically all the other organs and systems in the body and why osteoporosis now constitutes a global epidemic.

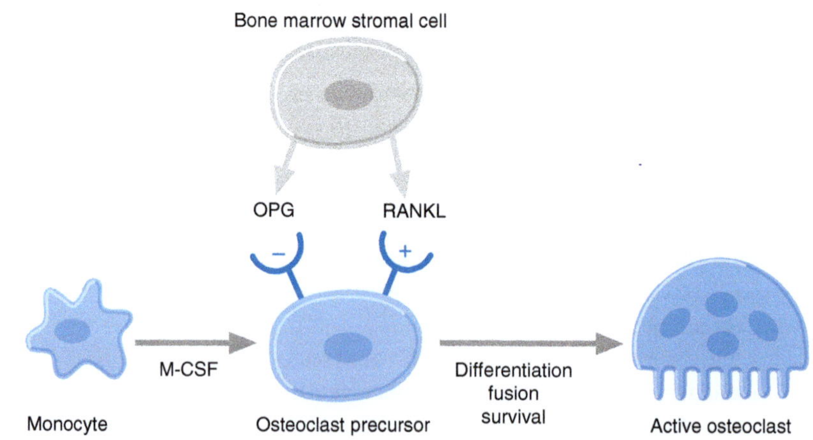

Fig. 4.4 The OPG/RANK/RANKL system and its control of osteoclastic resorption of bone

4.3 RANK/RANKL/ Osteoprotegerin System

The *RANK/RANKL/osteoprotegerin cytokine system* plays a key role in the regulation of and in "coupling" within the processes of remodelling. The discovery of this cytokine system was a milestone for understanding osteoclastogenesis and the regulation of bone resorption as well as other processes involved in local bone remodelling. Osteoprotegerin (OPG) is an important member of the tumour-necrosis factor-receptor family which is produced by osteoblasts and which blocks the differentiation of osteoclasts from their precursor cells and thus inhibits resorption of bone. RANKL (receptor activator of NF-kb ligand also known as OPG ligand, OPGL) and its receptors RANK and OPG are the key components of the regulation of bone remodelling units. RANKL, a member of the TNF family, is the main stimulus for osteoclast maturation and is essential for osteoclast survival. The processes of local remodelling are graphically illustrated in Fig. 4.4.

An increase in the expression of RANKL leads directly to increased resorption and loss of bone. RANKL is produced by osteoblastic cells and by activated T-lymphocytes. Its specific receptor RANK is located on the surface membranes of osteoclasts, dendritic cells, smooth muscle cells and endothelial cells. The production of RANKL by T-lymphocytes and the consequent activation of dendritic cells represent a connection between the immunoregulatory system and osseous tissues. The close collaboration between bone and haematopoiesis is reflected by the fact that M-CSF is required for osteoclastic differentiation.

The effect of RANKL is regulated by OPG, which is secreted in various organs including bone, skin, liver, stomach, intestine, lungs, kidneys and placenta. It also acts as a soluble endogenous receptor antagonist. Numerous cytokines, hormones and drugs may stimulate or inhibit the effects of RANKL or of OPG and thereby sway the results to the advantage or to the detriment of either of these two cytokines as follows:

- TGF-β increases production of OPG.
- PTH increases RANKL/decreases OPG production.
- Vitamin D_3 increases production of RANKL.
- Glucocorticoids increase RANKL/decrease OPG production
- Oestrogen increases production of OPG

Other stimulators of OPG production are vitamin K, leptin, genistein, raloxifen, statins (e.g. atorvastatin), bisphosphonates and mechanical forces. Moreover, new facets of these mechanisms are constantly being elucidated by ongoing research, for example, the suppression of osteoclastogenesis by alpha-lipoic acid. In addition, it has become clear that the relationship between RANKL and OPG contributes to preservation of the balance between resorption and formation in bone, i.e. "coupling" of these activities, and that the relative concentration of RANKL and OPG in bone is one of the main determinants of bone mass and strength.

Animal experiments have also demonstrated the important part played by OPG in the regulation of bone resorption. Genetically manipulated mice, which overexpress OPG, develop osteopetrosis, while OPG knock-out mice develop severe osteoporosis. These experiments indicate that OPG functions as a "brake" for the effects triggered by RANKL. Quite possibly, in the not-so-distant future, OPG may well be introduced as a therapeutic agent in numerous disorders characterised by increased resorption, such as:

- Postmenopausal osteoporosis and osteoporosis of the elderly
- Disorders with locally increased resorption
- Paget's disease of bone
- Periodontitis

- Rheumatoid arthritis
- Bone marrow oedema syndrome
- Osteoporosis in various immunologic disorders
- Haematologic disorders, e.g. multiple myeloma
- Carcinomatosis of bone
- Hypercalcaemic syndrome

During the last few years the significance of the OPG/RANKL/RANK system has been elucidated, not only in primary disorders of bone but also in secondary skeletal-related and vascular conditions which include such common diseases as diabetes, atherosclerosis, rheumatoid arthritis and metastases (Table 4.2). This confirms that the RANKL/OPG system is a cytokine system with widespread, far-reaching systemic effects. In a recent study, a substantially increased risk of hip fracture in women was demonstrated after the onset of a cardiovascular disease (CVD), a finding compatible with the concept of common pathologic pathways for osteoporotic fractures and CVD. The MINOS study, a long-term prospective trail, showed that aortic calcification is a considerable and independent risk factor for incident fractures in older men. Significantly, in all the conditions mentioned above, there are windows of opportunity for the inclusion of bisphosphonates in therapeutic interventions– some are already being explored and applied.

Table 4.2 OPG/RANKL/RANK system in the pathogenesis of bone, immune and vascular diseases

Metabolic bone diseases
Postmenopausal osteoporosis
Glucocorticoid-induced osteoporosis
Hyperparathyroidism
Sporadic Paget's disease of bone
Immune-mediated bone diseases
Rheumatic arthritis
Periodontal infection
Malignant diseases
Multiple myeloma
Bone metastases
Hypercalcaemia of malignancy
Inherited skeletal diseases
Familial expansile osteolysis
Familial Paget's disease of bone
Idiopathic hyperphosphatasia
Cardiovascular diseases
Atherosclerosis
Peripheral vascular disease
Coronary artery disease

4.4 Leptin

The observation that overweight individuals are less susceptible to osteoporosis hints at a link between obesity and the bone. It was first suggested that the effects of increased weight-bearing might protect bone mass. However, experimental studies have implicated leptin: a hormone produced by fat cells and which interacts with neurons in the brain and thereby influences weight. It was then discovered that in mice, leptin is also antiosteogenic, and it was speculated that increased bone mass in obese people may result from resistance to leptin's antiosteogenic activity. Leptin is released into the bloodstream in proportion to the amount of body fat. It regulates the body's energy balance and bone mass by binding to certain receptor proteins of specific neurons in the hypothalamus of the brain, which in turn activate sympathetic nerves. These extend into the bone, where they stimulate release of the neurotransmitter noradrenaline, which then stimulates beta-2-adrenergic receptors on osteoblasts, inhibiting osteoblastic activity. Leptin inhibits bone formation through its action on already differentiated osteoblasts and has no overt effect on osteoclast differentiation or function. These results seem to suggest that the millions of patients who have been treated with "beta-blockers" such as propranolol for hypertension should have increased bone mass – an argument for reassessing these clinical studies with respect to changes in bone density. The identification of leptin as a powerful inhibitor of bone formation definitely has potential therapeutic implications in the future.

5 Growth and Ageing of Bone

5.1 Types of Ossification

Osteoblasts derive from mesenchymal cells and produce osteoid, the organic matrix of bone, in two ways:

- *Intramembranous ossification:* Osteoid is directly secreted in loose vascular connective tissue. Mineralisation of the osteoid occurs shortly after deposition, and the newly formed bone tissue is called "primitive bone". Examples of this type of ossification are the flat bone of the skull as well as parts of the mandible and the clavicle. Furthermore, intramembranous ossification beneath the periosteum is a mechanism for increasing the diameter of long bones.
- *Endochondral ossification:* Most of the skeleton is formed by this process, whereby osteoid is deposited on pre-existing cartilage. Continuous endochondral ossification at the epiphyseal plate is responsible for longitudinal bone growth. The complex of newly formed bone with a core of calcified cartilage is called "primary spongiosa" and later replaced by mature lamellar bone.

At the *epiphyseal plate*, endochondral bone formation is highly regulated, and *four distinct morphologic zones* can be distinguished:

- Reserve or resting zone
- Zone of proliferation
- Zone of hypertrophy
- Zone of endochondral ossification

The epiphyseal plates close at different times during adolescence (distal femur and proximal tibia close between ages 16 and 19 marking the end of growth in height). The last plates to close are the iliac crest and the medial clavicle.

5.2 Growth of the Embryo in the Uterus

Genetic and environmental factors are involved in the normal growth and development of the embryo in the uterus as well as in growth retardation. In addition, recent studies that followed the trajectories of growth from birth to adulthood have demonstrated that size at birth and postnatal growth both effect the risk of and are associated with the development of a number of chronic diseases in adulthood. These include hypertension, coronary heart disease, stroke, diabetes and disturbances of renal function. Moreover, adverse maternal and other environmental factors are also involved. The most recent studies have shown that circumstances during the foetal period and early childhood may have life-long programming effects on different physical functions.

Intrauterine growth restriction has now been positively associated with low bone mass in infancy and with increased risk of development of osteoporosis in adulthood. Importantly, in the context of this book, it is now believed that osteoporosis is, at least partly, programmed in utero and that nutritional and other environmen-

R. Bartl, C. Bartl, *Bone Disorders*, DOI 10.1007/978-3-319-29182-6_5

tal factors in the pre- and postnatal period exercise a profound influence on skeletal development, which, in turn, has considerable consequences in adulthood. And there is no racial discrimination, because this applies equally to blacks and whites, as demonstrated in an investigation of bone size and bone mass in both black and white South African children. Moreover, not only organs such as the skeleton, but also cell systems may be modulated by the intrauterine metabolic environment as shown by intrauterine epigenetic modification of beta pancreatic cells towards a prediabetic phenotype, but this could be corrected by early intervention, i.e. supplementation of the maternal diet. However, many other studies have now demonstrated that the adverse pre- and postnatal effects listed above can and should be modified by application of appropriate measures (nutrition, supplements, possibly medications, exercise and lifestyle) during childhood, adolescence and adulthood into old age.

5.3 Peak Bone Mass

The skeleton acquires the maximal bone density – *peak bone mass* – at 25–30 years (Fig. 5.1). Consequently, the periods of growth before that provide the maximal opportunities for building the peak bone mass, 60–80 % of which is determined by genetic factors, but the rest 20–40 % by other determinants such as nutrition and exercise. Thereafter, beginning at about 30 years, a negative bone balance sets in, so that on average 1 % of bone is lost every year, independent of sex. Measurements of trabecular bone density between the ages of 20 and 80 years have shown reductions of approximately 50 % in density (Fig. 5.2). This bone loss is apparently genetically programmed. Marked racial differences in peak bone mass occur, with higher values in American blacks than in Caucasians and the lowest values in Asians and the Japanese. Some of the multiple pathogenic mechanisms and factors that contribute to subsequent loss of bone ("osteoporosis"), after the acquisition of peak bone mass, include the following:

- Genetic factors
- Foetal and neonatal factors
- Factors during growth
- Inadequate peak bone density
- Nutritional and lifestyle factors
- Menopause and reduction of oestrogen in women
- Age and deficiency of testosterone in men
- Reduction of about 80 % in adrenal steroids during ageing
- Comorbidities
- Other effects of ageing on the body and on the activities of daily living

Race and diet interactions are also involved in the acquisition, maintenance and loss of bone. Some of the genes that may influence

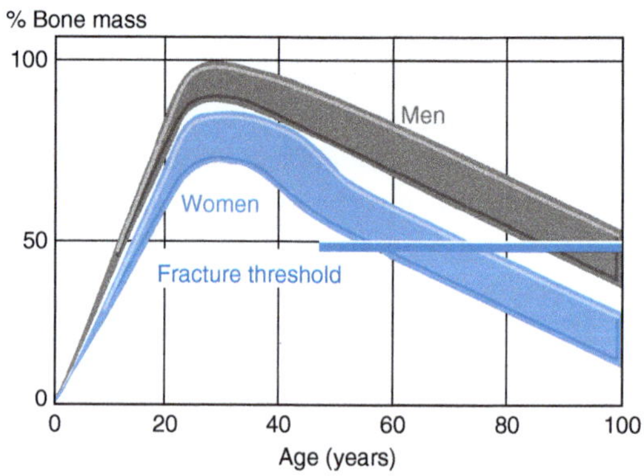

Fig. 5.1 Age-related changes in bone mass

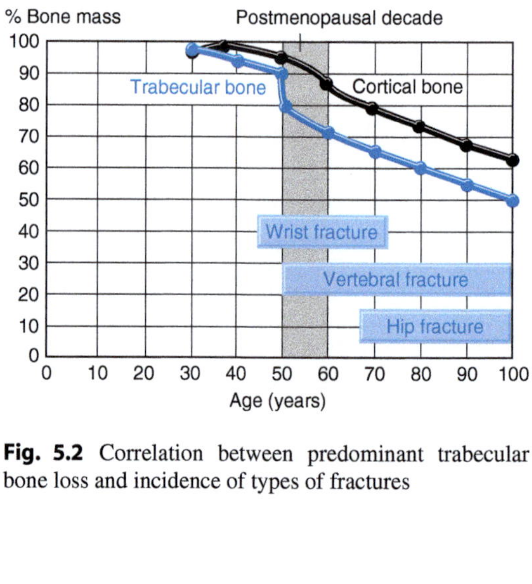

Fig. 5.2 Correlation between predominant trabecular bone loss and incidence of types of fractures

bone mass and rates of bone loss include the *genes* responsible for:

- Vitamin D receptor
- Oestrogen receptor
- Parathyroid hormone receptor
- IL-1 receptor antagonist
- TGF-β
- Sp1 site in α1chain of type I collagen

The bones are like a bank savings account for calcium. If the calcium supply is adequate, savings deposits are made and the calcium bone bank account builds up. If the dietary calcium intake is too low, then withdrawals of calcium are made from the "bone bank" itself, i.e. the skeleton. The peak bone mass attained in early life is a major determinant of subsequent bone mass and of fracture risk in later life. Peak bone mass is greater in men than in women, although these differences are reduced or even reversed if bone mass is expressed as volumetric bone density.

Calcium tends to be stored in the osseous tissue during the day and slowly released during the night. A bone biopsy study has shown that the loss of bone occurs fairly equally in all regions of the skeleton, perhaps slightly more in the vertebral bodies and the proximal femur. In postmenopausal women, the decline in oestrogen is accompanied by an increase in the loss of bone of up to 4 % annually. This implies that women may lose 40 % of their bone mass from 40 to 70 years. During the same period, men lose only about 12 %.

Part II

The Spectrum of Bone Disorders

6 Osteoclast: The Leading Actor in Bone Disorders

Bones are not inert, amorphous, rocklike substances, but are alive, sensible and dynamic like other tissues of the body. As indicated in the previous chapter, bone is subject to constant stress, maintenance, adaptation and repair. They get atrophic when they are not used, they die if they have no sufficient blood supply, they develop inflammations and tumours, they respond to various systemic and local influences and, especially, they can heal themselves. Considering the dynamic behaviour and pathologic consequences, one cell type of the osseous tissue is almost always involved and plays a major role both in normal and pathologic reactions: the *osteoclast*, belonging to the monocyte-macrophage-system. Anomalies and alterations in activity of this specific cell result in localised or systemic disorders of the bone and can manifest as:

- Skeletal deformities
- Restriction of movement
- Pathologic fractures
- Bone pain
- Hypercalcaemic syndrome

Hyperactive, abnormally activated osteoclasts are characterised by a high resorptive capacity and therefore a high destructive potential (Fig. 6.1a, b), so that numerous osteoblasts need months to repair an osteolytic lesion accomplished by a few osteoclasts within a week. The rate of radial erosion of an active osteoclast is about 12 μm/day, while the resorption cavity is carved out in about 8 days. In Paget's disease of the bone, for example, a single osteoclast can grow into a giant cell with more than 100 nuclei and correspondingly increased osteolytic activity (Fig. 6.2). Why and how osteoclasts, e.g. in Paget's and in Gorham's disease, are able to evade the established "coupling" mechanisms and independently, randomly resorb bone is still a mystery. The average life span of a labelled nucleus in osteoclasts is 11 days. Dysregulation of osteoclasts is the main cause of nearly all bone disorders (about 90 %), such as osteoporosis (systemic) or osteolysis (local), accompanied by spontaneous fractures and hypercalcaemia. The dysregulated and hyperactive osteoclasts are the key to over 90 % of all progressively destructive disorders of the bone, e.g. osteolytic bone metastases (Fig. 6.3)

There are only two osteopathies in which increased osteolytic activity is not involved:

- *Osteopetrosis* (osteosclerosis) due to osteoblastic bone formation with inadequate resorption
- *Osteomalacia* due to inhibition of mineralisation by lack of vitamin D

However, even in osteomalacia, osteoclasts are indirectly involved through secondary hyperparathyroidism (HPT). In osteopetrosis, various genetic and other factors inhibit

R. Bartl, C. Bartl, *Bone Disorders*, DOI 10.1007/978-3-319-29182-6_6

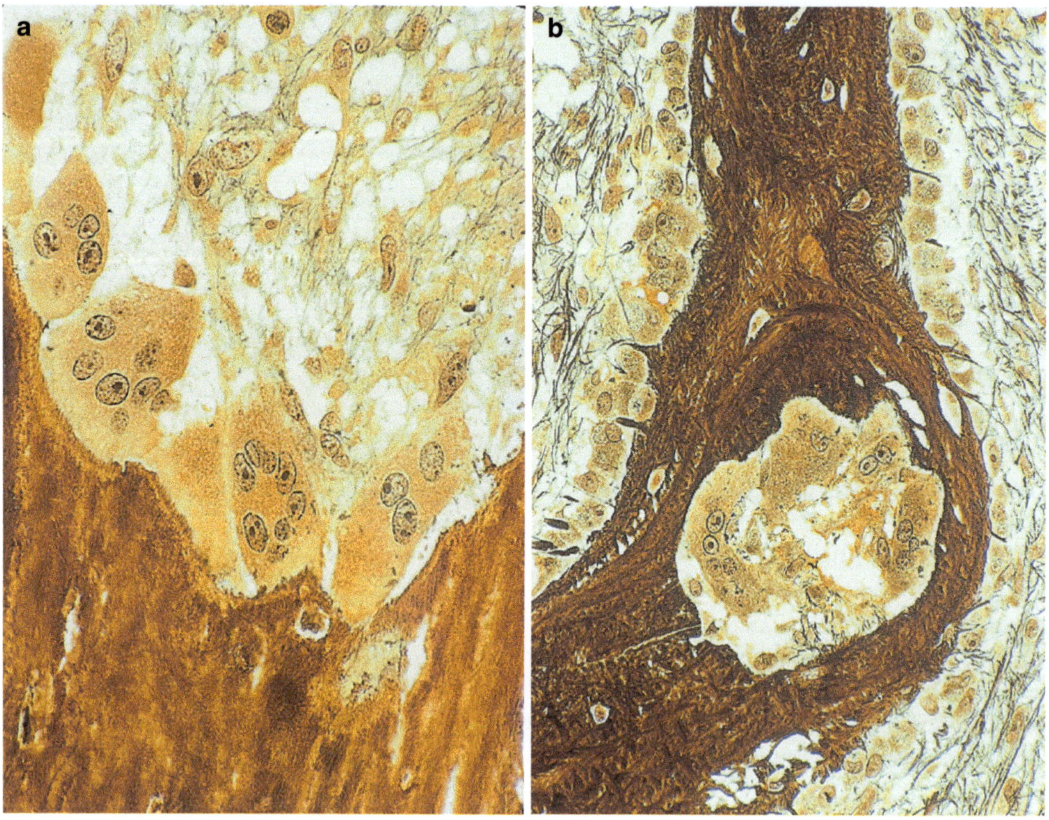

Fig. 6.1 Inordinate osteoclastic activity. (**a**) Numerous hyperactive osteoclasts and disorganised resorption of the bone in Paget's disease of the bone. (**b**) Classic appearance of dissecting osteoclastosis in HPT. Gomori staining

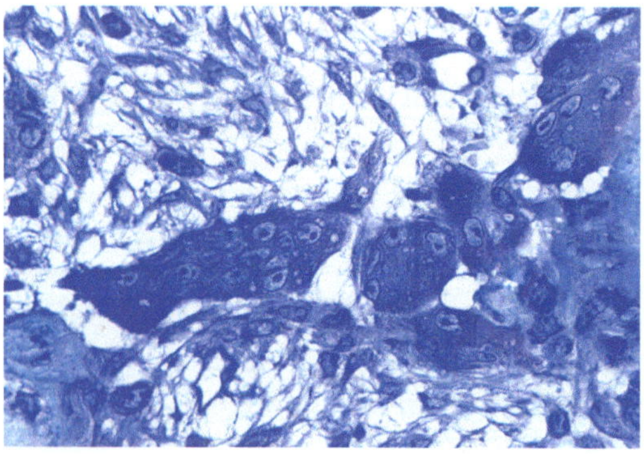

Fig. 6.2 Giant multinucleated and nucleolated osteoclasts within loose connective tissue but far from any osseous surface. Bone biopsy from a patient with Paget´s disease. Giemsa staining

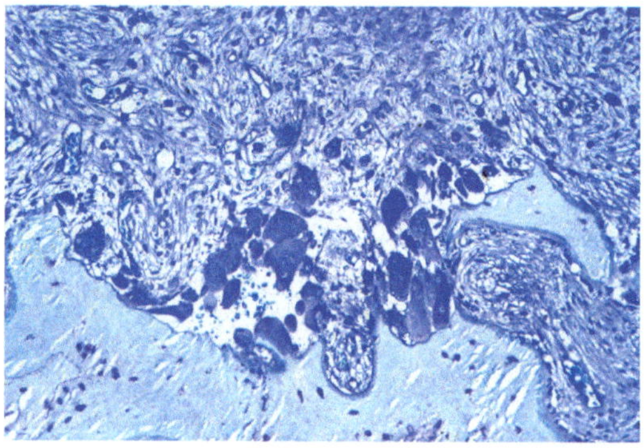

Fig. 6.3 Active osteoclasts activated by adjacent tumour cells and resorbing trabecular bone. Giemsa staining

osteoclast development and function and lead to an increase in bone mass and finally to osteosclerosis/osteopetrosis. But the dense bone produced is not proportionately strong and is therefore liable to fracture.

Dysregulation of the following factors/activities is involved in osteopathies:

- Intracellular signalling
- Cellular receptors

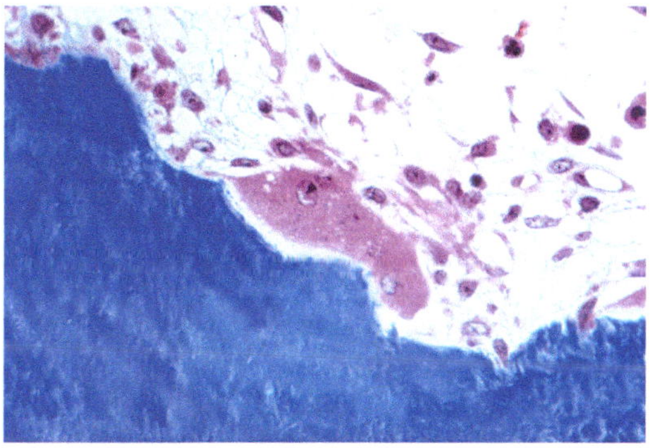

Fig. 6.4 Inactive osteoclast with cytoplasmic *bubbles* and complete loss of the ruffled border, under intravenously administered zoledronate. Ladewig staining

- Cellular attachment
- Cytokine production
- Activities of various enzymes
- Various non-genomic factors, systemic hormones and others

Today, first and foremost, hormones and drugs that decrease osteoclastic activity are required for the prevention and treatment of bone disorders. There are four possible approaches to correct the increased and unbalanced osteoclastic activity:

- Inhibition of recruitment of precursors – prevention of osteoclast formation
- Decrease in survival of osteoclasts – induction of apoptosis
- Inhibition of osteoclastic activity – prevention of resorption/osteolysis
- Interference with the interaction between osteoclasts and the surface of the bone – prevention of osteoclast attachment

Bisphosphonates (BPs), due to their high degree of efficacy and few side effects, have become the agents of choice for the inhibition of osteoclastic activity (Fig. 6.4). *Denosumab* is a new and potent inhibitor of osteoclastic differentiation and is meanwhile used in treatment both of osteoporosis and bone metastases. *Calcitonin* is now mainly used for fast relief of bone pain. Other substances are also utilised for their inhibitory effect on osteoclastic activity, but each has its own limitations. These agents include the following:

- Oestrogen and analogues
- Selective oestrogen receptor modulators (SERMs) (e.g. raloxifene and lasofoxifene)
- Testosterone
- Vitamin D and ipriflavone (a synthetic isoflavonoid)
- Anti-cytokines (IL-1, Il-6, TNFs)
- Osteoprotegerin
- Proton (H^+) pump inhibitors
- Calcium receptor modulators
- Nitric oxide modulators
- Statins
- Enzyme inhibitors (metalloproteinases, cathepsin K)
- Adhesion molecule inhibitors (RGD peptides)
- Intracellular signalling targets (c-src, TRAFs, NF-kB).

These are dealt with in the appropriate chapters. However, it must be clearly stated that none of these has the “global applicability” of BP, which can be given to any patient, at any age, for any condition to inhibit bone resorption (possibility not to pregnant and lactating women; see appropriate chapter), although studies have not revealed adverse or teratogenic effects on the fetus.

7 Classifying Bone Disorders According to Spread (Topography)

Two types of bone disorders are distinguished:

- *Generalised metabolic and genetic osteopathies* such as osteoporosis and osteomalacia. These affect the skeletal system as a whole, and typical for this group are osteoporosis, osteogenesis imperfecta, osteosclerosis and osteomalacia. Bone marrow metastases also belong to this group even though initially they manifest as focal lesions, solitary or multiple.
- *Localised focal osteopathies* such as Paget's disease of the bone, fibrous dysplasia and, initially, metastases. Bone scans are particularly useful in distinguishing monostotic from polyostotic involvement. Due to the differences in structure of the bone and bone marrow between the axial skeleton and extremities, there are also differences in metastatic spread and in the osseous and medullary reactions to the malignant cells. Osteopathies of the cranium, spinal column, flat bones, tubular bones as well as bones of the hands and feet are distinguished. Variable changes occur in the epi-, meta- and diaphyses of the tubular bones.

> There is one particularly decisive question for the treatment of osteopathies (as in oncology), namely, *Is the condition localised or systemic?*

R. Bartl, C. Bartl, *Bone Disorders*, DOI 10.1007/978-3-319-29182-6_7

8 Classifying Bone Disorders According to Underlying Pathologic Anatomy

Five main osseous manifestations, singly or in combination, occur in all disorders of the bone (Fig. 8.1):

- *Abnormal bone remodelling:* Balanced bone resorption and formation is abrogated, i.e. the two processes are decoupled – too much bone is resorbed or too little is produced, leading to alteration and weakening of the architecture of the involved bone and to a tendency to fracture. The inevitable consequence of a negative bone balance is a progressive loss of bone. Mixed pictures of both lytic and sclerotic areas, as well as local thickening, may also occur. Highly active remodelling is seen in hyperparathyroidism (Fig. 8.2), Paget's disease, Gorham's disease, fibrous dysplasia, osteomyelitis and some malignancies in the bones. Functionally inadequate osteoclasts or insufficient numbers of osteoclasts result in osteosclerosis. When osteoclastic hypo-/aplasia is congenital, then the bone marrow spaces are not laid down – "modelled" – in the first year of life. The end result is total ossification of the bone – marble bone disease – with a tendency to fracture and insufficient haematopoiesis with life-threatening pancytopaenias. Bone marrow transplantation with reconstitution of the normal monocyte-macrophage system is currently the only effective treatment. In summary, deviations from the normal level of bone turnover and "decoupling" are the two main pathophysiologic abnormalities encountered in osteopathies.
- *Abnormalities of bone mass*: Osteopenia and *osteoporosis* are defined as conditions with a decreased bone mass and an increased fracture risk (Fig. 8.3). The direct cause is a relative or absolute increase in osteoclastic activity in the absence of a corresponding osteoblastic reaction, leading to a negative bone balance, i.e. a reduction in the total amount of the bone – trabecular bone volume and cortical thickness are both reduced. High- and low-turnover variants occur. Osteopenia may be widespread as in the generalised osteoporosis of ageing; confined to the axial skeleton, as in the osteopenia/osteoporosis of young adults; or focal as in inflammatory or neoplastic processes. *Osteosclerosis* signifies expansion of bone volume at the expense of the bone marrow, resulting in poor bone quality (in spite of the greatly increased density) and thereby an increased risk of fractures (Fig. 8.4).
- *Abnormalities of the bone matrix*: A healthy bone matrix is required to maintain bone quality necessary for rigidity and strength. Synthesis of defective collagen with loss of lamellar structure as in osteogenesis imperfecta (Fig. 8.5a, b) or in Marfan syndrome, inadequate cross-linkage as in vitamin C deficiency and defects in other matrix proteins all reduce bone quality and increase the risk of fractures.

R. Bartl, C. Bartl, *Bone Disorders*, DOI 10.1007/978-3-319-29182-6_8

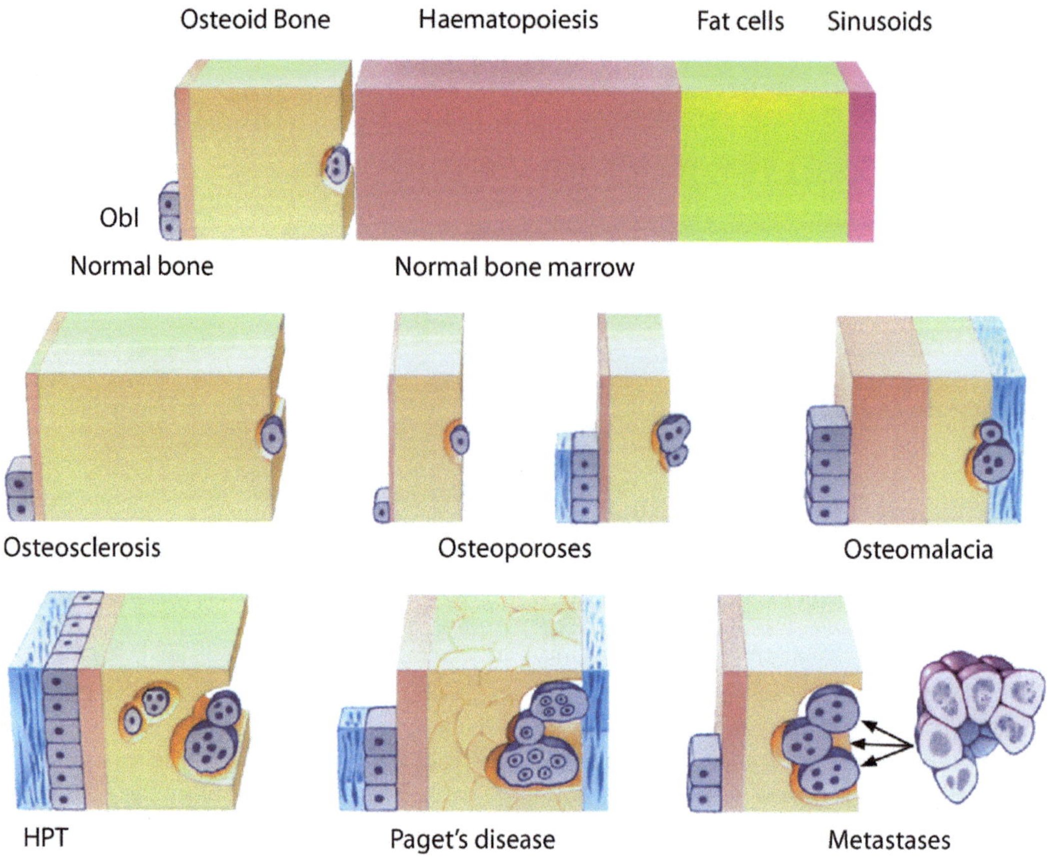

Fig. 8.1 Common osteopathies with examples of the anomalies of bone mass, mineralisation and bone remodelling caused by them

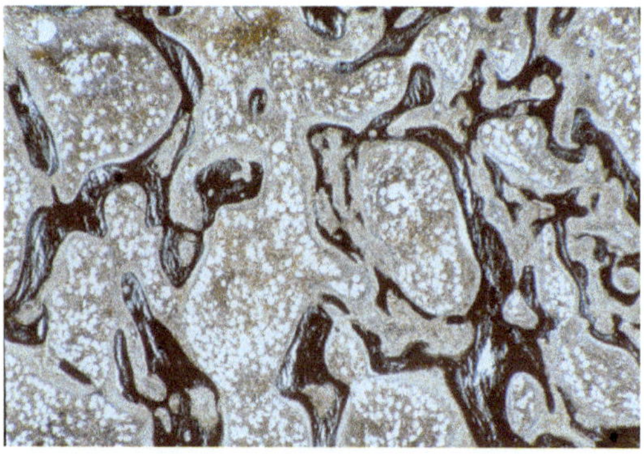

Fig. 8.2 Massive bone remodelling with dissecting osteoclasia and substitution of a large part of the trabecular network by fibrous connective tissue in a patient with primary hyperparathyroidism. Gomori staining

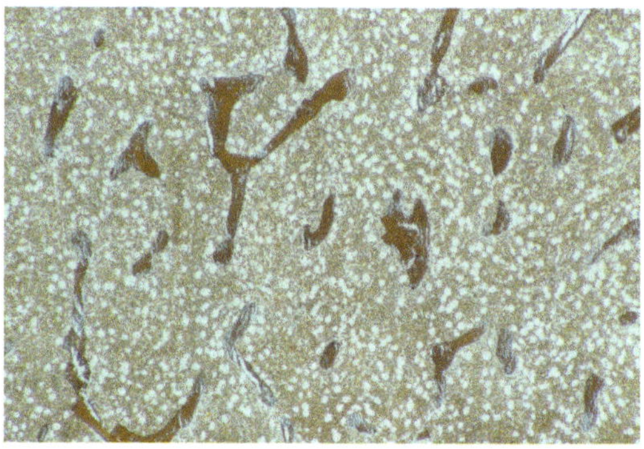

Fig. 8.3 Osteoporosis with decreased bone mass, thin trabeculae and small "buttons". Gomori staining

- *Abnormal mineralisation:* Vitamin D is required for normal mineralisation of the newly produced osteoid. Deficiency or absence of vitamin D leads to increased osteoid production – hyperosteoidosis – which is inadequately mineralised, known as osteomalacia in adults and rickets in children (Fig. 8.6a, b). Increased formation of osteoid with normal calcification may occur in conditions associated with high bone turnover as in primary HPT.
- *Architectural abnormalities:* These are due to disturbances in modelling, remodelling and in structure. They include macroscopic changes, microscopic changes and anomalies occurring at the molecular level. Woven bone, mosaic structures (Fig. 8.7), alterations of trabecular shape and size, discontinuities in the trabecular network, decrease in the number of trabecular connections known as the "nodes", microcracks and fractures all affect the architecture, strength and weight-bearing capacity of the bone.

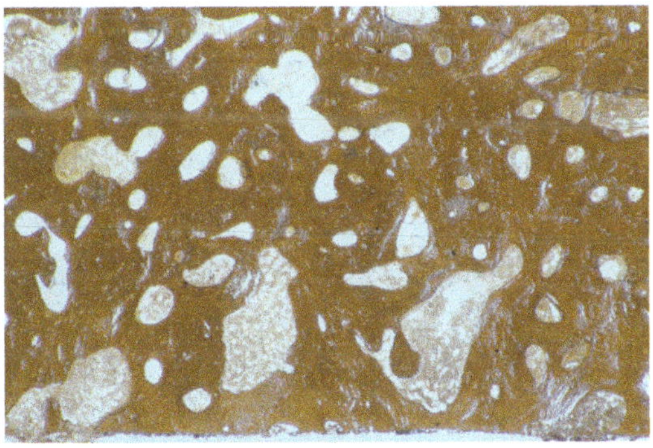

Fig. 8.4 Osteosclerosis illustrating almost complete obliteration of the marrow cavities. Gomori staining

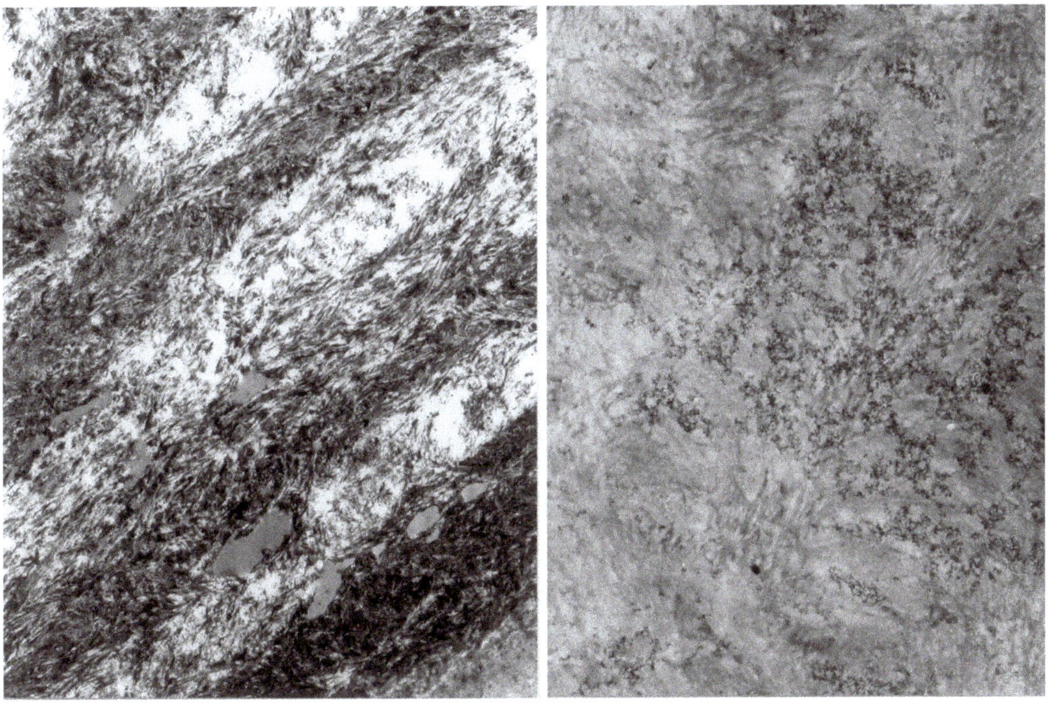

Fig. 8.5 (**a**, **b**) At the electron microscopic level, osteogenesis imperfecta is characterised by trabeculae without any organised microarchitecture (*right*), in contrast to trabeculae with lamellar structure in normal bone tissue (*left*)

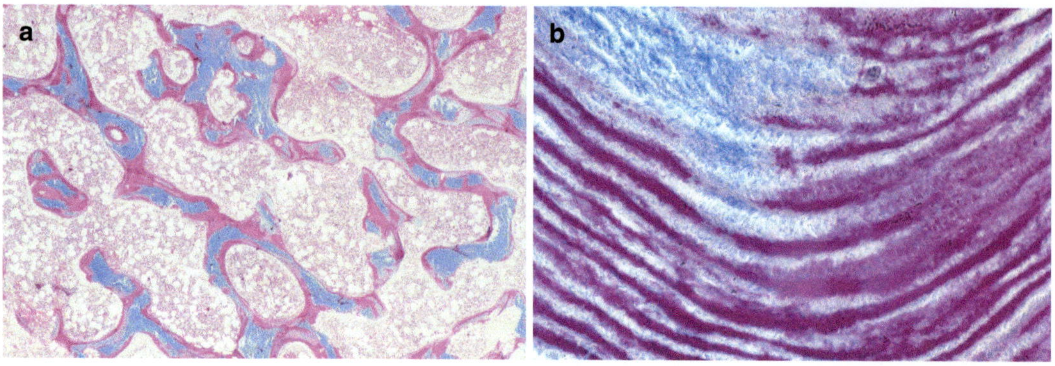

Fig. 8.6 (**a**, **b**) Iliac crest biopsy (**a**) revealing increased extent of osteoid surfaces (*red*) on the trabecular bone; (**b**) higher magnification shows patchy, irregular demineralisation of the lamellar trabecular bone. Ladewig staining

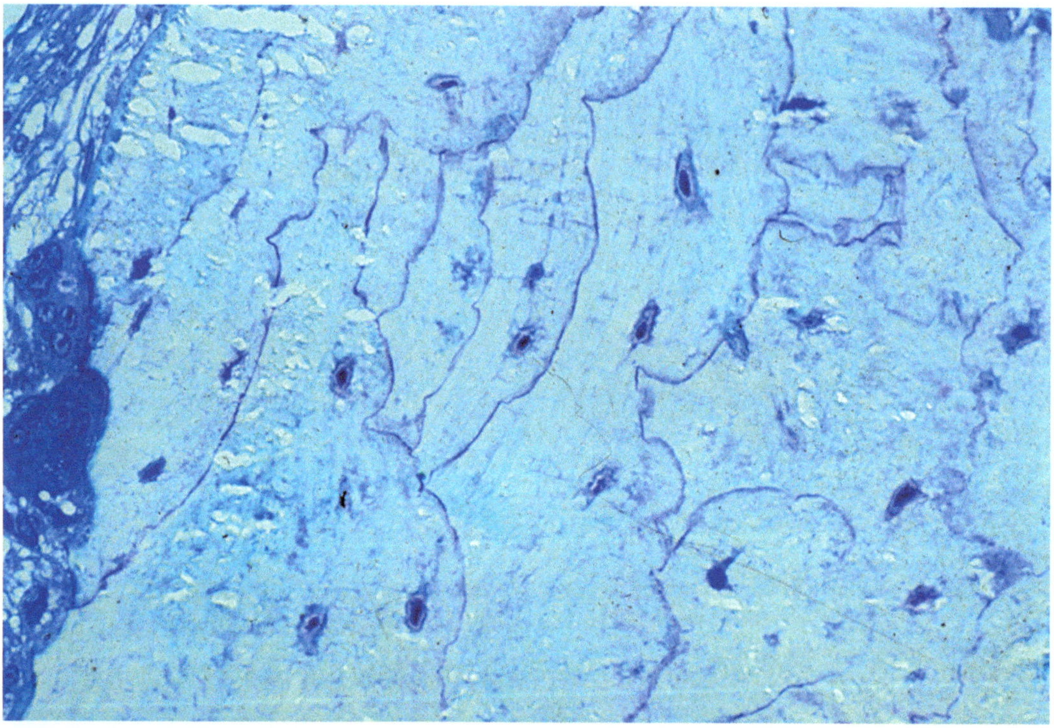

Fig. 8.7 Architectural abnormalities with abnormal bone remodelling and mosaic structures. Note multinucleolated osteoclasts (*left*). Giemsa staining

9 Classifying Bone Disorders According to Pathophysiology

An initial approach to diagnosing a bone disorder is to place the lesion in one of six major groups (categories):

- Congenital
- Metabolic
- Traumatic
- Circulatory
- Infectious
- Neoplastic

9.1 Congenital Bone Disorders

This group is due to gene mutations and usually manifest in childhood. *Skeletal dysplasias* are caused by mutations in numerous genes that control growth and development of the bone, cartilage and connective tissue. These bone dysplasias manifest in three ways:

- Short stature
- Abnormally shaped bone
- Bone fractures

A characteristic feature of these manifestations is their symmetry in the skeleton. Skeletal dysplasias are usually diagnosed and classified by radiologic features, but final diagnosis is based on genetic investigations. Skeletal dysplasias such as osteogenesis imperfecta show a wide range of clinical severity. Severe variants are evident in utero or at birth and are incompatible with life. Less severe dysplasias become manifest in childhood or may be asymptomatic throughout a patient's life. Since skeletal dysplasias usually affect only bones and cartilage, patients have normal intelligence and a normal life span. However, their abnormally shaped bones often lead to physical disability and require orthopaedic surgery. In addition to skeletal dysplasias, genetic disorders targeting other tissues can secondarily affect the bone. One example is neurofibromatosis with development of neural tumours and "café au lait" spots, as well as scoliosis and pseudoarthrosis.

9.2 Metabolic Bone Disorders

Metabolic bone disease results from alterations in the chemical environment of the body, namely, hormones, vitamins, minerals, cytokines and neuronal influences. Disturbances in this regulation system affect three components of the bone, bone mass, bone mineralisation and bone turnover, causing generalised decrease in bone mass (osteopenia and finally *osteoporosis* with fractures and bone pain), a defect in mineralisation of the bone (*osteomalacia* with weak bones and bone pain) or increased bone remodelling (hyperparathyroidism and finally *osteodystrophia fibrosa generalisata* with dissecting osteoclasia (Fig. 9.1) and hypercalcaemia).

R. Bartl, C. Bartl, *Bone Disorders*, DOI 10.1007/978-3-319-29182-6_9

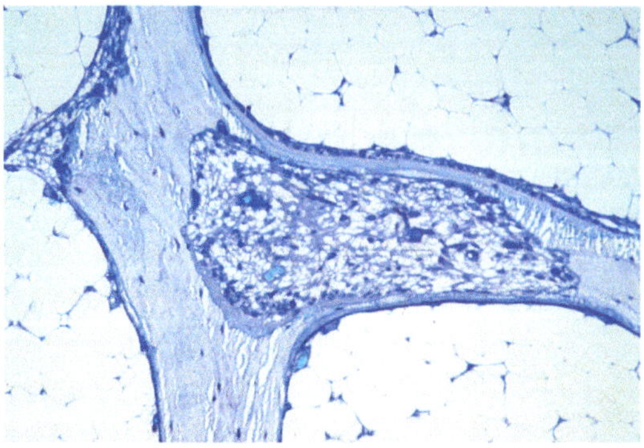

Fig. 9.1 Dissecting osteoclasia in a patient with hyperparathyroidism. Giemsa staining

9.3 Traumatic Bone Disorders

Fractures are by far the most common and severe bone complication. However, the bone has a remarkable healing ability. Whereas other tissues such as the brain, liver or heart heal with a fibrous scar, the bone heals completely with a new bone. A fracture takes a few weeks or months for the bone ends to unite, but it takes years for the bone to remodel to its original shape and strength. However, various complications occasionally occur at fracture, resulting in osteonecrosis, nonunion or pseudoarthrosis, and surgery is required for stabilisation or bone grafting.

Abnormal bone fractures with little trauma are known as *pathologic fractures* or *fragility fractures* in osteoporosis or in patients with bone metastases. One special type of bone injury often presents diagnostic problems, the *stress fractures*. They represent reactions of the bone to repetitive trauma. This cumulative effect weakens the bone by stimulating increased bone remodelling and producing a discrete line of rarefaction – the stress fracture. Because stress fractures are painful and cause only subtle radiographic changes, they are usually diagnosed only by MRI ("bone marrow oedema syndrome") (Fig. 9.2a, b) and often mistaken for bone tumours or other local bone disorders. *Avulsion injuries*, most commonly in children, result from repetitive muscular activity that pulls off the periosteum from the bone surface, resulting in adjacent bone marrow oedema. Most frequently the medial femoral condyle is involved.

9.4 Circulatory Bone Disorders

The bone is a highly vascularised tissue and receives about 10–20 % of the cardiac output. Blood supply of the bone comes from large nutrient arteries penetrating the diaphysis, epiphysis and metaphysis as well as from small arteries from the periosteum. Regional interruption of blood flow to the bone is mainly caused by fractures, infections or intravascular occlusions (*aseptic or avascular necrosis*). The disease appears to occur more frequently in males than in females (ratio of 8.1). The age of onset is variable; in the majority of cases, the patient is less than 50 years old. Bones particularly susceptible for *fracture-related osteonecrosis* are the displaced femoral neck, the humeral head, the talus and the carpal navicular. Also *osseous infections* may isolate a segment of the bone from blood supply. The isolated dead bone fragment (sequestrum) harbours virulent microorganisms and isolates them against the defence mechanisms and antibiotics. *Bone infarction* (Fig. 9.3) is mainly caused by intravascular coagulation, fat embolisation, haemorrhage and only rarely by arteriosclerosis. The most common site is osteonecrosis of the femoral head. Dead bone is brittle, and as a result, the articular surface collapses, and secondary osteoarthritis develops in the joint. Risk factors are steroid therapy, alcohol abuse and hypercoagulable blood. Infections, nicotine abuse, some drugs (e.g. bisphosphonates and denosumab) and dental trauma appear important factors in the aetiology of ONJ (osteonecrosis of the jaw). In the early stage of osteonecrosis, plain radiographs will be normal, but MRI will be diagnostic in 60–80 % of cases. Laboratory investigations will generally be normal.

9.5 Infectious Bone Disorders

Also bone tissue can become infected, a condition known as *osteomyelitis*. Although most patients with bone infections present systemic signs of inflammation, the clinical and radiological patterns vary considerably. Therefore, osteomyelitis must always be considered in the

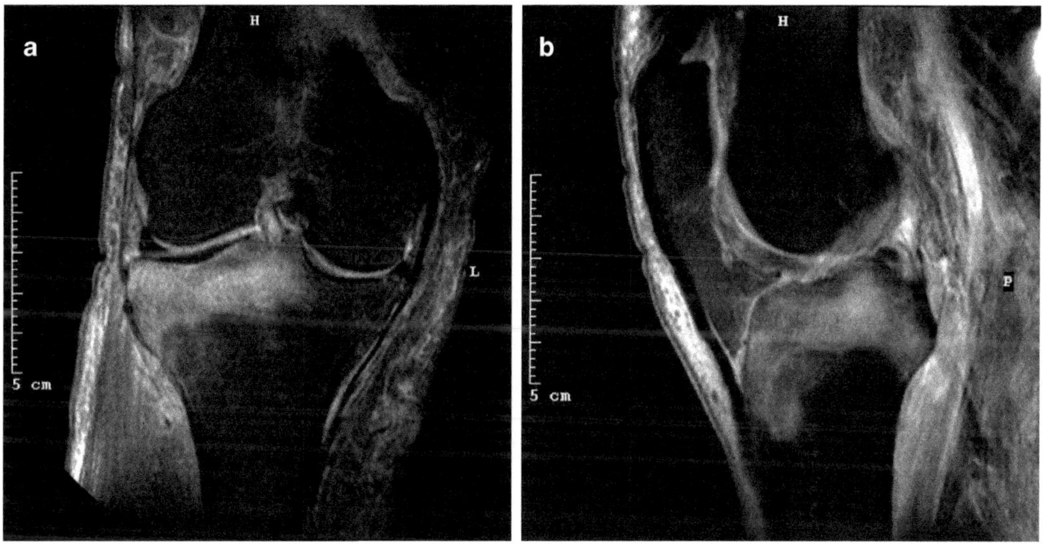

Fig. 9.2 (**a**, **b**) Painful bone bruise with adjacent massive bone marrow oedema in the tibia plateau (MRI)

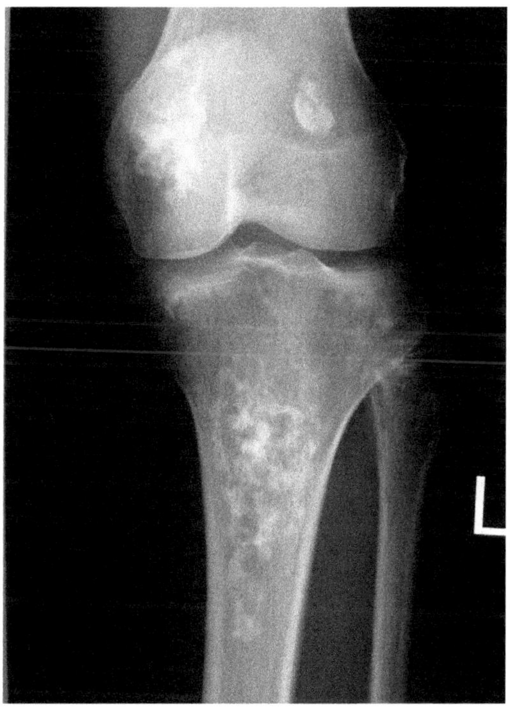

Fig. 9.3 Asymptomatic multiple bone (marrow) infarctions

diagnostic evaluation of any bone lesion, especially in children.

Osteomyelitis develops by two situations:

- Direct invasion of organisms (e.g. open fracture)
- Haematogenous spread of organisms to the bone from an infection elsewhere in the body

Primary osteomyelitis is usually a paediatric disease, and *Staphylococcus aureus* is the most common infectious organism. In adults the spine is the most common site. Incomplete eradication of *acute osteomyelitis* occurs in 5 % of the cases and finally leads to *subacute and chronic osteomyelitis*, extremely difficult to treat and to cure. Chronic osteomyelitis is defined by long-term interaction of the bone with the infecting organism. Radiographs show areas of bone loss mixed with regions of increased density. Although most bone infections are caused by bacteria, any type of microorganism can cause osteomyelitis (fungal or mycobacterial organisms especially in immunosuppressed patients, viruses and parasites).

9.6 Neoplastic Bone Disorders

Bone neoplasms can be divided in two major groups:

- Primary bone tumours, arising in the bone and may be benign or malignant
- Bone metastases, metastasised to bone from neoplasms elsewhere, which are always malignant, indicating an advanced stage of cancer

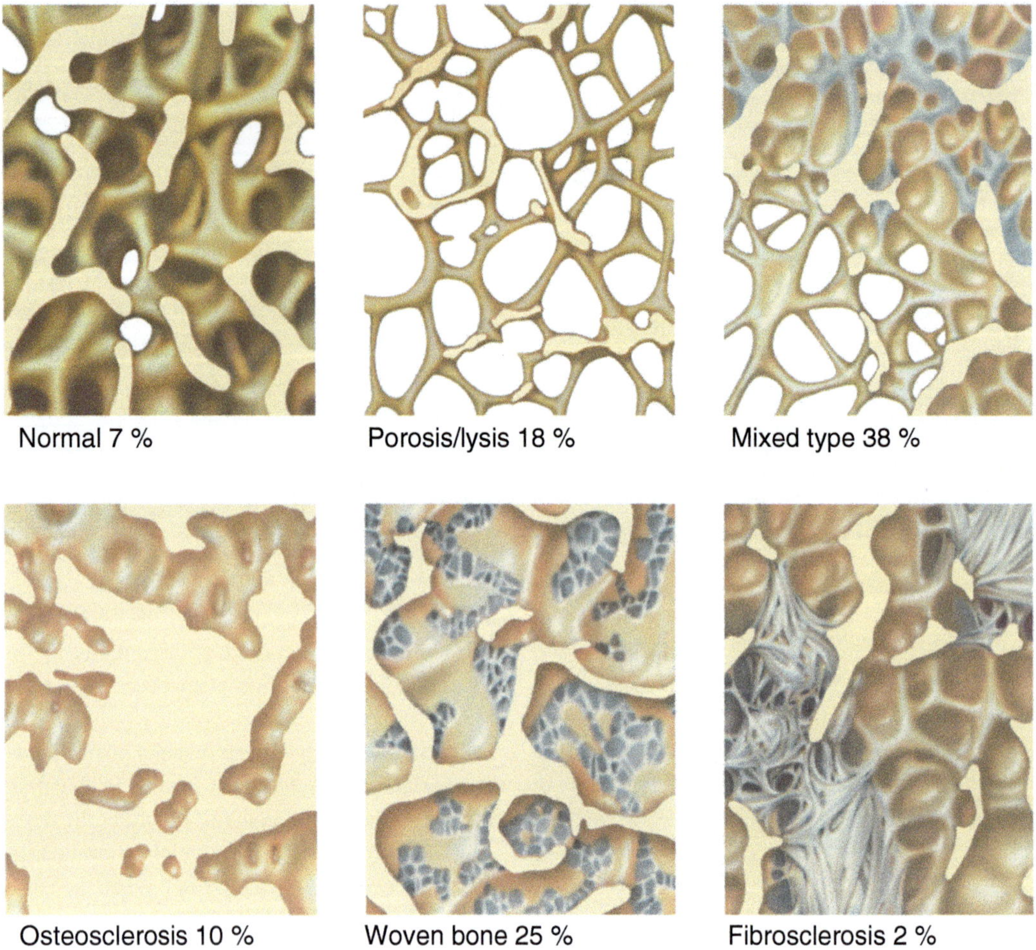

Fig. 9.4 Range and frequency of osseous reactions in metastatic bone disease

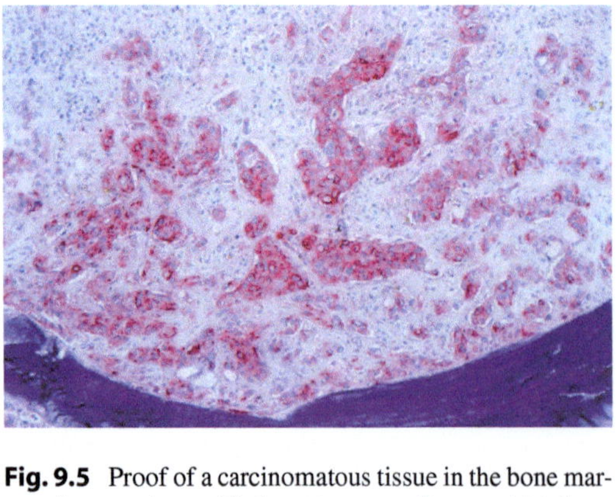

Fig. 9.5 Proof of a carcinomatous tissue in the bone marrow in a patient with breast cancer. Immunohistology, methacrylate-embedded iliac crest biopsy

Metastatic carcinoma of the bone shows a wide range of radiographic patterns (Fig. 9.4), ranging from radiodense (osteosclerotic metastases) to radiolucent lesions (osteolytic metastases). They usually develop in the axial skeleton and are most common in the spine and the pelvis. Although metastatic carcinoma may present in rare cases in one site, most patients develop multiple lesions. Some patients with a metastatic bone lesion have no history of a primary tumour, and finding the primary may be a major clinical problem. The second and more common presentation of bone metastases, however, occurs in patients with a known primary (Fig. 9.5). After metastatic carcinoma of the bone, multiple myeloma is the most common bone neoplasm (Fig. 9.6).

Unlike metastatic bone tumours, *primary bone tumours* begin in the bone and show several characteristic features:

- They exhibit a wide spectrum of tissue differentiation (chondrogenic, osteogenic, osteoclastic giant cell, fibrohistiocytic, vascular and notochordal lesions, with benign and malignant versions of each).
- They occur most often in adolescents and young adults. The probable cause of this age predilection is the susceptibility of growing bone to neoplastic transformation.
- They each have specific radiographic presentations. Thus, primary bone tumours may be regarded as radiographic-histologic entities.
- They show a wide variety of clinical behaviour. Some tumours are not neoplastic at all and grow very slowly, e.g. enchondromas and osteochondromas which are developmental lesions and cease growing after full skeletal maturation.

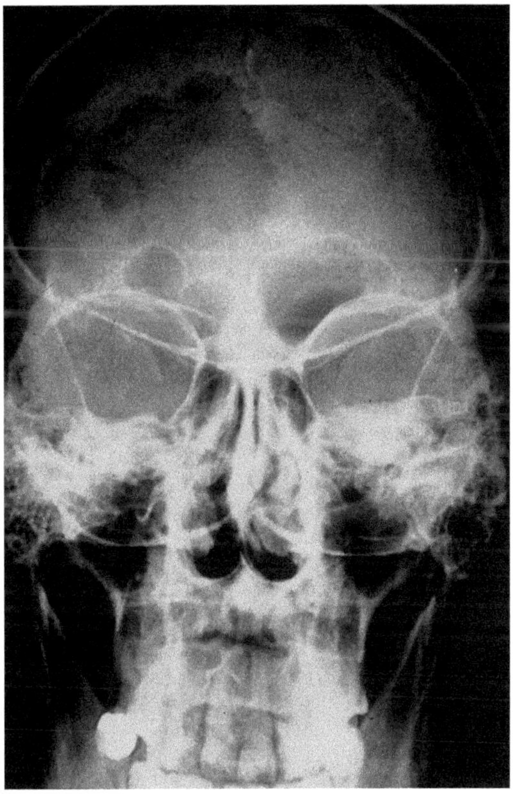

Fig. 9.6 X-ray of the skull illustrating a large osteolytic lesion in a patient with multiple myeloma

Part III

Diagnostic Tools in Bone Disorders

Diagnosis and management of bone disorders depends on the close teamwork of the clinician, the radiologist, the clinical chemist and the pathologist. Four principal sources of information are crucial to the process of judging and diagnosing bone problems, bone complications or bone lesions, gained by

- Clinical evaluation
- Skeletal imaging
- Laboratory studies
- Histologic investigations

10 Clinical Evaluation

The clinical presentation of a bone lesion helps to place it in one of the disease groups shown in the previous chapter. A careful and detailed clinical history and physical examination initiate the diagnostic investigation. Crucial information is frequently gained by careful interrogation of the patient. Important considerations are age of the patient, location of the lesion, type and site of pain, swelling and bone deformity, the patient's symptoms, general state of health, risk factors and additional illnesses. Co-morbidities as well as medications are assessed, as these may also influence the state of the bones. Special attention is paid to the oral cavity and the teeth in particular when i.v. therapy with the new more potent bisphosphonates is contemplated.

10.1 Age and Location

Although any lesion may occur at about any age, most bone lesions are more frequent in certain *age groups*. For example, eosinophilic granuloma usually occurs in children, while a lytic and painful lesion in an older adult is a metastatic tumour or a multiple myeloma until proven otherwise. Also *location* is an important diagnostic clue, and many lesions occur almost exclusively in certain sites of the bones. For example, a giant cell tumour almost always involves the epiphysis and an osteoblastoma favours the spine. When multiple lesions are present, their distribution is extremely important. Symmetrically distributed lesions usually indicate a systemic or congenital disease, whereas asymmetrically distributed lesions often indicate a metastatic neoplasm.

10.2 Bone Pain

Pain as a primary symptom must be thoroughly investigated with respect to its localisation, duration, intensity, characteristics and sensitivity. Meticulous palpation of the skeleto-muscular system in the affected areas can greatly aid this clarification. The physical examination should include inspection of the skin, eyes, teeth, spine, ribs, cranium and limbs. Observation of the patient's gait, coordination and other movements is required. Specific details are given in the appropriate chapters. Pain usually indicates that a lesion is growing and results from the stimulation of unmyelinated nerves in the bone tissue or from expansion of the periosteum.

> Bone pain is a dull aching pain and is characteristically worse at night.

Often, a painful joint calls attention to a nearby unrelated bone lesion. Unlike bone pain, joint pain eases at night or with immobilisation of the joint and disappears with an intraarticular injection of an analgesic. In painful stress fractures, an MRI is usually diagnostic.

R. Bartl, C. Bartl, *Bone Disorders*, DOI 10.1007/978-3-319-29182-6_10

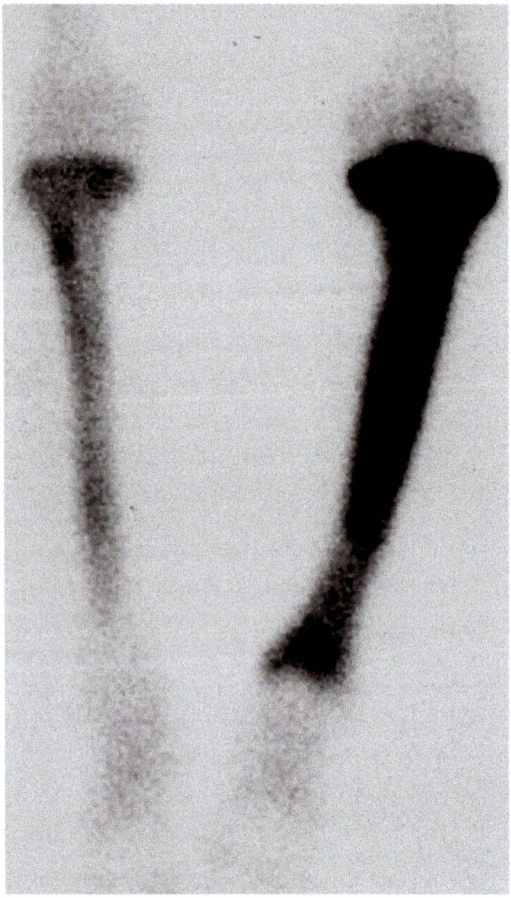

Fig. 10.1 Involvement and bowing deformity of the tibia in a patient with Paget's disease. Bone scan

10.3 Swelling and Deformity of Bone

Swelling is usually caused by the expansion of a surface lesion, such as a parosteal osteosarcoma. The duration and rate of swelling reflect the speed of the lesion's growth. Inflammation in the surrounding soft tissue or bursae and muscles may further increase their size. Therefore, the clinician should compare the amount of swelling with the radiographs to avoid misinterpretation. In children, lesions near the epiphyseal plate may stimulate or retard bone growth. *Deformities* of involved bones are characteristic of Paget's disease (Fig. 10.1), fibrous dysplasia and some other rare bone disorders.

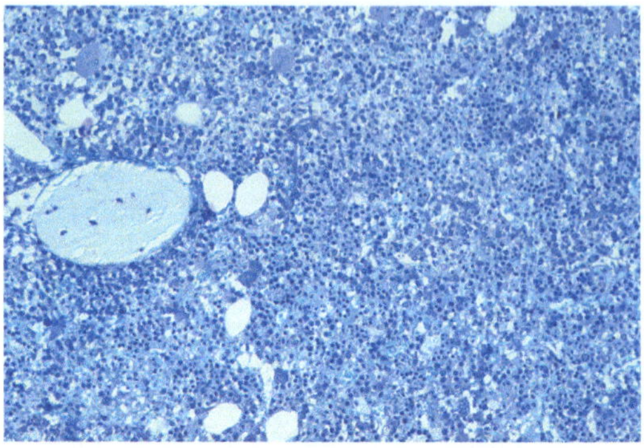

Fig. 10.2 Severe osteoporosis with "button phenomenon" (*left*) and expansion of hyperactive erythropoiesis in a patient with haemolytic anaemia. Giemsa staining

10.4 Systemic Signs and Basic Systemic Diseases

A further question in the evaluation of a bone lesion is whether it is a manifestation of a *basic systemic disease*. Because the bones are sensitive to almost all systemic factors, a careful history must be taken. Renal, endocrine, haematologic (Fig. 10.2), pulmonary, infectious, immunologic, hepatic and gastrointestinal disorders may all influence the bone and explain the bone lesion. In the presence of fever, a leukocytosis and an elevated CRP increase the suspicion of an osteomyelitis or a rapidly growing neoplasm with tumour necrosis.

> Even a large tissue biopsy from a necrotic or inflammatory portion of a neoplasm in the bone (e.g. Ewing's sarcoma or Hodgkin's disease) may be histologically mistaken for chronic infection.

11 Skeletal Imaging

11.1 Conventional Radiography (X-Rays)

Conventional X-rays are indispensable for diagnosis of skeletal disorders. X-rays of the spine are essential for the investigation of unexplained back pain, suspected secondary osteoporosis and the differential diagnosis.

> High-quality X-ray pictures taken under professional guidance are one of the cornerstones of osteology.

Characteristic changes are observed in the following conditions:

- Degenerative, inflammatory changes in joints
- Established osteomalacia
- Advanced osteoporosis
- Bone lesions due to malignancy
- Hyperparathyroidism (HPT)
- Osteosclerosis

11.2 Morphometry of X-Ray Films

X-rays of different skeletal regions are carefully aimed and taken according to the patient's symptoms and presumptive diagnosis. Quantitative morphometry of the X-ray pictures is applied especially in investigations of thoracic and lumbar vertebrae and of the hips and the femur. The following calculations are used:

- Vertebral deformation score
- Singh index
- Length of the femoral neck

11.3 Computed Tomography (CT)

CT is suited for the evaluation of osseous structures and soft-tissue calcification. It is widely used for detailed evaluation of *fracture assessment*. The exquisite bone detail allows evaluation of focal bone metastases (lytic, sclerotic and mixed). CT also provides important information regarding cortical and trabecular structure of the spine and long bones and therefore potential

R. Bartl, C. Bartl, *Bone Disorders*, DOI 10.1007/978-3-319-29182-6_11

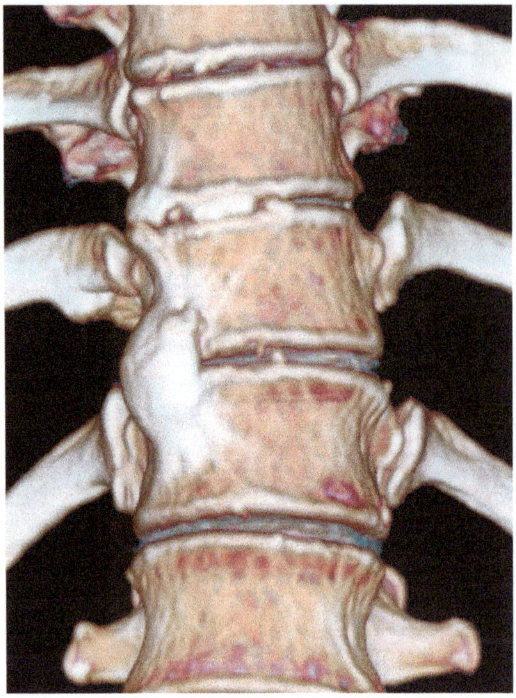

Fig. 11.1 Degenerative disc with spondylarthritis, three-dimensional CT

fracture risk. Dual-energy CT also has been shown to demonstrate bone bruising due to changes in marrow composition (bone marrow oedema). In addition to imaging thin body slices, CT software allows three-dimensional reconstruction of the slices. This three-dimensional image can be rotated on the computer screen and studied from all directions (Fig 11.1).

11.4 Ultrasound (US)

In clinical practice US has now an important role in the management of musculoskeletal disorders. It provides high-resolution assessment of soft tissues. Though investigation of the bone is limited; US gives information regarding the bone surface, ligaments, tendons and periosteum. Abnormalities such as tendon subluxation and impingement may be clinically suspected, but confirmation using US can be diagnostic and helpful. US can differentiate between solid and cystic structures, and *soft-tissue calcification* is evident earlier on US than on X-rays. The anatomy of the spine and the extremities allows excellent *needle visualisation*, as it is nearly always possible to position the needle parallel to the transducer.

11.5 Scintigraphy (Bone Scans)

These are performed after administration of technetium 99, gallium or a bisphosphonate labelled with technetium 99. The advantage of a bone scan lies in the rapid assessment of the whole skeleton. Focal *hot spots* especially in the spine indicate fractures, as well as degenerative, inflammatory or neoplastic lesions. Locally increased uptake may be seen within two days of a bone fracture. However, due to the poor structural detail in a hot spot targeted X-rays or other films are required for clarification. Lytic lesions without increase in osteoblastic activity such as multiple myeloma are occult. Furthermore, the radiation dose of the injected radiotracer is high compared to radiography and is applied to the entire body rather than limited to the region under review. Though appearances are nonspecific, scintigraphy provides a functional display of skeletal metabolism, it is highly sensitive for lesion location, and it gives a rapid evaluation of the total skeleton.

11.6 Magnetic Resonance Imaging (MRI)

This method does not involve radiation; it highlights the bone marrow and differentiates between yellow adipose tissue and red haematopoietic bone marrow.

> MRI is the method of choice for investigation of suspected malignant lesions or local oedematous processes. It is also the ideal method for distinguishing between osteoporotic and metastatic fractures of the spine.

When MRI is applied together with the latest methods of fat saturation, diffusion and perfusion, the diagnostic specificity is greatly increased so that MRI is now considered essential in the evaluation of soft tissue and of the bone marrow. Tissue contrast can be enhanced by the prescan administration of *gadolinium*. This technique is particularly effective in T1-weighted images in which the fat signal has been suppressed. Because the gadolinium concentrates in richly vascular regions, viable, necrotic and neoplastic tissues may be differentiated.

12 Essentials of Skeletal Radiology

12.1 Imaging Techniques

12.1.1 Conventional X-Ray

- Primary imaging technique for the diagnosis of bone disease: traumatology (fracture diagnostics, position control), evaluation of structural bone disease
- Standard: X-ray examination of the bone section in two plains
- Linear propagation of X-rays, same geometric laws like the shadow cast by the light. Summation images:
- If necessary, pitched or targeted images in different positions. For example, rib hemithorax
- Assessment of cortical and cancellous bone structure
- Advantages of conventional X-ray: wide availability, low radiation dose, low cost
- Disadvantages of conventional X-ray: the use of ionising radiation, overlay and summation effects
- If necessary, images of the contralateral side for comparison

12.1.2 Computed Tomography (CT)

- Computed tomography (CT): cross-sectional imaging with the best representation of cortical bone, cancellous bone and soft tissues. Method of choice for displaying complex or subtle bone trauma, certain bone tumours or imaging in the context of interventions (e.g. CT-controlled facet joint infiltration)
- Advantages of CT: widespread and high availability, short examination time, good representation of calcified bone constituents and soft tissue calcifications, three-dimensional multiplanar reconstructions
- Disadvantages of CT: use of ionising X-rays
- Contrast agent: contains iodine
  - Check the need for the administration of contrast medium prior to the investigation! Allergy or intolerance of contrast agents (premedication with antihistamines, and if necessary, consider cortisone directly before the administration of contrast agents) → Outpatients: after premedication limited responsiveness, no active participation in traffic!)
  - Side effects: hyperthyroidism (functional diagnosis of the thyroid or radioiodine therapy not possible after administration of iodinated contrast agents for weeks to months), renal dysfunction (tubulotoxicity, especially in patients with pre-existing renal failure, in this case reduce dosage, i.v. isotonic saline solution, i.v. acetylcysteine), hypersensitivity reactions/allergies (typical symptoms:

The authors of this chapter: Andrea Baur-Melnyk and Tobias Geith.

R. Bartl, C. Bartl, *Bone Disorders*, DOI 10.1007/978-3-319-29182-6_12

nausea, vomiting, erythema, urticaria, bronchoconstriction/laryngospasm, convulsions, anaphylaxis)

Practical Advice: CT Scans with Contrast Agents Required laboratory tests: TSH (if TSH decreased: fT3, FT4), creatinine.

Patient history regarding contrast media hypersensitivity/allergy

In case of hypersensitivity reactions: documentation for necessary future investigations

In case of slight symptoms (nausea, vomiting, erythema, itching): i.v. antihistamines and corticosteroids; if necessary, medical monitoring

In case of pronounced symptoms (laryngospasm, circulatory reaction): intensive care monitoring (ventilation, shock therapy)

12.1.3 Magnetic Resonance Imaging (MRI)

- Magnetic resonance imaging (MRI): cross-sectional imaging with the best soft tissue contrast (tumours, bone marrow, muscles, tendons, ligaments, intervertebral discs). Cortical bone and calcifications only produce weak signal and assessment is limited (→ computed tomography)
- Advantages of MRI: no use of X-rays, excellent soft tissue contrast, representation in different plains, isotropic sequences allow three-dimensional multiplanar reconstructions
- Disadvantages of MRI: claustrophobia (depending on the severity, if necessary premedication, e.g. with Tavor®)
- Risks of MRI: strong static magnetic field → possible dislocation and warming of magnetisable implants/foreign bodies in the patient (e.g. metal splinters, certain makeup pigments, non-removable piercings); in certain cases possible with specially manufacturer-approved pacemakers or cochlear implants, obtain written individual or general release of the manufacturer prior to the examination and discuss with radiologists questions about indications, technical and personnel requirements to carry out the investigation or alternative imaging possibilities!
- Contrast media: gadolinium chelates (MRI contrast agent contains no iodine), relatively low allergic potential, no known relevant nephrotoxicity in normal renal function, very low risk of developing nephrogenic systemic fibrosis in patients with renal impairment (Table 12.1)

Table 12.1 Signal intensity of tissues in musculoskeletal MRI

Tissue	T1w	PDw fs	T2w
Blood vessels	↓	↓	↓ or ↑
Bone marrow	↑	↓	↔
Fat	↑	↓	↑
Fibrocartilage	↓	↓	↓
Hyaline cartilage	↔	↔	↑
Ligaments and tendons	↓	↓	↓
Muscles	↔	↔	↔
Nerves	↔ lower than muscle	↔ lower than muscle	↔ lower than muscle

Practical Advice: MRI Examinations with Contrast Media

Required laboratory tests: creatinine, depending on patient age/risk factors

Patient history regarding contrast media hypersensitivity/hyperallergy

In case of hypersensitivity reactions: documentation for necessary future investigations

In case of slight symptoms (nausea, vomiting, erythema, itching): i.v. antihistamines and corticosteroids; if necessary, medical monitoring

In case of pronounced symptoms (laryngospasm, circulatory reaction): intensive care monitoring (ventilation, shock therapy)

12.1.4 Nuclear Medical Examination Techniques

- Scintigraphy: radiopharmaceuticals (e.g. 99 m technetium) gamma ray dissolves in scintillation light flashes, which are amplified by a photomultiplier tube and then recorded. Distinction of cold spots (areas of inactivity, e.g. cysts) and hot spots (areas of increased activity, e.g. inflammations, tumours).
- SPECT (single-photon emission computed tomography): several gamma cameras rotate around the patient, similar to the CT reconstruction of slice images in multiple planes (spatial resolution about 1–1.5 cm).
- PET (positron emission tomography): During beta decay, electrons and positrons recombine immediately afterwards while releasing energy. Two photons then spread in exactly the opposite direction. The coincidence circuit of exactly opposite detectors of a closed detector ring registers almost simultaneously arriving photons and allows the reconstruction of an activity distribution pattern in axial, sagittal and coronal layers (spatial resolution approximately 3–6 mm). Frequently used positron emitter is 18-fluoro-deoxyglucose (half-life 109 min).
- Combination of PET and CT in one device (PET-CT): advantages of nuclear medical functional diagnostics combined with the high spatial resolution of computed tomography. Exact allocation of pathological activity and CT image in an identical plain position.

12.1.5 Bone Densitometry

- DXA (dual X-ray absorptiometry): measurement of bone mineral density at the spine and femoral neck. Plain value in mg/cm^2 as measured by X-ray absorption. Calculation of *T*-value (comparing the measured value with young healthy adults) and *Z*-value (compared with age-matched persons).
  - Normal BMD: T-score > −1.0
  - Osteopenia (moderate bone loss): T-score between −1.0 and −2.5
  - Osteoporosis (severe bone loss): T-score < −2.5

Indications for drug therapy in synopsis of the bone density values with age and other risk factors.

- Problems of DXA: falsely increased values by overlying structures (aortic calcifications) or degeneration (osteochondrosis with sclerosis of vertebral endplates, spondylophytes, facet joint osteoarthritis, fractured vertebrae).

Practical Advice
To exclude falsely high values by superimposing or degeneration, an X-ray of the lumbar spine should be done at the first DXA measurement. If only one or two vertebral bodies are affected, exclude them from evaluation.

- Q-CT (quantitative CT): (unit "mg calcium hydroxyapatite/ml") calculation of volume value in three lumbar vertebral bodies.
  - Normal bone density: >120 mg Ca-HA/ml
  - Osteopenia (moderate bone loss): 80–120 mg Ca-HA/ml
  - Osteoporosis (severe bone loss): <80 mg Ca-HA/ml

Practical Advice
Perform QCT when the DXA is not available or if the DXA does not give sufficient values (e.g. due to strong degenerative changes).

12.2 Aspects of Imaging of Selected Tissue Disorders

12.2.1 Fractures

Fractures are breaks in the continuity of bone substance independent of location and extent. The spongiosa or cortical substance (alone or together) can be involved. Aetiologically, distinction is traumatic, stress (fatigue fractures in normal bone and overuse, insufficiency fractures in weakened bones and normal stress) and pathological fractures (insufficiency fractures: destruction of bone tissue, e.g. by metastases, multiple myeloma).

The elasticity of the bone in childhood allows strong deformations without complete discontinuity, resulting in typical fracture forms, such as greenstick fracture (cortical break on the tension side, bending on the compression side), bead or torus fracture (metaphyseal compression) or avulsion fractures (epiphyseal avulsion fractures of tendons). Another special feature in childhood is the injury of the epiphysis and growth plate (classification by Salter and Harris type IV or by Aitken) (Fig. 12.1).

Primary radiological fracture diagnosis:

- Radiographs in two mutually perpendicular planes (type, extent, dislocation?). If necessary, additional oblique projections.
- In fractures of the long bones always display the adjacent joints.

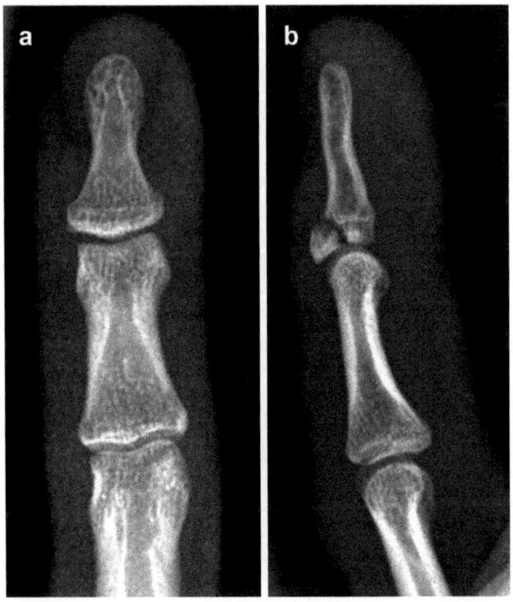

Fig. 12.1 A 27-year-old patient. Avulsion fracture of the extensor digitorum tendon. (**a**) Conventional radiograph in AP view is inconspicuous. The lateral projection (**b**) shows the avulsion fracture. Two planes are mandatory in fracture diagnostics

- In cases of more complex anatomy (e.g. craniofacial, skull base) or clinical relevance (e.g. intracerebral haemorrhage after traumatic brain injury) primary CT.

Supplementary radiological diagnostics:

- Follow-up X-ray: in cases of initially radiographically occult fracture (e.g. lamellar periosteal reaction, sclerotic lines)
- CT with unclear fracture or articular surface involvement, for a more precise representation of complex fractures or complex anatomy (e.g. spine, pelvis, tarsus)
- MRI for the detection of a "bone bruise" with radiographically occult fractures and for the clarification of capsule tendons and ligaments. Representation of osteochondral defects, cartilage flakes

Additional nuclear medical examinations:

- Bone scan is already showing initial posttraumatic increased radionuclide uptake, which can last for several years. In children, physiologically high activity possible.

12.2.2 Osteoporosis

Decreased bone mass with impairment of the microarchitecture of the bone and increased tendency to break. Typical osteoporotic fractures are vertebral fractures, femoral neck fractures, distal radius fractures and subcapital humeral fractures. These fractures are regarded as insufficiency fractures. A reduction in bone mineral density can be depicted in X-ray with a loss of bone mass of at least 30–50 %.

Method of choice: DXA (dual energy X-ray absorptiometry) and QCT (quantitative CT, more sensitive because separate evaluation of the cancellous bone of the vertebral bodies is possible).

Radiographic features of osteoporosis:

- Increased transparency for X-rays, accentuation of tension trabeculae or accentuation of cortical bone (frame vertebrae)
- Fish and wedge shape of vertebrae

DD: Any fracture above level Th7 must be regarded as tumour-suspicious. An inhomogeneous bone structure should also rise the suspicion of a tumour (e.g. multiple myeloma or metastatic). MRI is the method of choice for clarification. Differentiation of fresh/old fracture: MRI shows bone marrow oedema in acute fractures.

12.2.3 Other Systemic Bone Disease

12.2.3.1 Osteomalacia and Rickets

Vitamin D deficiency in children (rickets) or adulthood (osteomalacia) with lack of mineralisation of the osteoid.

Osteomalacia:

Method of choice: conventional radiographs of thoracic and lumbar spine and pelvis overview and femurs (a.p.).

Radiographic features of osteomalacia:

- Increased transparency of the bone in faded spongiosa (Matt glass phenomenon corresponds to non-calcified osteoid)
- Looser zones (cortical insufficiency fractures) typical at the femoral diaphysis, but also insufficiency fractures of the ribs, pubis, ischium, scapula
- Skeletal deformations (e.g. heart-shaped pelvic bone with acetabular protrusion, biconcave fish vertebrae, kyphoscoliosis, bell-shaped thorax, bending of the bones)

Rickets:

Radiographic features of rickets:

Method of choice: conventional radiographs of distal femurs (a.p.), distal ulna (a.p.), pelvis overview, possibly thoracic and lumbar spine in scoliosis.

- Increased radiolucency of the bone by impaired mineralisation
- Widened epiphyses of distal ulna and distal femurs
- Swollen metaphyses
- Bending of the long bones, scoliosis, heart-shaped pelvic bone
- "Rachitic rosary" (swellings of bone-cartilage boundaries of the ribs)

12.2.3.2 Hyperparathyroidism

Primary hyperparathyroidism

Autonomy due to parathyroid adenoma or hyperplasia or carcinoma. High serum calcium.

Secondary hyperparathyroidism

Overactive parathyroid gland as a result of chronic hypocalcaemia, e.g. due to chronic renal failure (renal osteodystrophy) or malabsorption.

Method of choice: plain radiography of the spine and hands (a.p.)

Radiographic features of hyperparathyroidism:

- Subperiosteal radial side resorptions in particular on the cortical bone of the fingers, also on the distal phalanges, medial proximal tibia, humerus, femur, cortical bone of the ribs. Subchondral resorptions at the joints may resemble rheumatoid arthritis
- Spine: "rugger jersey spine" (poorly defined densifications of vertebral endplates) Schmorl's node through subchondral resorption of the vertebral endplates
- Skull: granular atrophy ("salt and pepper skull")
- Osteolytic "brown tumours" at an advanced stage mainly in the pelvis, ribs, femurs, craniofacial
- Chondrocalcinosis

12.2.3.3 DISH (Diffuse Idiopathic Skeletal Hyperostosis)

DISH is a diffuse idiopathic skeletal hyperostosis.

Method of choice: X-ray of the spine

Diagnosis of coarse bridging ossifications of the anterior longitudinal ligament at least four segments (especially thoracolumbar junction).

Radiographic features:

- Coarse bridging spondylophytes to the spine at least four vertebrae, no significant degenerative disc space height reductions
- Fibroostoses, e.g. iliac crests

12.2.3.4 SAPHO Syndrome (Synovitis, Acne, Pustulosis, Hyperostosis, Osteitis)

The "SAPHO syndrome" = acquired hyperostosis syndrome = pustular arthroosteitis (PAO) is a chronic nonbacterial inflammation of the bone in adults, which often goes hand in hand with psoriasiform and acne-like pustular lesions. It shows predominantly sclerotic hyperostotic changes and periosteal new bone formation.

Method of choice: X-ray, CT, scintigraphy (pathognomonic findings, looking for further foci)

Radiographic features:

- Enthesitis (inflammation at the fibro-osseous junction)
- Sclerosis and hyperostosis, mostly sternoclavicular junction (bull horn sign in scintigram)
- Sclerotic involvement of single vertebrae (Fig. 12.2)

12.2.3.5 CRMO

Chronic recurrent multifocal osteomyelitis (CRMO) occurs as a nonbacterial inflammation of the bone in children and adolescents. Often several bones are successively attacked and painful over time. Depending on the stage of disease, X-ray offers a different picture:

- First 3 weeks: osteolysis as in acute osteomyelitis
- Later: sclerotic seam around osteolysis, mixed lytic-sclerotic and sclerotic lesions can occur simultaneously. Later pure sclerosis
- Diagnosis: the three-phase bone scintigraphy allows the display of a clinically silent focus; MRI shows early-stage appearance like acute osteomyelitis. DD bone infarcts, tumours, bacterial osteomyelitis

12.2.4 Local Bone Disease

12.2.4.1 Osteomyelitis

Osteomyelitis is an infection of the bone or bone marrow mostly with bacterial pathogens (30 % *S. aureus*). The cause is either a direct infection from neighbouring structures, open fractures, surgeries or haematogenous spreading.

Method of choice: X-ray/CT and MRI

Radiographic features:

- X-ray:
  - Acute: up to 14 days after onset of clinical symptoms, detectable changes can be missing, initially often oedematous soft tissue swelling. After 2–3 weeks, cancellous and cortical destruction, lamellar or spicular periosteal reactions, sequestra.
  - Chronic: mostly osteoproliferative changes with sclerosis and cortical thickening.
- CT: depiction of osseous destruction and sequestration without overlay. Detection of fistulas: instillation of iodinated KM into the fistula via a blunt probe. Detection of bone and joint contact. If necessary, CT-controlled biopsy.
- MRI: much earlier detection than conventional X-ray (in STIR and T2 hyperintense in T1 hypointense bone signal, significant contrast enhancement, surrounding soft

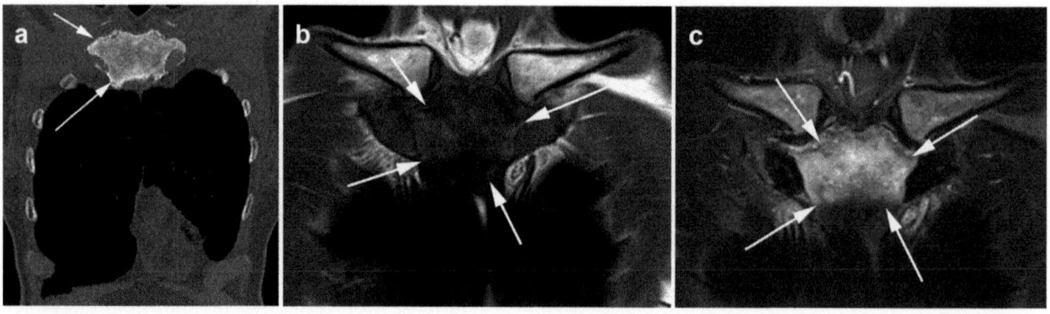

Fig. 12.2 A 41-year-old patient with SAPHO syndrome. (**a**) Diffuse sternal sclerosis in CT. Diffuse sclerosis with erosive inflammatory changes. MRI T1w (**b**) and T1w fs with contrast (**c**) show inflammation with contrast uptake. *Arrows* diffuse sclerosis and the corresponding area with contrast-uptake in MRI

tissue), detection of intraosseous abscesses (centrally in STIR/T2 hyperintense, with marginal contrast enhancement) and necrotic sequesters (centrally without signal, no contrast enhancement). Detection of soft tissue inflammation, abscesses, sinus tracts.

- Scintigraphy: also earlier detection than plain radiography. Inflammation scintigraphy with 99mTc-labelled diphosphonates (increased radionuclide enrichment in arterial phase, the blood pool phase and static phase), leukocyte (unphysiological pattern of tracer uptake).

Practical Hint
Osteomyelitis

In suspected acute osteomyelitis, conventional radiography is the primary diagnosis of choice. However, a negative radiograph does not exclude osteomyelitis! → complementary MRI!

To assess the activity of chronic osteomyelitis, comparison with X-ray images is crucial. Emergent destruction or progressive findings indicate an active event.

Healing characteristics: increasing sclerosis, decreasing scintigraphic activity, decreasing oedema and soft tissue swelling in MRI, decreasing contrast uptake over time (Fig. 12.3).

12.2.4.2 Paget Disease

Paget's disease is a disease of unknown aetiology, which leads to increased bone resorption and remodelling. Mostly men >40 years. Preferred sites are the femur, pelvis, tibia, skull and vertebral bodies.

Method of choice: X-ray or CT

Radiographic features:

- *Stage I (osteolysis):* wedge-shaped hypertransparent zones
- *Stage II (mixed):* simultaneous osteolyses and scleroses, coarse bone structure, increasing of the bone
- *Stage III (burnt-out stage):* mostly coarse trabecular sclerosis

Diagnostics with conventional X-ray usually sufficient. Mostly a mixed stage is present. CT for evaluation of complications (e.g. cranial nerves, compression of the spinal canal or nerve root).

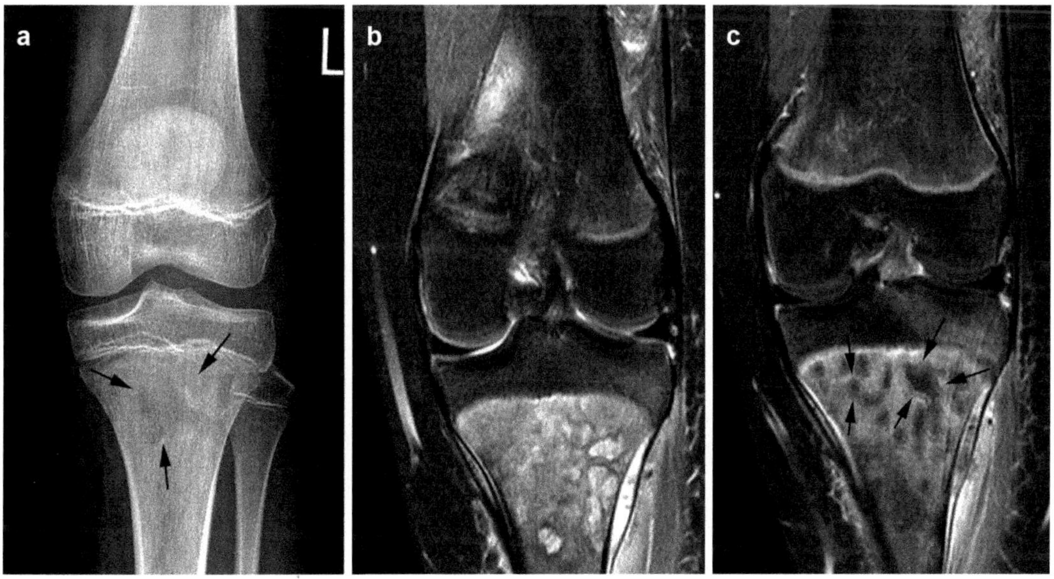

Fig. 12.3 A 12-year-old patient with osteomyelitis. Conventional radiograph (**a**) shows hypertransparent area in the tibial metaphysis. MRI shows bone marrow oedema (**b**, STIR) and abscesses with peripheral contrast enhancement (*arrows*) (**c**, T1WPS after contrast). Also note the surrounding inflammatory soft tissue oedema with contrast uptake

MRI: MRI shows an inconspicuous bone marrow or residues of fatty marrow within the lesions. Coarsened trabeculation of thickening of the compact bone.

Practical Hint

Malignant alteration: Newly occurring osteolysis and pain (Fig. 12.4).

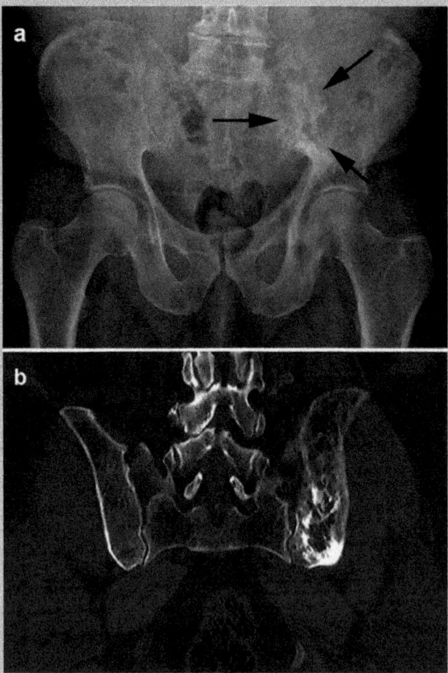

Fig. 12.4 A 58-year-old patient: swollen bone structure in the left posterior os ilium with Paget's disease in conventional radiograph (**a**) and CT (**b**)

12.2.4.3 Bone Marrow Oedema

The bone marrow oedema syndrome is a diagnosis by exclusion! Various diseases can cause bone marrow oedema (inflammation, tumour, fracture, etc.). Here the clinical constellation and image interpretation by an experienced musculoskeletal radiologist is important.

Method of choice: MRI
Radiographic features:

- Conventional X-ray: can show an osteopenic decrease of density in the subchondral lamella a few weeks after the onset of symptoms; the width of joint space is maintained. After 4–10 months possible patchy sclerosis due to remineralisation.
- MRI is the diagnostic tool of choice: oedematous signal changes (T1 blurred hypointense, T2 usually isointense, PD fs or STIR hyperintense, homogeneous contrast uptake) often with joint effusion. Positive MRI about 48 h after onset of symptoms. In particular useful to distinguish bone marrow oedema syndrome from a stress fracture or insufficiency fracture (with fracture line) and osteonecrosis but not always certainly possible (subchondral microfractures in bone marrow oedema possible). Healing usually after 3–6 months.
- Bone scan due to low specificity not suitable for routine diagnosis.
- Outlook: newer MRI techniques (e.g. diffusion and perfusion sequences) have the potential for follow-up assessment of treatment response and the differentiation from tumour (Fig. 12.5).

12.2.4.4 Osteonecrosis, Bone Infarcts

Osteonecrosis is caused by hypoperfusion of the subchondral epiphyseal bone. Bone infarcts are ischaemic foci in the meta- and diaphyseal area. Risk factors include smoking, alcohol abuse, cortisone and pregnancy.

Method of choice: X-ray and MRI
Radiographic features of osteonecrosis:

- Conventional X-ray initially mostly inconspicuous, later stages show subchondral radiolucent lines (crescent sign), contour changes of the articular surface, intrusion of the

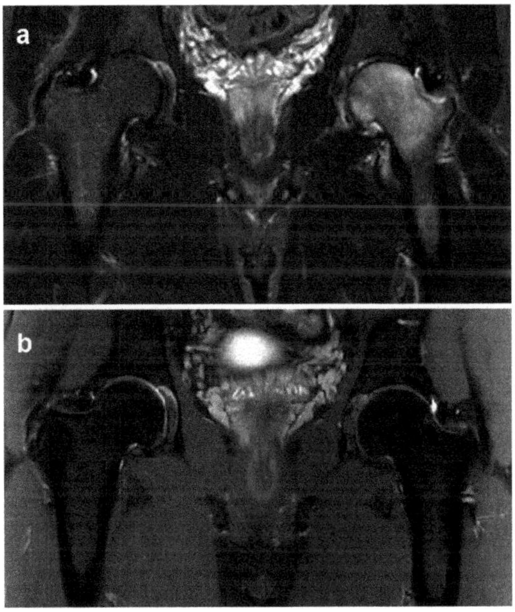

Fig. 12.5 A 40-year-old patient with bone marrow oedema. Significant oedema (STIR sequence) in the left femoral head and neck shortly after the onset of symptoms (**a**). The follow-up after 8 weeks shows a clear decrease of the oedema (**b**)

articular surface and secondary osteoarthritis (femoral head necrosis: classification of Ficat and Arlet and ARCO).

- CT: subchondral fractures displayed free of superimposition → crucial for further treatment (drilling versus joint replacement)
- MRI: higher sensitivity and specificity. Bone marrow oedema in STIR with additional epiphyseal hypointense line in T1-weighted SE image that clearly demarcates the necrotic area

Radiographic signs of bone infarcts:

- X-ray: usually incidental finding; linear to serpiginous central calcification figures in the bone
- MRI: early oedema with high signal intensity in STIR/proton density/T2, later demarcated border zone (T1-weighted hypointense demarcation line, T2 hyperintense granulation tissue adjacent to the necrosis and hypointense sclerosis/fibrosis towards the healthy bone, peripheral zone with contrast uptake)
- Scintigraphy: initial decreased uptake in necrosis (cold spot); after some time, edge zone with increased enrichment (cold in hot spot)
- DD enchondroma: central popcorn-like calcifications, where applicable; MRI for safe differentiation

12.2.4.5 Soft Tissue Calcification

The causes of soft tissue calcification are multiple. The decisive factors are the clinical constellation and laboratory findings.

Method of choice: X-ray

- CPPD: calcium pyrophosphate deposition disease.
  - Four types: (1) Asymptomatic chondrocalcinosis. (2) CPPD arthropathy: joint degeneration at atypical places with line-shaped calcifications. (3) Pseudogout: pseudo gouty attacks with joint effusion and pain. (4) Pseudotumourous form
- CHA: calcium hydroxylapatite depositions in tendons and around joints. Degenerative disease, e.g. tendinosis of the supraspinatus tendon
- Ossifying myositis: calcifications in an old haematoma, e.g. posttraumatic. Typical: calcifications begin peripherally. DD osteosarcoma (relatively vague calcifications of central starting)
- Bursitis calcarea: calcified bursae (typical localisations, e.g. bursa trochanteric)
- Pseudotumourous calcinosis
- Old avulsion fractures
- Synovial chondroma (typical configuration, roundish smoothly limited calcification in the joint) (Fig. 12.6)
- Soft tissue calcification due to impaired calcium metabolism

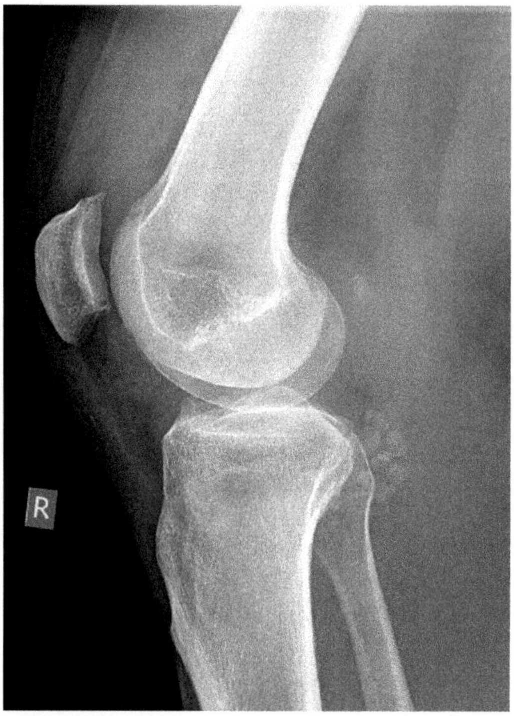

Fig. 12.6 A 53-year-old patient: calcified synovial chondroma in the dorsal part of the knee in conventional radiograph

12.2.5 Bone and Bone Marrow

12.2.5.1 Myelogenous Osteopathies

Various haematopoietic neoplasms and bone marrow diseases lead to osseous involvement in the form of a diffuse osteoporosis or osteolysis.

Method of choice: X-ray/CT for the detection of osseous involvement; MRI for the detection of bone marrow infiltration.

Osteomyelofibrosis/osteomyelosclerosis.

Ranks among the myeloproliferative disorders.

Method of choice: X-ray and MRI.

Radiographic features:

- X-ray/CT: mostly no changes, advanced stage of disease with diffuse bone sclerosis
- MRI: typical diffuse signal decay of the bone marrow on T1- and T2-weighted sequences. Variable after contrast administration, initially often significant accumulation in the bone marrow. Extramedullary haematopoietic foci and bone marrow reconversion in the periphery

12.2.5.2 Storage Diseases

Certain products of metabolism are stored in the bone marrow or in the reticulohistiocytic system because of enzyme deficiency, e.g. glucocerebrosidosis in Gaucher's disease due to lack of glucocerebrosidase (= lipid storage disease, autosomal recessive trait).

Method of choice: MRI

Radiographic features:

For example, Gaucher's disease (glucocerebrosidosis):

- X-ray: osteoporosis with increased susceptibility to fractures, relative constriction of the diaphysis and flaring of the metaphysis (Erlenmeyer flask deformity), osteonecrosis
- MRI: diffusely decreased signal intensity in T1-weighted SE; no signal increase when fat saturation is applied (in contrast to multiple myeloma or leukaemia). MRI is suitable for assessing the extent of the infiltration and detection of complications such as osteonecrosis, occult osteoporotic fractures and osteomyelitis.
- Outlook: quantitative determination of the fat content in the bone marrow by means of chemical shift method in MRI for assessing the degree of disease [Hollak, C., M. Maas, et al. (2001). "Dixon quantitative chemical shift imaging is a sensitive tool for the evaluation of bone marrow responses to individualized doses of enzyme supplementation therapy in type 1 Gaucher disease." Blood cells, molecules and diseases 27 (6): 1005–1012].

12.2.5.3 Lymphomas

There are primary (3 %) and secondary bone lymphomas. Primary lymphomas of the bones are rare. Often there is a secondary manifestation in the context of non-Hodgkin's lymphoma. Typical localisation is the axial skeleton.

Method of choice: X-ray + MRI and FDG PET-CT for therapy assessment

Radiographic features:

- X-ray/CT: Mostly osteolytic lesions or radiographically occult. Partially mixed lytic-sclerotic shaped; rarely pure sclerotic
- MRI: Direct representation of bone marrow infiltration, representation of the degree of infiltration. Whole-body MRI for the detection of additional foci (most sensitive method). Depiction of soft tissue components
- FDG-PET-CT
  - (1) For baseline assessment! Lymphomas significantly accumulate FDG. Early detection of treatment response (no/reduced FDG uptake). Positive MRI is often delayed. The foci often disappear in MRI after up to 1 year.
  - (2) Exact depiction of the osseous destruction.

12.2.5.4 Multiple Myeloma

Multiple myeloma is a malignant bone marrow neoplasia with bone marrow infiltration by atypical monoclonal plasma cells. There is a secondary destruction of bone by osteoclasts. Typical paraproteins in electrophoresis (M-peak).

Method of choice: whole-body CT and MRI

Radiographic features:

- X-ray: skeletal status (skull, spine, arms, pelvis, chest, thighs and arms). Often with coexistence of different forms of destruction: diffuse osteoporosis, well-circumscribed osteolysis, endosteal thinning of the cortical bone in long bones. Overall, low sensitivity and specificity.
- CT: more sensitive than plain radiography. At least 16-slice CT necessary for whole-body CT. This replaces the X-ray skeletal status. Sharply circumscribed osteolytic lesions with density values of 40–80 HU in trabecular bone. Extraosseous manifestations (homogeneous contrast-enhancing soft tissue tumours without necrosis or calcifications). The medullary involvement in the long bones should be viewed in the soft tissue window because osseous changes are often missing!
- PET/PET-CT: shows high activity of bone and soft tissue involvement due to glucose utilisation. Good for assessment of treatment response. Disadvantage: low availability.
- MRI: inconspicuous bone marrow does not exclude plasma cell infiltration (infiltration <20 %). These patients have a significantly better prognosis than patients with >1 focus or diffuse infiltration. Focal myeloma (hyperintense STIR, hypointense in T1-weighted, contrast media uptake). Diffuse infiltration (diffusely decreased signal intensity in T1 image and hyperintensity in STIR, contrast uptake). Often combined focal and diffuse infiltration. A special type of infiltration is the "salt-and-pepper pattern" (T1w, T2 very inhomogeneous signal pattern; however, corresponds to a low plasma cell infiltration of <20 % with circumscribed spots of fatty bone marrow). MRI whole-body imaging: possibility of direct visualisation of the entire bone marrow.

12.2.5.5 Systemic Mastocytosis

Mastocytosis is characterised by a mastocyte proliferation in the bone marrow. This results in a trabecular destruction and reactive formation of new bone. The secreted heparin induces osteopenia.

Method of choice: X-ray; MRI if applicable

Radiographic features:

- X-ray/CT: focal or diffuse osteopenia or osteosclerosis
- MRI: partly hypercellular bone marrow as in leukaemia or lymphoma. Focal or diffuse, depending on the distribution pattern (Fig. 12.7).

12.2.6 Bone and Joints

12.2.6.1 Degenerative Joint Diseases

Osteoarthritis

Osteoarthritis of the joints has a great socio-medical importance. It affects up to 80 % of over 65s. Common sites are the hip, knee, hand (STT,

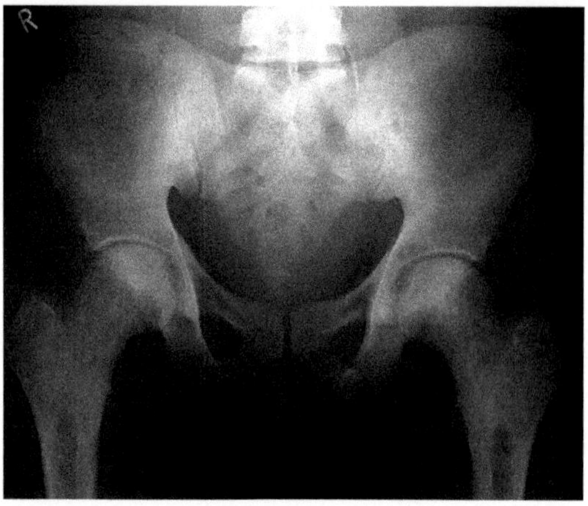

Fig. 12.7 A 56-year-old patient with mastocytosis. The conventional X-ray image of the pelvis shows diffuse osteosclerosis

rhizarthrosis, Heberden's and Bouchard's osteoarthritis), ACG joint, and spine. Can be primary idiopathic (cause has not yet been precisely clarified) or secondary (altered biomechanics, e.g. *varus gonarthrosis*) posttraumatic, inflammatory, neuropathic. There can be an inflammatory oedematous component=erosive osteoarthritis. Usually there is a primary cartilage injury with secondary changes in the joint capsule and/ligaments. Most patients complain of stress-related pain or start-up pain. However, the clinical symptoms do not necessarily correlate with the imaging findings!

Method of choice: X-ray in two planes, possibly with load; MRI

Practical Hint
Images of the lower extremity (particularly the knee) should always be with load, i.e. while standing. The true joint space may differ substantially compared to a prone radiograph. It is advisable to include a radiograph of the leg alignment to detect a malposition of the legs axis (varus/valgus). The clinical symptoms do not necessarily correlate with the imaging findings!

- X-ray:
- Typical signs of osteoarthritis are an asymmetric joint space narrowing, subchondral sclerosis, osteophytes and subchondral cysts. Secondary findings can be loose bodies and reactive synovitis with joint effusion and malalignment.

Table 12.2 Staging of osteoarthritis by Kellgren and Lawrence

KL degree	Osteophytes	Joint space narrowing	Sclerosis
0	–	–	–
1	Doubtful	–	–
2	Slight	Possible	–
3	Moderate	Present	Possible
4	Large	Marked	Marked

Table 12.3 Adapted MRI classification of cartilage injury according to Outerbridge

Stadium	Imaging findings
I	Chondromalacia, cartilage oedema
II	Fibrillation, incipient fragmentation, max. 50 % loss of cartilage height
III	Fibrillation, fragmentation, more than 50 % loss of cartilage height
IV	Exposed subchondral bone

Classification of osteoarthritis:

There are several X-ray staging systems. A common classification is by Kellgren and Lawrence (Table 12.2).

- CT: depiction of the X-ray signs without superposition, possibly as an adjunct in search for loose bodies or in complex joints (sacroiliac joint/atlanto-dental joint)
- MRI: direct depiction of chondromalacia as the earliest change in osteoarthritis on T2-weighted FSE or fat-saturated proton-weighted images (PDW fs) → signal heterogeneties in T2-weighted images. Loss of cartilage volume. Subchondral cysts hyperintense on T2. Painful reactive subchondral bone marrow oedema, Synovitis (contrast enhancement of the synovium) and joint effusion in activated osteoarthritis

Stages of cartilage lesions in MRI according to the arthroscopic classification of Outerbridge (Table 12.3).

Table 12.4 Stages of erosive osteochondrosis by Modic

Stage	Imaging findings
I	Oedema along the endplates: hypointense in T1w, hyperintense on STIR, with contrast uptake
II	Subchondral fatty marrow conversion: hyperintense on T1w and hyperintense on T2w
III	Subchondral sclerosis: hypointense in T1w and T2w (see also X-ray/CT)

Osteochondrosis

Degeneration of the intervertebral disc with endplate changes of adjacent vertebral bodies.

Method of choice: X-ray and MRI

- X-ray: reduction in height of the disc space, subchondral sclerosis, spondylophytes. Possible spondylolisthesis. Osteoarthritis of the facet joints, sometimes hypertrophic with narrowing of the neural foramina (oblique views of the cervical spine or CT).
- CT: accurate depiction of the narrowing of the spinal canal and the neuroforamina by disc tissue, spondylosis, osteoarthritis of the facet joint and ligaments. Thickening of the yellow bands (ligamenta flava).
- MRI: earliest sign is the loss of water signal (signal reduction) in T2-TSE image. Then height reduction of the intervertebral disc, possibly disk protrusion or prolapse. Reactive bone marrow (usually very painful) in micro-instability (= erosive osteochondrosis). Staging according to Modic (Table 12.4).

> **Practical Hint**
> Erosive osteochondrosis is usually caused by a micro-instability and often very painful. It usually heals after months or years. Sometimes spondylodesis is necessary. Herniated discs can be asymptomatic. They must be correlated to clinical symptoms and to sensomotoric functions!

12.2.6.2 Chronic Polyarthritis

Chronic inflammatory disease of the joints. The synovium is primarily involved, which secondarily destroys the capsule-ligament apparatus, the cartilage and bone by proliferation (pannus). In particular, the metacarpophalangeal (MCP) and proximal interphalangeal joints (PIP) are involved.

Method of choice: X-ray in two planes (often initially occult) and contrast-enhanced MRI

- X-ray:
  - Soft tissue swelling
  - Juxta-articular osteoporosis
  - Symmetrical joint space narrowing
  - Erosion in the area of "bare areas", destruction by pannus
  - Subchondral cysts
  - Joint destruction and malalignments
  - Late stages: possibly ankylosis
  - HWS: atlantoaxial dislocation
- Ultrasonography: depiction of soft tissue swelling and effusions, erosions (e.g. phalanges, metacarpals).
- CT: depiction of bone destruction (if not exactly shown in X-ray, e.g. at the spine and pelvis).
- MRI: early detection of bone marrow oedema (hyperintense on STIR, contrast uptake) and synovitis (contrast uptake of synovium), which have prognostic significance. Later, erosion and cartilage destruction. Detection of joint effusion. T1-weighted sequences with fat saturation show the pannus approximately 4–6 min after contrast administration. Dynamic contrast-enhanced sequences show the activity of the inflammatory pannus. Tendovaginitis.

12.2.6.3 Seronegative Spondyloarthritis/Ankylosing Spondylitis

Inflammatory rheumatic disease that primarily affects the spine and sacroiliac joints. Typical HLA B27 positive. Deep-seated nocturnal back pain in young men is typical.

Method of choice: X-ray and MRI
Radiographic features:

- X-ray:
  - Anterior spondylitis (= Romanus' lesion): inflammatory erosive changes in the anterior edge of the vertebral body, later in healing "shiny corners" = sclerosis
  - Box-shaped vertebrae (loss of anterior concavity)
  - Syndesmophytes (ossification of the annulus fibrosus)
  - Andersson's lesion: nonbacterial discitis
  - Osteoporosis with fractures
  - Late stage: bamboo spine
  - Sacroiliac joints: erosive changes, later sclerosis and ankylosing
  - Peripheral joints: arthritis-like changes
  - Tendons: enthesitis, erosion below the tendon insertions
- CT: subordinate role, possibly in some cases better representation of bone destruction and proliferation
- MRI: anterior spondylitis (oedema on the anterior and posterior parts of the vertebral bodies, in STIR hyperintense, contrast uptake). Oedema of the costovertebral joints. Discitis with inflammatory oedematous changes along the vertebral endplates. Inflammation of the facet joints. Sacroiliac joints: oedema; later fatty degeneration while healing of the acute inflammation

12.2.6.4 Infectious Spondylitis/Spondylodiscitis

Mostly bacterial infection of the vertebrae with involvement of the intervertebral disc. Often haematogenous spread with *Staphylococcus aureus* or gram-negative pathogens. Rarely tuberculosis. Other causes: postoperatively iatrogenic infection. CRP usually increases but may be inconspicuous or only slightly increased in the elderly.

Method of choice: MRI

- X-ray: 3–8 weeks after the start of the symptoms, first bony changes can be seen (blurred erosive changes in vertebral endplates, height reduction of the intervertebral space).
- Note: MRI should be performed in cases of suspected spondylodiscitis. X-ray is often normal or simulates osteochondrosis.
- Contrast-enhanced MRI: method of choice for early diagnosis. Detection of fluid-like signal intensity in the vertebral disc with contrast enhancement as a sign of the abscess in the intervertebral disc. Contiguous oedema/inflammation along the endplates. Paravertebral epidural abscesses. Signs of healing: decrease of oedema, conversion to normal fatty marrow, regressive contrast uptake, often lag behind clinical findings. The differential diagnosis is an erosive osteochondrosis Modic type I, sometimes difficult to distinguish.
- CT: indicated only if MRI is not feasible (e.g. in patients with cardiac pacemaker). CT-controlled biopsy!
- Scintigraphy: two- or three-phase scintigraphy in contraindications for MRI. Unspecific increased uptake at all stages (Tables 12.5 and 12.6).

12.2.7 Bone and Tumour

12.2.7.1 General Diagnostic Approach for Tumours in the Peripheral Skeleton

A. Determination of localisation:
   - Conventional radiograph in two planes (→ Lodwick classification), also in soft tissue tumours, radiographs needed to evaluate calcifications
   - CT in complex anatomy (e.g. pelvis, spine, sternum, skull base) and stability assessment
   - Bone scintigraphy for the detection of multifocal infestation and in metastases, assessment of biological activity

B. Diagnostic assignment:
   - Assessment according to patient age, tumour localisation, growth rate
   - MRI for determination of contrast enhancement, signal characteristics, medullary infiltration, always entire affected bone and adjacent compartments for the

Table 12.5 Differentiation of pyogenic and tuberculous spondylodiscitis

	Pyogenic spondylodiscitis	Tuberculous spondylodiscitis
Clinical findings	Acute, high inflammatory markers	Chronic, low inflammatory markers
Segments	Usually monosegmental	Often several segments
Intervertebral disc involvement	Early	Late
Soft tissue	Epidural abscesses	Large paravertebral abscesses, possibly with calcification

Table 12.6 Differentiation of spondylodiscitis and erosive osteochondrosis

	Spondylodiscitis	Erosive osteochondrosis
Endplates	Blurred in T1w	Continuous in T1w
Bone marrow oedema	Large parts of the vertebral body	Narrow along the endplates
Vertebral disc	Fluid signal in the disc, contrast uptake within the vertebral disc!	Usually hypointense on T2, no intradiscal contrast uptake
Intradiscal vacuum phenomenon (CT)	No, because abscess is present	Very specific, if present
Phlegmons/abscess	Usually	No
Soft tissue	Paravertebral soft tissue mass or epidural abscess	Mostly no or only slight soft tissue reaction

detection of locoregional metastases or skip lesions
- Decision on radiological follow-up or biopsy

C. Tumour staging:
- MRI to assess the extension in bone and soft tissue (nerve/vascular/muscle infiltration)
- Recurrence diagnostics: MRI, PET-CT possibly scintigraphy in metastases or multifocal disease

Lodwick classification: assessment of aggressiveness and growth rate

The width of the transition zone between the tumour and normal bone correlates with the aggressiveness of the tumour.

12.2.7.2 Bone Metastases

After the liver and lungs, the third most common place for metastatic infestation. Each new bone lesion in patients >40 years is primarily suggestive of a metastasis.

Method of choice: X-ray and MRI

- Osteolytic metastases: lung cancer, thyroid cancer, breast cancer, malignant melanoma, colorectal cancer, Ewing's sarcoma, renal cell carcinoma, adenocarcinoma (visible in X-ray: >30 % reduction in bone mass)
- Osteoblastic metastases: prostate cancer, breast cancer, rarely neuroblastoma, bronchial carcinoid, head and neck tumours, gastric cancer, metastases under/after therapy
- Mixed osteolytic and osteoblastic metastases

Diffuse manifestation at an advanced stage; possible DD multiple myeloma

Peripheral metastases: lung cancer; renal carcinoma

- CT:
  - Best method for the detection of osteodestruction (fracture risk?)
  - In complex anatomy (e.g. spine, skull base)
- MRI:
  - Is the most sensitive method for the detection of bone metastases
  - Typical signal behaviour: significantly hypointense on T1-weighted SE, hyperintense STIR/proton density/T2 FSE depending from the degree of calcification (the more calcified, the less signal)
  - Contrast uptake (except purely osteoblastic metastases)

Table 12.7 Criteria for the differentiation of benign osteoporotic and metastatic vertebral body fractures

Benign osteoporotic fracture	Malignant fracture
Localisation in middle thoracic and upper lumbar spine below Th 7	Localisation above Th 7
Concave posterior border – retropulsion of bony fragments	Convex posterior border (bulging)
Intravertebral vacuum (CT) or fluid sign (MRI)	No intravertebral vacuum (CT) or fluid sign (MRI) – soft tissue density
Symmetric infraction (in a.p. view), wedge-shaped or fish-like vertebra, no involvement of the pedicles and the neural arch	Asymmetric infraction (in a.p. view), involvement of the pedicles (vanished "eyes of the vertebra")
Homogeneous osseous structure in X-ray and CT	Inhomogeneous osseous structure with osteolyses and sclerotic areas
Band-like sclerosis adjacent to vertebral end plate	Fractures of the posterior part of the vertebra
Spared normal bone marrow, incomplete or band-like signal changes	Complete replacement of normal vertebral bone marrow, diffuse hyperintense signal on STIR
Isointensity after Gd on T1w images (*"return to normal signal intensity"*)	High/inhomogeneous SI after Gd on T1w images
No or only thin surrounding paraspinal mass	Epidural soft tissue mass – focal paraspinal mass
Further (old) osteoporotic fractures	Other spinal metastases

- Scintigraphy:
  - Osteoblastic metastases strongly positive in phase of mineralisation; osteolytic metastases may be unnoticed due to reduced tracer uptake
  - Positive in accompanying osseous reaction at the tumour edge of osteolytic metastases
- FDG-PET (-CT):
- FDG-PET-positive when metabolic rate is elevated, depending on the primary tumour (purely osteoblastic metastases can also be FDG-negative! Small metastases <1 cm can escape detection) (Table 12.7).

13 Bone Densitometry

The early diagnosis of osteoporosis, before occurrence of fractures, can only be made by means of bone density measurements (bone mineral density, BMD, test) (Table 13.1). These measure bone density at various skeletal sites and thereby enable a prediction of risk of later fracture. A 10 % decrease in bone density doubles the fracture risk for the vertebral body and trebles it for the hip joint. If a fracture has already occurred, this test is used to confirm the diagnosis of osteoporosis and determine its degree of severity. BMD provides the following information:

- Detects osteopenia and/or osteoporosis before occurrence of a fracture
- Predicts risk for later development of osteoporosis
- Indicates the rate of bone loss – progression – in sequential measurements
- Documents the efficacy or failure of therapy
- Increases compliance of both doctor and patient

The relation between BMD and fracture risk is well established. The association between bone density (measured at hip and lumbar spine) and hip fracture is three times stronger than that between cholesterol levels and heart disease. Currently, a bone density measurement remains the best and most readily quantifiable method for assessing fracture risk and skeletal response to different treatments.

13.1 Methods for Measurement

The *bone mineral content (BMC)* is measured in g and the *bone mineral density (BMD)* in g/cm^2 (area) or g/cm^3 (volumetric). The precision and accuracy of a measurement depend on:

- Type of instrument (pencil or fan beam techniques)
- Regular (daily) check and setting of the instrument
- Cooperation of the patient (must keep still)
- Exact adjustment of the instrument by the investigator
- Degree of osteoporosis: the less the bone mass, the more inaccurate the measurement!

Dual Energy X-Ray Absorptiometry (DEXA, DXA, Rarely Also Called QDR, DPX, DER) Today DEXA is the most completely developed, reliable and popular method in use, the "gold standard" (Fig. 13.1). DEXA was developed in the 1980s and its widespread use began in 1988. The skeletal site is exposed to two X-ray beams of different intensity, and the mineral content of the bone is calculated by means of computer programs from the amount of radiation. Using the results of the two measurements, the effects of the soft tissue components (different quantities of muscle and fatty tissue) can be calculated and discarded. DXA can measure central (hip and spine) (Fig. 13.2a–c)

R. Bartl, C. Bartl, *Bone Disorders*, DOI 10.1007/978-3-319-29182-6_13

Table 13.1 Techniques for measuring bone mineral density (BMD)

Method	Precision (%)	Accuracy (%)	Scan time (min)	Radiation dose (mrems)
Dual-energy X-ray absorptiometry (DXA)	1–2	3–5	2–8	1–3
Lumbar spine AP				
Lumbar spine lateral				
Proximal radius				
Distal radius				
Proximal femur				
Total body				
Quantitative computed tomography (QCT)	2–10	5–20	10–15	100–1000
Lumbar spine				
Radius				
Quantitative ultrasound (QUS)	–	2–8	5–10	0
Calcaneus Phalanges Patella				

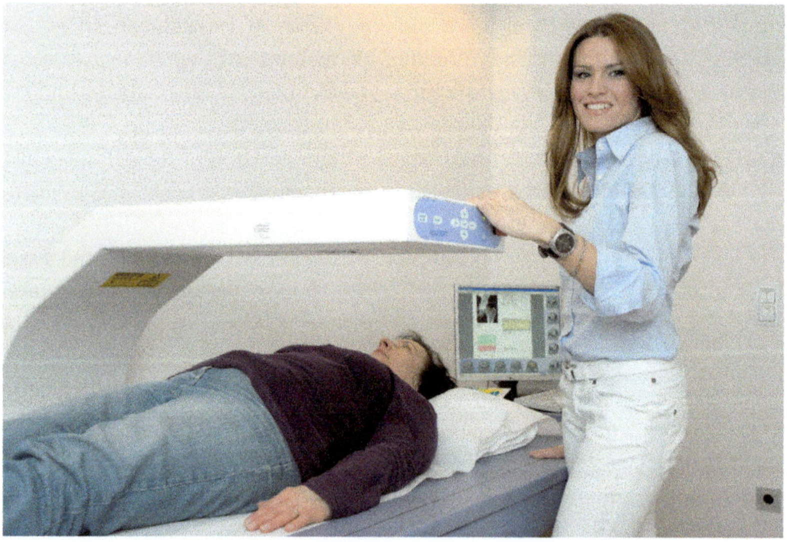

Fig. 13.1 Modern DXA unit (Hologic) for measurement of bone density in the lumbar spine and the hips

and peripheral (forearm) sites and can even perform a total body scan ("full-body DXA scanner"). Advantages and limitations of the DXA methods are summarized in Table 13.2.

The hip joint and the lumbar spine are routinely measured from the front (AP) or the side (lateral). The combined evaluation of these two measurements improves the assessment of a patient's bone mineral status and the fracture prediction, especially in cases with anatomic variations, severe degenerative changes or fractures. The measurements of the lumbar spine are not confined to the vertebral bodies; they also include the arches and spinous processes which have a considerable quantity of compact bone. The International Society of Clinical Densitometry (ISCD) suggests

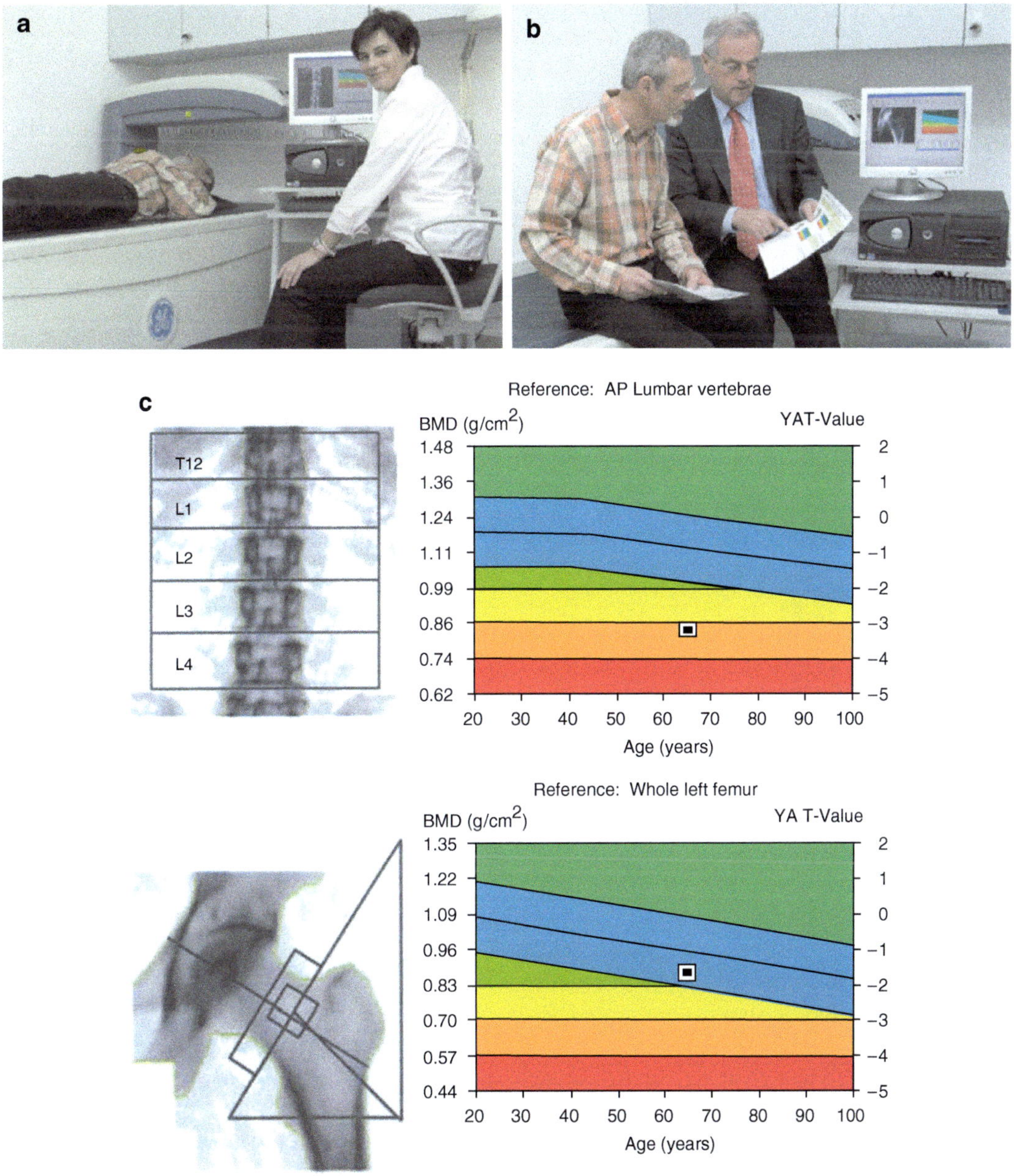

Fig. 13.2 (**a–c**) Measurement of bone density of the hip and lumbar vertebrae using the DXA method (Lunar, GE) (**a**), and the following discussion of the results with the patient (**b**), and DXA of the lumbar spine (L1–L4) and left hip of a male patient showing different BMD values in the two skeletal areas measured (**c**)

measurement of at least two sites if possible and recommends that diagnosis is based on the lowest T-score. It suggests using the L2–L4 average measurement rather than a single vertebra if possible. In measurements of the hip, either the total hip or the femoral neck measurement is used, whichever is the lowest standard deviation.

The results of the measurement of the lumbar vertebral bodies 1–4 are expressed separately as well as in combination, by which single, possibly defective, vertebrae can be excluded. Many factors dealing mainly with variations in density in the spine and/or in neighbouring soft tissues can give misleading values and must be considered in

Table 13.2 Advantages and limitations of the DXA method

Advantages	
	Consensus that T-scores of BMD results can be interpreted
	BMD results can predict fracture risk
	BMD results are used in the FRAX® algorithm for predicting 10-year fracture risk
	BMD results are decisive for starting anti-fracture risk
	Good precision
	Effective in monitoring response to treatment
	Widely available
	Effective quality control procedures
	Short scan times
	Rapid set-up of the patients
	Low ionising radiation dose
	Reliable reference ranges
Limitations	
	2D projection measurement influenced by bone size and shape
	Errors caused by heterogeneity in soft tissue composition
	Discordant findings between different sites measured
	Degenerative changes affect spine BMD in older patients
	Cannot differentiate between osteomalacia and osteoporosis

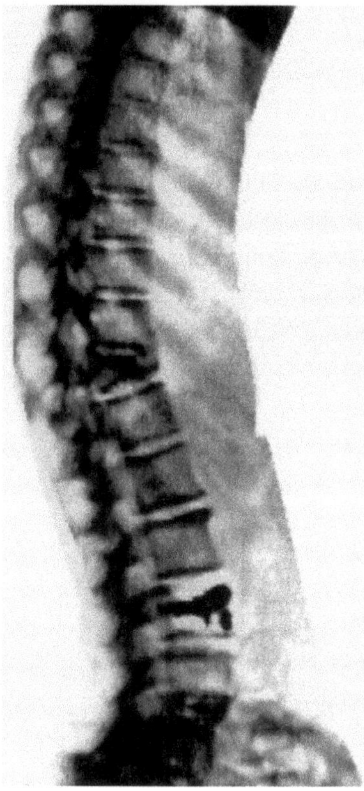

Fig. 13.3 Lateral measurement of the whole spine using a modern DXA machine in order to document or to exclude any vertebral fractures

the results. In really difficult cases, measurement of the lumbar spine may have to be abandoned and only the bones of the hip joint measured. But there may also be variations in density in the proximal femur so that great care must be taken to measure the same areas in sequential investigations. The only real disadvantage of DEXA is that everything in the selected area is included. Sometimes it may be difficult to decide what an ossification is due to, for example, the aorta, calcified lymph nodes or muscles, spondylophytes, etc. Other X-ray dense substances such as metal fasteners on clothes, X-ray dense contrast media or calcium tablets may also be included in the overall measurement. These "pitfalls" can be recognised and subsequently avoided by a prior X-ray of the skeletal area to be measured.

Recent developments in instrumentation enable lateral measurement, and by means of picture enhancement, the vertebral bodies and the hip are clearly displayed (Fig. 13.3). Because of its high precision, it is wise for premenopausal women to get a baseline DEXA scan that can serve as a reference value to determine loss of bone density after menopause.

Two terms, T-score and Z-score, are commonly used to report DXA results, and both of these rely on a *standard deviation (SD)* for the measurement. SD represents the normal variability in a measurement in a population: the difference between the 5th and the 95th percentile of a group covers about 4 SDs. 1 SD of the hip or spine BMD corresponds to about 10–15 % of the mean value.

- *Z-score* is the number of SDs below (minus) or above (plus) the mean BMD value for people of the same age ("age- and sex-matched" controls).

- *T-score* is the number of SDs below or above the mean value of BMD for young (20- to 30-year-old) adults ("peak bone density").

Because BMD declines with age at all sites, after age 30, the T-scores are lower than the *Z*-scores, and the differences increase with age. By definition, diagnosis of osteoporosis is based on a T-score of <–2.5 SD.

Single Energy X-Ray Absorptiometry (SXA) This method is still used today to measure the bones of the ankle because of the paucity of surrounding soft tissue.

Quantitative Computed Tomography (QCT) This is an established technique to measure BMD of the lumbar spine and appendicular skeleton. Moreover, it provides cross-sectional images and therefore separate measurements of the trabecular and cortical bone as well as true volumetric mineral density in g/cm^3. In clinical studies, QCT has been used for assessment of vertebral fracture risk. The method is usually applied to the spine to measure trabecular bone in consecutive vertebrae (Th12–L4). The measurement takes about 20 min and has a relatively high radiation exposure of about 100–1000 mSv. The region of interest (ROI) is either manually or automatically positioned. QCT can be performed in single-energy (SEQCT) or dual-energy (DEQCT) modes, which differ in precision, accuracy and radiation exposure. The presence of marrow fat in the vertebral bodies may cause an underestimation of BMD by 10–15 %. The values obtained by direct measurement and by means of a "calibration phantom" should not be reported as T-score, but they are calculated as hydroxyapatite mass per volume:

- Normal >120 HA/cm^3
- Osteopenia 120–80 HA/cm^3
- Osteoporosis <80 HA/cm^3

Special, small instruments are used to measure bone density in the fingers and the wrist (*pQCT*). The values obtained, however, cannot be considered as representative to the skeleton as a whole, even though they do give accurate values for the bones measured. For example, cancellous bone in the radius may show osteoporosis in density measurements but may be nowhere near that of the lumbar vertebrae or the hips. The future of computed tomography lies in the field of direct visualisation of the trabecular bone architecture by high-resolution and three-dimensional (volumetric) imaging – *3D-CT*. However, this development does entail a greater amount of radiation.

Quantitative Ultrasound (QUS) This is already used successfully in many different conditions. The FDA has approved QUS of the bone for its diagnostic value in osteoporosis and related fractures. The behaviour of these ultrasound waves in the bone differs greatly from that of X-rays. The absorption, the speed and the reflection in the bone and from its surface are all measured. Two major parameters are used in measuring the bone by QUS:

- Speed of sound through the bone (transit velocity, SOS)
- Attenuation of sound as it passes through the bone (broadband ultrasound attenuation, BUA dB/MHz).

Some instruments combine SOS and BUA to formulate a clinical index (quantitative ultrasound index, QUI). The skeletal part to be measured is placed between the ultrasound transmitter and receiver. Consequently, this method is very suitable for easily accessible bones: calcaneus, radius, tibia and phalanges. It is currently accepted that the QUS results are influenced mainly by three parameters:

- Microarchitecture of the bone
- Mineral constituents of the bone matrix
- Elastic modulus

Recent studies have shown that QUS of the calcaneus is a predictor of hip fracture risk, independent of femoral BMD, and that this technology can discriminate between normal and osteoporotic subjects. For every SD decrease in BUA of the calcaneus, the risk of hip fracture increases twofold, comparable with the results of DEXA. QUS is becoming increasingly popular because of the absence of exposure to radiation and the simplicity of application. An additional advantage is that the cortical and cancellous bone is described separately. These advantages account for the fact that QUS is now widely applied as a screening test, though it cannot yet replace DEXA measurements of the spine and hips. It must be emphasised that normal values for the fingers using QUS do not rule out the possibility of a severe osteoporosis of the spine or hips. Conversely, if the phalanges show osteoporotic values, then this should be regarded as a manifestation of generalised osteoporosis, and DEXA of the lumbar spine and/or hips should be carried out for clarification and WHO classification. Measurements of the fingers are especially indicated in patients with rheumatic disorders involving the hands. At present, QUS is not recommended for monitoring of treatment.

13.2 Skeletal Sites of Measurement

A fundamental rule states that "the result of a bone density measurement applies only to the particular site measured". Osteoporosis does not affect the bones of the skeleton to the same degree. Bones with a high proportion of cancellous (trabecular) bone such as the vertebrae and hip bones are the first victims, and these bones are also the first to suffer fractures. Concordance of bone mass between different skeletal sites in individual patients increases in the elderly population. However, even in the elderly female population, measuring only the hip to make a diagnosis of osteoporosis (<–2.5 SD) will detect slightly less than 50 % of the affected people, whereas measuring multiple skeletal sites in this population will detect nearly 80 % of the affected people. Therefore, the lumbar vertebrae and hip bones are always measured according to a precise, topographical plan. The more sites measured, the higher the likelihood that a diagnosis of osteoporosis will be made. Of course, also the reverse is true: if only one peripheral site is measured, there is a much higher probability of missing osteoporosis. The peripheral techniques are quick and easy to use, but they are not appropriate for initial diagnosis or to measure response to therapy.

Lumbar vertebrae are measured individually and together, but fractured or otherwise deformed vertebrae are excluded.

Five areas are measured in the *hip joint*:

- Femoral neck
- Trochanter
- Intertrochanteric region
- Ward's triangle
- Total

Subsequently, when the bone density is checked for monitoring therapy or progression of disease, it is crucial to measure exactly the same areas again.

The *ankle* is also a good site to measure, because of its content of trabecular bone and its accessibility. When done by QUS, differences in rarefaction of the trabecular network along stress lines must be taken into account, and the exact same area must be measured for subsequent monitoring. DEXA does not have this drawback since the whole ankle is measured and the exact area is illustrated.

In the past, the *radius* was frequently measured, but the significance of the results is reduced because of the variable amounts of cancellous and cortical bone and of surrounding soft tissues. The same applies to pQCT and QUS of the radius. However, one advantage of pQCT is that the architecture of the distal radius is displayed.

Worried patients frequently come into the outpatient clinic and produce the results of density measurements of the fingers together with the diagnosis of "severe osteoporosis with very high risk of fractures". Subsequent density measurement of the spine and hip may reveal normal values. The opposite may also occur – normal bone density in the fingers with severe osteoporosis in the axial skeleton and multiple fractures of the vertebral bodies. Such situations simply indicate different bone density in different parts of the skeleton! The lesson to be drawn from this is that the diagnosis of generalised osteoporosis must never be based on the result of a peripheral bone density measurement. In addition, DEXA density measurements to monitor therapy must always be made on the same skeletal site, preferably by the same instrument (DEXA) at yearly intervals.

Investigations of the *whole skeleton* to determine bone mineral content are only made in clinical trials.

13.3 Indications for Measurement

Until recently the diagnosis of osteoporosis was largely based on history, X-rays and clinical symptoms, especially fractures. The clinical relevance of quantitative bone density measurements is based upon two important assumptions:

- That bone density is related to fracture risk
- That treatments to increase bone mass can be given

And indeed, with the introduction of quantitative techniques of bone densitometry, the diagnosis of osteoporosis can now already be established in the early asymptomatic phase of the disease. Low bone density is accepted as the most important predictor of fragility fractures, comparable with blood pressure and cholesterol as reliable predictors of subsequent cardiovascular disease. Nevertheless, density measurements are not yet recommended as a screening procedure. However, for health-conscious individuals, this test is just as important as other generally established investigations. It is cheap and simple to perform and facilitates subsequent diagnosis and monitoring.

13.4 Exposure to Radiation

Low bone mass is the most important objective predictor of fracture risk, and BMD measurement is simple to perform for the patient. Considering that the "natural" exposure to radiation is about 2400 μSv, for example, 100 μSv during a transatlantic flight, then the 10 μSv of a DEXA measurement is so low that it is the most suitable for monitoring. For comparison, radiation doses of currently used techniques are listed:

- X-ray, lateral lumbar spine 1000 μSv
- QCT 100 μSv
- DXA PA pencil beam 10 μSv
- DXA PA fan beam 1 μSv
- pQCT 1 μSv
- QUS 0 μSv

14 Laboratory Investigations

14.1 Recommended Tests

These should be carefully chosen in the light of the clinical picture and results of the imaging techniques outlined above (Table 14.1). It is worth mentioning that relatively few routine tests are diagnostically specific; exceptions are the acid and alkaline phosphatases and of course the specific markers of bone resorption and formation (see below). Nevertheless, laboratory screening, including the following blood tests, has proved its value in clarification of bone disorders:

- Erythrocyte sedimentation rate (ESR)
- Complete blood count
- Calcium and phosphate (serum)
- Alkaline phosphatase (serum)
- Glucose (serum)
- Transaminases and gamma-GT (serum)
- Creatinine (serum)

In addition, when specifically indicated:

- T3, T4, TSH
- Oestrogen and/or testosterone
- Vitamin D metabolites (1,25-hydroxyvitamin D and calcitriol)
- Parathyroid hormone (PTH)
- Electrophoresis and immunoelectrophoresis
- Tumour markers (PSA, CEA, CA 15-3 and others as clinically indicated)

It is important to note that 20 % of women and up to 64 % of men with osteoporosis also suffer from diseases linked to osteoporosis (comorbidities), hence the importance of the analyses listed above.

14.2 Significance of Markers of Bone Turnover

The measurements of collagen metabolism and bone turnover in daily practice are essential for the diagnosis and monitoring of progressive bone diseases such as skeletal metastases or Paget's disease of the bone (Table 14.2). However, bone markers cannot be used to diagnose osteoporosis, though they may help to answer some important clinical questions:

- Predicting the future rate of bone loss (high or low bone turnover)
- Predicting the risk of osteoporotic fractures
- Monitoring response to therapy

The metabolites of bone remodelling, i.e. of resorption and formation, as well as the products of bone matrix metabolism such as collagen type 1, pass into the blood stream and from there into the urine. These products can be identified biochemically, and their levels in the blood and urine indicate "high-turnover" or "low-turnover" osteoporosis. But it should be noted that bone markers

R. Bartl, C. Bartl, *Bone Disorders*, DOI 10.1007/978-3-319-29182-6_14

Table 14.1 Laboratory tests for the evaluation of secondary osteoporoses

Basic tests	Diseases	Additional tests to include
Complete blood count	Malabsorption Multiple myeloma Leukaemia Bone metastases	PTH, vitamin D, calcium (S) Ferritin, vitamin B12 Bone marrow biopsy Protein electrophoresis (S,U) Blood smear PSA, Ca15-3, CEA
Thyroid-stimulating hormone (TSH)	Hyperthyroidism	Thyroxine (T4), T3
Glucose (S,U)	Diabetes mellitus	Oral glucose tolerance test
Cortisol (S)	Cushing's syndrome Addison's disease	ACTH, dexamethasone test ACTH
HIV antibody	AIDS	Infection diagnosis
HLA B-27	Ankylosing spondylitis	CRP
Testosterone in men	Hypogonadism	SHBG, LH, FSH, Prolactin
Calcium (S)	Hyperparathyroidism Malabsorption Morbus Crohn Celiac disease Osteomalacia	PTH Complete blood count PTH, vitamin D Alkaline phosphatase, gliadin PTH, vitamin D Alkaline phosphatase
Alkaline phosphatase	Chronic renal failure Osteomalacia	PTH, calcium, phosphate (S) PTH, vitamin D Calcium (S)
Protein electrophoresis	Multiple myeloma	Complete blood count Bone marrow biopsy
Liver enzymes	Haemochromatosis Alcoholic liver disease Primary biliary cirrhosis	Iron, ferritin (S) Antibodies
Creatinine	Chronic renal failure	PTH, calcium, phosphate (S)
Histamine 24 h U	Mastocytosis	Bone marrow biopsy

do not replace bone density measurements for the diagnosis of osteoporosis. However, these markers do provide information about the future risk for bone loss and fragility fractures. Changes in bone formation in response to therapy are relatively slow, starting after some weeks and reaching a plateau after several months, in contrast to bone resorption which decreases rapidly a few days after initiation of antiresorptive therapy with, for example, a bisphosphonate, and reaches a nadir a few weeks later. These characteristics of bone remodelling must be taken into consideration when evaluating the significance of the levels of markers of bone remodelling in the blood and urine. However, large-scale studies have shown that serial evaluation of markers of bone turnover in the serum does identify people at the highest risk of loss of bone and osteoporosis.

Parameters of bone formation are bone-specific alkaline phosphatase (bone ALP), osteocalcin and osteonectin. These are produced by osteoblasts (possibly also by endothelial cells), and their levels in the peripheral blood reflect osteoblastic activity. ALP is also produced in various tissues including the liver and kidney; but bone-specific ALP can be distinguished by immunoassays with high specificity. Osteocalcin (OC) shows a diurnal rhythm, and only about 50 % is released into the circulation, while the remaining 50 % is incorporated into hydroxyapatite. OC reflects total bone turnover, i.e. the sum of both resorption and formation. The serum concentrations of the C- and N-terminal propeptides of type I procollagen (PICP and PINC) reflect changes in synthesis of new collagen, produced by osteoblasts in the bone and by fibroblasts in other connective tissues. All the PICP and PINC produced are secreted into the circulation.

Parameters of bone resorption: these consist primarily of collagen degradation products such as "cross-links" which are released into the blood stream and then excreted into the urine (Fig. 14.1). They appear to predict the risk of hip fracture in elderly women independently of bone density. Studies have shown that women with high levels of markers of bone resorption have about a 1.5- to 3-fold increased risk of hip or non-vertebral fractures. Desoxypyridinoline and cross-link telopeptides of type I collagen are the two markers of resorption most frequently investigated. Telopeptides are distinguished by their terminals: amino- (*NTX-OSTEOMARK*) and carboxy- (*CTX-CROSSLAPS*). Variations in diurnal rhythm and the effect of meals must be taken into account when results of these tests are evaluated. Both NTX and CTX show a significant response to antiresorptive therapy and are currently considered to be the most reliable parameters of bone resorption. However, serum NTX concentrations are elevated in chronic renal failure, and this must, of course, be taken into account, i.e. by investigation of renal function.

Table 14.2 Biochemical markers of bone turnover

Bone resorption	Bone formation
Blood:	*Blood:*
Tartrate-resistant acid phosphatase (TRAP)	Total or bone-specific alkaline phosphatase
Free pyridinoline or deoxypyridinoline	Osteocalcin
N- or C-telopeptide of type I collagen	Procollagen I C- and N-terminal extension peptides
Cross-links	Osteocalcin
Urine:	
Fasting urine calcium-to-creatinine ratio	
Pyridinoline and deoxypyridinoline	
Glycosides of hydroxylysine	
Pyridinoline and desoxypyridinoline	
N- and C-telopeptides of type I collagen	

Bone sialoprotein (BSP) also appears to be a sensitive marker of bone turnover. Furthermore, BSP is thought to play an important role in attraction and growth of tumour cells in the bone marrow, e.g. in multiple myeloma, and metastases of breast cancer.

Hydroxyproline should no longer be used as a marker of bone metabolism because of its lack of specificity. Its level in the urine is influenced by the breakdown of collagen in sites other than the skeleton, as well as by dietary intake of collagen.

Excretion of *calcium* in a 24 h urinary specimen is also not an accurate reflection of bone resorption, because it depends on the renal threshold for calcium reabsorption and the dietary calcium intake.

Results of bone markers before starting a treatment are not useful predictors of response to the treatment. It is also not clear if patients with

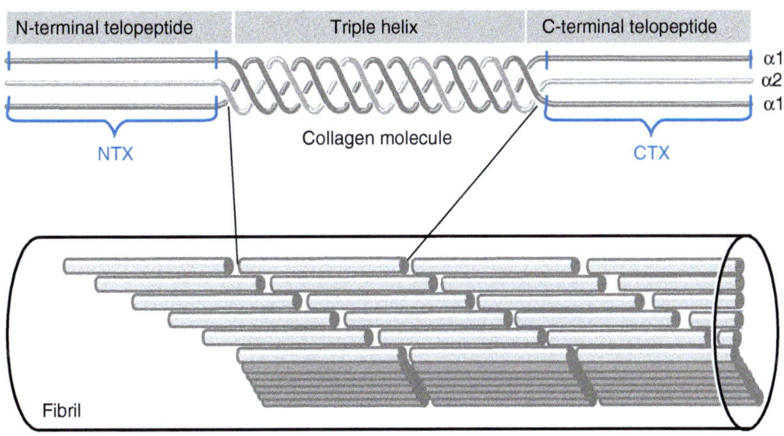

Fig. 14.1 Molecular structure and organisation of collagen into fibrils. Note position of end terminal CTX and NTX, used as biochemical markers of collagen breakdown products in the serum

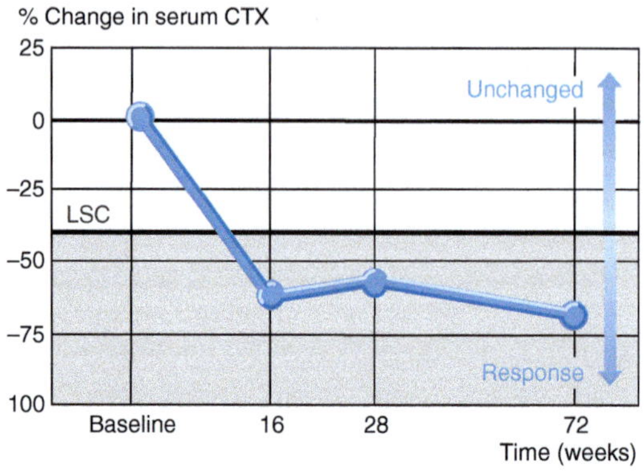

Fig. 14.2 Response of bone markers to antiresorptive agents. A decrease below the least significant change (*LSC*) is regarded as statistically significant

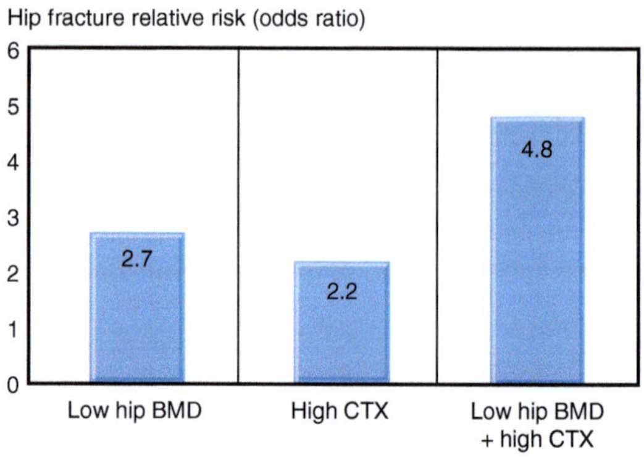

Fig. 14.3 The combination of a low hip BMD and a high serum CTX have a greater predictive value than either low hip BMD or high serum CTX alone (Modified from Garnero et al. 1996)

high bone turnover are more likely to gain bone under therapy. Some studies have demonstrated that patients with the largest decreases in markers of bone resorption during treatment with alendronate tend to have the greatest increases in BMD. Nevertheless, changes in markers during treatment must be interpreted with caution. The results of each patient must be compared with the *least significant change* (LSC) (Fig. 14.2). The LSC is the minimum change that must be seen in an individual patient to be at least 95 % sure that the change is "real" and not caused by biological or laboratory variations. The LSC is about 25 % for most formation markers and 40–65 % for most resorption markers. About 65 % of patients treated with oestrogen or bisphosphonates have changes in bone resorption markers that are greater than the LSC. In contrast, raloxifene and calcitonin are associated with smaller changes in these markers. However, patients may benefit from a decrease in risk of fractures even if they do not have reductions in bone markers or improvements in bone density. In these cases, with little or no change while on antiresorptive medication, it is important to check carefully:

- If the patient is taking the medication
- If the patient is taking the drug as prescribed
- If there are secondary causes of osteoporosis

The advantage of monitoring treatment with markers is that changes in levels can be observed within weeks of starting therapy, and evidence of its efficacy is psychologically important at a time when patients are most likely to discontinue their medications (Fig. 14.3). It is necessary to emphasise that the specimens for investigation should always be taken at about the same time of day and with the patient fasting. Furthermore, indices of bone turnover may show seasonal and circadian variations.

When using bone markers, one should keep in mind that:

- They are not unique to the bone.
- They may reflect both formation and resorption.
- They are influenced also by nonskeletal diseases.

When using bone markers in the monitoring of antiresorptive therapy:

- Always compare the same marker.
- Use only markers validated for assessing bone resorption/formation.
- Collect the samples at the same time (8.00–10.00), if necessary after an overnight fast.
- Keep reasonable intervals between the controls (about 3–6 months).
- Use cut-off values to identify responders (–30 % for urinary DPD, –65 % for urinary NTX and CTX, –40 % for serum bone-specific AP).

15 Bone and Bone Marrow Biopsy

In recent years there has been a great increase in the number of bone and bone marrow biopsies (BMB) taken because the indications have broadened in direct proportion to improvements in:

- Biopsy needles
- Methods of processing and therefore diagnostic reliability
- The number and range of additional investigative techniques available and applicable to bone and bone marrow sections

Consequently, the indications for taking biopsies have increased especially in internal medicine, haematology, oncology and osteology. Biopsies can be obtained from patients of all ages, and therefore the differences in skeletal structure and bone marrow in different bones as well as the age-related alterations in both osseous and haematopoietic components must be taken into account, particularly with respect to histomorphometric measurements.

15.1 Potential of Bone Biopsy in Clinical Practice

Many clinicians still maintain that clinical history and examination combined with a biochemical profile, radiology and a bone scan provide sufficient information in most cases to make the diagnosis of osteoporosis and other osteopathies. However, the limitations of the radiologic and densitometric examinations in this disorder have been described in detail above. It is therefore reasonable to take a bone biopsy (Fig. 15.1) under the following circumstances:

- When the diagnosis is in doubt
- When confirmation of a specific process is sought, for example, metastases, multiple myeloma and systemic mastocytosis, among other possibilities
- When further categorisation is required for therapeutic decisions (e.g. different subtypes of renal osteopathy)
- When follow-up of a specific process is necessary, as after therapy for osteomalacia or metastases

Moreover, the unique attraction of a bone biopsy is that it allows direct visualisation of both cortical and trabecular bone and the bone cells, as well as the bone marrow and its constituents: haematopoiesis, mesenchyme and adipose tissue. In addition, when the biopsy has been embedded in plastic, the histologic sections permit reliable identification of both calcified bone and osteoid, enabling quantification of various morphologic parameters, i.e. *histomorphometry*. These measurements reflect the mount and "metabolic state" of the bone and its cells by providing information on both osteoclastic resorption and osteoblastic formation of bone. Finally, the dynamics

R. Bartl, C. Bartl, *Bone Disorders*, DOI 10.1007/978-3-319-29182-6_15

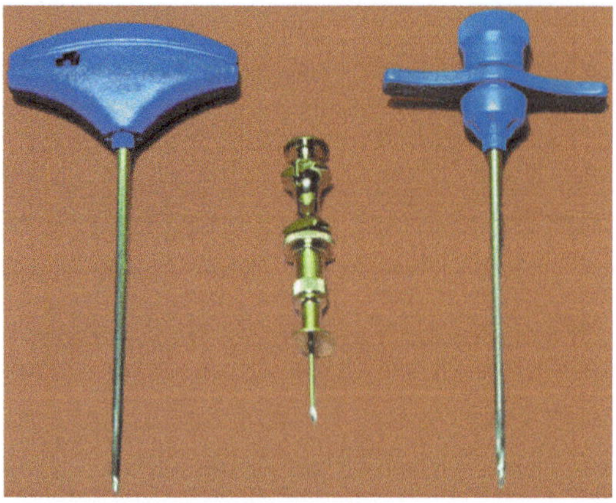

Fig. 15.1 Different manual trephines for bone biopsy and aspiration of bone marrow

of the formation of osteoid and its calcification can be studied by double labelling with tetracycline.

To *summarise,* though bone histomorphometry has contributed little to the diagnosis of osteoporosis, it has provided unique information on the heterogeneity of bone cell behaviour in osteoporosis: low turnover versus high turnover states. In addition, analysis at the level of the basic bone remodelling unit, and possibly mini-modelling of the trabecular bone, permits a more critical choice of therapeutic regimens in individual cases. In the future, there may well be more widespread use of bone biopsies for the immunohistochemical demonstration of osteotropic factors and their receptors on bone cells.

15.2 Biopsy Sites

The posterior and occasionally the anterior iliac crest is the preferred site from which bone and bone marrow biopsies are obtained under local anaesthesia (Fig. 15.2). Bone biopsies can be obtained in the operating theatre under radiologic guidance from almost any skeletal area, depending on the patient's condition, the indications and the diagnostic requirements. There are differences in the amounts of cortical and trabecular bone and marrow in different regions of the ilium, but these have no practical significance. Likewise, the proportions of bone, parenchyma and fat vary in different parts of the bone containing red haematopoietic marrow, but the basic constituents are the same.

15.3 Biopsy Needles and Electric Drill

- The needle most commonly used (especially by the haematologist) is the 11 to 8 gauge "disposable" needle ("Jamshidi needle") which provides biopsies 2 mm in diameter while the length varies (1–6 cm) according to the depth to which the needle is introduced in the posterior iliac crest (Fig.15.3).
- The transilial needle used for horizontal cortex-to-cortex biopsies, 8 mm in diameter, and taken from the anterior iliac crest is often used by the osteologist (Fig. 15.3).
- The electric drill used for vertical biopsies from the anterior iliac crest is used by some clinicians when the bone is expected to be very soft or very hard and is suitable for histomorphometric requirements (Fig. 15.3).

Once the sterile pad is removed, an aspiration needle is introduced, preferable at about 1 cm from the spot where the bone marrow biopsy was taken, and the marrow is aspirated into sterile test tubes with the appropriate anticoagulant or culture media.

Biopsies may be cut and pieces used for different purposes: fixation for both plastic and paraffin embedding and fresh frozen for cryostat sections and immunohistology (Fig. 15.4). In our laboratory the following *stainings* were used: Giemsa (haematopoiesis, cells, osseous structures), Gomori (fibres, osseous structures), PAS (PAS-positive tumour cells, deposits, vessels) and Ladewig (osteoid).

15.4 Biopsy Evaluation

A systemic survey is made, beginning with a scan of the whole biopsy section at low power and ending with examination at high power, under oil if necessary, of individual cells and structures

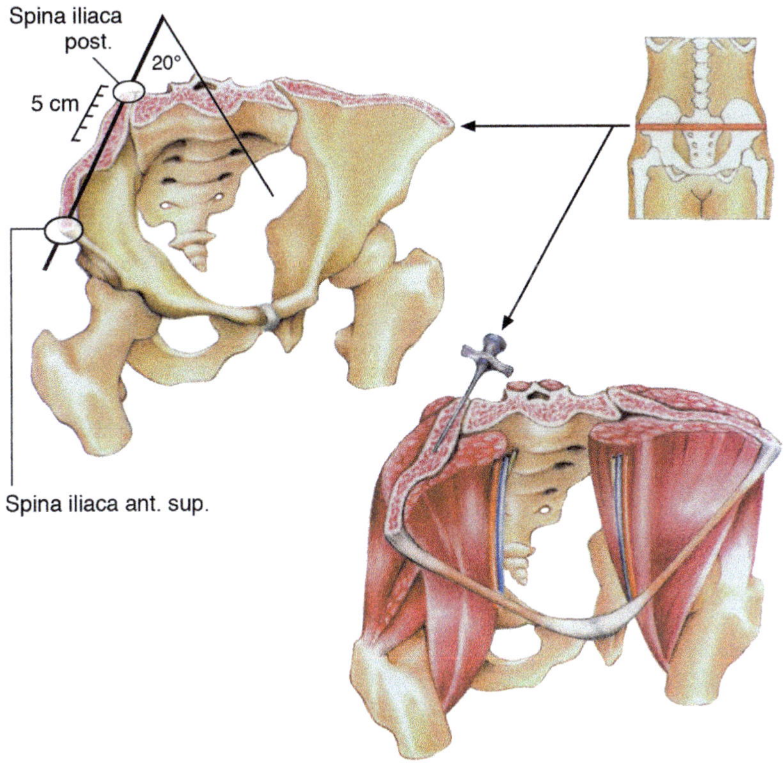

Fig. 15.2 Anatomy of the pelvis at the level of the usual biopsy site (manual trephine)

(Fig. 15.5). Though this book is concerned with the bone marrow, it is important to consider the bone and bone marrow together as a single system, because alterations in one are almost invariably accompanied by changes in the other. Diagnostic evaluation is made, first with respect to the histological and histopathological findings and, where appropriate, immunohistological results, second, take into account patient's clinical status and the results of other diagnostic procedures (CT, MRI, scans) and, third, the peripheral blood picture and the smears of the bone marrow aspirate. Occasionally chromosome analysis, enzyme and marker studies are useful in the confirmation of a diagnosis.

15.5 Indications for Taking a Bone Biopsy

Before dealing with this question, it should be clearly stated the diagnosis of most osteopathies is based on clinical findings and bone density measurements. In addition, it should be pointed out that normal bone histology in an iliac crest biopsy does not exclude osteoporosis elsewhere, for example, in the axial skeleton. Nevertheless, a bone biopsy is sometimes required for investigation of other disorders of bone. A long *list of indications* has now been established in osteology, haematology and internal medicine and can be summarised as follows:

- In all conditions that might affect the bone, either primarily or secondarily, when the diagnosis is in doubt, or when confirmation is sought of a specific process, e.g. metastases, multiple myeloma or systemic mastocytosis.
- In all cases where aspiration of the bone marrow is considered as a diagnostic procedure, there are advantages in taking a biopsy at the same time: aspiration and biopsy are complimentary procedures.
- Clarification of numerous other disorders, such as infections, toxo- and histoplasmosis, granulomatous disorders, amyloidosis, vascular

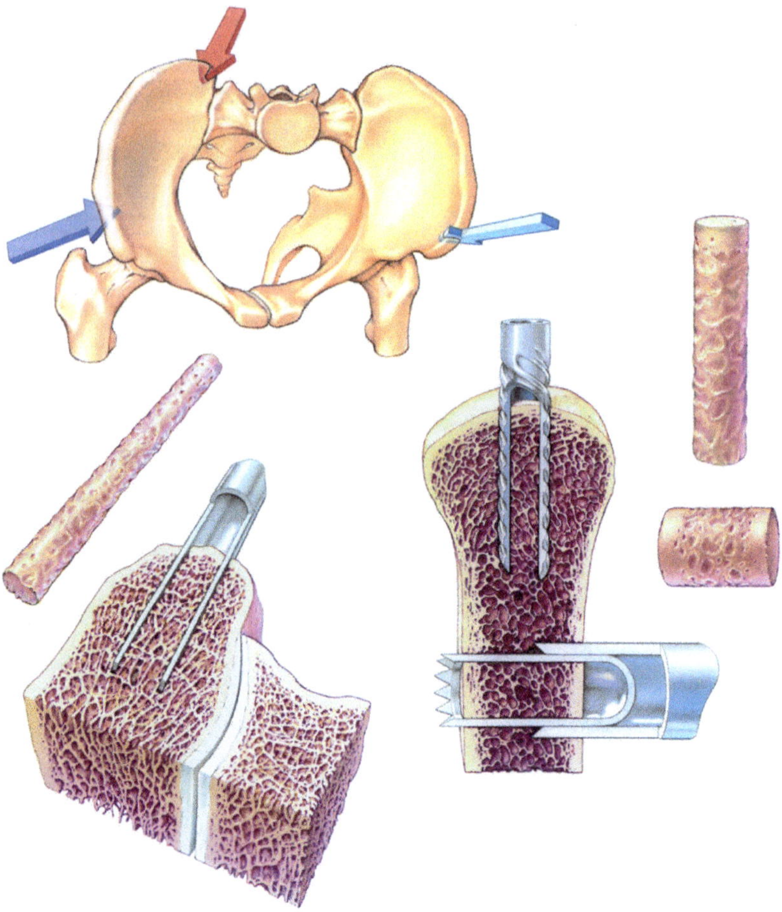

Fig. 15.3 Sketch illustrating the three sites on the iliac crest from which bone biopsies are generally taken. Electric drill and manual transilial trephine in situ in the anterior ilium, manual trephine ("Jamshidi needle") in situ in the posterior ilium

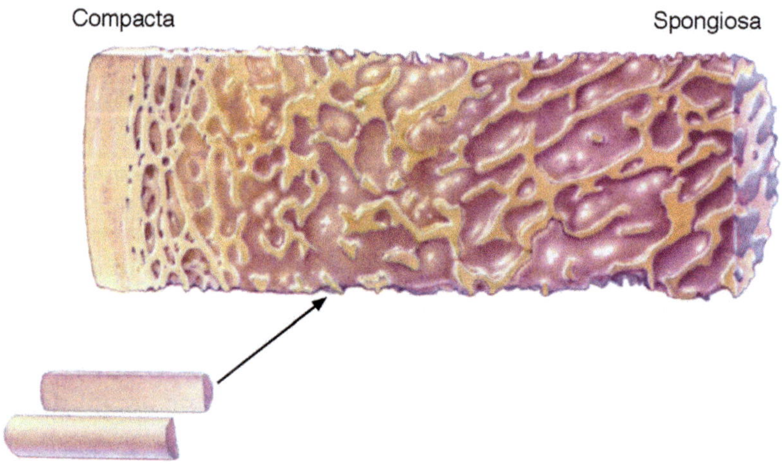

Fig. 15.4 Biopsy longitudinally halved and cut to enable multiparameter studies: plastic histology, cryostat sections, mineral analysis and electron microscopy. Imprints of the cut surface of one biopsy half are also made for cytology

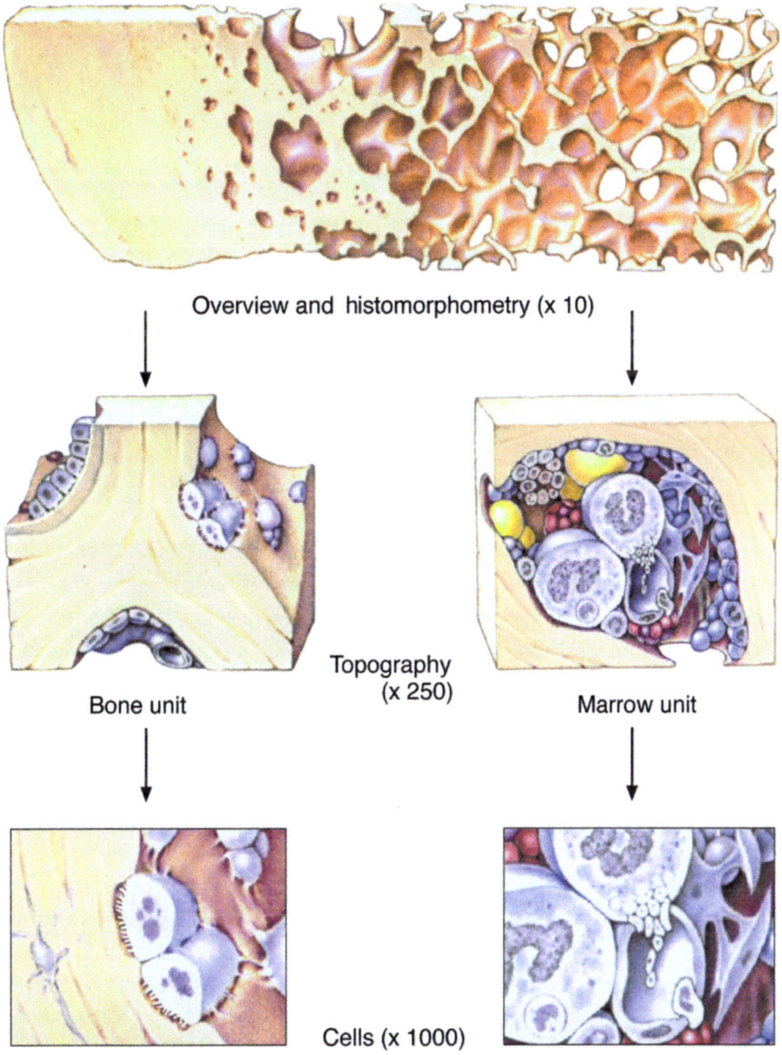

Fig. 15.5 Sequence of biopsy evaluation: overview of the biopsy core, bone and marrow topography and cellular details

disease, pyrexia of unknown origin, storage disorders and effects of metabolic disturbances.

- Whenever a dry tap or insufficient material is obtained on aspiration.
- Staging and classification in malignant lymphomas multiple myeloma and Hodgkin's disease. Pattern of involvement, quantification of the tumour cell burden in the bone marrow and bone reactions.
- Suspected minimal lesions and hypocellular variants of haematologic malignancies and other conditions (e.g. aplastic anaemias).
- Evaluation of fibrosis and other stromal reactions and manifestations, e.g. iron depletion or overload, serous atrophy and inflammatory reactions (e.g. bone marrow oedema).
- Monitoring of therapy, remission, relapse, disease progression or transformation (as in ML, MPD and MDS) and recognition of concomitant disorders in the bone marrow.
- There are many other indications in oncology, in osteology and in internal medicine, for example, clarification of anaemia, fever of unknown origin (FUO), unexplained weight loss and elevated erythrocyte sedimentation rate. Note that when an aspirate is taken, it is known exactly what was taken out, but there is no knowledge of what was left inside!

Obtaining a bone biopsy nowadays is a relatively simple procedure and nearly always without complications. The vast majority of bone biopsies are taken from the posterior iliac crest with an 8-gauge manual trephine (3 mm width). This needle technique is less invasive, can be performed relatively easily and is particularly suitable for outpatients. Manual anterior transilial trephines are recommended when detailed histomorphometric measurements of bone are necessary, but at the cost of greater invasiveness and rate of complications. There are a number of new improved biopsy needles available, as well as up-to-date techniques for processing bone biopsies from fixation and embedding to *histology* and *immunohistology*. These methods provide optimal biopsy sections for evaluation of the overall structure of the cortex and the trabecular network, demonstration of the bone cells and their activities in remodelling, distinction between and quantification of osteoid and calcified bone and, last but not least, state of the bone marrow, from the proportion of adipose tissue to haematopoiesis and mesenchyme, to the visualisation of all the stages of differentiation of the haematopoietic cell lineages. Immunohistochemistry using undecalcified sections identifies proteins specific to various types of tissue differentiation. Stains with antibodies identify metastatic carcinomas, lymphoma cells, macrophages, inflammatory cells and many other specific cells. In clinical trials any of these parameters can be evaluated quantitatively by *histomorphometry*. Quantitative histology of bone comprises four main types of primary measurement:

- Surface
- Volume
- Thickness
- Number

Other more sophisticated parameters can be derived from combinations of these primary variables. Quantitative evaluation of the components of a normal iliac crest biopsy shows the following volumes:

- Osteoid 5 vol.%
- Bone tissue 25 vol.%
- Haematopoiesis 47 vol.%
- Fatty tissue 22 vol.%
- Sinusoids 1 vol.%

Bone biopsies are indicated in the investigation of secondary osteoporosis. In these conditions they frequently provide essential information. When a disturbance of mineralisation is suspected, histologic evidence of undecalcified bone can be obtained by means of bone biopsies. In renal osteodystrophy (ROD), bone biopsies provide essential information required to determine the type and severity of ROD. PTH levels in serum, though widely used, are not necessarily predictive of the underlying bone disease, which can, however, be readily assessed by bone biopsy. In addition, estimation of the histologic aspects of bone and its cells enable correlation with the measurable parameters of bone remodelling and with age. Disorders of the bone marrow and suspected metastatic processes are additional indications.

To *summarise*, a bone biopsy is no longer necessary for the demonstration of uncomplicated bone loss in primary osteoporosis; it has been replaced by the non-invasive BMD measurements. However, when other underlying causes are suspected or established, a bone biopsy may provide essential information. Finally, in trials on the therapeutic efficacy of specific, possibly newly developed drugs, the data in a bone biopsy may be necessary for comprehensive evaluation. In this connection, a novel method of tetracycline labelling allows longitudinal (i.e. sequential) evaluation of short-term effects of hPTH therapy, for example, during one month, on bone formation in a single bone biopsy. It also has been postulated that improvements in trabecular microarchitecture, as seen in iliac crest biopsies, can be correlated with increases in BMD in patients on teriparatide therapy. In contrast, a comprehensive histological analysis can also be applied to analyse adverse effects of, for example, alcohol or drugs as well as beneficial effects of antiresorptive and osteoanabolic therapies.

Part IV

Epidemiology and Diagnosis of Osteoporosis

16 Epidemiology of Osteoporosis

A young healthy adult can hardly imagine that he/she will ever suffer from osteoporosis.

Moreover, when an older individual sustains a fracture or notices a gradual decrease in height, the first reaction is: "This cannot be true, this can't be happening to me. Why should I have osteoporosis? I never had a single problem with my bones in all my life!" And that is just the problem! Osteoporosis slowly but surely nibbles away at the bones, possibly unnoticed for years, until finally it is exposed by the occurrence of a fracture almost without cause!

Osteoporosis: a silent thief!

And so the vicious cycle begins, and the patient is suddenly confronted by many psychological, social and possibly financial problems, which at times may appear overwhelming: starting from the fracture itself, leading to pain, possibly deformities, anger, anxiety, frustration, depression, loss of self-esteem, decreased mobility and finally even social isolation.

One of the most appropriate and effective sources of help is the local osteoporosis support group, where patients can learn from other patients who have had a similar experience how best to cope with their new challenges.

Unfortunately, many people who are at risk are unaware of it, and have not yet adopted preventive measures or received treatment. Some estimates suggest that less than 30 % of women with osteopenia/osteoporosis are correctly diagnosed, and less than 15 % of those diagnosed receive treatment for prevention in cases of ; or for therapy in established osteoporosis. The situation is even worse for men, because it has only recently been recognised that osteoporosis has no gender discrimination – it only attacks men later than women, that is, at the time of the andropause when the levels of male hormones start to decrease and androgen deficiency occurs, from about 50 to 60 years of age onwards. It has now been calculated that men >50 years have a 13 % lifetime risk for fractures!

R. Bartl, C. Bartl, *Bone Disorders*, DOI 10.1007/978-3-319-29182-6_16

Regrettably, some doctors still regard osteoporosis as a "normal" aspect of ageing, a process whereby organisms gradually "lose the capacity to deal with life's stresses effectively".

The "ageing process" includes pathophysiological changes such as decreases in muscle and bone mass, and these in turn are brought about by quantitative, structural and functional alterations in mechanisms participating in control of all the systems in the body.

These changes may affect the structure of individual cells and their constituents such as mitochondria, as well as changes in the cytokines and other factors the cells produce. However, many of these mechanisms can be favourably influenced by outside interventions!

We can no longer accept osteoporosis as a "normal component" of ageing, which impinges on or even ruins the active life of more than half of all women over 50 years of age and nearly as many men over 70 years!

The purpose of the following sections is to unmask the bone robbers and to provide guidelines for early prevention, correct diagnosis and successful treatment of osteoporosis. Today many in the medical profession and in healthcare authorities have come to the realisation that osteoporosis can affect everybody from newborn babies to the oldest old and, significantly, that both sexes are equally prone and vulnerable, and under similar conditions, the difference is mainly a temporal one!

Osteoporosis is now identified as one of the ten most important conditions affecting the entire human race, along with others such as cardiovascular disorders, hypertension, stroke and diabetes mellitus, and it is essential to take into consideration that each of these disorders is itself a risk factor for osteoporosis!

An estimated 44 million people suffer from osteoporosis in the USA alone; 1.5 million fragility fractures were occurring each year and equally high percentages of the populations in many other countries in the Americas, in Europe and in Asia. Moreover, it has been estimated that the numbers of people with osteoporosis in the USA will increase to 61 million by the year 2020. Other calculations claim that there are already over 200 million osteoporotic people in the world today: one in three women and one in eight men!

One in three women older than 50 years suffers an osteoporotic fracture.

Fracture of a bone is the most significant consequence of osteoporosis. For comparison, while every eighth woman suffers from breast cancer, every third woman sustains a fracture due to osteoporosis. Although osteoporosis can attack any bone in the body, the typical sites of osteoporotic fractures are the hip, the spine and the wrist. 70 % of the fractures that occur annually in the USA in patients aged more than 45 years are attributable to osteoporosis. From the age of 50 years onwards, a woman has the following risk for a fracture:

- Vertebral 32 %
- Lower arm 16 %
- Hip 15 %

Furthermore, a hip fracture poses an increased risk of mortality (Fig.16.1a, b) related to possible co-morbidities such as rheumatism, chronic cardiovascular disease, stroke, chronic lung disorders, as well as the complications secondary to surgical treatment of the fracture itself.

> Nearly 50 % of the patients with hip fractures never fully recover the mobility and the independence they previously had, and an additional 25 % require a long-term nursing facility or home care. Mortality after a hip fracture is estimated to range from 12 to 35 % which is higher than that expected in the general population.

The highest mortality typically occurs within the first 6 months after a fracture, but some studies have shown a sustained effect over a longer period. It has been estimated that the respective figures for men are worse than these given for women. Monetary costs associated with osteoporotic fractures are tremendous: about 40 million US dollars daily in the USA. The total cost for medical and hospital expenses, possibly nursing home care, and lost productivity reached 17 billion US dollars in 2005 (Fig. 16.2a, b)! Hip fractures alone account for about 60 % of these costs, and fractures at other sites about 40 %.

> Global demographic changes are expected to increase the incidence of hip fractures nearly fourfold by the year 2050. Each year, osteoporotic fractures affect more women than heart attacks, strokes and breast cancer combined. Indeed, the economic costs of osteoporosis are as significant as those of chronic obstructive pulmonary disease, myocardial infarction, strokes and breast cancer.

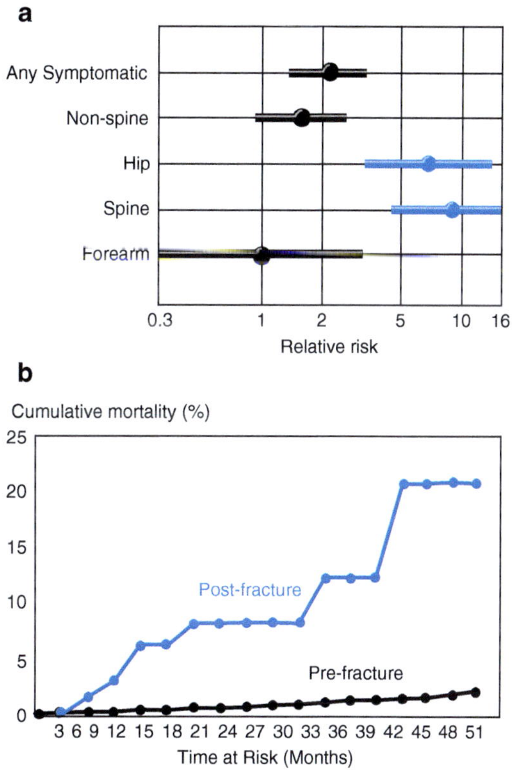

Fig. 16.1 (**a**) Risk of mortality following clinical fractures (Modified from Cauley et al. 2000). (**b**) Risk of mortality in the pre- and post-fracture situation

Another highly significant aspect of osteoporosis is the fact that numerous disorders in most medical disciplines have deleterious effects on the bones, primarily involving osteoporosis. Examples of some such conditions are infections and inflammatory disorders, e.g. AIDS and inflammatory bowel disease, cardiovascular disorders, diabetes mellitus and the metabolic syndrome and neurologic conditions such as Parkinson's disease and epilepsy. Cancers of the breast, prostate, lung and colon, congenital disorders such as osteogenesis imperfecta and interdisciplinary causes such as effects of drugs – a notable example are the glucocorticoids – and last but not least transplantations of cells and of organs all may be associated, directly or indirectly, with decrease in bone mass and bone

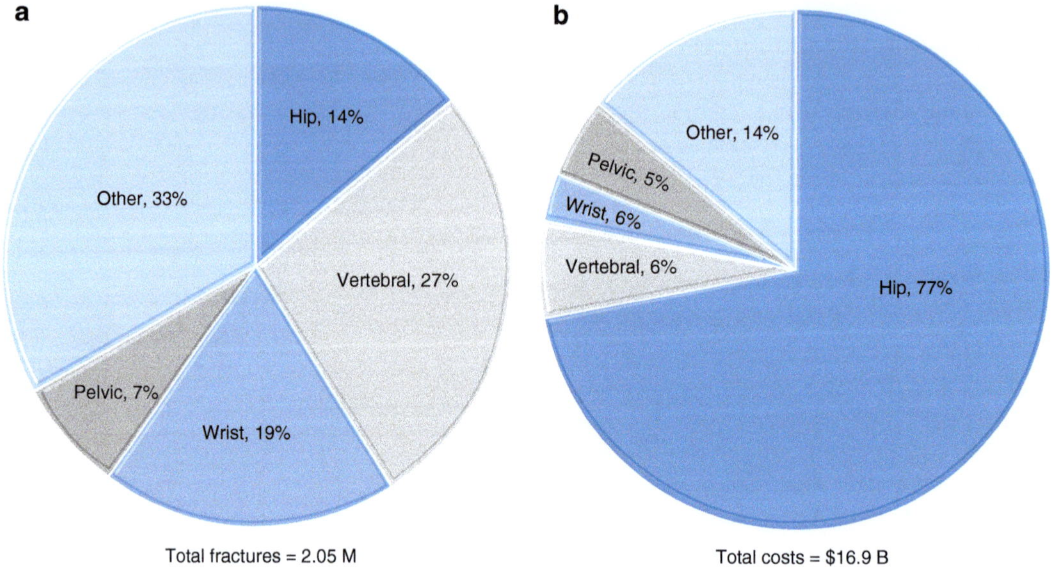

Fig. 16.2 (**a**) Fracture distribution by type in the USA, 2005. (**b**) Cost distribution by type in the USA, 2005 (Modified from Burge et al. 2007)

density. In this context, it should also be stressed that metabolic conditions that cause intrinsic biochemical alterations and thereby also damage the bones have initiated the concept and the classification of metabolic bone diseases. Included under this heading are rickets (osteomalacia), renal osteodystrophy, hyperparathyroidism and osteoporosis.

It is now abundantly clear that osteoporosis is globally a common condition and poses a major public health burden, and arresting this disorder should be a primary goal of our preventive efforts in the coming decade.

17 Definition of Osteoporosis

The word "osteoporosis" literally means porous bone, indicating that the bone density is low and the bones are thin. But bone does not fracture due to thinness alone. In the early 1990s, a consensus meeting of the World Health Organization (WHO) defined osteoporosis as

> "a systemic skeletal disorder characterised by a low bone mass and by microarchitectural deterioration of bone tissue, with a subsequent increase in bone fragility and susceptibility to fracture".

The first Consensus Conference on Osteoporosis of the new millennium proposed a new definition of osteoporosis as:

> "A skeletal disorder characterized by compromised bone strength predisposing to an increased risk of fracture".

However, in order to better understand the aetiology of osteoporotic fractures and the effects of therapy on risk of occurrence of fractures, it is essential to recognise the factors that govern *bone strength*. The strength of an individual bone (and of the whole skeleton) depends on its mass, shape and the quality of the bone itself (Fig. 17.1). Numerous large studies have already confirmed the connection between bone density, bone strength and fracture risk. Density is responsible for 60–90 % of the strength of bone. From the outside however, osteoporotic bones may even have the same size and look like normal bones, but inside they are brittle, with a thin cortex and a disrupted (or even localised lack of) trabecular network.

Low bone mass has proved to be the most important objective predictor of fracture risk. The lower the bone mass, the weaker the bone and the less force is required to cause a fracture. Therefore, according to the *WHO* (The WHO Study Group 1994), osteoporosis in postmenopausal women was also defined in terms of bone density measurement and based on a comparison of the patients' measurement to the standard adult peak bone mass (PABM) as follows:

> "Osteoporosis is present when the bone mass is more than 2.5 standard deviations (SD) below that of healthy premenopausal adult females, the T-score".

However, taking into consideration the multifactorial nature of bone fragility, an updated position paper was issued by the WHO and the International Osteoporosis Foundation (2007).

R. Bartl, C. Bartl, *Bone Disorders*, DOI 10.1007/978-3-319-29182-6_17

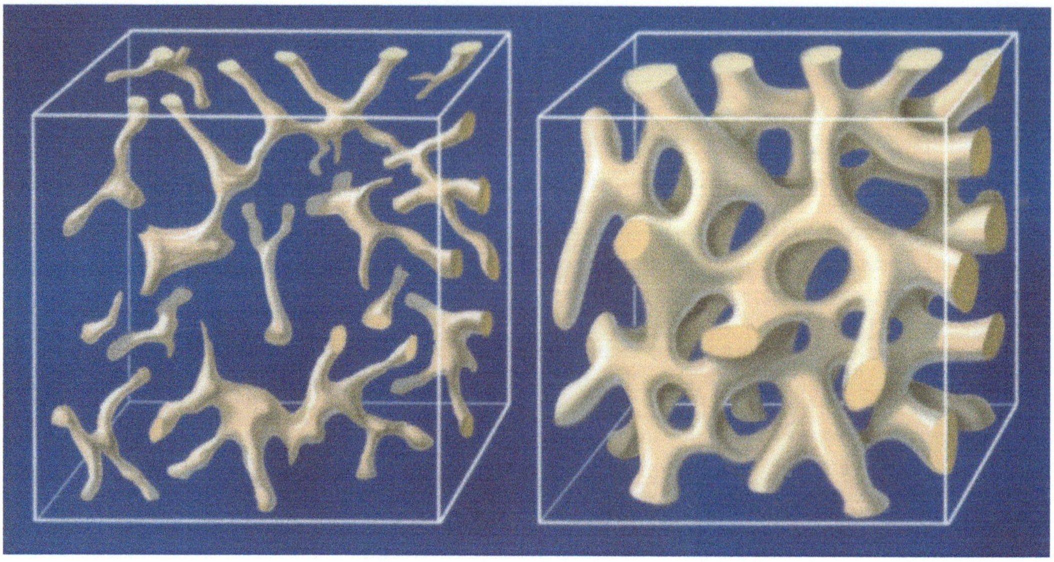

Fig. 17.1 Progressive architectural deterioration of cancellous bone: marked attenuation of the cancellous bone and disconnected trabeculae, no longer a network (*left*)

This proposed that "osteoporosis" is no longer diagnosed as such, but by a total individual 10-year fracture risk on the basis of independent risk factors. Nevertheless, the T-score as obtained by measurements at the femoral neck is utilised internationally as an accepted criterion for osteoporosis. The hip and/or the lumbar spine are measured by the DXA method to obtain the T-score. Low bone mass in any individual is still the most important factor in the determination of fragility fractures. In the new European guidelines, from 2008 onwards, only measurements of DXA at the femoral neck are accepted as diagnostic criteria for osteoporosis.

Osteopenia has now been defined by a T-score between −1.0 and −2.5.

As the emphasis on skeletal health shifts from treatment to prevention, the diagnostic term of *osteopenia* may take on increasing importance, especially in combination with the evaluation of the major risk factors. Hence, postmenopausal women with osteopenia should be targeted for prevention strategies to preserve their skeletal mass. Patients with osteopenia and relevant risk factors should be treated early with effective drugs to prevent fragility fractures!

18 Pathogenesis of Osteoporosis

Where and how does bone resorption occur? The bone cells carry out their remodelling preferably on the inner surface of the bone, the endosteum (Fig. 18.1). Bones with a large component of cancellous bone present the largest surface area to bone cells for remodelling: these bones include the vertebral bodies, the femoral neck, the ribs, the wrist and the heel. Due to their immense surface, these cancellous bones are resorbed five times as fast as the cortical bone of the long bones (Fig. 18.2a, b). Considered sequentially the ossicles in the middle of the bone disappear first, especially those at the horizontal "stress" lines. The vertical "pillars" which carry greater loads remain intact for longer periods and are seen as vertical stripes on X-ray (Fig. 18.3). In vitro and in vivo studies have shown that bone density is indeed responsible for 50–80 % of the strength of the bone and therefore constitutes a very important risk factor particularly in postmenopausal women. As numerous prospective studies have demonstrated, the risk of a fracture increases exponentially with the decrease in density: a reduction of 10–15 % in bone density doubles the fracture risk.

The bone does not break only because it is thin – as indicated by the fact that half of all people with decreased bone density never sustain a fracture. The recognition that osteoporosis is far more complex than previously thought suggests that factors in addition to bone mineral density may contribute to bone fragility and therapeutic effectiveness. Recent studies have shown that osteoporosis is also a question of the quality of the bone, which, in many disorders, is adversely affected even more than the BMD (Fig. 18.4).

Perforations, "microfractures" of trabeculae occur constantly throughout life and normal activity, and these lead to a decrease in bone strength and weight-bearing ability – and of course require immediate repair. Moreover previous thinning of the trabeculae because of decreased osteoblastic activity accelerates the destruction of the microarchitecture. Disconnected trabeculae are functionally useless and are rapidly resorbed. Should a situation arise in which numerous microfractures are not completely repaired, a critical point will eventually be reached at which the bone will break. Should the bone structure be qualitatively inferior to begin with, bones of even normal thickness may break. This is an important point to take into account and has already been demonstrated in osteoporosis in hypogonadal men. Studies on mineral density by magnetic resonance microradiography have shown a marked deterioration in microarchitecture in the spine and hips of these patients – more than would be expected from the results of densitometry. Moreover at the nanoscale level, it has been demonstrated that interactions between collagen fibres and mineral crystals can affect bone quality.

An important (even crucial) aim of osteoanabolic therapy is to re-establish the microarchitecture. This goal could probably be achieved in the not-too-distant future by sclerostin antibodies.

R. Bartl, C. Bartl, *Bone Disorders*, DOI 10.1007/978-3-319-29182-6_18

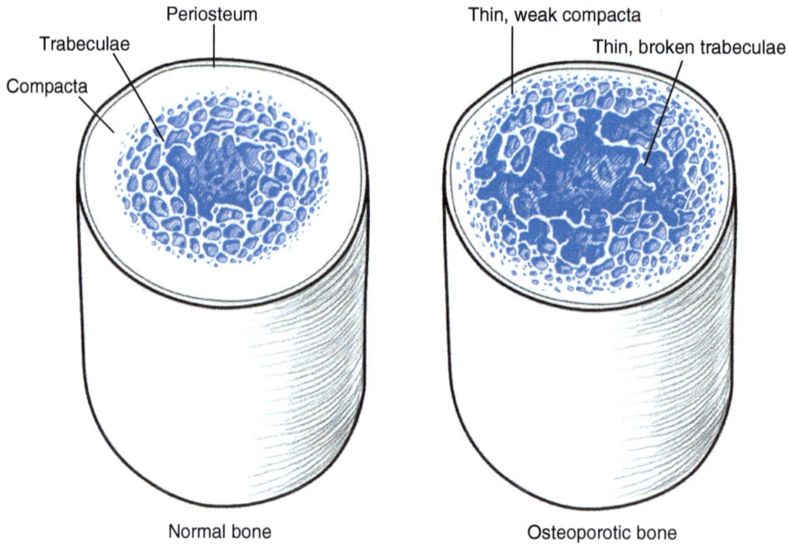

Fig. 18.1 Osteoporotic tubular bone: shrinkage of cortical width; rarefaction and discontinuity of trabecular network

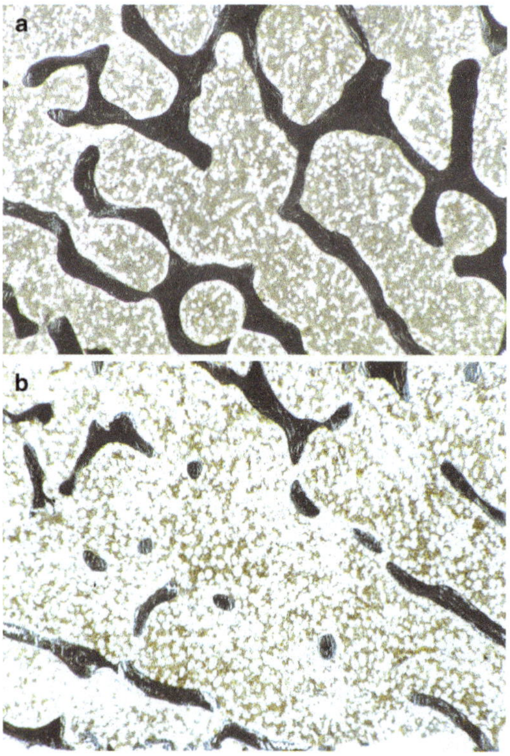

Fig. 18.2 Normal (**a**) and osteoporotic (**b**) trabecular network. Note "button" phenomenon with disruption of the trabecular network in (**b**). Gomori staining

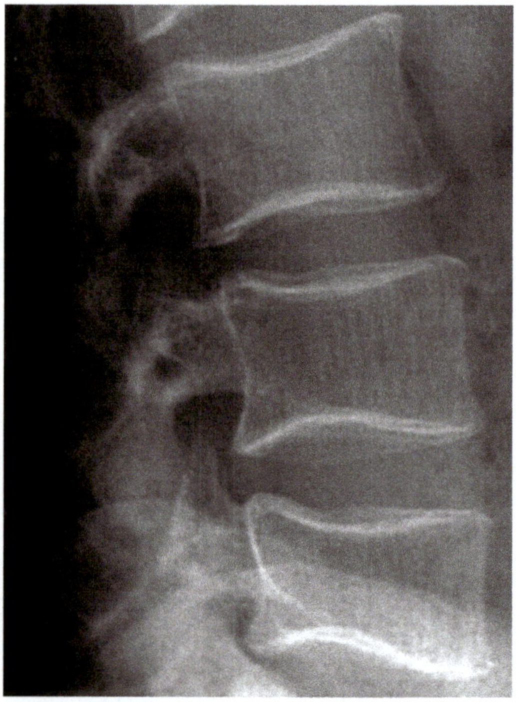

Fig. 18.3 Osteoporosis of the vertebrae: note relative preservation of the stress-bearing vertical trabeculae

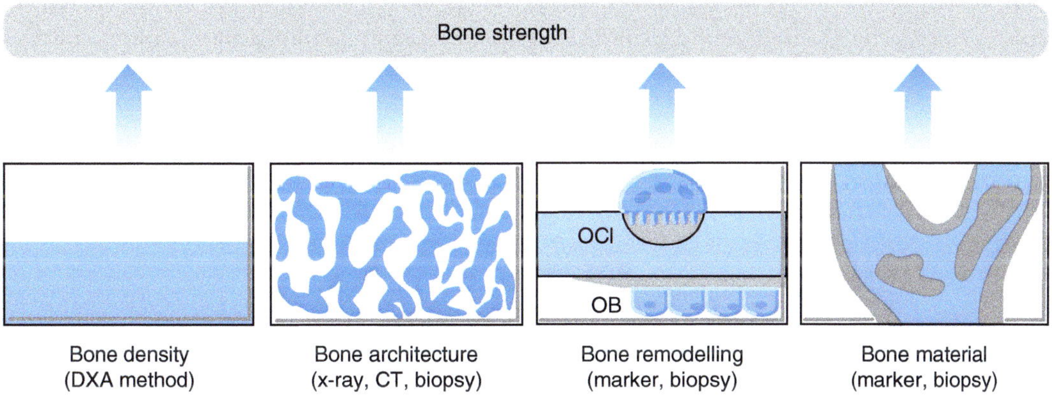

Fig. 18.4 The four main structural factors of bone strength are bone density, bone architecture, bone remodelling and bone material

Generally speaking, osteoporotic fractures are caused by *eight different abnormalities of the bone*:

- Reduced thickness (density)
- Unequal proportions of compact and cancellous bone
- Decrease in number of "nodes" in the cancellous bone
- Transection of trabeculae caused by osteoclasts
- Inadequate bone formation
- Inadequate mineralisation of bone matrix (osteoid)
- Anomalies of structure and binding of collagen molecules ("cross-linking")
- Faulty repair mechanisms

How can fragility be reduced? There are two ways to make bones stronger:

- Increase bone mineral density and distribute bone mass more effectively, i.e. increase bone tissue where the mechanical demands are greatest ("extrinsic biomechanical properties").
- Improve the material properties of bone tissue, from the microscopic to the molecular level ("intrinsic biochemical properties").

An effective treatment for bone fragility should improve the extrinsic biomechanical properties of the bone but at the same time should not substantially impair the intrinsic properties. Strong inhibitors of bone resorption such as bisphosphonates can reduce bone turnover by 70–90 %, causing a gain in bone mineral density. Due to reduced bone remodelling, the mean tissue age of the bone is increased as is bone mineralisation. Properly mineralised bone has the best combination of stiffness and brittleness, while poorly mineralised bone tends to be very weak with increased displacement, and hypermineralised bone is too brittle with decreased displacement. Consequently, in treating osteoporosis, attention must be paid to bone density, to improvement of the microarchitecture, to mineralisation and to the repair mechanisms. Today, with the modern bisphosphonates, it is no longer a problem to fill up resorption lacunae, to increase mineralisation and to thicken attenuated trabeculae. At present there is no convincing evidence that microdamage accumulation occurs under intravenous treatment with bisphosphonates. But it is not yet possible – as far as we know from experimental studies – to restore completely the trabecular network (restitutio ad integrum) or the shape of the bone that has been destroyed.

19 Subgroups of Osteoporosis

Osteoporosis has traditionally been categorised as primary or secondary. *Primary osteoporosis* occurs together with and as a result of the major physiological condition known as ageing (senescence) and its causes and consequences. *Secondary osteoporosis* develops as a consequence of the major physiopathological effects on the bones, by numerous disorders of other organs and tissues in the body.

19.1 Grouping According to Spread

Osteoporosis may be *localised* to one or more skeletal regions, i.e. focal or regional osteoporosis, as distinct from the classic *generalised* osteoporosis (systemic). The most important causative factors responsible for bone loss are:

- *Inactivity* (immobilisation osteoporosis): A classic example is the regional osteoporosis which occurs when an extremity is immobilised either because of a fracture or a motor neuron injury. The lack of use and movement results in increased osteoclastic resorption which, if sufficiently extensive, is also accompanied by hypercalciuria and hyperphosphaturia. On cessation of immobilisation and resumption of activity, the process can be reversed and the bones normalised, especially those of children and young people.
- *Complex regional pain syndrome* (CRPS, Sudeck's disease, algodystrophy, sympathetic reflex dystrophy): This affects mainly the hands, knees and ankles and is characterised by swelling, pain, hyperaesthesias and vasomotor reactions.
- *Transient (transitory) osteoporosis*: Transient osteoporosis is a regional process first described in the pelvic bones in pregnant women. Since then, it has also been observed in knee and ankle joints in both young men and young women. The pain appears to start spontaneously without apparent prior trauma. The diagnosis is established by means of MRI (magnetic resonance imaging) which shows extensive oedema of the bone marrow around the painful joint. Clinically, the process is self-limiting with complete restitution within a year. Together with CRPS, this disorder is now summarised under the heading of "bone marrow oedema syndrome" and can be treated effectively with intravenous bisphosphonates (complete remission in about 80 % of the cases). See Chap. 31.
- *Gorham-Stout syndrome* ("vanishing bone disease"): The cause of this rare bone disease has not yet been elucidated, though a vascular and lymphatic connection has been suggested, mainly by way of activated endothelium. It begins with completely uncoupled osteoclastic resorption of a bone and spreads to adjoining bones. Progression is variable.

R. Bartl, C. Bartl, *Bone Disorders*, DOI 10.1007/978-3-319-29182-6_19

Severe or life-threatening complications may occur when bones of the thorax or the vertebrae are involved. So far, the only effective therapy is administration of bisphosphonates as early as possible to prevent extensive loss of bone (see Chap. 31).

- *Other osteolytic syndromes*: These may be due to a variety of different causes, including infections, tumours, trauma as well as metabolic, vascular, congenital and genetic aberrations.
- *Generalised (systemic) osteoporosis*: This is far more frequent than localised osteoporosis. In spite of its name, generalised osteoporosis is rarely manifest in the whole skeleton, but it does have a symmetrical distribution. Juvenile and postmenopausal osteoporoses generally affect the axial skeleton, while the age-related form also attacks the tubular bones, especially in men. Consequently, presence of a normal bone density in bones of the extremities does not rule out osteoporosis (possibly even severe) of the axial skeleton. This is important to bear in mind in evaluation of local measurements of BMD, which only represent the bone measured, and cannot be extrapolated to the rest of the bones in the skeleton.

19.2 Grouping According to Age and Sex

- *Idiopathic juvenile osteoporosis*: This is a rare self-limiting disease of prepubertal children, usually occurring between 8 and 14 years of age. It generally manifests as compression fractures of the vertebrae accompanied by severe back pain. The differential diagnosis includes osteogenesis imperfecta, Cushing's syndrome and diseases of the bone marrow which are diagnosed by analysis of peripheral blood and bone marrow and by bone biopsies.
- *Idiopathic osteoporosis of young adults*: This affects primarily men between the ages of 30 and 50 years, and it is also characterised by fractures of the vertebral bodies. Biochemical parameters and bone biopsy findings show increased resorption of the bone. Frequently the patients are heavy smokers, which have been implicated as a possible contributory factor. A mild form of osteogenesis imperfecta, not previously diagnosed, must be excluded in these patients.
- *Postmenopausal (type I) osteoporosis* (Fig. 19.1): This is the most common form of osteoporosis, and it occurs in women between 51 and 75 years of age as a consequence of cessation of ovarian function. The loss of bone actually starts years beforehand and increases at the time of the menopause (perimenopausal). About 30% of all women develop osteoporosis after the menopause. Cessation of oestrogen secretion leads to a decrease in IL-6 and other cytokines, which in turn leads to increased recruitment and activation of osteoclasts. In addition, the bone becomes more sensitive to the resorption-stimulating action of parathyroid hormones. As a consequence, there is increased resorption of cancellous bone in the vertebrae and in the hip bones with a corresponding increase in the risk of fractures. Obviously this postmenopausal form of osteoporosis occurs only in women, but men are also subject to increased bone resorption as a consequence of testosterone deficiency, though at a later stage in life, from 50 to 60 years onwards.
- *Involutional (age-related, type II) osteoporosis* (Fig. 19.1): Postmenopausal, in women, and postandropausal, in men, osteoporosis merge imperceptibly into the involutional, age-related type which represents part of the ageing process and which can lead to frailty. This is characterised by many factors common to osteoporosis including sarcopenia, falls, decreased physical activity, cognitive decline, changes in many hormones, vitamins and cytokines. The bone is mainly affected by the increased osteoclastic activity. A study of bone biopsies taken from normal individuals (i.e. without any known metabolic, endocrine or osseous disorders) of different age groups has shown that the number of osteoclasts and osteoblasts increases from the age of 50 years. This indicates that the bone, far from being a

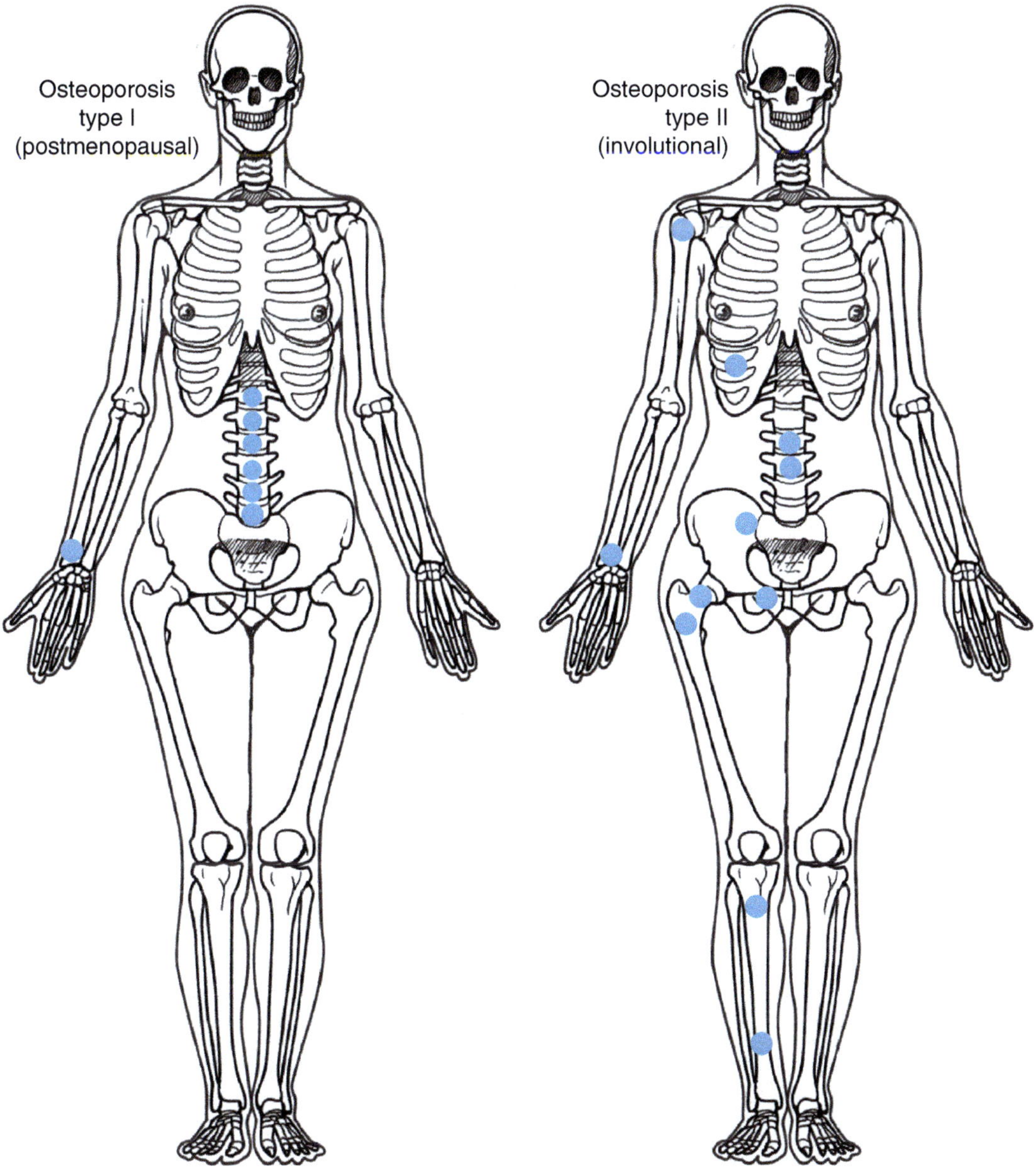

Fig. 19.1 Topographic differences in skeletal involvement between type I and type II osteoporosis

slow, inactive and atrophic tissue in the older age groups, presents the picture of increased osseous remodelling. Other causative factors for involutional osteoporosis are decreased mobility, defective vitamin D metabolism, insufficient calcium and mild secondary hyperparathyroidism. Osteoporosis type II develops after 70 years of age and is now only twice as frequent in women as in men (however they are catching up!). It has been postulated that a major factor in the mechanism of osteoporosis, especially severe osteoporosis, in the elderly, in both men and women, is the adipogenic shift, i.e. the predominance of adipogenesis over osteoblastogenesis in the bone marrow, due to the increased differentiation of mesenchymal stem cells into adipocytes. Studies have indicated that osteogenic and adipogenic differentiation in the mesenchymal stem cells is parallel until a late stage in the process. The cortical bone, especially that of the femoral neck, the radius and the pelvic bones, is then also involved in involutional osteoporosis, especially in males. About 80% of all osteoporotic fractures occur at this time, i.e. after 70 years.

19.3 Grouping According to Severity

In daily clinical practice, the *degree of severity* of a bone disorder must be accurately determined before decisions are made on urgency and strategy of therapy. In women osteoporosis can be diagnosed if the bone mineral density (BMD) is 2.5 SD below the mean of a young reference population. Kanis and co-workers commented on this definition and gave diagnostic categories that may be applied to white women:

- *Normal bone*: a BMD value that is higher than 1 SD below the young adult female reference mean (T-score greater than or equal to −1 SD)
- *Low bone mass (osteopenia)*: a BMD value more than 1 SD below the young female adult mean, but less than 2.5 SD below this value (T-score <−1 and >−2.5 SD)
- *(Preclinical) osteoporosis*: a BMD value 2.5 SD or more below the young female adult mean (T-score less than or equal to −2.5 SD)
- *Severe (manifest, established) osteoporosis*: a BMD value 2.5 SD or more below the young female adult mean value in the presence of one or more fragility fractures.

This definition uses the T-score of DXA at the femoral neck as a diagnostic criterion, which in fact has already long been done in bone densitometry (Fig. 19.2). Bone density results are compared to those of age-, sex- and race-matched controls. It is also evident that the T-score cannot be used interchangeably with different techniques and at different sites. Therefore, a reference standard must be adopted in terms of skeletal site and measurement technique, and measurements with DXA at the femoral neck have the highest predictive value for hip fracture, as established in many prospective studies. Data are also available for the total hip, but the evidence to date does not suggest any improvement in fracture

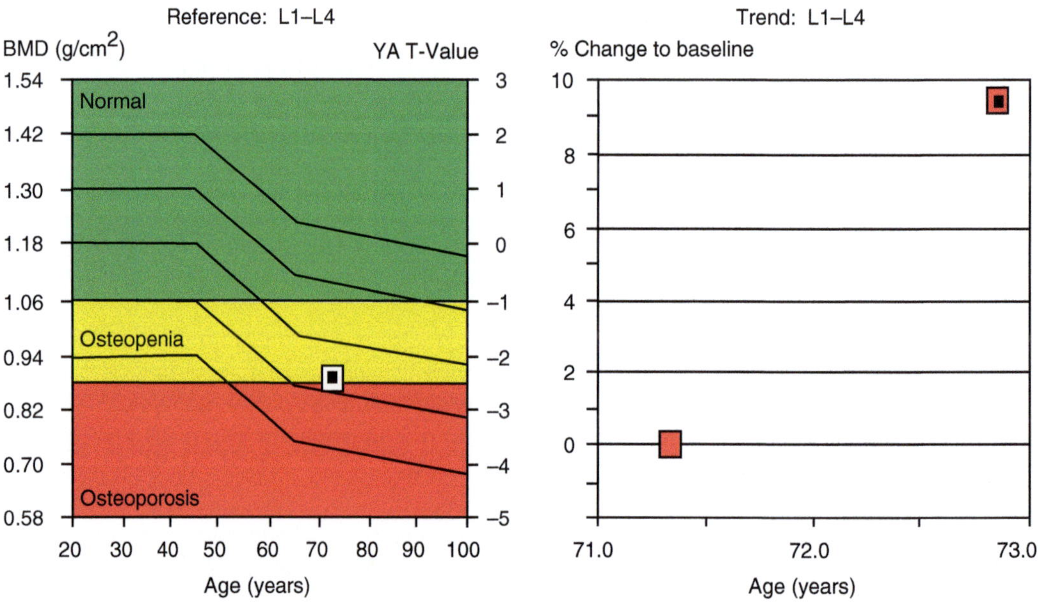

Fig. 19.2 Print of DXA measurement of the lumbar spine with definition of the T-score (*left*), and monitoring under treatment with zoledronate (*right*)

prediction. In lumbar spine BMD, an important source of accuracy error is aortic calcification and osteoarthrosis that increase progressively with age. Moreover, the hip is the site of highest clinical relevance, since hip fracture is the dominant complication of osteoporosis in terms of morbidity, mortality and cost.

19.4 Grouping According to Histology

The trabecular bone volume in iliac crest biopsies of normal adults comprises about 20–25 vol. % of the biopsy section. When this value drops to 16 %, "rarefaction" of the trabeculae has occurred. Other histologic parameters are also evaluated (Figs. 19.3 and 19.4):

- Cortical thickness and cortical porosity
- Disruption of trabecular network
- Trabecular width; type A = long and thin, type B = short and stout
- Quantity and distribution of osteoid (degree of mineralisation)
- Quantity and distribution of fat cells (atrophy in the endosteal region)
- Changes of the stromal elements (inflammatory reactions)
- Quantity and maturation of the haematopoietic cell lines
- Presence of foreign or malignant cells

When the trabeculae are surrounded by fat cells or layers of fatty tissue, then osseous remodelling is decreased and osteoid seams are absent (bone atrophy). This particular distribution of fat cells is a sign of incipient osteoporosis, the "low turnover" type as seen in sequential biopsies (Fig. 19.5a, b). Recent research has demonstrated that there is indeed a connection between fat cells and osteoblastic activity.

The volume, extent and width of osteoid seams are always noted in order to estimate the presence and degree of osteomalacia (Fig. 19.6). These data are required for estimating the therapeutic amounts of vitamin D required. The value for osteoid should not exceed 2 vol. % of the trabecular volume. However, in older patients values of 2–5 vol. % are frequently found, which indicate the presence of an "osteoporo-malacia", when a low trabecular volume % is also present. A *histologic diagnosis of osteomalacia* is based on three criteria:

- Periosteocytic demineralisation (an early sign!)
- Osteoid occupies more than 50 % of the trabecular surface
- Width of osteoid seams more than 10 % of the total trabecular volume (volume %)

Immunohistochemical evidence of bisphosphonates in bone biopsy sections is of particular interest (Fig. 19.7). A comprehensive description of the significance of bone biopsies in internal medicine can be found in the atlas *Biopsy of Bone in Internal Medicine* (Bartl and Frisch 1993). Moreover, with the introduction of improved biopsy needles and the latest immunohistological techniques as well as increasing interest in the bone and its cells, bone biopsies will also acquire greater significance in the investigation of disorders of bone including osteoporoses, especially secondary and drug induced.

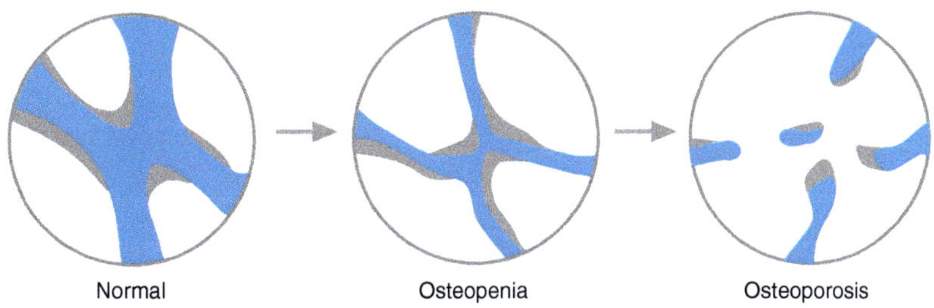

Fig. 19.3 Degrees of reduction in trabecular bone: osteopenia followed by osteoporosis with complete destruction of the trabecular network

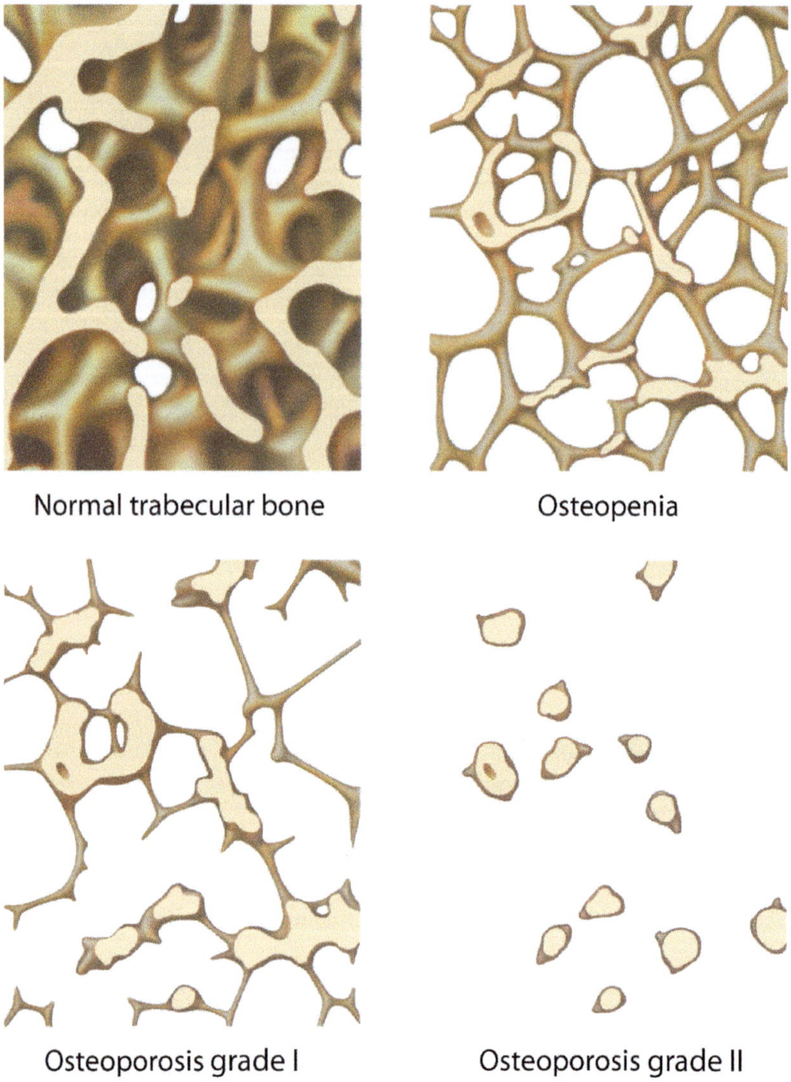

Fig. 19.4 Type and degree of rarefaction of the trabecular bone in patients with established osteopenia/osteoporosis

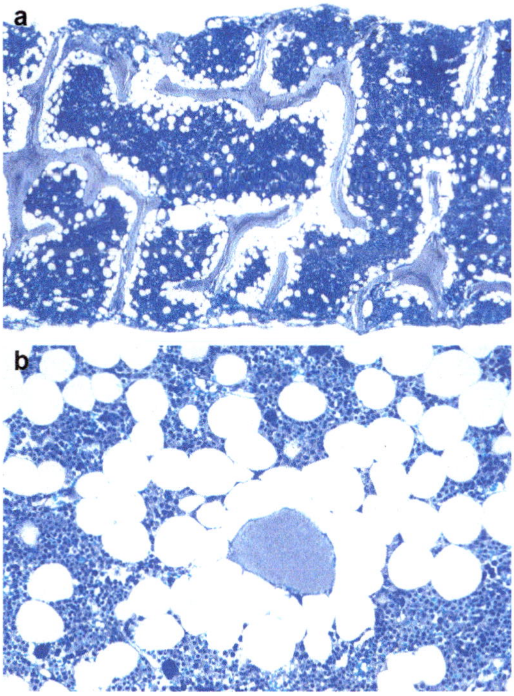

Fig. 19.5 (**a**) Low-turnover osteopenia with paratrabecular localisation of fat cells. (**b**) At higher magnification rim of fat cells around a button-like trabecula. Giemsa staining

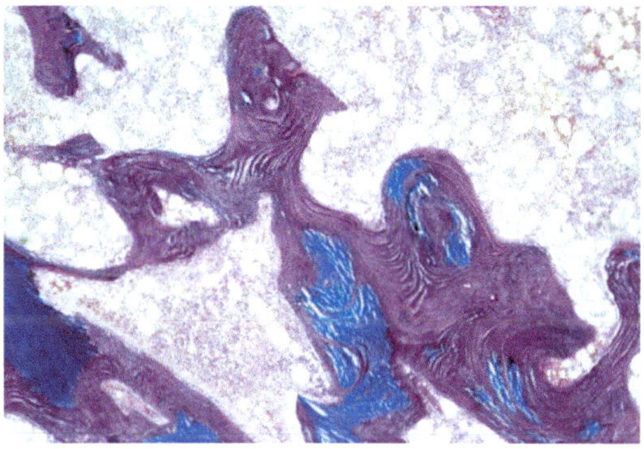

Fig. 19.6 Severe osteomalacia with irregular trabecular structure and increased trabecular volume due to increased amount of osteoid (*red*). Ladewig

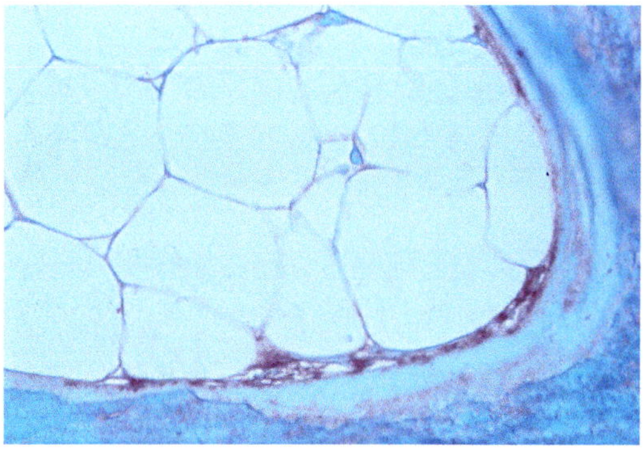

Fig. 19.7 Deposition of bisphosphonate (*red*) on the surface of a trabecula visualised by means of an antibody to ibandronate. Immunohistology

20 Clinical Evaluation of Osteoporosis

Early and correct diagnosis is essential for effective therapy. Reliable information concerning the state of bones is absolutely crucial especially if risk factors are already present. The following key questions must be accurately answered:

- What is the present bone mass (results of recent (and previous) measurements)?
- What is the present rate of bone loss (markers of remodelling in blood and urine)?
- Has physical damage already occurred (evidence of previous fractures on X-rays)?
- Are the changes (if present) reversible?

The aims of clinical investigations are:

- To exclude a disease that can mimic osteoporosis (e.g. osteomalacia, myeloma)
- To elucidate the causes of osteoporosis
- To define the severity and topography of osteoporosis and to determine the risk of subsequent fractures
- To select the most appropriate form of treatment
- To perform the baseline measurements required for the subsequent monitoring of any treatment given.

20.1 Indicative Symptoms

Back pain is one of the most frequent reasons for seeking medical advice, and every case of acute or chronic back pain must be thoroughly investigated. Since osteoporosis may be dormant and symptomless for extended periods, the onset of pain may indicate collapse or fracture of a vertebra. On the other hand, osteomalacia is characterised by widespread, early, systemic and severe bone pain – an important factor in differential diagnosis, which includes numerous other disorders:

- Vertebral diseases: inflammatory, degenerative, myelogenous and neoplastic
- Extravertebral diseases: visceral, neurological, muscular, psychosomatic and neoplastic (e.g. carcinoma of the pancreas)

A detailed *evaluation of back pain* comprises localisation, onset, duration, continuous, intermittent, extent, type, intensity, sensory/motoric disturbances and responsiveness to various stimuli and to drugs. Possible underlying causes include:

- Muscular contractions and tension
- Vertebral collapse
- Protrusion of disc
- Ankylosing spondylitis
- Bone metastases
- Pancreatic tumours
- Myocardial infarction

Clinical history and a careful physical examination (Table 20.1) must include the following:

R. Bartl, C. Bartl, *Bone Disorders*, DOI 10.1007/978-3-319-29182-6_20

- Loss of height
- Posture and bearing
- Pain on percussion of spinal processes
- Mobility of the vertebral column
- Presence of thoracic kyphosis or lumbar scoliosis
- Muscle tone and contractions
- Signs of congenital osteoporosis (e.g. blue sclerae)

Acute back pain in osteoporosis is caused by sudden collapse or fracture of a vertebra. Patients often report having heard a snapping or cracking sound in the back. In contrast chronic pain in osteoporosis is due to inability of the axial skeleton to match up to the demand made on it by muscles, joints and extremities.

> The following questions should be answered to make the most comprehensive diagnosis of the pain syndrome: location, nature, timing, radiation and severity of the pain as well as factors that make the pain worse.

Table 20.1 Medical history and physical examination in osteoporosis

Skeletal history	Fractures, pain, deformity, reduced mobility, height loss
Risk factor assessment	
Family history	Osteoporosis, fractures, renal stones
	Age, ethnicity, weight
Medical history	
Reproductive	Menarche > age 15 years, oligo-/amenorrhoea, menopause
Diseases	Renal, GI, endocrine, rheumatic, neurologic, eating, depression
Surgery	Gastrectomy, organ transplant, intestinal resection or bypass
Drugs	Glucocorticoids, anticonvulsants, cytotoxic agents, heparin, warfarin, GnRH agonists, lithium
Lifestyle and exercise	Smoking, poor nutrition and exercise, alcohol
Diet and supplements	Frequent dieting, calcium, vitamin D, caffeine, protein
Current medications	Hormones, sedatives, hypertensives, diuretics, nonprescription drugs
Physical examination	
Weight loss, diarrhoea	Malabsorption, thyrotoxicosis
Weight gain, hirsutism	Cushing's syndrome
Muscle weakness	Osteomalacia, Cushing's syndrome
Bone pain	Osteomalacia, fracture, malignancy, hyperparathyroidism
Tooth loss	Hypophosphatasia
Joint and lens dislocation	Collagen disorders
Skin pigmentation, stria	Mastocytosis, Cushing's syndrome
Nephrolithiasis	Hypercalciuria, primary hyperparathyroidism

Neurological features such a persistent nerve root pain or spinal cord syndromes are rare. The massive spinal shrinkage in osteoporosis (>4 cm) is mostly a consequence of the collapse of one or more of the thoracic vertebrae, but the distance from foot to hip remains constant. Other reasons for moderate decrease in height are poor posture, disc deterioration and muscle weakness. *Loss of height* can be approximated from the difference between the standing height and the arm span; loss of height occurs only in the spine, with hip-to-heel length remaining constant (Fig. 20.1a). When the height of the lumbar spine is reduced, the ribs may come to rest painfully on the bones of the pelvic girdle. A distinctly longer arm span indicates the degree of vertebral bone damage. Loss of height also entails characteristic folds in the skin of the back (*Christmas tree phenomenon*) as well as a forward bulge of the abdomen (*osteoporosis tummy*). Moreover the decrease in height of the vertebral bodies results in painful contact between the spinal processes (*Baastrup syndrome* or "kissing spine"). The body's centre of gravity is displaced forward, so that movements during walking become slow and unsure, with

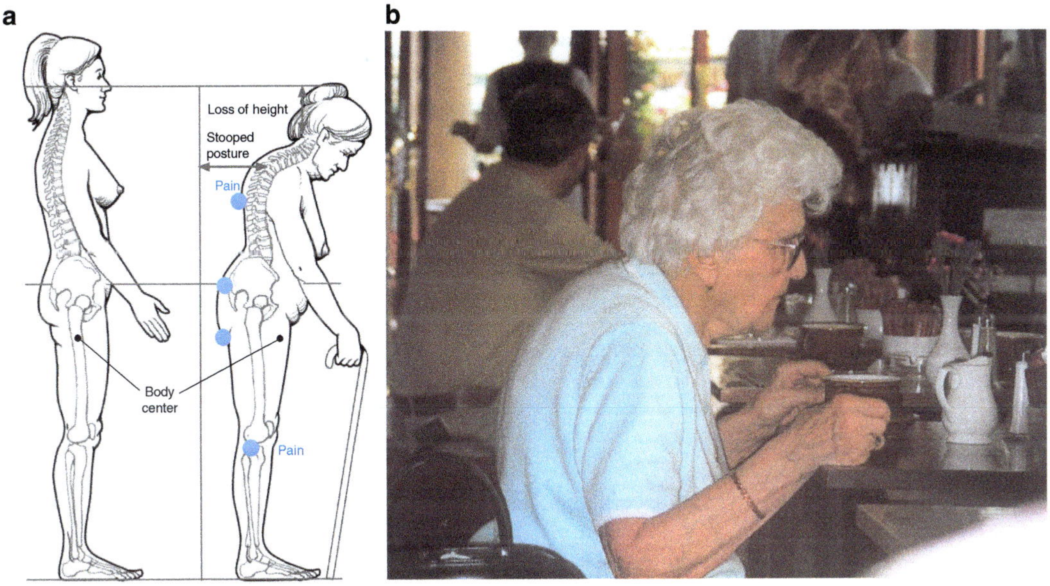

Fig. 20.1 (**a**) Changes in stature and posture due to generalised osteoporosis. (**b**) Typical rounding of the back ("dowager's hump") in a patient with osteoporosis

small steps to avoid transmitting shocks to the vertebral column. The resulting faulty weight-bearing in turn gives rise to arthroses of the knee joints (*gonarthrosis*). Moreover, the unsure gait carries with it an increased risk for falls and fractures. The collapse of the thoracic vertebra produces the typical "round" back (*dowager's hump*) (Fig. 20.1b). A good way to estimate the degree of "hump" is to measure the distance between the back of the head and the wall when the patient is standing straight up against it. When thoracic kyphosis is marked, the thoracic capacity may be reduced which impairs total lung volume, respiratory efficiency and exercise tolerance, and the patient's chin may come to rest on the sternum.

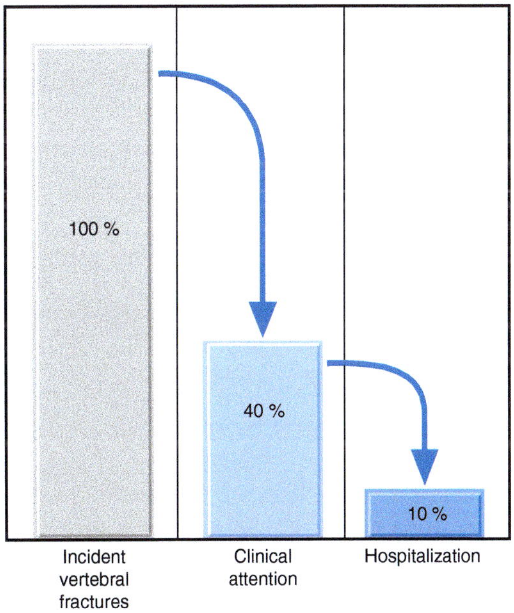

Fig. 20.2 Overall outcome of vertebral fractures (Data from Cooper C, Atkinson E, O'Fallon W et al. (1992)) Incidence of clinically diagnosed vertebral fractures: a population-based study in (Rochester, Minnesota, 1985–1989. J Bone Miner Res 7:221–227)

20.2 Role of Conventional X-Rays in Osteoporosis

Skeletal X-rays indicate bone loss only when the density has been reduced by 30–40 %; therefore, X-rays are not appropriate for early diagnosis. But they are very useful to reveal previous fractures or compressions (Fig. 20.2). The *vertebral bodies* exhibit various changes in shape which occur when the cancellous bone is resorbed while the cortex remains intact. Loss of trabecular bone occurs in a predictable pattern. The non-weight-bearing trabeculae are resorbed first, and therefore the vertebral bodies typically show a rarefication of the horizontal trabeculae accompanied by a relative accentuation of the vertical trabeculae (*verticalisation, vertical striation*) and the presence of reinforcement lines. Furthermore, the cortical rim of the vertebral bodies is accentuated, while the vertebral bodies demonstrate a *picture frame*, *empty box*, *ghost-like* appearance. Another useful criterion is the *ballooning* of the intervertebral spaces, an indication of the incipient compression of the roof and ground plates (biconcavity of the vertebrae). Schmorl's nodes, which are caused by protrusions of the intervertebral disc into the vertebral body, are common in osteoporosis, although not pathognomonic. The *criteria* used to suggest the presence of osteoporosis on lateral X-rays of the spine include:

- Increased radiolucency
- Prominence of vertical trabeculae
- Presence of reinforcement lines
- Thinning of the vertebral endplates
- Presence of compression fractures

Figure 20.3 shows the various types of vertebral deformities in osteoporosis

For a semiquantitative evaluation of vertebral deformities, Genant has published a grading scheme, based on reductions of the anterior, middle or posterior height of vertebral bodies:

- Grade 0: normal
- Grade 1: mild deformity, 20–25 % reduction of any vertebral height
- Grade 2: moderate deformity, 25–40 % reduction of any vertebral height
- Grade 3: severe deformity, >40 % reduction of any vertebral height

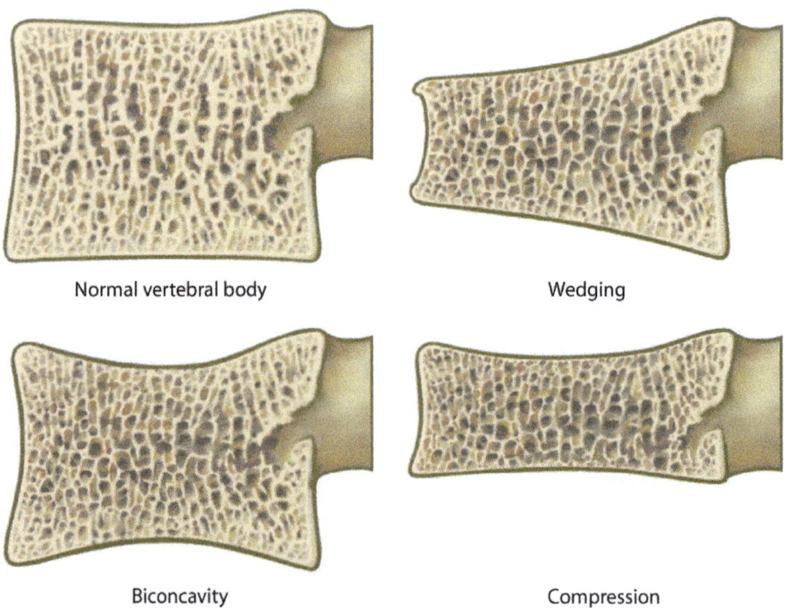

Fig. 20.3 Types of vertebral deformities in osteoporosis: wedge-shaped, biconcave and compressed

20.3 Other Useful Imaging Techniques

Other Parameters of the Proximal Femur The length of the femoral neck (hip axial length) correlates with the fracture risk at this site independently of the cancellous and compact bone of the proximal femur. Each cm increase in length doubles the fracture risk. The following radiological parameters are useful to calculate the fracture risk in the proximal femur:

- Thickness of the medial femoral shaft 3 cm below the trochanter minor
- Thickness of the medial cortex at the centre of the femoral neck
- Femoral head width
- Intertrochanteric region width
- Acetabular bone width

Bone Scan ^{99m}Tc-labelled bisphosphonate is used to detect focal bone lesions and fractures. The whole skeleton can be scanned quickly by this method. Foci of increased uptake in the spine indicate fractures, degenerative, inflammatory or neoplastic lesions. Two days after a fracture, an increased uptake at the site can be expected. However, because of the limited structural details, additional imaging techniques are required for further identification.

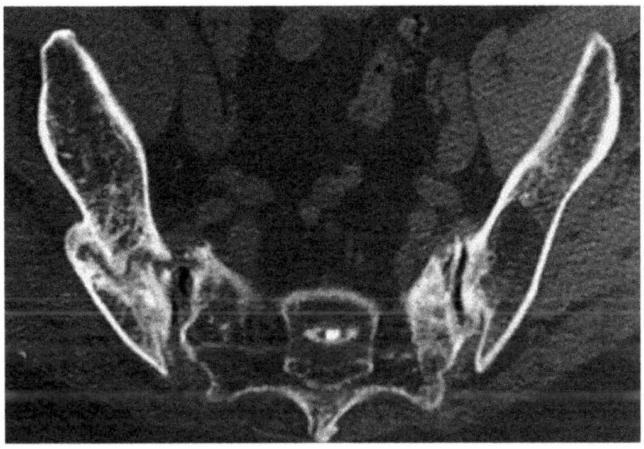

Fig. 20.4 Fractures of the pelvic girdle demonstrated in CT

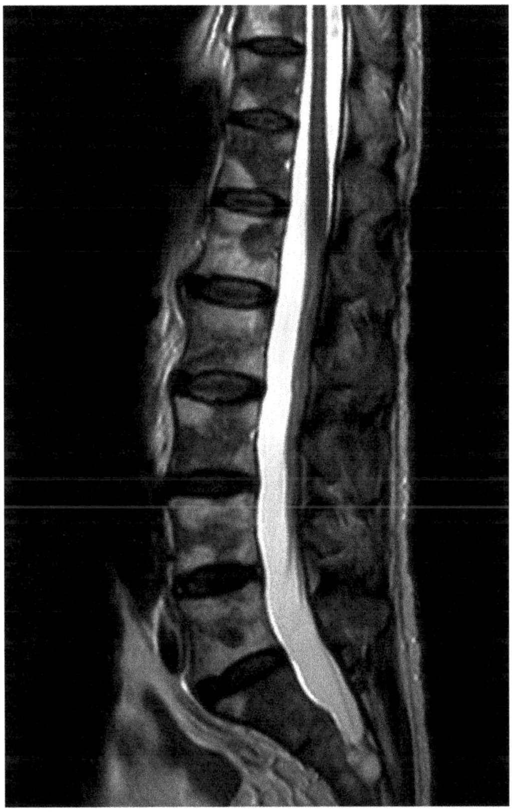

Fig. 20.5 Spondyloarthritis with bone marrow oedema syndrome of the whole spine

Computed Tomography (CT) This technique is particularly useful for analysis of bones and cancellous bone (Fig. 20.4). However, this can only be done with modern high-resolution instruments using sections 0.5 mm thick, together with special picture enhancing facilities, but at the cost of higher exposure to radiation.

Magnetic Resonance Imaging (MRI) This method involves no exposure to radiation and is especially adapted for demonstration of the bone marrow. It offers the possibility of identifying both haematopoietic and fatty bone marrow and inflammatory and neoplastic infiltrates (Figs. 20.5 and 20.6). It is the method of choice for demonstration of myeloma, lymphoma and metastases, as well as localised oedematous processes (transient osteoporosis and early stages of Sudeck's disease). It is the ideal method to distinguish between an osteoporotic fracture and one due to spinal metastases. In addition, the diagnostic

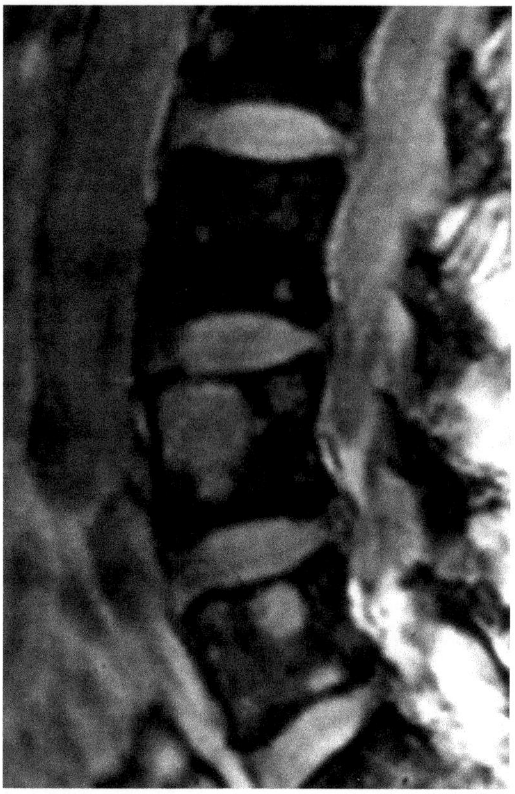

Fig. 20.6 Nodular metastatic process in the spine in a patient with breast cancer and secondary osteoporosis

capability is greatly enhanced by application of special gradient echo sequences and by the use of contrast media.

20.4 Bone Densitometry in Osteoporosis (DXA Method)

The early diagnosis of osteoporosis, before occurrence of fractures, can only be made by means of bone density measurements (bone mineral density tests, BMD) (see Chap. 13). These measure bone density at various skeletal sites and thereby enable a prediction of risk of later fracture. A 10 % decrease in bone density doubles the fracture risk for the vertebral body and trebles it for the hip joint. If a fracture has already occurred, this test is used to confirm the diagnosis of osteoporosis, to determine its degree of severity and to establish the indication for treatment (Fig. 20.7). BMD provides the following information:

- Detects osteopenia and/or osteoporosis before occurrence of a fracture
- Predicts risk for later development of osteoporosis
- Indicates the rate of bone loss – progression – in sequential measurements
- Documents the efficacy or failure of therapy
- Increases compliance of both doctor and patient

Currently, a bone density measurement remains the best and most readily quantifiable method for assessing fracture risk and skeletal response to different treatments. Today *dual energy X-ray absorptiometry* (*DEXA*, *DXA*) is the most completely developed, reliable and popular bone densitometric technique in use, the "gold standard" and the "reference standard". It is versatile and can be used to assess bone mineral content of the whole skeleton as well as of specific sites, especially those most vulnerable to fractures.

Important advantages of DXA are:

- It is not invasive, the patient remains clothed, and it is therefore not a burden to the patient.
- It is very quickly carried out (5–10 min).
- It is cost-effective.
- It has a very low radiation dose (1–3 mRem equivalent to 1/10–1/100th of a normal X-ray film).
- It measures those skeletal areas most vulnerable to osteoporosis and to fractures – the lumbar spine and the hips.
- It has a documented strong gradient of risk for fracture prediction. The risk of hip fracture increases 2.6-fold for each standard deviation decrease in BMD at the femoral neck.
- The measurements are accurate and therefore ideal for follow-up and control investigations (accuracy error 1–10 %, precision 1 %).
- It is recognised by the WHO as the standard method for diagnostic definition of osteoporosis.
- It is recognised by the ESCEO and the IOF as the "reference standard" in the diagnosis of osteoporosis (2008).

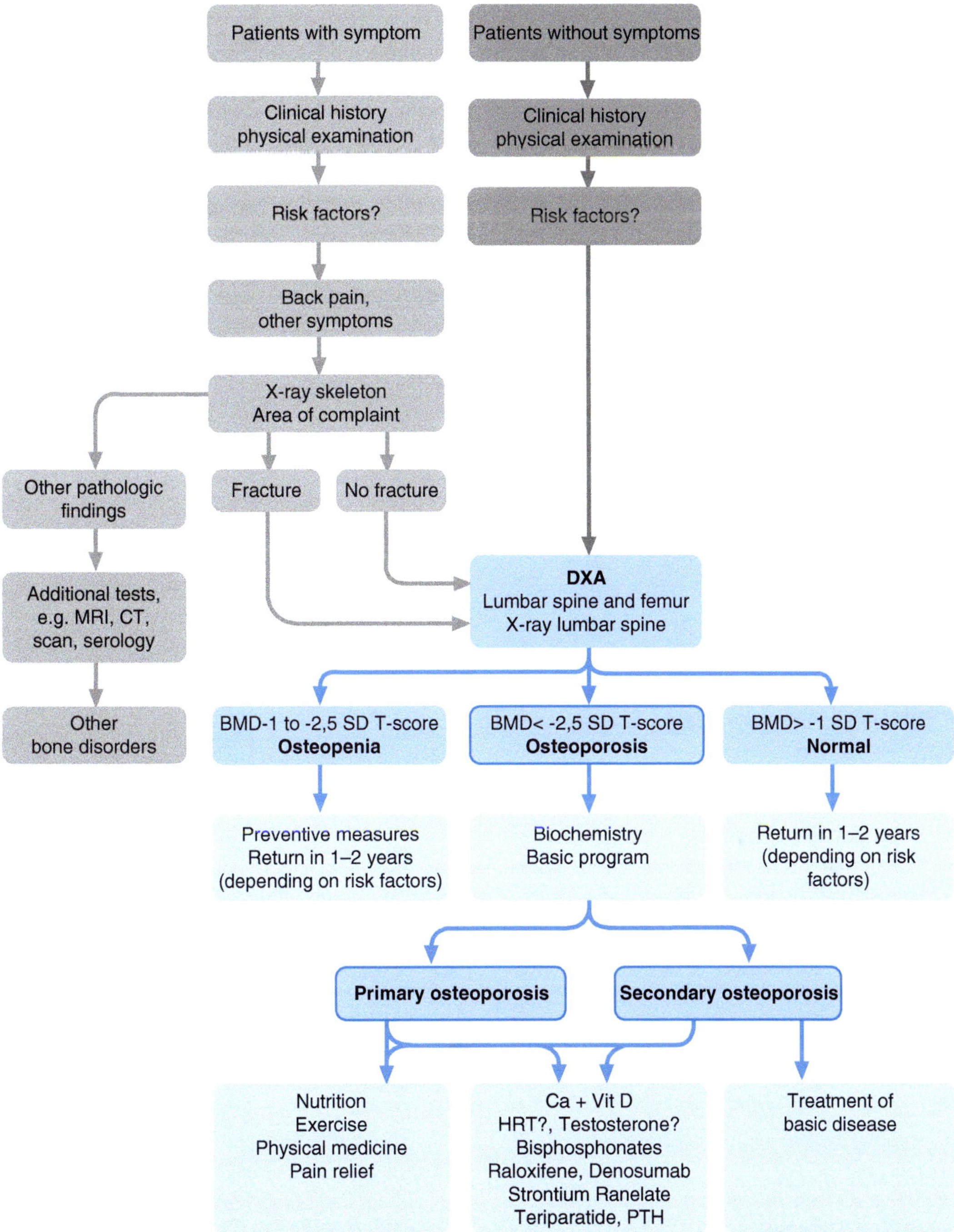

Fig. 20.7 Algorithm for diagnostic investigation and treatment of osteoporosis

Indications for Bone Density Measurements The simplest way to determine who should have a bone density test is to decide in each case whether the results will influence a clinical decision. Any individual with risk factors should have a bone density measurement, for example, a postmenopausal woman who does not take HRT or its equivalent, a woman with early menopause or a woman with a family history of osteoporosis or men with decreased levels of androgens.

According to the National Osteoporosis Foundation (NOF), a BMD measurement is recommended for:

- All women >65 years regardless of additional risk factors
- All women <65 years with one or more risk factors
- All postmenopausal women with fractures
- All women contemplating osteoporosis therapy and whose decision depends on the result of BMD
- All women undergoing protracted hormone therapy

Additional Indications Anyone who has a disease or a condition or is taking certain drugs with the potential to induce bone loss is a candidate for a bone density measurement (DXA preferred)

- Age-related decrease in height
- Back pain of obscure origin
- Slim smokers
- Previous fractures
- Diseases of joints which limit movement
- Long-term use (>6 months) of drugs such as cortisone, warfarin, heparin or antiepileptic drugs
- Hyperthyroidism and hyperparathyroidism
- Post-transplantation, especially of the kidney, liver, heart and lungs
- Chronic diseases and operations which can lead to bone loss, e.g. gastric and intestinal resections
- Anorexia nervosa
- Chronic renal insufficiency
- Neoplasias, pre and post therapy

Measurements in children are problematic for a number of reasons:

- There are inadequate reference data for children.
- There is a broad variability in developmental age at any given chronological age.
- DXA has inherent limitations for paediatric use because of its inability to measure the bone size in three dimensions.

To ameliorate this problem, whole-body bone mineral content (BMC) is sometimes recommended for paediatric measurements. Also, the Z-score rather the T-score is the appropriate criterion for assessing the bone mineral status. BMC is preferable to BMD, because of the problems posed by changing bone size and shape during growth.

Bone density measurement by DEXA is currently the only reliable method to document the effects of therapy on osteoporosis (*monitoring*). Decrease in the incidence of fractures is another. Moreover, annual BMD measurements increase the patient's compliance. Clinical trials have documented significant increases in bone density under therapy with bisphosphonates after 3 months in the vertebrae and 1 year in the hips. Biannual measurements should be carried out in high-risk patients, for example, those on corticoid therapy or patients with rapid bone loss (as indicated by biochemical parameters).

20.5 Recommended Laboratory Tests

The parameters usually tested in blood and urine are within normal limits in primary osteoporosis in the absence of co-morbidities. The significance of laboratory tests therefore lies mainly in recognising secondary osteoporosis (Table 20.2). Consequently the following "basic" laboratory screening tests should be carried out at diagnosis and regularly thereafter:

- Erythrocyte sedimentation rate
- Complete blood count
- Calcium and phosphate (serum)
- Alkaline phosphatase (serum)
- Glucose (serum/urine)
- CRP
- Transaminases and gamma GT (serum)
- Creatinine (serum), GFR

And when the appropriate indications are present:

Table 20.2 Laboratory tests for the evaluation of secondary osteoporoses

Basic tests	Diseases	Additional tests to include
Complete blood count	Malabsorption	PTH, vitamin D, calcium (S)PTH, vitamin D, calcium (S)
		Ferritin, vitamin B12
	Multiple myeloma	Bone marrow biopsy
		Protein electrophoresis (S,U)
	Leukaemia	Blood smear
	Bone metastases	PSA, Ca15-3, CEA
Thyroid-stimulating hormone (TSH)	Hyperthyroidism	Thyroxine (T4), T3
Glucose (S,U)	Diabetes mellitus	Oral glucose tolerance test
Cortisol (S)	Cushing's syndrome	ACTH, dexamethasone test
	Addison's disease	ACTH
HIV-antibody	AIDS	Infection diagnosis
HLA B-27	Ankylosing spondylitis	CRP
Testosterone in men	Hypogonadism	SHBG, LH, FSH, prolactin
Calcium (S)	Hyperparathyroidism	PTH
	Malabsorption	Complete blood count
	Morbus Crohn	PTH, vitamin D
	Celiac disease	Alkaline phosphatase, gliadin
	Osteomalacia	PTH, vitamin D
		Alkaline phosphatase
Alkaline phosphatase	Chronic renal failure	PTH, calcium, phosphate (S)
	Osteomalacia	PTH, vitamin D
		Calcium (S)
Protein electrophoresis	Multiple myeloma	Complete blood count
		Bone marrow biopsy
Liver enzymes	Haemochromatosis	Iron, ferritin (S)
	Alcoholic liver disease	
	Primary biliary cirrhosis	Antibodies
Creatinine	Chronic renal failure	PTH, calcium, phosphate (S)
Histamine 24 h U	Mastocytosis	Bone marrow biopsy

- T3, T4 and TSH
- Oestrogen and/or testosterone levels.
- Vitamin D metabolites.
- Vitamin K has recently been introduced as a new biochemical marker.
- Parathormone (PTH).
- Protein electrophoresis and immuno-electrophoresis.

It is important to note that 20 % of women and up to 64 % of men with osteoporosis also suffer from diseases linked to osteoporosis (co-morbidities), hence the importance of the analyses listed above.

In summary, every patient should be investigated according to the personal risk profile indicated by medical history and lifestyle factors, which determine the appropriate tests and examinations. Subsequent management will depend on the results, i.e. whether or not there is osteopenia/osteoporosis, presence of co-morbidities, current medications, etc.

20.6 Significance of Markers of Bone Turnover

The measurements of collagen metabolism and bone turnover in daily practice are essential for the diagnosis and monitoring of progressive bone diseases such as skeletal metastases or Paget's disease of bone (Table 20.3). However, bone markers cannot be used to diagnose osteoporosis, though they may help to answer some important clinical questions:

- Predicting the future rate of bone loss (high or low bone turnover)
- Predicting the risk of osteoporotic fractures
- Monitoring response to therapy

The metabolites of bone remodelling, i.e. of resorption and formation, as well as the products of bone matrix metabolism such as collagen type 1 pass into the bloodstream and from there into the urine. These products can be identified biochemically, and their levels in blood and urine indicate "high turnover" or "low turnover" osteoporoses.

> It should be noted that bone markers do not replace bone density measurements for the diagnosis of osteoporosis. However, these markers do provide information about the future risk for bone loss and fragility fractures.

Table 20.3 Biochemical markers of bone turnover

Bone resorption	Bone formation
Blood:	*Blood*:
Tartrate-resistant acid phosphatase(TRAP)	Total or bone-specific alkaline phosphatase
Free pyridinoline or deoxypyridinoline	Osteocalcin
N- or C-telopeptide of type I collagen	Procollagen I C-and N-terminal extension peptides
Cross-links	Osteocalcin
Urine:	
Fasting urine calcium-to-creatinine ratio	
Pyridinoline and deoxypyridinoline	
Glycosides of hydroxylysine	
Pyridinoline and desoxypyridinoline	
N- and C-telopeptides of type I collagen	

Changes in bone formation in response to therapy are relatively slow, starting after some weeks and reaching a plateau after several months, in contrast to bone resorption which decreases rapidly a few days after initiation of antiresorptive therapy with, for example, a bisphosphonate and reaches a nadir a few weeks later. These characteristics of bone remodelling must be taken into consideration when evaluating the significance of the levels of markers of bone remodelling in blood and in urine. However, large-scale studies have shown that serial evaluation of markers of bone turnover in the serum do identify people at the highest risk of loss of bone and osteoporosis.

Parameters of bone formation are bone-specific alkaline phosphatase (bone ALP), osteocalcin, and osteonectin. These are produced by osteoblasts (possibly also by endothelial cells), and their levels in the peripheral blood reflect osteoblastic activity. ALP is also produced in various tissues including the liver and kidney; but bone-specific ALP can be distinguished by immunoassays with high specificity. Osteocalcin (OC) shows a diurnal rhythm, and only about 50 % is released into the circulation, while the remaining 50 % is incorporated into hydroxyapatite. OC reflects total bone turnover, i.e. the sum of both resorption and formation. The serum concentrations of the C- and N-terminal propeptides of type I procollagen (PICP and PINC) reflect changes in synthesis of new collagen, produced by osteoblasts in bone and by fibroblasts in other connective tissues. All the PICP and PINC produced are secreted into the circulation.

Parameters of bone resorption consist primarily of collagen degradation products such as "cross-links" which are released into the bloodstream and then excreted into the urine (Fig. 20.8). They appear to predict the risk of hip fracture in elderly women independently of bone density.

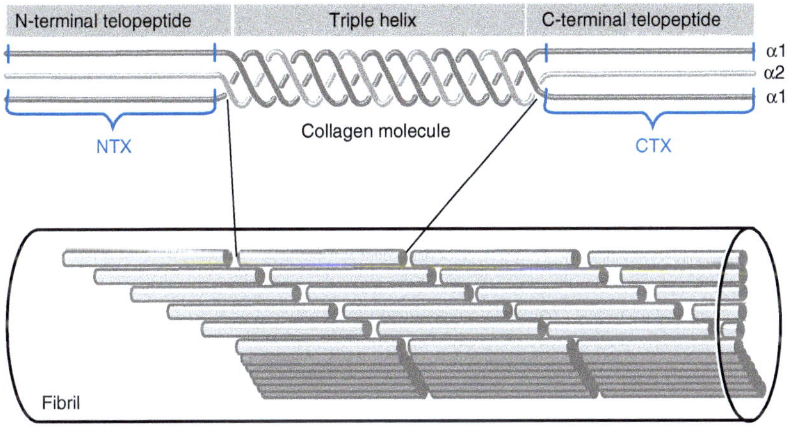

Fig. 20.8 Molecular structure and organisation of collagen into fibrils. Note position of end terminal CTX and NTX, used as biochemical markers of collagen breakdown products in the serum

Studies have shown that women with high levels of markers of bone resorption have about a 1.5–3-fold increased risk of hip or non-vertebral fractures. Desoxypyridinoline and cross-link telopeptides of type I collagen are the two markers of resorption most frequently investigated. Telopeptides are distinguished by their terminals: amino (NTX-OSTEOMARK) and carboxy (CTX-CROSSLAPS). Variations in diurnal rhythm and the effect of meals must be taken into account when results of these tests are evaluated. Both NTX and CTX show a significant response to antiresorptive therapy and are currently considered to be the most reliable parameters of bone resorption. However, serum NTX concentrations are elevated in chronic renal failure, and this must, of course, be taken into account, i.e. by investigation of renal function.

Bone sialoprotein (*BSP*) also appears to be a sensitive marker of bone turnover. Furthermore, BSP is thought to play an important role in attraction and growth of tumour cells in the bone marrow, e.g. in multiple myeloma, and metastases of breast cancer.

Hydroxyproline should no longer be used as a marker of bone metabolism because of its lack of specificity. Its level in the urine is influenced by the breakdown of collagen in sites other than the skeleton, as well as by dietary intake of collagen.

Excretion of *calcium* in a 24 h urinary specimen is also not an accurate reflection of bone resorption, because it depends on the renal threshold for calcium reabsorption and the dietary calcium intake.

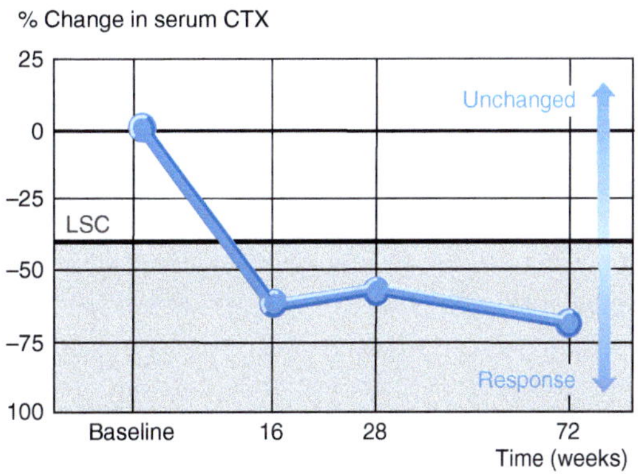

Fig. 20.9 Response of bone markers to antiresorptive agents. A decrease below the least significant change (LSC) is regarded as statistically significant

Results of bone markers before starting a treatment are not useful predictors of response to the treatment. It is also not clear if patients with high bone turnover are more likely to gain bone under therapy. Some studies have demonstrated that patients with the largest decreases in markers of bone resorption during treatment with alendronate tend to have the greatest increases in BMD. Nevertheless, changes in markers during treatment must be interpreted with caution. The results of each patient must be compared with the *least significant change* (LSC) (Fig. 20.9). The

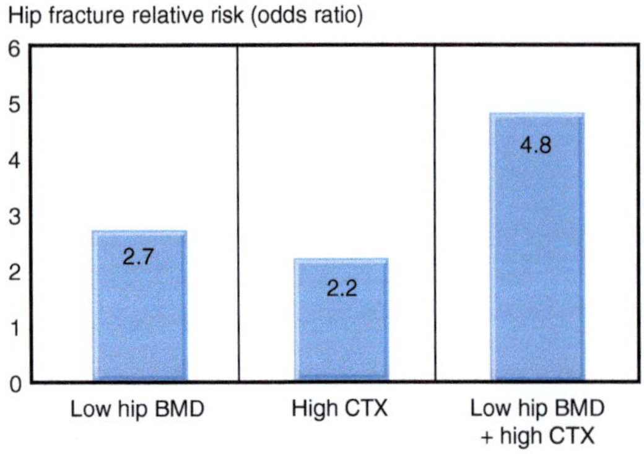

Fig. 20.10 The combination of a low hip BMD and a high serum CTX have a greater predictive value than either low hip BMD or high serum CTX alone (Modified from Garnero et al. 1996)

LSC is the minimum change that must be seen in an individual patient to be at least 95 % sure that the change is "real" and not caused by biological or laboratory variations. The LSC is about 25 % for most formation markers and 40–65 % for most resorption markers. About 65 % of patients treated with oestrogen or bisphosphonates have changes in bone resorption markers that are greater than the LSC. In contrast, raloxifene and calcitonin are associated with smaller changes in these markers. However, patients may benefit from a decrease in risk of fractures even if they do not have reductions in bone markers or improvements in bone density. In these cases with little or no change while on antiresorptive medication, it is important to check carefully:

- If the patient is taking the medication
- If the patient is taking the drug as prescribed
- If there are secondary causes of osteoporosis

The advantage of monitoring treatment with markers is that changes in levels can be observed within weeks of starting therapy, and evidence of its efficacy is psychologically important at a time when patients are most likely to discontinue their medications (Fig. 20.10). It is necessary to emphasise that the specimens for investigation should always be taken at about the same time of day and with the patient fasting. Furthermore, indices of bone turnover may show seasonal and circadian variations.

Recommendations for practical use of bone markers:

When using bone markers, one should keep in mind that:

- They are not unique to bone.
- They may reflect both formation and resorption.
- They are influenced also by nonskeletal diseases.

When using bone markers in the monitoring of antiresorptive therapy:

- Always compare the same marker.
- Use only markers validated for assessing bone resorption/formation.
- Collect the samples at the same time (8.00–10.00), if necessary after an overnight fast.
- Keep reasonable intervals between the controls (about 3–6 months).
- Use cut-off values to identify responders (–30 % for urinary DPD, –65 % for urinary NTX and CTX, –40 % for serum bone-specific AP).

Part V

Risk Factors and Prevention of Osteoporosis

21 Risk Factors for Osteoporosis and Fractures

Until recently, the diagnosis of osteoporosis was made only when the patient presented with painful fractures. Today, with a greater consciousness of health and healthy living, we realise that recognition and avoidance of risk factors can prevent many chronic illnesses. A 50-year-old postmenopausal woman who goes to her physician for a yearly "check-up" expects to have her blood pressure taken, her cholesterol measured and a mammography performed – that is good medical practice. Likewise, she should ask for a bone mineral density measurement to investigate her risk for developing osteoporosis (Fig. 21.1). Results of studies even suggest that low bone mass density is a better predictor of fracture risk than increased cholesterol is of having a heart attack and high blood pressure of having a stroke (Fig. 21.2). We are now aware of many genetic and acquired factors which are responsible for and/or contribute to the development of osteoporoses. Furthermore, a low bone mineral density is associated with a lower risk of breast cancer: stimulating effects of oestrogen on both trabecular bone and mammary cells may be responsible for this correlation. Another study has shown that bone density changes might be related to the progression of atherosclerosis, or vice versa, in haemodialysis patients.

21.1 Risk Factors Which Cannot (yet) Be Influenced

Genetics The saying "as mother so daughter" applies especially to osteoporosis. A family history of an osteoporotic fracture in a first-degree relative is a powerful indicator that genetic factors may play a role in the development of osteoporosis. We know that the "peak bone mass" and the subsequent later loss of bone are genetically programmed. Studies of twins have shown that genetic factors account for up to 80 % of the variance in bone mineral density, the best known predictor of the risk of osteoporosis.

A heritable component has been found in the determination of peak bone mass, femoral neck geometry, markers of bone turnover, age of menopause and muscle strength, all of which contribute to osteoporotic fracture.

Some loci such as for vitamin D and oestrogen receptor genes as well as the collagen type Iα1 locus are promising genetic determinants of bone

R. Bartl, C. Bartl, *Bone Disorders*, DOI 10.1007/978-3-319-29182-6_21

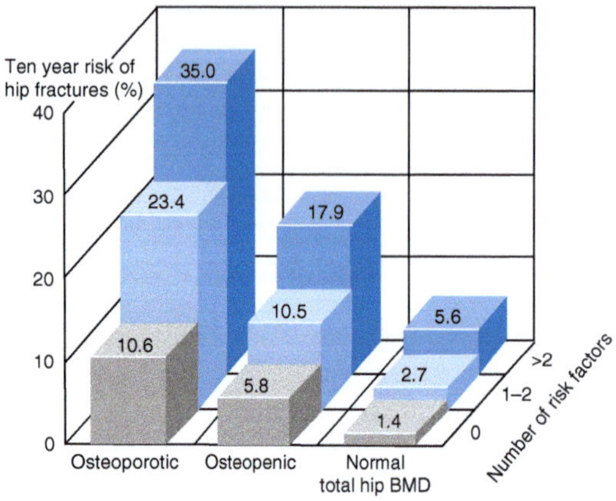

Fig. 21.1 Ten-year risk of hip fractures relative to the total hip BMD (normal, osteopenic and osteoporotic) and to the number of risk factors (Modified from Taylor B et al. 2004)

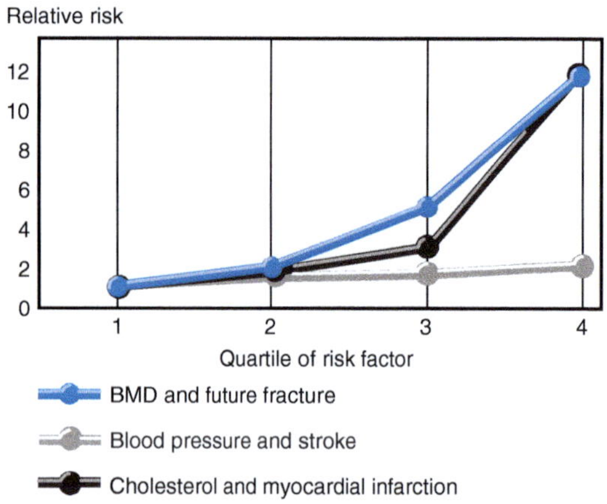

Fig. 21.2 Risk factors for three selected chronic disorders

Table 21.1 Genetic syndromes featuring osteoporosis

Syndrome	Clinical features
Turner (XO)	Short stature, primary amenorrhoea
Klinefelter (XXY)	Tall stature, gynecoid features
Osteogenesis imperfecta	Blue sclerae, dental abnormalities
Ehlers-Danlos	Joint hypermobility, dislocations
Cutis laxa	Lax skin, premature-aged appearance
Marfan	Tall stature, lens dislocation, aortic root dilation
	"Floppy valve syndrome"
Homocystinuria	Tall stature, thrombosis, lens dislocation
Cleidocranial dysplasia	Sloped shoulders, dental abnormalities
Osteoporosis-pseudoglioma	Poor vision, early fractures
Werner	Short stature, premature ageing
Hereditary sensory neuropathies	Insensitivity to pain

mass, but the molecular basis of osteoporosis still remains largely undefined. Experts have also implicated gene-gene and gene-environment interactions as significant determinants of bone density and risk of osteoporosis. As yet there are no tests available to evaluate the genetic risk of osteoporosis. Nevertheless, a proper diet and exercise in childhood and youth can go a long way to ensure a peak bone mass in adulthood. Part of the heterogeneity of osteoporosis may be due to the presence of osteoporosis in a number of genetic syndromes ("syndromic osteoporosis") or as a consequence of a congenital syndrome, such as Down's, in which skeletal changes including a low bone mass already occur in childhood. Information derived from genetic studies is being used to developed markers for assessment of fracture risk and new drugs for osteoporosis. Genetic syndromes causing osteoporosis can be distinguished by careful physical examination (e.g. stature, as well as abnormalities of the teeth, skin and eyes). These features are common to a number of the syndromes listed in Table 21.1. Although there is a genetic component to osteoporotic fractures, it is much smaller than that of BMD. As fracture is the end result of a number of factors including BMD, bone turnover, body size and shape, muscle function and the risk of falling, all of which are all controlled by different genetic pathways, it is difficult to disentangle the underlying genetics of fracture. However, genetics also influence other aspects of the metabolism of the bones such as the PTH signalling pathways, by way of single nucleotide polymorphisms (SNPs) and various haplotypes, some of which are associated with risk of fractures, independently of BMD in certain populations.

Many factors control the development and growth of the bones, including the deposition, accrual and retention of mineral in bone from the embryonic stage onwards throughout life. Numerous epidemiological studies, published towards the end of the last century, demonstrated a relationship between weight and length at birth and during infancy, with the bone mass, stature and height at adulthood. It soon became evident that heredity, i.e. genes, contributes to control of physical traits such as bone mass and density, height and obesity, and this realisation has stimulated a massive increase in research into the genes involved in these processes. It has been estimated that about 60–70 % of the variability in bone mineral mass or density (BMD) is due to genetic variation, while other environmental factors account for the remaining 30–40 % of the phenotypical variation. Another hereditary factor, more strongly expressed in female than in male offspring, is paternal skeletal size. At the biochemical level, a cohort study of 966 men and women provided evidence of an interaction between a single nucleotide polymorphism (SNP) in the calcium-sensing receptor gene (CASR) and birth weight and in the determination of bone mass in a female population. Correlations between the growth hormone gene, weight in infancy and adult bone mass have also been described. Numerous studies, and from various aspects, have addressed the question of bone growth in infancy and childhood and its effects on peak bone mass, on bone strength and on fracture risk later in life. To date, up until now in the first decade of the new millennium, many large-scale studies have been published on the genetics of both physiological and pathological aspects of skeletal development, modelling and growth as well as on remodelling, repair and maintenance of the bones. In addition, linkages between mechanisms controlling metabolism of bone and a variety of chronic disorders prevalent in adulthood and in the elderly have also been elucidated, particularly with respect to osteoporosis. Polymorphisms have been identified in many genes active in different aspects of osseous metabolism and their associations with osteoporosis clarified. Moreover, identification of specific genetic loci, for example, loci connected to height, has revealed new biological pathways in human growth, and these could well indicate targets for the design of future drug therapies.

Additional large-scale analyses have now been reported on the effects on osteoporosis of the association of *genomic polymorphisms and other factors* in osseous metabolism. Examples include polymorphisms of the oestrogen receptor ESR1, vitamin D receptor variations and polymorphisms in the transforming growth factor B1 gene and in the LRP5 and LRP6. Today, one novel aspect of genetics is the ongoing investigation of genes in so-called causation, i.e. the relationships of genotypes to phenotypes, which are extremely complicated and conclusive observations are awaited.

> A substantial number of genes involved in osteoporosis are known influencing three biological pathways: the oestrogen pathway, the Wnt-β-catenin signalling pathway and the RANKL-RANK-OPG pathway.

In addition, the patient's family history must also be taken into account, since it has been shown that family history is an important risk factor for osteoporosis in women in the USA. Patients with developmental difficulties, congenital or acquired, are also liable to osteoporosis and fragility fractures. The passage of time sets in motion many processes such as mitochondrial dysfunction and apoptosis which, in various organs and tissues, gradually lead to reduction in mass as in the skeletal muscles: *sarcopenia*. This in turn leads to a decrease in BMD. It has been postulated that the detection of sarcopenia at the time of the DXA could be used as a screening test for women who require special exercises to restore the muscles and the BMD values. Another age-related process that induces changes in bone cells and thereby promotes osteoporosis is *telomere shortening* with replicative ageing of osteoblast precursors:

Race Caucasians tend to have the lowest bone mass, and hip fractures are far more common among whites than non-whites. Age-adjusted hip fracture incidence rates are higher among Scandinavian residents than other comparable populations. Afro-American women tend to have the highest bone density and lose bone less rapidly as they age.

Gender Women have a greater risk for most fractures than men. In general, the rate of spine and hip fractures in women is two or three times greater than in men. These sex-related differences in osteoporosis-associated fractures have been attributed to higher bone mineral density in men than in women, to differences in body size, bone size and width, while differences in geometry of the bones and in (possibly accumulated) microarchitectural damage may also contribute. In addition, male and female hormones may differentially alter the mechanostat set points, by which bone tissue is added to a particular location when and where it is mechanically needed.

Age Between 30 and 35 years of age osseous remodelling, i.e. resorption and formation are balanced. Thereafter the genetically determined loss of bone sets in, somewhat greater in women than in men, at a rate of approximately 0.5–1 % per year after the age of 30. With onset of the menopause and the drop in oestrogen secretion, the rate of osteoporosis and of fractures in women increases steadily (Fig. 21.3). Early menopause is also an important risk factor for osteoporosis. Moreover, it is worth remembering that now that HRT is no longer acceptable, most of these women are subject to other hormone-dependent conditions, affecting their general health and the bones. In men the risk of fractures increases steadily with the decline in testosterone secretion from about 60 years onwards. The risk increases even more with each decade of increasing age. The elderly also have an increased tendency to fall: one third of individuals over 65 years of age will fall at least once a year. About 6 % of falls for individuals over age 75 result in a fracture. Additional risks for developing osteoporosis are due to:

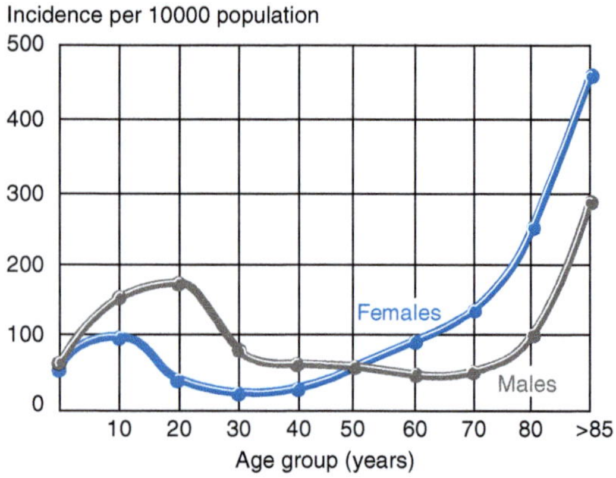

Fig. 21.3 Incidence of fractures according to sex and age. Notice the time lag of about 10 years in elderly men

- Increasing occurrence of co-morbidities together with the necessity of taking various medications,
- Deficiencies of calcium and vitamin D
- Decrease in physical activities that possibly potentiate the age-related decrease in muscle mass, i.e. sarcopenia
- Unbalanced osseous remodelling because of the decline in osteoblastic activity

Height and Weight Women with hip fractures have been reported to be taller than those without, whereas there was no effect of height on male hip fractures. Clearly, body weight and BMI are positively related to BMD and inversely related to osteoporosis and fracture rates. Investigations have demonstrated that low body weight and BMI are predictive of low BMD and increased fracture risk in women aged 40–59 years. It should be stressed that the maintenance of an appropriate weight is an important factor for the prevention of osteoporosis. Obese persons need to lose weight to reduce the risk of co-morbid conditions. However, clinicians must be aware of the fact that marked weight loss can be detrimental to bone in the absence of appropriate precautionary measures. In addition, it is very important to take into account that osteoporosis in obese postmenopausal women is almost invariably associated with co-morbidities that may affect the bones. Moreover, there is a high prevalence of micronutrient deficiency (vitamin D included!) in morbidly obese people for which they should be checked and treated, also prior to and after bariatric surgery to avoid insufficiencies due to possible postoperative complications such as inadequate diet and malabsorption, including that of calcium and vitamin D.

Previous Fractures Even if the cause is unknown, the risk of sustaining another fracture is doubled when one has already occurred. Possibly individuals with one fracture tend to fall and develop subsequent fractures at a greater rate than individuals with no history of fractures. It has been estimated that a single spontaneous vertebral fracture raises the risk of further vertebral fractures by five, while two or more fractures increase the risk by a factor of 12.

Family History It has transpired from the comprehensive data on the patients and their relatives, taken for the many trials on osteoporotic fractures, and which have now accumulated, that the family history is also a significant and independent risk factor for osteoporosis.

Pregnancy and Lactation A woman nursing a baby secretes about 500 mg calcium daily into the milk. After nursing five babies, she will have secreted some 300 g of calcium – about a third of the amount of bound calcium incorporated in the bone. To some extent, the high levels of sex hormones during pregnancy stimulate a greater absorption of calcium from the gastrointestinal tract and a greater uptake by the bones. However, there are additional risks for osteoporosis when several weeks' bed rest is required and also if muscle relaxants and sedation are administered during pregnancy. In some cases corticosteroids are also given. In these circumstances, a massive excretion of calcium and loss of bone are the inevitable result, and the pregnant women must be given calcium and vitamin D to compensate for the loss. In general, there is a decrease in bone density during pregnancy and breast-feeding, but the bone density is restored to normal after birth and weaning. Only a few women suffer fractures during this temporary decrease in bone mass, mainly due to nutritional inadequacies.

21.2 Risk Factors Which *Can* Be Influenced

Chronic Inactivity Insufficient physical movement is the single most important risk factor for osteoporosis. This applies also to younger, bedridden patients who may lose up to 30 % of their bone mass in a few months, but may require years to regain their original bone density. When an arm is immobilised in plaster for 3 weeks because of a wrist fracture, the bones involved lose 6 % of their density. A study of patients restricted to bed rest showed that trabecular bone was lost at the rate of about 1 % per week! It has been suggested that trabecular bone increases at about 1 % per month, so that restoration of bone mass is much slower than bone loss.

Examples of immobilisation with rapid bone loss are:

- Paralysis after spinal injuries
- Hemiplegia after cerebrovascular events
- Paraplegia of the lower half of the body
- Immobilisation after fractures of the lower extremities at any age
- Weightlessness in astronauts

Patients with osteoporosis who are confined to several weeks' bed rest after a fracture frequently sustain more fractures during the subsequent period of mobilisation. A prolonged period of postoperative bed rest should therefore be avoided by implementation of new surgical techniques, early mobilisation and the bones protected by administration of the appropriate drugs readily available today (e.g. aminobisphosphonates). In addition, there is a close relationship between muscle and bone mass. Moreover, with advancing age, many diseases could be avoided or at least positively influenced by regular exercise and physical activity. It is regrettable that the conveniences of civilisation are exploited at the cost of our bones and that we play a dangerous game in ignoring the increasing trends towards physical inactivity in our children, as witnessed by the well-nigh global epidemic of juvenile obesity!

Microgravity Healthy astronauts must perform special exercises before and while they are in outer space, because of the lack of gravity. Nevertheless, they lose about 1 % of their bone mass every month. Under spaceflight conditions, astronauts experience a loss in bone density at a rate up to ten times faster than that of earthbound patients with osteoporosis. Experimental studies have shown that weightlessness induces osteocytic apoptosis, and this in turn attracts osteoclasts to the vicinity and thus initiates resorption. The decrease in bone during space flight has been extensively studied and used a model for the decrease in BMD in osteoporosis on earth, for example, immobilisation due to fractures or paralysis and bone loss due to decline in hormones in the menopause, the andropause, and in involutional osteoporosis. Two mechanisms observed in spaceflight under microgravity, i.e. the demineralisation of bone and the inhibition of osteoblasts, also characterise bone loss here on earth.

Excessive Sport Female athletes in particular are liable to osteoporosis later in life. Constant and lengthy training and strict control of diet and weight both lead to an extreme reduction in body fat and a drop in levels of oestrogen, so that menstrual periods become irregular or cease altogether; consequently, the risk of fractures is clearly increased.

Low Body Weight (Low Body Mass Index) "Slim women, thin bones" – all large studies of risk factors for osteoporosis have confirmed this saying. Underweight women have a high risk of fractures, while overweight women are rarely affected by osteoporosis. This is because the increased weight strengthens the bones, while the oestrogen metabolites produced by the fat cells further protect the bones from osteoporosis. After the menopause, the hormones produced by the adrenal cortex – androstenedione, for example – are metabolised by the fat cells by means of their aromatases and converted to bone-protecting oestrogen. On the negative side however, overweight has deleterious consequences such as deformities of the vertebrae and "wear and tear" of the joints especially the knees and ankles. Low body weight with its decrease in bone density and increase in fracture risk affects both men and women equally. For decades, our society has broadcast the message to women that to be thin is attractive, beautiful and desirable. Embroiled in this "thinness mania", millions of women still persist in following misguided attempts at attaining and maintaining thinness, at the cost of their bones. It is impossible to consume adequate amounts of the nutrients required for bone growth and bone maintenance on a low-calorie diet alone. Patients with anorexia nervosa are particularly prone to the development of osteoporosis. In some countries 1–3 % of women are subject to eating disorders, the consequences of which include osteoporosis. There are several potential mechanisms to explain the increased fracture risk in individuals with low body weight:

- Decreased mechanical loading of the bone
- Hypogonadism
- Reduced production of oestrogen by fat cells (adipocytes)
- Low insulin and IGF-I levels
- Less impact-absorbing fatty padding over the greater trochanter (hip fracture)

Obesity It was previously believed that obesity and osteoporosis were two unrelated diseases, but recent studies have shown that both diseases share several common genetic and environmental factors. Normal ageing is associated with both a high incidence of osteoporosis and with bone marrow atrophy, i.e. reduction in haematopoietic tissue and a corresponding increase in fat cells (adipocytes). Bone remodelling and adiposity are both regulated via the hypothalamus and the sympathetic nervous system, and adipocytes and osteoblasts derive from a common mesenchymal precursor cell. But, based on the present state of knowledge, it is still unclear whether the fatty tissue has beneficial effects on bone. However, relationships have already been demonstrated between adiposity and adipocyte dysfunction and adverse effects on many systems, which in turn can also adversely affect the bones. Obesity is also closely related to insulin and diabetes, which in turn are part and parcel of the metabolic syndrome which also affects the metabolism of bone. The increased risk of osteoporosis posed by morbid obesity has now been demonstrated by the results of measurements of BMD, BMI and other parameters, such as bone turnover markers, taken before and after bariatric surgery. Risk factors for osteoporosis, if not already present, are increased after bariatric surgery, due to various factors including difficulties with nutrition, absorption and periods of decreased physical activity. A comprehensive programme for a change in lifestyle is required, including nutrition, physical exercise and appropriate medication, possibly i.v. bisphosphonates to avoid gastrointestinal problems and vitamin supplements as required.

From a practical point of view, the adverse metabolic consequences of obesity can best be avoided, or managed if already present, by scrupulous attention to lifestyle factors! And, as recently pointed out, not only during the work days of the week, but especially during the weekends, the temptation to indulge must be resisted!

Low Lifelong Calcium Intake The average adult ingests about 500 mg calcium daily. If there is a decreased calcium intake over years, increased parathyroid hormone levels stimulate bone to release calcium from its stores, and this causes osteoporosis. The greater the calcium intake in childhood and adolescent years, the higher the peak bone mass, and this makes the bone less susceptible to fracture with normal ageing in women as well as in men.

State of Depression Depression by itself is most probably not a main cause of osteoporosis, but the accompanying circumstances are. Studies have shown that women with severe long-standing depression have 6 % less bone mass than matched controls without depression. The main contributory factors linking depression, low BMD and fracture risk are:

- High levels of stress hormones
- Low levels of gonadal steroids
- Various antidepressant drugs
- Lack of appetite and inadequate nutrition
- Increased alcohol abuse
- Co-morbid medical conditions
- Most importantly reduced physical activity
- Lack of motivation

Cigarette Smoking: The "Bone Terrorist Number One" Cigarette smoking has a negative influence on BMD independent of differences in weight and physical activity. Smoking doubles the risk of osteoporosis and therefore constitutes an important risk factor. Women who smoke one pack a day during adulthood have 5–10 % less BMD at the age of menopause than do non-smokers. Swedish studies report that the BMD of a 70-year-old woman who smokes is equivalent to an 80-year-old non-smoker. According to the results of recent studies, it is estimated that smoking increases the lifetime risk of vertebral fractures by 13 % in women and 32 % in men. The figures for hip fractures are 31 % for women and 40 % for men. It is suggested that 10–20 % of all hip fractures in women are attributable to smoking. The exact mechanism is not known, probably various chemical substances in the cigarette smoke are responsible. Nicotine inhibits oestrogen secretion, stimulates oestrogen breakdown in the liver and accelerates onset of menopause. Smoking also depletes the body of certain nutrients such as vitamin C, which are essential for bone building. Smoking seems to impair the bone-protective effects of nutritional calcium in postmenopausal women, more clearly in the lumbar spine than in the femoral neck. In addition, smoking increases the body's toxic burden of cadmium, lead and many other toxic substances which interfere with calcium absorption and mineralisation. It has been demonstrated that smoking impairs the protective effects of nutritional calcium on bone. Finally, smoking also inhibits osteoblasts and diminishes blood circulation in bone. Cigarette smokers also tend to be thinner than their non-smoking counterparts, which may play a role as well. No BMD differences were found between former and never-smokers. Reducing current smoking would help prevent many fractures, including hip and spine fractures, and may also improve the healing of fractures.

Excessive Alcohol Intake Many physicians believe that alcohol intake is bad for bone. However, studies have shown that modest intake is associated with increased estradiol concentration and therefore with higher bone density and a lower risk of fractures. Consequently, there is no reason to advise individuals who drink alcohol in moderate amounts to stop for reasons of preventing osteoporosis. However, no study published so far has given the definition of "moderate amounts" in measured quantities of alcohol; the amount is usually given as "1/2–1.0 drinks per day". Genuine alcoholism, however, increases the risk of osteoporosis and of fractures and substantially delays the healing of fractures. But, in assessment of patients with chronic alcoholism, it should be noted that decisive factors are the accompanying poor nutrition, lower weight, hepatic damage, lower calcium absorption and decreased levels of oestrogen. Chronic alcoholism induces cardio -, hepato- and splenomegaly which contribute to the adverse consequences and poorer outcome of patients with chronic alcoholism. Chronic alcoholism may be five to ten times more frequent among patients with fractures than among those without fractures. The negative effects of excessive alcohol on bone are seen in women as well as in men.

Excessive Lipid Intake Hyperlipidaemia and an increased susceptibility to lipid oxidation may also constitute risk factors for osteoporosis. In addition, dietary lipids have now been implicated in calcium exclusion, fatty acid metabolism and osteoblast function.

Nutritional Deficiency Nutrition is an essential factor in the maintenance of bone health, and the following factors are known to be important:

- Minerals: calcium, phosphorus, magnesium, zinc, manganese, copper, boron and silica
- Vitamins: D, C, K, B_6, B_{12} and folic acid
- Proteins
- Essential fatty acids

A number of articles published since 2008 have stated clearly that hypovitaminosis D is widespread, regardless of geographic location. The far-reaching consequences include osteoporosis, falls, altered glucose and lipid metabolism and increased risk of cancer on an international scale.

We frequently underconsume most of these key bone-building nutrients. In a recent survey, not a single person consumed 100 % of the recommended daily allowance (RDA) for the nutrients listed above. As mentioned previously, when insufficient calcium is absorbed from food, it is mobilised from the bones by parathyroid hormones, causing a negative bone balance with respect to remodelling (i.e. more resorption than formation). In childhood, youth and pregnancy, it is particularly important to meet the needs of the growing bones by strict attention to appropriate nutrition. On the other hand, too much of certain substances should also be avoided; to give but one example: daily consumption of chocolate by 70–85-year-old women resulted in a reduction in BMD and in bone strength.

Hormones For women, an early menopause (natural or surgical) is an important risk factor. Likewise insufficient *testosterone* in men also leads to osteoporosis. Moreover, alcoholism and anorexia nervosa can both contribute to testosterone deficiency. Therefore, testosterone levels in the serum should always be investigated in young men with osteoporosis of unknown aetiology to detect hypogonadism or testosterone deficiency. Oral *contraceptives* contain a combination of oestrogen and progesterone, and both may increase bone mass. Indeed there is some evidence that women who have used birth control pills for a long time have stronger bones than those who have not. Oral contraceptives may especially protect some women athletes against the risk of stress fractures.

Medications Many drugs weaken the bones, and the most important are *cortisone* and its derivates, the glucocorticoids. These are used systemically in many diseases: bronchial asthma; allergies; rheumatic, haematologic, intestinal and immunologic diseases; and after transplantations. Adult and elderly patients with co-morbidities are very likely to be at risk for medication-induced osteoporosis. Patients who are treated with cortisone (or its derivates) for more than a year develop osteoporosis with a high risk of fractures. There is another long list of medications which weaken the bones on long-term use including lithium; isoniazid, carbamazepine and other antiepileptic drugs; heparin, warfarin and other anticoagulants; antacids containing aluminium; and in particular immunosuppressive drugs such as cyclosporine A. However, thyroid hormone when given in daily doses of 75–125 μg probably does not harm the bones. Warfarin competitively inhibits vitamin K, but concern about osteoporosis should not deter use of anticoagulants for prevention of thromboembolic disorders. In contrast, thiazide diuretics and beta-blockers, however, both appear to exert some skeletal benefit as indicated by higher BMD values, less bone loss and lower fracture rates. A recent study has demonstrated that the use of ß-blockers is associated with a reduced risk of fracture in middle-aged and older subjects. It should also be noted that occasionally therapy of comorbidity has a beneficial effect on bone, as observed in patients treated with ultraviolet light B for psoriasis. On the other hand, patients treated with radiotherapy localised to one particular site in the body may develop osteoporosis in adjoining skeletal areas.

Homocysteine Increased plasma homocysteine levels have been suggested as an independent risk factor for osteoporosis, bone loss and fragility fractures, perhaps by interfering with collagen cross-linking and stimulating osteoclast activity. Although some of the risk may be related to low serum levels of folate and vitamin B12, it is now acceptable to consider an elevated level of homocysteine as a marker of elevated fracture risk.

Imbalance, Tendency to Fall and Obstacles Almost a third of elderly people fall at least once a year, but only 10 % break a bone. Obviously, in addition to the degree of severity of osteoporosis, the type of fall also determines whether or not a fracture is likely to occur. Protective reflexes – such as stretching out the arms to break a fall – are reduced in older people who also have less energy absorbing soft tissue around the hip joints, resulting in an increased tendency to break the hip bone on falling. Similar considerations apply to lateral or forward falls. Moreover, cognitive or visual impairment, dizziness and syncopal events and various rheumatic disorders may further diminish the capacity to prevent and or to mitigate a fall. A very simple test can be used to evaluate a patient's coordination and thereby the risk of falling and of fracture: the *rise and walk test.* The patient gets up from a chair, walks to a wall 3 m away, touches it and returns to sit on the chair again. If this takes longer than 10 s, then there is an increased risk of fracture. Examples of physiologic changes found in frequent fallers include impaired proprioception and motility, impaired visual acuity, impaired ankle dorsiflexion, decreased reaction time and increased body sway. Protection against blows to the hip is afforded by *pads* sewn into the underwear or worn underneath it. The pads disperse the impact of the fall and thus protect the hip joint (Fig. 21.4a, b). When osteoporosis is already established, various other factors – either health related as listed above or in the environment – increase the fracture risk. These include muscular weakness, poor coordination, awkward movements and inadequate protective reactions, excitement, dizziness, brief fainting attacks,

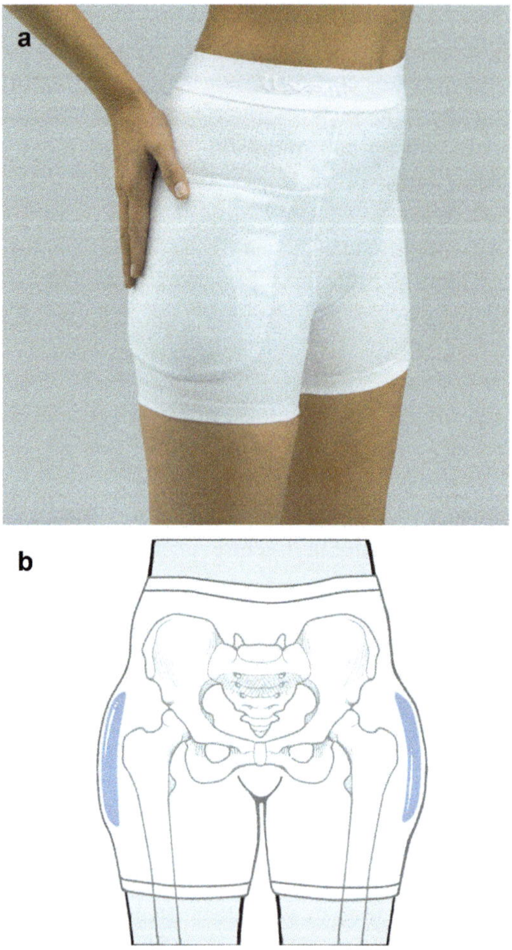

Fig. 21.4 (**a**, **b**) Hip protectors to absorb the energy of a fall and to redistribute the load to the surrounding tissues

Parkinson's disease and alcoholism, and fatigue, which may be drug-induced and possibly due to antidepressive or antihypertensive medication or to a variety of sleeping tablets which entail a high risk of falling, while simultaneously decreasing the body's protective mechanisms. Cardiac medications and analgesics have also been implicated as risk factors. Other culprits are obstacles in the home such as telephone and other wires and cables, stairs, loose carpets, slippery bathroom mats, lack of grab bars and poor lighting.

A Previous Fracture Patients who have already sustained a fracture in the past are at increased risk of another fracture in the future; therefore, preventive care is especially important, and all the considerations outlined above apply equally to these patients.

21.3 Education and Knowledge

Many of the risk factors listed above could be avoided by proper information and emphasis on how the patients themselves could contribute to a reduction in risk factors. The emphasis should be on aspects of daily living, especially in the elderly, who could probably also benefit from a device, such as a picture, sketch or other graphic reminders which would be constantly displayed in their rooms (homes). Finally, it should be remembered that, even in the absence of osteoporosis, falls and fractures may occur. One such example is fracture of the ankle, which may occur as a consequence of a heavy fall or an accident which caused multiple injuries. Results of the National Osteoporosis Risk Assessment (NORA) study of 158,940 postmenopausal, 50–98-year-old women showed a positive association between a previous wrist fracture and future osteoporosis- related fractures within the next 3 years. Consequently, a previous wrist fracture can be considered as an independent risk factor for postmenopausal women, regardless of the presence or absence of other risk factors.

21.4 Fracture Risk Assessment Tool (FRAX®)

The main goal of treating or preventing osteoporosis is to reduce fractures. However, no current medication is free of side effects, and most available drugs are still expensive. It is therefore important to target patients at risk of sustaining fractures to maximise potential benefits and cost-effectiveness and to minimise side effects of drugs. The WHO guidelines for osteoporosis are based entirely on bone mineral density (BMD), and a T-score cut-point of −2.5 has been chosen to identify the population the individuals most likely to get a fracture. However, the majority of patients with fractures do not have densitometric evidence of osteoporosis. There is therefore a need to better identify individuals at risk of fractures.

There are two groups of risk factors with increased risk of fractures:

- Factors reducing bone density and strength
- Factors increasing the risk of falls

The most important single factors affecting fracture risk are:

- Bone mineral density (BMD)
- Bone geometry (e.g. hip axis length and angle)
- Bone turnover
- Age and sex
- Many other factors (e.g. smoking, immobility, drugs, various disorders)

In 2008 the WHO published the first version of a fracture risk assessment tool (FRAX®). It is freely available on the web and has been included in the reporting software of several DXA manufacturers. FRAX® estimates the patient's 10-year probability of sustaining a hip or other major osteoporotic fracture. Results of FRAX® can be used for treatment decisions and reimbursement purposes. One of the advantages of FRAX® is that it can be calculated without BMD. Disadvantages of FRAX® are that it uses the BMD of the femoral neck and not the lumbar spine, and it does not take into consideration the patient's tendency to fall, a major risk factor. Even with all these limitations, FRAX® remains a useful tool to identify patients with increased fracture risk. But like all diagnostic tools, it needs to be used skilfully, carefully and critically.

A Step-by-Step Programme for Healthy Bones

22

Maintenance of healthy bones and thereby avoidance of osteoporotic fractures can be achieved by the institution of, and the adherence to, a specific *plan of action*, a programme of ten specific steps for the prevention of loss and the maintenance of the structural and functional integrity of the bones. These *self-help measures* are specifically intended for people who do not have osteoporosis, because their implementation unequivocally reduces the risk of developing the disease. But there is one absolute condition for success of the plan – a sine qua non! – the individual person must have the will power to start and the perseverance to continue!

22.1 Step 1: First of All a Calcium-Rich Diet!

Calcium is the most important mineral for prevention and treatment of osteoporosis (Table 22.1). An adult has over 1 kg of calcium in the body, 99 % of which is in the bone. A fifth of total bone mass is calcium:

- Prevention of osteoporosis begins in *childhood*. M. Drugay defined osteoporosis as a "paediatric disease with geriatric consequences". As the bone develops and grows, a calcium-rich diet provides the building blocks required to attain a peak bone mass at about 25 years. During this period, children and young people need about four times as much calcium as adults per kilogramme of body weight, which means that 500–1000 mg of calcium should be ingested daily, depending on age.
- Even weight-conscious *teenagers* can achieve this goal by means of a calcium-rich, fat-poor diet composed mainly of low-fat milk, cheese and yogurt, bread and calcium-rich drinks such as fruit juice. Just one large cup of yogurt provides nearly a third of their daily calcium requirement. The early to mid-teens are a critical time in bone formation, as demonstrated in one clinical trial which found that by the age of 16 young women had already reached about 95 % of their mothers' premenopausal bone density.
- The requirement for calcium is particularly high during *pregnancy* and *lactation*, about 1200–1500 mg a day.
- It is not too late to start a bone-conscious diet even after the *menopause*, especially since there is a dramatic increase in bone loss at this time. Clinical trials have demonstrated that 80 % of postmenopausal women require more than 800 mg calcium daily in food, but during the perimenopausal period of increased resorption, the daily intake should be 1500 mg to prevent the drastic increase in bone loss. In other words, preventive measures should be instituted before cessation of ovarian function and continued thereafter.
- Likewise, calcium intake should be adjusted to the decline in male sex hormones – the andropause – and continued indefinitely, as one of the preventive measures for involutional osteoporosis.

R. Bartl, C. Bartl, *Bone Disorders*, DOI 10.1007/978-3-319-29182-6_22

Table 22.1 Suggested calcium intakes

Age groups	Amount mg/day
Infants	
0–6 months	210
6–12 months	270
Children	
1–3 years	500
4–8 years	800
9–18 years	1500
Adults	
19–50 years	1200
51 years and older	1500
Pregnant and lactating women	1500

Table 22.2 Major dietary sources of calcium (approximate values)

Nutrient	Calcium mg/100 g
Primary food sources of calcium	
Milk, whole	111
Milk, skimmed	124
Yogurt	134
Cheese	600–1000
Ice cream	120
Secondary food sources of calcium	
Beans	65
Nuts	75
Almonds	250
Salmon, canned with bones	200
Sardines, canned with bones	300
Broccoli, cooked	130
Spinach, cooked	160
Rhubarb, cooked	300
Kale, cooked	200
Parsley	100

Sufficient calcium can be obtained by means of a *bone-friendly diet* (Table 22.2):

- *Milk and milk products* are rich in calcium, especially low-fat milk and hard cheeses. The harder the cheese, the more calcium it contains. Soft cheeses also frequently have supplementary calcium. Low-fat cheeses are especially recommended. Moreover, lactose in milk facilitates absorption of calcium by the gut. Some people avoid milk and dairy products because of several misconceptions, for example: Milk makes you fat! It weakens bone! It causes allergies! It is full of antibiotics and hormones! Unfortunately, these people are depriving themselves of foods that provide important nutrients, especially calcium.
- *Fresh green vegetables, fruits and wheat products* are important sources of calcium. However, it should be pointed out that oxalate in some vegetables inhibits its absorption. Wheat products are also good sources of calcium except for white bread and some other processed varieties. Likewise, addition of sugar, salt, phosphate, fat and protein can substantially decrease calcium absorption (see below).
- *Mineral water*: This can contribute to a positive calcium balance when the water is enriched with calcium. But the amount in each type of mineral water varies and may range from 10 to 650 mg/l. The exact amount is always stated in the label on the bottle.
- *Fruit juices*: These are particularly useful for patients with allergies to milk or milk products, especially if the juices have been fortified by addition of calcium. Moreover, the vitamin D in the fruit juice increases absorption of calcium from 30 % (milk and milk products) to 40 %. Addition of vitamin D to various food products may further increase intestinal absorption of calcium.

Calcium Tablets Additional calcium in the form of tablets should only be taken on medical advice. There are some dangers if excessive amounts of calcium are taken, including the possibility of kidney stones and adverse cardiovascular events; the results of studies published so far have not reached definitive conclusions but do flag cardiac health as an area of concern in relation to excessive calcium intake. Calcium carbonate is the least expensive and most commonly used compound, but only some 200 mg calcium is absorbed when a tablet containing 500 mg calcium carbonate is taken. Calcium citrate has been found to dissolve more easily than carbonate, phosphate, lactate or gluconate and has about 60 % more bioavailability in the body. While calcium carbonate and calcium phosphate must be taken with food, because gastric acid is required for absorption, calcium citrate can be taken with or without food. It also has the advantage of not producing gas or causing constipation, but it is more expensive. The following hints may help to get the maximum benefit from calcium tablets.

- A single dose should not exceed 500 mg, so the daily amount should be taken in divided doses as necessary, with sufficient fluid.
- One dose before bedtime makes up for withdrawal of calcium from bone during the night.
- Calcium should be taken with meals. Absorption in the gut is also improved by vitamin C as well as a little fat and protein together with the tablets.
- Absorption is inhibited by foods rich in fibres and in fat.
- Calcium should not be taken together with iron as these combine to form insoluble compounds and so are lost to the body. This is important for patients taking iron supplements.

Other Useful Minerals Numerous minerals, necessary for absorption of calcium and other activities, include magnesium, boron, copper, manganese, zinc, silicon, strontium, fluoride and phosphorus. They are also essential for normal growth of bones and play an important role in bone metabolism and turnover.

The best way to ensure the correct balance is through a variety of foods, as these minerals may be dangerous if taken in too large amounts.

Magnesium especially is essential for bone health. Summary of its actions:

- Activates osteoblasts.
- Increases mineralisation density.
- Activates vitamin D.
- Enhances sensitivity of bone tissue to PTH and active vitamin D.
- Facilitates the transport of calcium in and out of bone.
- Magnesium is highly effective for the prevention of painful muscle cramps.

About 60 % of magnesium is stored in bone, the rest in muscles and other tissues. The recommended dosages are 300–500 mg daily, with an appropriate calcium/magnesium ratio of 2:1. Since high single doses of magnesium may cause diarrhoea, it is best to distribute the total amount throughout the day. However, there is little evidence that magnesium is needed to prevent osteoporosis in the general population.

Taking the above recommendations into consideration must be done with adequate attention to age, especially the young and the old, because of their different physiological functions and therefore also nutrient requirements. Moreover, interactions between race/ethnicity and diet have also been demonstrated in studies of areal bone density in different populations, e.g. African, Hispanic and Asian Americans, as well as American white populations and Chinese Americans. However, there are still ongoing studies regarding interactions between race and diet, and results are awaited.

22.2 Step 2: Ensure an Adequate Supply of Vitamins!

Vitamin D promotes bone formation by improving intestinal absorption of calcium and phosphate and by stimulating maturation and mineralisation of osteoid – the ground substance of bone. A daily allowance of 1000–2000 IU is required for healthy bone. A daily 15-min sunbath would be required for an individual to produce an equal quantity of vitamin D by way of the skin. But this is not a practical option for the majority of people under today's living conditions. In addition, there is the fear of skin cancer caused by too much exposure to the sun. Moreover, the conversion of sunlight into vitamin D in older people is only half that of younger people. Consequently, a daily intake of

800–1000 IU of vitamin D in the form of tablets with meals is reasonable and cost-effective. Different segments in any population may have inadequate intake of vitamin D, and recent investigations have emphasised that hypovitaminosis D can be considered a widespread epidemic, regardless of geographical location at all ages and in both sexes. Therefore, take heed and take the supplements, and don't join the deprived populations!

Vitamin C, another relatively new player in bone health, is required for maturation of collagen (cross-linking); it stimulates the osteoblasts and improves absorption of calcium. 60 mg of vitamin C is the minimal daily requirement, enough to prevent scurvy, but not enough to reap all the possible benefits. The best sources are citrus fruits. Ideally 1000 mg should be taken daily as calcium ascorbate. Epidemiologic studies have shown a positive association between vitamin C and bone mass. There is also a connection between vitamin C and immunology, as shown by its beneficial effects in infections such as the common cold.

Vitamin K is now recognised as a "new" bone-building vitamin. Though better known for its part in coagulation, it plays a significant role in synthesis of osteocalcin, one of the building blocks of bone. Vitamin K mediates the attachment of calcium to proteins for their incorporation into hydroxyapatite crystals in bone matrix formation. Vitamin K is also required for fracture healing. Observational studies have shown that women with high intake and serum levels of vitamin K tend to have high bone densities and patients who sustain fractures have been reported to have low serum vitamin K levels. 100–300 μg of vitamin K is required daily, taken with meals. It is produced by bacteria normally found in the intestinal tract (menaquinone). Dark-green vegetables (e.g. spinach or broccoli) also contain large amounts of vitamin K (phylloquinone). Since this is a fat-soluble vitamin, it is helpful to consume vitamin K-rich foods with a little fat or oil.

Vitamin A is a fat-soluble vitamin and so can be stored by the body. It influences the development of bone cells. The recommended daily allowance is 5000 IU.

Vitamin B_{12} and folic acid are necessary for formation as well as maintenance of healthy bones. Vitamin B_{12} protects the bones against the effects of homocysteine, the levels of which decrease with age. The recommended daily dose of vitamin B_{12} is 1 mg.

Other elements, such as boron, are also important for bone health, and they require a well-balanced diet, rich in fruits and vegetables.

The significance of proteins and the quality of the proteins ingested should also not be overlooked, as these are essential for good quality bones.

22.3 Step 3: Protect the Spine in Everyday Living!

Thoracic and lumbar vertebrae are composed largely of cancellous bone and therefore highly susceptible to fracture – caused by the combined effects of a reduction in trabecular bone without a decrease in weight-bearing. Osteoporosis usually induces collapse of the upper and lower plates of the vertebrae and their protrusion into the vertebral bodies. When the BMD shows osteoporotic values, everyday life should be adapted to ensure protection for the spine and hip joints (Table 22.3):

- *Activity while upright*: Upright posture in front of a working surface adapted to the height of the worker.
- *Activity while sitting*: The back of the chair should provide support for the spine from 15 to 12 cm above the seat of the chair. The spine should not be curved (danger of wedge fractures!). One should never stay for long in the sitting position, but every now and then get up, stretch and move around.
- *Load lifting and carrying*: Do not bend down with a curved back and straight legs! This may damage the lumbar discs and cause vertebral body compression. Rather bend the knees, lift up the load and rise up keeping the spine straight. This applies especially to heavy objects such as cartons of drinks.

Table 22.3 Guidelines for safe movement for osteoporotic patients

Proper posture and alignment when standing, sitting or walking: lift breastbone, keep head erect, look forward, keep shoulders back, gently tighten abdominal muscles, maintain small hollow in the lower back
Standing for a long time: point feet straight ahead, periodically switch from one foot to the other
Sitting: use a pillow at the small of the back, maintain upright alignment, rest feet flat on the floor or on a small footstool. Sit on chairs with backs, not on stools
Standing from a chair: move hips forward to front of the chair, shift weight over the feet leading with a lifted chest, stand by pushing down into the floor using leg muscles; the arm muscles can assist by pushing down on arm rests of the chair
Walking: hold chin in and head upright, point feet straight ahead
Bending: keep feet shoulder width apart, maintain straight back, bend at the hips and knees (not the waist), avoid twisting and bending together, use one hand on a stable support devise
Lifting: keep object close to the body, first kneel on one knee and stand with the object close to the waist, use lightly packed plastic grocery packages with handles and carry one in each hand. Following acute vertebral fracture, limit weight to 4.5 kg
Tying shoes: first, sit in a chair, cross one foot over the opposite knee or rest one foot on a stool
Getting in and out bed: in – sit on the edge of the bed, lean trunk towards head of bed and lower body down with the help of one arm, while lowering trunk to the bed, bring legs and feet on to the bed, roll on to the back with knees bent; reverse for getting out of bed
Coughing and sneezing: gently tighten abdominal muscles to support back, and place one hand on the back, or press back into chair or wall for support

From "boning up on osteoporosis: a guide to prevention and treatment". Washington DC National Osteoporosis Foundation 2003

- *Housework*: During the daily performance of household activities, bending or curving the spine should be avoided, better to go down on one's knees or to crouch.
- *Lying down and sleeping*: Soft mattresses should be avoided, but a flexible mattress on a hard frame is recommended as it gives equal support to the whole body. Also recommended is a small flat pillow, just to provide support for the head and neck.

22.4 Step 4: Regular Physical Activity, for Preservation of Strong Bones!

With ageing, there is a continuous and significant reduction in axial muscle strength. Men lose as much as 64 % and women as much as 50 % of the peak muscle strength in the fourth decade to the lowest muscle strength in the ninth decade. Bone, muscles and joints are all strengthened by movement. Exercise also has the benefit of improving flexibility and balance and therefore has a positive effect, i.e. a decrease in the number of falls and fractures in the elderly.

The theory that putting stress or forces of gravity onto the skeletal system causes it to form more bone is known as *Wolff's law*. Physical fitness ensures confidence both in locomotion and coordination. Physical activity stimulates blood flow and stabilises blood pressure which in turn decreases attacks of dizziness in older people, a common cause of falling. In the event of a fracture, anybody who exercises regularly will have shorter periods of pain as well as of recovery. Training and exercise should be regular rather than irregular and then exaggerated. Comparative studies have shown that women who walk daily for half an hour have stronger bones than those who do not. The relationship between mechanical loading and bone strength is curvilinear, with a much steeper slope at very low levels of loading (complete immobility, weightlessness or spinal cord injury).

Immobilised patients may lose 40 % of their initial bone mass within a year.

Studies have shown that standing upright for as short as 30 min each day prevents bone loss. However, increasing the level of exercise of active people results in very small gains in bone (about 1 % per year) (Fig. 22.1). In postmenopausal women, the lumbar spine BMD increased by 1.3 % per year for impact programmes and 1 %

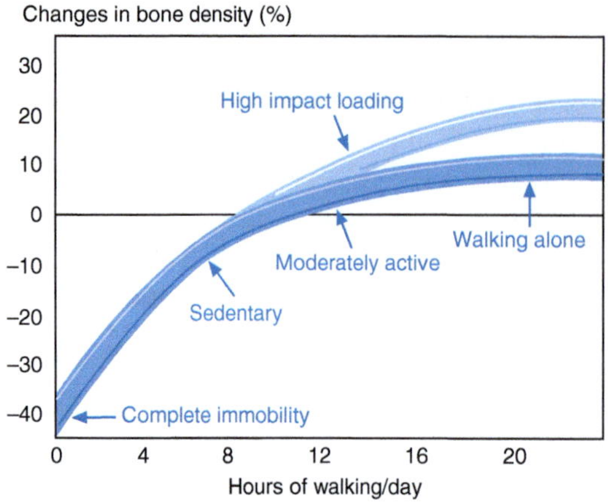

Fig. 22.1 Relationship between mechanical loading and bone mass. There is a greater gain in bone density at the lowest levels of activity than at the highest

per year for non-impact programmes. Femoral neck BMD increased 0.5 % per year to 1.4 % per year in the impact and non-impact groups. In premenopausal women, there was no difference in femoral neck BMD between exercise and control groups. A meta-analysis of fall prevention trials found a modest but significant reduction in the risk of falling (10%) associated with general exercise. It is worth stressing that the age-related decrease in muscle mass and strength (sarcopenia) can be modified by exercise and calorie restriction (if the intake is above the recommended amount).

The optimal exercise regimen for preventing osteoporosis and related fractures is not known. A recent Swedish study of randomly selected elderly women could not confirm an effect of previous and present everyday physical activity on bone mass. However, any exercise is better than none, and consistent activity is associated with the greatest long-term benefit. Weight-bearing exercises, those which counteract the force of gravity, such as climbing mountains or stairs (instead of taking the elevator) and walking, running and jumping, are the most effective in strengthening the bones. Take the car or the bus only when absolutely necessary! Moreover, regular sport – in one form or another – improves the quality of life. But it must be stated that if the person concerned does not enjoy a particular activity, it will not be carried out regularly – if at all – and therefore the exercise sport or activity chosen must be in tune with the patients' wishes and abilities. In addition, it is advisable to choose a sport or activity which involves as many muscle groups as possible, as well as not causing physical complaints and pain. Today sport-oriented institutions and clubs offer a whole variety of activities in a friendly and social environment. There are no age limits. For the sedentary or the frail elderly, a programme of walking, low-impact aerobics or possibly light gardening, in addition to muscle strengthening programmes, is recommended. Training-induced gains in strength are initially rapid but tend to plateau after more than 12 weeks, even with progressive increases in training loads. When correlating mechanical load with bone mass, there is greater gain in bone mass when starting at the lowest levels of activity (complete immobility to sedentary) than at the higher levels from moderately active to walking with high-impact loading. Tai chi may have beneficial effects on balance, prevention of falls and non-vertebral fractures, but there is no convincing evidence for any influence on the prevention or treatment of osteoporosis.

Though exercise is usually considered with respect to muscles and bones, it also has a beneficial effect on a wide range of diseases associated with increased reactive oxygen species (ROS), which in turn may be related to osteoporosis. The diseases include cardiac conditions, type 2 diabetes, rheumatoid arthritis, Alzheimer's and Parkinson's diseases and various cancers. It would appear that exercise strengthens the body's resistance to certain types of diseases.

It has been shown that in *childhood and adolescence*, bone responds more favourably to mechanical loading than at other ages, presumably because this is part of the period in which active growth takes place. A study of female tennis players showed that when training was started before the menarche, differences in bone mineral density in the humerus ranged from 17 to 24 % compared to 8–14 % when training began after menarche. In 15–20-year-old Olympic weightlifters, the mean distal and proximal forearm BMD was 51 and 41 % above that of the age-matched controls, respectively. Swimming, on the other hand, did not increase bone mass as measured by DXA. Although elite swimmers undertake intense training programmes, their BMD is similar to that of control subjects, clearly this is because the water supports the weight of the body. There is some evidence that higher levels of bone mass and density attained in childhood are maintained in gymnasts, but whether childhood physical activity influences the rate or timing of adult bone loss is not known. It should be pointed out that there is a peak fracture incidence in young people – 10–14 years in girls and 15–19 years in boys. These fractures are not related to osteoporosis, but are the result of falls or trauma sustained during intense physical activity – possibly "extreme sports" – and the fractures occur in completely healthy, well-nourished young people with no deficiencies whatsoever. With the right therapeutic care and management, healing and "restitutio ad integrum" are also rapid.

More attention must be devoted to the role of exercise for *osteoporotic patients* or those who have already sustained fractures. Studies have shown that the rehabilitation of patients after hip fractures, for example, is frequently inadequate. Usually these patients show reluctance to participate in an exercise programme because they may have pain or fear of additional fractures. This attitude must be overcome, in order to facilitate the patient's recovery and to prevent additional complications. Moreover, avoidance of any activity will aggravate further bone loss. Bed-bound bones rapidly lose bone mass, and a bed rest study showed that trabecular bone was lost at a rate of about 1 % per week and cortical bone at a rate of about 1 % per month. Restoration of bone mass is much slower than bone loss: about 1 % per month for trabecular bone. An exercise programme should increase the ability to carry out routine daily activities while minimising the risk of falls or subsequent fractures. Patients with vertebral fractures should avoid activities that place an anterior load on vertebral bodies, such as back flexion exercise. However, studies have shown that significantly fewer refractures occur in patients who practice back extensor-strengthening exercises. When advising patients with osteoarthritis or associated conditions, patients who have been previously sedentary and frail elderly patients, physicians should consider referring the patients to physical therapists to start with a moderate exercise programme and for instruction in proper exercise techniques. Patients with cardiovascular diseases require cardiologic consultation for risk evaluation before starting an exercise programme.

To summarise, exercise is potentially crucial for prevention and reduction of osseous fragility in later life (Fig. 22.2). The favourable effects of physical activity and exercise on bone strength, and on muscular strength and balance, apparently contribute to the 20–70 % reduced risk of hip fracture among people who engage in regular physical activity, compared to their sedentary counterparts. The positive effects of exercise on falls and fractures have been demonstrated even in osteopenic women, who are already in a high-risk category. Primary prevention of fragility fractures focuses on regular weight-bearing (high-impact) activity, starting in childhood and continued throughout life. Management of an elderly individual with low bone mass and increased risk for falling includes lower-impact exercises designed to improve balance, lower limb strength, posture and gait. In this respect, brisk walking, Nordic pole walking, climbing upstairs and downstairs, dancing, modified tennis and adult-aged gymnastics can be recommended. Among elderly persons with a high risk for falling, gait-stabilising devices and external hip protectors are useful additions to the list of measures for prevention of falls and fractures. In addition, not to forget that exercise training has general beneficial effects on health, as demonstrated by the reduction in oxidative stress levels in postmenopausal women. Exercise training also has a positive effect on the actions of HRT (even in the small doses given today) in postmenopausal women.

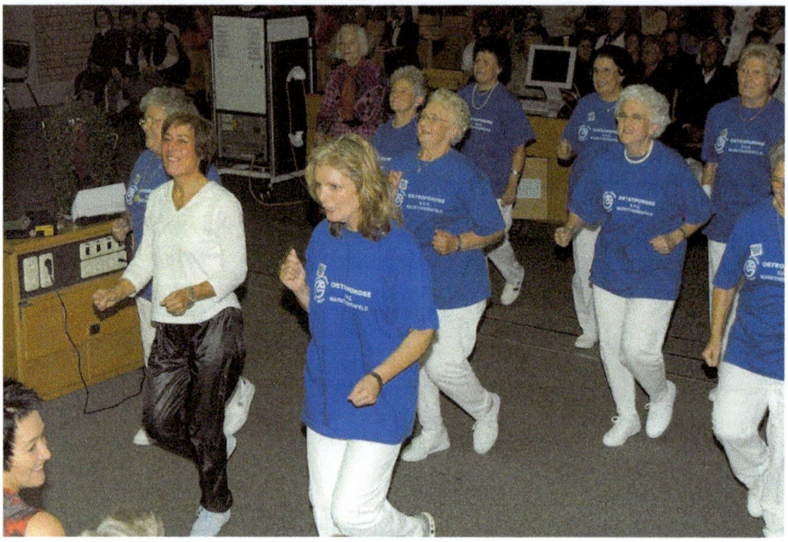

Fig. 22.2 Exercise training in a group – not only beneficial effects on bone and health!

22.5 Step 5: No Smoking, Please!

Every smoker has the power – in the truest sense of the word – to stop smoking and thereby reduce by half the risk of osteoporosis. Smokers have almost double the risk of hip fractures compared to non-smokers. Up to 20 % of all hip fractures are attributed to cigarette smoking. Women who smoke a pack a day have 10 % less mineral bone density at the menopause than non-smokers. Studies have shown that smokers sustain fractures of the vertebral bodies earlier and more frequently than non-smokers, while fracture healing is delayed or prolonged (or both). Smokers also experience menopause 1 or 2 years earlier than non-smokers.

Smoking produces a number of *effects* harmful to bone:

- Decreases production of oestrogen in women
- Increases breakdown of oestrogen in the liver
- Decreases production of testosterone in men
- Reduces conversion of adrenal androgens to estrogens
- Damages bone and bone cells by means of many toxic substances
- Decreases blood flow through bone and bone marrow circulations
- Affects pulmonary function and causes decreased uptake of oxygen
- Creates free radicals

Some experts are convinced that the anti-oestrogen effects of smoking are enough to cancel the effects of oestrogen therapy in the menopause.

In men, smoking causes a significant reduction in testosterone levels which (as in women) results in decreased mineral bone density, i.e. accelerated loss of bone. This loss occurs primarily in trabecular bone and particularly in the vertebral bodies of the spine. Moreover, smokers harbour a higher concentration of substances harmful to bone: these include cadmium, lead and other toxic substances. It should be noted that today, there are many successful programmes and strategies available to help people to stop smoking, but none can succeed without the one crucial requirement – the will power to do so!

22.6 Step 6: Reduce Nutritional "Bone Robbers"!

These are substances in food that require calcium for their metabolism, neutralisation and elimination. These substances are usually not recognised as damaging and therefore not avoided, which enables them to withdraw calcium from bone and thereby increase bone loss unobserved. *Bone robbers* include the following:

High Alcohol Intake This inhibits absorption of important building blocks for bone and damages the liver, an organ required for activation of vitamin D. Moreover, manifest hepatic cirrhosis also causes malabsorption by reducing the flow of bile. In addition, alcohol damages the bone cells directly. Many male alcoholics suffer from androgen deficiency which in turn aggravates osteoporosis. Alcohol also has a negative effect on the immature bone.

> In contrast, small quantities of alcohol (a drink a day) have been shown to have a beneficial effect on bone in older women.

Caffeine and Other Potentially Harmful Drinks Caffeine acts as a diuretic causing an increased urinary excretion of calcium and magnesium. People with a low-calcium intake are especially vulnerable to this loss. It would be prudent to avoid excessive intake >4 cups daily, but patients who do not – for one reason or another – limit their consumption of coffee are advised to drink a glass of milk for each cup of coffee to restore the calcium balance. Phosphate is the culprit in drinks made with cola, because the high content of phosphate binds calcium in the gut and thereby reduces its absorption. Many medicines, including aspirin and other pain relievers, diet aids and diuretics, also have caffeine as an ingredient.

> On the other hand, tea – though also a caffeine-containing drink – is associated with a decrease in femoral neck fractures possibly because tea contains flavonoids.

Sugar Consumption of sugar has increased 1000-fold during the past 100 years. About half of the intake of carbohydrates consists of sugar. Furthermore, the metabolism of sugar in the body utilises vitamins and augments the renal excretion of valuable substances such as calcium, magnesium and other minerals. In addition sugar also inhibits uptake of calcium in the intestines as well as stimulating the secretion of acids in the stomach – another "bone robber".

> In particular the combination of coffee and sugar, as in very sweet black strong coffee or in "soft drinks" such as Coca-Cola, is a veritable "bone gobbler".

Consequently it is not surprising that healthy teeth and strong bones are characteristic of countries with a low overall consumption of sugar.

Salt It has long been established that a high intake of salt is associated with an increased risk of high blood pressure and its associated disorders. In contrast to patients with normal blood pressure, hypertensives have a higher loss of calcium in the urine with its attendant risk of osteoporosis. In addition, some people seem to be more sensitive to the effects of salts than others. A sodium intake of less than 2400 mg/day is recommended. Every additional 500 mg of salt takes another 10 mg of calcium out of the bones, because sodium competes with calcium for reabsorption in the renal tubules. The latest studies have shown that limiting salt intake is directly associated with a decreased risk of osteoporosis.

Proteins Acids, especially phosphoric and sulphuric acids, are produced during the metabolism and breakdown of proteins. These acids must first be neutralised – buffered – by combining with calcium before they are eliminated by the kidneys; otherwise, the body would be "acidified". Meat protein is more acidic during digestion than protein from fish, beans, nuts and seeds, because these consist of different amino acids and different kinds of fatty acids. When protein intake is high while that of calcium is low, a "negative calcium balance" is created, and the required calcium is mobilised from the bones. So, avoiding excessive protein intake (>60 g/d) will improve calcium balance and overall health.

Vegetarians with their low consumption of animal proteins always show a positive calcium balance and stable bones.

On the other hand, Eskimos with their high intake of animal protein and low consumption of calcium suffer a 20 % greater loss of bone than Europeans.

Phosphate Combined with calcium, it produces a strong crystalline substance which gives teeth and bones their hardness. Ideally, one part phosphate should combine with one part calcium.

Our diet contains far more phosphate than is required.

This in turn triggers secretion of PTH to neutralise the excess phosphate by mobilisation of calcium and magnesium from the bones. Meat products, soft drinks and many prepared "ready to eat" and "fast foods" contain high levels of phosphate, and their intake should be correspondingly restricted.

Lipids Prior to absorption into the bloodstream, calcium is dissolved in the acidic gastric juices and combined with lipids. Only in this form can calcium be taken up by the gastric mucosa and pass into the circulation. But when too much fat is present, the opposite effect occurs – calcium and magnesium are lost and bone is lost too. The deleterious effect of fat on bone is illustrated by comparison of the incidence of osteoporosis in the "low-lipid countries" of the Far East, with that of the USA, where it is significantly higher.

Overacidification In actual fact, our bodies are swamped by acids produced by the body itself or absorbed with food (proteins, sugars, fats) in large quantities. The acids have to be neutralised, and this is accomplished in the bone. The bones harbour a large quantity of alkaline salts such as calcium, potassium, sodium and magnesium which are mobilised immediately to neutralise any acids in the blood.

The connection between an acidic pH value and osteoporosis is well known and is taken into consideration in any programme for prevention of osteoporosis.

These observations underline the importance of sufficient quantities of basic vegetables and fruits in order to supply the body with these alkaline substances as well as with vitamins. It is clear therefore that vegetables and fruits are required for neutralisation of acids and milk and its products for an adequate supply of calcium.

22.7 Step 7: Strive for an Ideal Body Weight!

All large osteoporosis studies have demonstrated the close connection between osteoporosis and low body weight. Underweight individuals consume insufficient calories and insufficient materials to maintain their bodies in particular the skeletal system. A low body weight and a low muscle mass result in less stimulation of the bones, hence lower bone mass. Women with less body fat also tend to produce less oestrogen. However, obesity should not be encouraged because of its many harmful effects on overall health, by way of the many possible co-morbidities which, in turn, also affect the bones. The best course is to aim for a weight that is normal for height and body build.

Anorexia nervosa is an eating disorder triggered by an overwhelming fear of weight gain. It affects young women and disrupts the menstrual cycle, lowers oestrogen levels and so inhibits a normal peak bone mass. As many as 50% of patients with anorexia nervosa have low bone density in their lower spine.

22.8 Step 8: Identify Drugs that Cause Osteoporosis and Take Appropriate Steps to Counteract Them When Possible and Necessary!

A comprehensive list of drugs associated with increased risk of osteoporosis in adults has been outlined by the National Osteoporosis Foundation. The most commonly used groups of drugs are given in Sect. XIV.

Glucocorticoids Excess of exogenous glucocorticoid is the most frequent cause of secondary osteoporosis. This group includes all substances derived from cortisone, such as prednisone and dexamethasone. Bone loss may be rapid, particularly in children and in women over 50 years. The BMD should be measured in all patients before starting long-term therapy with glucocorticoids and subsequently every 6 months thereafter during the whole course of treatment. Patients with a low bone mass or fractures should be considered for simultaneous therapy with antiresorptive agents. A study on the epidemiology of glucocorticoid adverse events noted that these may occur even under low-dose therapy, depending on dose and especially duration and possibly also presence of other risk factors. However, short-term local application of cortisone derivatives such as ointments or sprays is not damaging to bone. Not all patients experience the same degree of bone loss even with the same or similar medications and amounts of the drugs. Two major factors influence bone loss: the quantity and the length of the period during which the medication is taken. Therefore, the daily dose and the period of administration should be kept to a minimum. When prednisone is unavoidable, the patient should be advised to stop smoking, to take calcium and vitamin D tablets and to undertake (or to continue) regular sport or other physical activity.

Thyroid Hormones These have two applications: to prevent development of struma and to treat hypothyroidism. Overdosage, which might occur with prolonged administration, should be avoided, as this may also lead to osteoporosis and fractures.

Anticoagulants Heparin and warfarin given over long periods (years) may cause severe osteoporosis, as shown in some studies, but not confirmed in others. Therefore, as with glucocorticoids, the bone density is taken before starting therapy and at regular intervals thereafter. The patient is advised on preventative measures, also with consideration of co-morbidities.

Anticonvulsants These include carbamazepine, phenytoin and barbiturates. They can damage bone over time and cause disturbances in mineralisation as well as bone loss ("osteoporomalacia").

Many *other medications* also weaken the bones on prolonged use. This list includes antidepressives, lithium, antibiotics, isoniazid, antacids containing aluminium, cytostatic drugs and certain diuretics. Pain medications: the effects on bone vary from none to an increased risk of fracture. Any medication to be taken by a patient must first be checked for its potential to effect bone adversely, so that precautions may be taken in advance. Alternatively, a different medication may be substituted, but of course, the same precautions apply.

22.9 Step 9: Recognise Diseases Which Damage Bones!

Primary chronic polyarthritis (PCP) is probably the most important representative of this group. Over the years PCP has consistently caused osteoporosis and fractures. Damage to bones is further aggravated by three additional factors: patients are treated with corticoids, they are limited in their movements, and they are underweight. All three factors must be addressed by the physician in charge.

Chronic *pulmonary diseases*, especially the bronchitis and emphysema caused by smoking, increase the risk of osteoporosis, which is further enhanced by the drugs often given as therapy. Chronic obstructive pulmonary disease (COPD) carries an increased risk of vertebral fractures.

Chronic Cardiac Insufficiency This leads to increased resorption of bone because of limitations in mobility and secondary hyperparathyroidism. Consequently when a heart transplant is considered, it is advisable to institute bisphosphonate therapy months in advance to avert the otherwise inevitable loss of bone.

Diabetes Mellitus This in itself constitutes a considerable risk for osteoporosis. The lack of insulin causes an increase in bone resorption as well as a decrease in production of collagen. This affects mainly patients who are treated with oral insulin tablets.

Inflammatory bowel disorders and gastric/intestinal operations. These conditions almost inevitably lead to a decreased absorption of calcium and vitamin D; therefore, particular attention must be paid to an adequate diet and sufficient vitamin intake, with supplements if required.

Renal Insufficiency The pathogenesis of renal bone disease is complex, multifactorial and as yet incompletely understood.

22.10 Step 10: Management of Patients Who Have Already Sustained a Fracture

Many reports have investigated the conditions and states of patients in the immediate and long-term post-fracture periods, and the overall conclusion was reached that the management of these patients could be much more effectively implemented with the aim of improving the quality of life and most importantly of preventing further fractures. In fact, the Interactive Trial has recommended special nutritional and exercise strategies for early intervention in the post-fracture period especially for older and vulnerable people, in particular by taking the individual risk profile of each of the patients into consideration. One retrospective study of patients after vertebroplasty demonstrated that significantly fewer fractures recurred if the patients had participated in a targeted exercise programme. Wide application of such programmes is highly recommended. A recent follow-up study of 215 fracture patients has demonstrated the efficacy of such a programme and that the patients really took it seriously!

Five Main Steps to Preserve Bone Health

- *Don't smoke.*
- *Be active.*
- *Eat well.*
- *Think positive.*
- *Take vitamin D.*

23 Physical Activity and Exercise Programmes

The human body is equipped with an impressive apparatus to overcome the forces of natural gravity on planet earth and that can adapt to varying demands.

From an evolutionary perspective, we were born to run!

This apparatus consists of the bones and the joints of the skeleton, together with the tendons and muscles. Moreover, the physical stimuli of pressure, weight and the "push and pull" of movements – controlled and uncontrolled, sudden and slow and continuous and interrupted – directly stimulate the bone cells to form new bone and thereby increase bone mass. Without adequate physical activity, 5–10 % of the muscle mass may be lost per annum. And this in turn leads to a decrease in bone mass. It should be noted that physical activity is just as, if not more, important for prevention of osteoporosis as the medications.

Strong muscles make and maintain strong bones!

Immobilisation, bed rest, spinal cord injury and a sedentary lifestyle inevitably induce rapid bone loss. The ultimate test of evaluating the effects of weight-bearing activity on bone occurred in space, where there is zero gravity. Before preventive measures were introduced, post-flight bone density of astronauts showed significant decrease in density after only 4–14 days in outer space!

In order to benefit the bones, exercise must be *weight-bearing* together with special training to strengthen the muscles. Weight-bearing exercise is any type of exercise in which the bones must support the weight of the body against gravity. The most effective activities are those which challenge gravity such as climbing, walking, jogging, running, volleyball, basketball and especially going up the stairs. Therefore, use the legs and not the lift. Whoever does not manage at least 30 min walking daily should at least do some regular exercises at home. Giving up a half-hour of TV every day is all that it takes! The importance of sustained exercise, especially with high-impact loading, cannot be overemphasised for the prevention of osteoporosis as well as for its therapy, which has been extensively documented in various studies. No matter how you look at it, an effective exercise programme takes approximately 3 h per week. Everybody should be able to manage that! As the age-old saying has it – "where there's a will, there's a way!"

R. Bartl, C. Bartl, *Bone Disorders*, DOI 10.1007/978-3-319-29182-6_23

Muscle strength of older individuals responds dramatically to resistance exercise. Strength gains vary from 30 % to more than 100 % in various muscle groups. Training-induced strength gains are initially rapid but tend to plateau after 3 months, even with progressive increases in training loads. Thus, muscle strength can be improved and can also be maintained in older people without high-intensity training schedules.

The sense or the automatic ability to keep one's *balance* is gradually but systematically reduced from about 30 years onwards. However, the body is able to compensate, so that this deficit only becomes noticeable if and when other senses such as sight and hearing are also impaired. In osteoporotic patients, the consequences of the decreased ability to balance include falls and possibly fractures. Clearly, appropriate measures must be taken to avoid this. Balance can be tested with the *get up and go test*: get up from a chair without using your arms. Walk several steps. Turn around and walk back to the chair. Sit without using your arms. If this is accomplished successfully, balance is not a problem. Randomised clinical trials have shown that exercise can reduce the risk of falls by as much as 25 %. Prospective observational studies suggest a U-shaped relationship of an increased risk of falls among people who are either very frail or sedentary or extremely active. Trials have also shown that current or past physical activity is associated with a 20–60 % reduction in hip fractures, but only a modest reduction in vertebral fractures.

23.1 The Muscle-Bone Unit and Sarcopenia

There is one aspect of the muscle-bone unit which has global consequences and on which there is global agreement: *sarcopenia*! sarcopenia is the age-related loss of skeletal muscle mass with concomitant decrease in muscle strength leading to a reduction in physical activity, which with advancing age is a major cause of osteoporosis and other disabilities (Fig. 10.1). Sarcopenia is internationally recognised as a major feature of human senescence. The mechanisms of this muscle loss are still under investigation, but various aspects and pathways have been described. These include biochemical aspects such as reduction in myosin heavy chain protein synthesis, changes in hormonal and neural activities, impaired post-traumatic regeneration, oxidative stress, mitochondrial abnormalities and dysfunctions and myositic apoptosis, as well as apoptotic loss of single nuclei in multinucleated cells. A sedentary lifestyle does have an effect on telomere length and may accelerate the ageing process! So that at least is one physiological risk factor that can be controlled!! Just get up and do it! Also important is endocrine-immune dysfunction involving both inflammatory and other cytokines, lifestyle factors, i.e., smoking, and, most significantly, nutritional deficiencies such as inadequate dietary protein and vitamins particularly vitamin D. In addition to its function as a major regulator of calcium homeostasis, in the skeletal muscle actions of vitamin D are involved in protein synthesis and in the kinetics of muscular contractions. Clinically, vitamin D deficiency is extremely common in the elderly in many countries and is associated with neuromuscular functions and symptoms of osteoporosis. Recent studies have emphasised the positive effects of dietary supplementation, in particular amino acids and vitamins, vitamin D in particular, on muscle mass and strength. In contrast, moderate calorie restriction and exercise have favourable effects on skeletal muscles, but studies have shown that an increase in muscle mass occurs only after resistance exercise. At the biochemical level, the beta-adrenergic signalling pathway is involved, and it has been shown that beta-agonists increase muscle mass while decreasing body fat. Further investigations of such pathways could identify therapeutic targets and indicate new approaches to counteract the decrease in skeletal muscle mass in many disorders, including involutional osteoporosis and especially the sarcopenia of ageing.

23.2 Exercise Programmes: Preventive and Restorative

Without the excess stress caused by falls, even a fragile bone may cope well with normal living. Fractures due to falling among ageing people have become a serious problem, and therefore there is great interest in finding preventive strategies. Regular exercise is undoubtedly one of the most promising preventive options, with benefits for both bone strength and neuromuscular performance. Before undertaking an exercise programme at home, various aspects should be considered:

- Location: a place in the home which is suitable; this implies that there is enough free space, without furniture or appliances with sharp edges and no loose carpets or slippery surfaces.
- Clothing: use comfortable and non-restrictive clothing.
- Time: everyone has an individual biorhythm and daily schedule, so everyone should choose the most suitable time of day for himself/herself.
- Company: private or public, with a friend or a group, or with one of the many different commercial and other supervised facilities available today in many countries. However, these may involve cost.
- Grade of bone loss: when osteoporosis is already present, according to the bone density measurement or other imaging techniques, sports involving sudden or forceful movements and/or pressure on any skeletal area should be avoided. Such activities include volleyball, squash, jogging, cricket and others. Moreover, special care must be taken when physical activity involves bending the spine, in particular when the movement tends to be uneven – i.e. tilted more to one side than to the other. Examples of daily activities during which this may occur are filling and emptying washing machines and driers and dishwashers, lifting heavy cartons or boxes filled with bottles or other containers with drinks, carrying shopping or other heavy objects unilaterally on the arm or shoulder, bending unevenly when using the vacuum cleaner, etc. In contrast, walking, dancing and golf are suitable as they induce bone formation, whereas cycling, swimming and rowing are more suitable and advantageous for the vascular system and for the muscles than for the bones, as these exercises do not carry the body's weight. Before beginning any training programme, patients with severe osteoporosis must consult a doctor or an authorised trainer as to what kind of exercise and training they should or should not carry out. With improvements in the state of the skeleton over time, such recommendations may obviously be modified.

23.3 Implementation of a Training Programme

There are *five aspects* to consider:

- Warming-up period before doing the exercises, usually 5–10 min depending on the physical condition; slow movements using the shoulder, hip and knee joints
- Training for high-impact activities, e.g. volleyball, basketball or vertical jumping; risky for individuals with established osteoporosis!
- Training for strength (the stronger the muscles, the more powerful the stimulation of bone formation)
- Training for stretching (to avoid injuries and to improve flexibility)
- Training for balance (to prevent falls)

All of these can be carried out in *four positions*: Standing, sitting, supine on back and supine on all four limbs. The specific details of training programmes can be found in various books and manuals and of course are given by any authorised trainer of any group or organisation attended by the patient. As mentioned in the previous chapter, programmes for patients after the first fracture should not be neglected. And especially adapted programmes are required for the elderly.

> The effective dose of exercise for reducing the risk of hip fractures is at least 3 h per week. It is never too late to start exercising! The greatest challenge is to get younger and older people moving, keep them active and avoid sedentary lifestyle.

Part VI

Calcium, Vitamin D and HRT for Prevention and Therapy of Osteoporosis

24 Calcium and Other Minerals

Calcium is the most abundant mineral in the body, and most of it (about 99 %) is deposited in the bone (about 1 kg) (Fig. 24.1). There is no doubt that calcium is a fundamental factor in prevention and treatment of osteoporosis. However, there is less agreement regarding precise recommendations for appropriate calcium intake. The calcium recommendation for adults is about 1000 (800–1500) mg a day. The higher values are required by teenage girls, pregnant and lactating women, postmenopausal women who are not taking oestrogen and both men and women over age 50. Today we ingest far less calcium than our ancestors did. In fact, studies reveal that three quarters of Americans are deficient in calcium, with an average intake of only 500–600 mg a day in their diet. For adolescents and young adults, the National Institute of Health (NIH) consensus statement recommends 1200–1500 mg/day of elemental calcium.

Numerous studies have shown that calcium intake reduces postmenopausal bone loss and the risk of fractures, even in people who have already had fractures. However, some recent studies came to the conclusion that calcium and vitamin D provided no benefit for reducing risk for fractures and

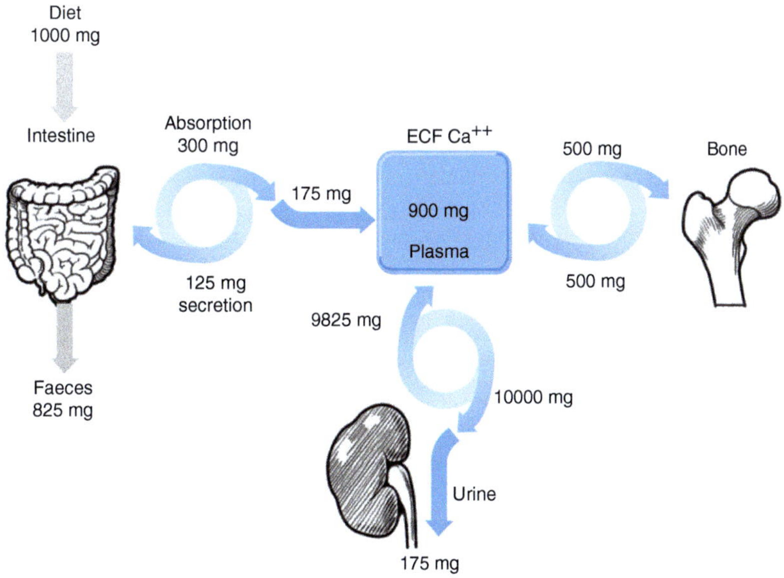

Fig. 24.1 Calcium metabolism in normal adult. Note distribution of calcium and excretion of large quantities in faeces and urine

R. Bartl, C. Bartl, *Bone Disorders*, DOI 10.1007/978-3-319-29182-6_24

possibly increased the risk for kidney stones. Three of these studies, however, had serious deficiencies, and there was poor compliance. Moreover, some evidence points to greater effectiveness of a high-calcium intake perimenopausally before the decline in oestrogen secretion by the ovaries has stimulated unbalanced bone resorption. Supplements of calcium (1000–1500 mg a day) and vitamin D alone have been shown to decrease the risk of fracture. Calcium supplementation at levels of 1000 mg a day will suppress bone breakdown, probably by decreasing parathyroid hormone secretion. Increased calcium intake during adolescence helps to build up the peak bone mass, and these mineral stores definitely decrease the risk of osteoporosis in later years.

Total calcium intake should be 1000–1500 mg/day, preferably from dietary sources. There is no reason to increase intake above 1500 mg/day.

While calcium by itself cannot treat or heal established osteoporosis, it appears to enhance the effectiveness of other treatments which inhibit resorption and/or promote formation of bone. In addition to calcium, sufficient *protein*, at least 1 g/kg body weight, is necessary to maintain the function of the musculoskeletal system. An adequate diet, together with the required supplements, can shorten the duration of the stay in hospital of elderly patients with hip fractures.

The best way to get sufficient calcium is to eat foods rich in it. Moreover, getting enough calcium with meals entails consumption of many other nutrients at the same time. Bottled mineral waters with high-calcium content, low-fat dairy products, green leafy vegetables and calcium-fortified juices will help to provide plenty of calcium.

However, experience has shown that most patients do not get the required amount of calcium by nutrition alone. In this situation, *calcium supplements* are recommended and are available in tablet, powder as well as in several other forms, each with its own advantages and disadvantages (Table 24.1):

- Naturally derived calcium (dolomite, bone meal, oyster shells): this type of supplement is inexpensive and easy to swallow, but is harder to absorb and may contain significant amounts of lead and other toxic minerals.
- Refined calcium carbonate is the least expensive form of calcium and has the highest percentage of elemental calcium, but it is poorly absorbed. It often causes constipation, and because it is an antacid, in the long run, it may lead to "rebound hyperacidity" and gastric irritation. It requires acid in order to dissolve. Taking calcium carbonate supplements together with vitamin C or with meals helps to some extent, because that is when the acid levels in the stomach are at their highest.
- Chelated calcium is calcium bound to an organic acid, including citrate, citrate malate, lactate, gluconate and others. Although chelated calcium is bulkier than calcium carbonate, it dissolves easily and therefore may be easier to absorb. In older patients, calcium citrate is preferred.

Calcium carbonate is a good source of calcium even for patients with achlorhydria or who take proton pump inhibitors (PPI) if it is taken with a meal. Furthermore, calcium carbonate binds dietary oxalate and reduces the risk for developing kidney stones.

Very few patients cannot take calcium or only under medical supervision. Patients with hypercalcaemia, nephrolithiasis and renal insufficiency belong to this group. The following *points* may help in the choice of calcium supplements:

Table 24.1 Amounts of elemental calcium in calcium salts used as supplements

Calcium salt	Calcium mg/1000 mg calcium salt	% calcium
Calcium carbonate	400	40.0
Calcium phosphate tribasic	388	38.8
Calcium lactate	184	18.4
Calcium gluconate	93	9.3
Calcium citrate	241	24.1

- Calcium is primarily absorbed in the small intestine, especially in the duodenum and proximal jejunum. Absorption of calcium is complete within 4 h. During periods of rapid skeletal growth, children absorb about 75 % of ingested calcium; this value decreases to 30 % in adults.
- Avoid taking more than 500 mg of calcium in one dose. Take one dose before bedtime to prevent bone loss at night. If more is needed, take several doses throughout the day.
- Calcium supplements should be taken with meals to boost their absorption, which is increased by lactose and proteins.
- Certain substances can hinder absorption of calcium: foods rich in fibres and fat, zinc, iron, spinach, coffee, alcohol and antacids. Therefore, calcium should not be taken together with these.
- Patients should be advised to aim for a calcium-phosphorus ratio of 2:1. The easiest way to achieve this is to avoid excess of cola drinks and foods with phosphorus additives – check the labels before buying the products!
- Calcium may interfere with certain drugs; these include thyroid medications, tetracycline, anticonvulsants and corticosteroids. Therefore, these should always be taken separately.
- There is no need to worry about development of kidney stones, if the correct dosage in the suitable form of calcium is taken together with sufficient fluid.
- The amount of calcium in blood and urine should be checked regularly when supplements are regularly taken.
- Calcium supplements can cause gas, abdominal distension and constipation in some individuals. In this situation it is reasonable to switch to a different preparation.

Phosphorus is an important mineral in skeletal development and mineralisation. Although 85–90 % of the 600 g phosphorus in the body is deposited in bone mineral, it is also a main intracellular constituent, both as the free anion and as a component of many organophosphate compounds (structural proteins, enzymes, nucleic acids and high-energy stores). In cells and in the extracellular fluid (ECF), phosphorus exists in several forms, mainly as H_2PO_4 or $NaHPO_4$, the mixture of anions referred as "phosphate". In serum, about 12 % of phosphorus is bound to proteins. Concentrations of phosphates in blood and ECF are expressed in terms of elemental phosphorus, the normal range in adults being 0.75–1.45 mmol/L (2.5–4.5 mg/dl). Serum concentrations are less tightly regulated than in the case of calcium, and serum phosphate levels vary by as much as 50 % on a normal day reflecting the effects of food intake and an underlying circadian rhythm. Daily net intestinal phosphate absorption varies widely according to the composition of the diet, generally in the range of 500–1000 mg/day. Changes in dietary intake are responsible for much of the variations in the serum. Phosphate is available in food and is efficiently absorbed (65 %) by the small intestine, even in the absence of vitamin D. Control of serum phosphate is controlled mainly by the rate of renal tubular reabsorption of the filtered load, which is about 4–6 g/day.

Further nutritional supplements for healthy bones are *magnesium* and four essential *trace elements*: boron, silicon, zinc and copper. Magnesium plays several roles in the metabolism of vitamin D and in the regulation of parathyroid hormone. Finally, osseous alkaline phosphatase is activated by magnesium. Some studies have found that higher magnesium intake are associated with higher BMD in the elderly. However, magnesium supplementation is only recommended in magnesium-depleted individuals. The recommended daily dose of magnesium is 200–500 mg.

Patients on osteoporotic medication, who do not respond to treatment, need to take an adequate amount of calcium and vitamin D.

25 Vitamin D and Other Useful Vitamins

25.1 The Concept of Vitamin D in the Twenty-First Century

The structure of vitamin D was identified in 1900. In the following decades till the end of the century, numerous studies elucidated its metabolism and its effects on calcium-phosphate homeostasis and its correlation to skeletal mineral metabolism. Indeed, some authors have claimed that the bone is an "intracrine organ" for vitamin D metabolism, based on its direct effects on the bone cells and on the fact that the bone cells themselves can convert 25D into 1,25D by means of the 25-hydroxyvitamin D 1-alpha-hydroxylase (CYP27B1), thereby participating in the autocrine and paracrine loops of vitamin D metabolism.

Moreover, with the start of the new century, an impressive accumulation of work has now established a role for vitamin D in multiple (if not all) organ systems and in their physiological (and pathological) molecular processes. This is accomplished by way of the cellular vitamin D receptors which are present in many organs and tissues. By attachment to its receptor(s), vitamin D initiates and/or participates in numerous processes such as proliferation and differentiation, inflammation in the immune system, as well as various functions in the endocrine systems, including the angiotensin system, in glucose and insulin metabolism and in the metabolism of lipids, to mention some of its more prominent activities.

With regard to the *reproductive systems*, vitamin D is a secosteroid hormone and affects pregnancy, the foetus and lactation. The association between ultraviolet B irradiance (UVB), vitamin D status and incidence rates of type 1 diabetes in children up to 14 years old was studied in 51 regions all over the world by the Diabetes Mondiale Project Group. The results demonstrated that the incidence rates approached zero in regions with high UVB, confirming the action of vitamin D in risk reduction for diabetes type 1 in children.

The far-reaching effects of vitamin D in *oncology* have only recently been recognised, as represented by some reports in the 1980s and 1990s, but numerous publications in the first decade of the twenty-first century. At the cellular level, these reports describe specific actions of vitamin D including pro-apoptotic, anti-metastatic, anti-angiogenic, anti-inflammatory, pro-differentiating and immunomodulating effects. These anticancer properties have been attributed to calcitriol, the "hormonal" form of vitamin D. Equally significant – probably even more so – is the preventive effect of an adequate amount of vitamin D in the daily food intake on the incidence of various cancers at the individual and at the population levels! And this is definitely not the present situation, because vitamin D deficiency is now recognised as a worldwide pandemic! The preventive effect of vitamin D has now been demonstrated by evidence-based investigations for a number of malignancies including

R. Bartl, C. Bartl, *Bone Disorders*, DOI 10.1007/978-3-319-29182-6_25

colon, pancreatic, renal and breast cancers. But so far, studies of vitamin D and risk of prostate cancer have not shown a protective effect, on the contrary. Apparently higher circulating 25(OH)D concentrations have been associated with an increased risk of a more aggressive type of prostate cancer. Recent results of the pooled data taken from 45 observational studies of 26,769 men on the effects of dairy products, vitamin D and calcium intake found no support for any association with risk of prostate cancer. However, the situation is more complex, because calcitriol and its analogues exert several anti-inflammatory actions in normal prostate cells, and it is thought that these reactions could contribute to a putative preventive or therapeutic effect in prostate cancer cells also. Investigations of the effects of calcitriol and its analogues are now underway on prostate cancer cells in animals. Moreover, there is also a genetic component, as polymorphisms of the vitamin D receptor (VDR) gene have been shown to affect the risk of, for example, renal cell carcinoma, while other polymorphisms in vitamin D receptor genes also appear to reduce the risk for recurrence of colorectal carcinoma.

Genetics has recently revealed the existence of another significant factor linked to *ageing* and also involved in mineral and vitamin D metabolism, namely, alpha-Klotho, an age-suppressing gene which participates in the regulation of $1,25(OH)_2D_3$ production and thereby in calcium homeostasis by maintaining the extracellular level of calcium in blood and body fluids. Studies have now demonstrated that Klotho-deficient mice exhibit multiple pathologic changes resembling human ageing. These findings have significant implications for musculoskeletal metabolism including involutional osteoporosis in humans. Animal studies have already demonstrated the involvement of Klotho in dentinogenesis and its mineralisation, which could also be significant in pathologic conditions of the jaw bones and teeth. One study in human elderly people has described downregulation of CD4(+) T lymphocytes especially in patients in association with rheumatoid arthritis. Further investigations of the functions of Klotho are expected also to indicate possible future therapeutic applications.

25.2 Functions, Sources and Deficiency of Vitamin D

According to the international literature, vitamin D is now considered an endocrine system. Vitamin D itself is the prohormone, which is converted into the active hormonal form: 1,25 $(OH)_2D$ in various tissues, for example, the skin, which is now considered the largest endocrine organ of the human body!

> Vitamin D: Don't rely on sunshine, take supplements.

Vitamin D as the most important regulator of calcium homeostasis (Fig. 25.1) has the following actions which affect the skeleton:

- Promotes absorption of calcium from the gut into the bloodstream
- Decreases the excretion of calcium in the kidney
- Promotes the recruitment, maturation and action of bone cells and protects osteoblasts from apoptosis
- Promotes the incorporation of calcium into bone (mineralisation)
- Protects microstructure of trabecular bone

Additional beneficial *actions of vitamin D* are:

- Increase of muscle mass and strength by support and maintenance of type 11 fibres.
- Improvement of coordination and balance.
- Lower risk of falling. Several meta-analyses revealed that vitamin D supplementation reduced the risk of falling by as much as 22 %.
- Lower risk for hypertension and heart failure.
- Lower risk of type 1 diabetes mellitus.
- Lower risk of breast, lung, colon, breast and possibly other cancers by its antiproliferative effect mediated by the vitamin D receptor (VDR). In a recent comprehensive study, the

chemopreventive effect of calcitriol on development of lung cancer was indicated.

- Anti-inflammatory action (immunomodulatory effects in immunological and autoimmune conditions, e.g. in gastrointestinal inflammations).
- Antithrombotic effect.
- Participation in the treatment of psoriasis, tuberculosis and Alzheimer's disease.
- Anti-ageing effect

The major source of vitamin D for children and young adults is *exposure to sunlight.* Ultraviolet B radiation enters the skin and is absorbed by 7-dehydrocholesterol in the keratinocytes resulting in its transformation into previtamin D_3. By diffusion, vitamin D_3 enters the surrounding capillaries and is bound to the vitamin D-binding protein in the blood. Now vitamin D can either enter fat cells to be stored or is transported to the liver for its first metabolism.

Patients who are vitamin D deficient are at higher risk for fractures due to decreased muscle strength and increased swaying.

Vitamin D deficiency is more common in obese children and adults due to the fact that vitamin D is stored in body fat.

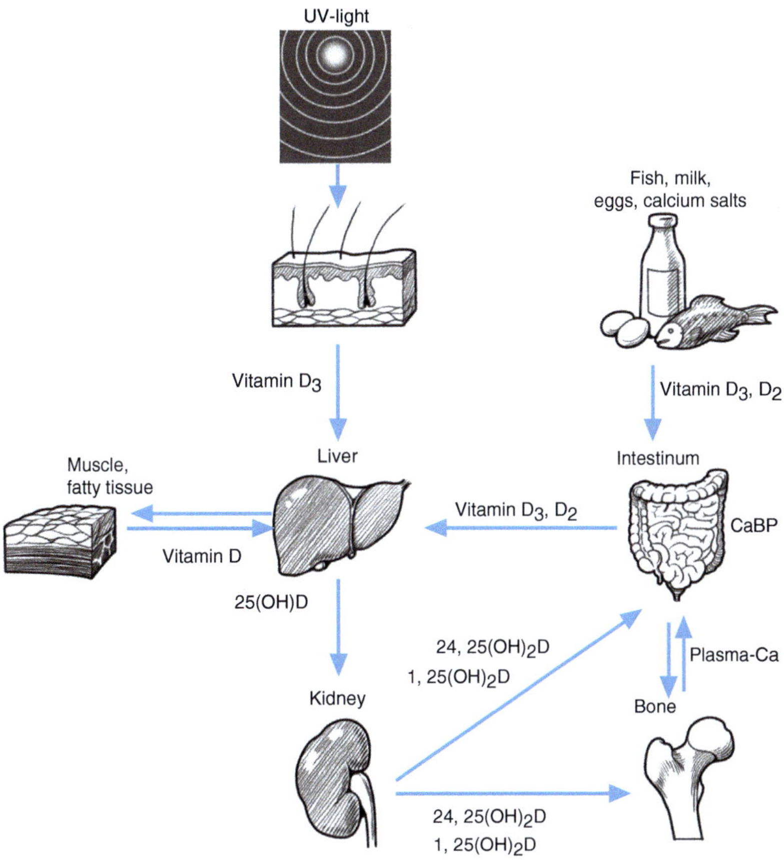

Fig. 25.1 Pathways of vitamin D metabolism

Vitamin D is measured in international units (IU). The recommended daily intake of vitamin D is 200–400 IU, but this is a maintenance dose; therapeutic applications require higher amounts, e.g. 400–1000 IU (10–25 μg), which is considered to be effective. These values may vary, depending on age, ethnic group, nutritional status and skeletal size. Most people with vitamin D deficiency readily agree to take supplements and not to rely on dietary intake. The best assay to determine vitamin D status is to check the level of 25(OH)D in the blood. The normal range for 25(OH)D in most laboratories is approximately 30–57 ng/ml. Controversy has arisen about the level of serum 25(OH)D that defines vitamin D insufficiency and deficiency. In 2011 the Endocrine Society defined insufficiency as 20–29 ng/mL.

Vitamin D deficiency 25(OH)D <20 ng/mL
Vitamin D insufficiency 25(OH)D 20–29 ng/mL

However, patients with levels of 25(OH)D between 8 and 25 ng/ml are most probably vitamin D deficient. Moreover, levels of vitamin D of <20–25 ng/ml have been shown to be associated with secondary hyperparathyroidism, which may result in bone loss over time. Serum 25(OH)D levels below or equal to 12 ng/mL were associated with an increased fracture risk in persons aged 65–75 years, as shown in a recent study. Although there are a variety of other metabolites of vitamin D in the circulation, the measurement of these has not proved to be of any significance.

Experts recommend a total calcium intake of 1000–1500 mg/day on average, preferably from dietary sources and 1000–2000 IU per day of cholecalciferol. There is little argument for the use of the active vitamin D metabolites, except in patients with renal failure.

25.3 Rickets and Osteomalacia

Rickets is a childhood disease resulting from vitamin D deficiency characterised by inadequate mineralisation of osteoid. In adults, the resulting disease is called *osteomalacia* or *osteoporomalacia* when there is component of osteoporosis. A relative vitamin D deficiency often occurs in the older age groups and in people with disorders of the gastrointestinal tract. Moreover, inadequate vitamin D levels are more common than has been previously appreciated. Based on many large studies, the prevalence of vitamin D insufficiency proved to be >25 %, and it has been as high as 70 % in studies done in northern latitudes in the winter. If vitamin D deficiency is suspected, the level of 25(OH)D in the serum must be checked.

The following factors contribute to a calcium/vitamin D deficiency in older people:

- Inadequate consumption of calcium-rich foods
- Reduced absorption capacity of the intestinal mucosa
- Reduced exposure to sunlight
- Reduced synthesis of vitamin D in the skin
- Reduced metabolism of vitamin D to its active form

As a consequence of these factors, most elderly patients have some degree of vitamin D deficiency and secondary hyperparathyroidism with increased bone resorption (Fig. 25.2). Consequently, correction of the deficiency by vitamin D supplements causes a decrease in the serum PTH concentration, a decrease in bone turnover and an increase in bone mineral density. Vitamin D and calcium supplements could reduce the incidence of hip and other peripheral fractures in an elderly nursing home population. Therefore, prescription of 1000 mg calcium and 1000 IU vitamin D daily for prevention of involutional,

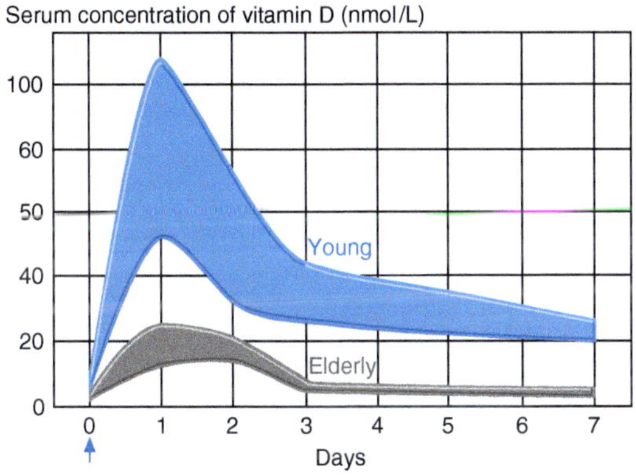

Fig. 25.2 Graph illustrating the decreasing ability of the skin to produce vitamin D in response to exposure to sunlight (Modified from Holick et al. (1989))

age-related osteoporosis is indicated and highly recommended. Alternatively 50,000 IU i.m. every 6 months may be used if there are difficulties in compliance or in order to avoid them. Calcium and vitamin D should always be considered as adjuncts together with other specific treatments for osteoporosis and osteomalacia.

> There is a variety of drugs that may alter metabolism of vitamin D:
>
> - Antiepileptic drugs
> - Glucocorticoids
> - AIDS drugs (HAART)

Vitamin D is especially important in *childhood* during growth. Growing children need vitamin D for:

- Increased absorption of calcium from food.
- Recruitment, maturation and activation of bone-forming cells.
- Mineralisation and hardening of newly formed bone (osteoid).
- An adequate supply of vitamin D (recommended dose of 1000 IU daily) is therefore extremely important for normal development of the skeleton.

Vitamin D belongs to the group of fat-soluble vitamins such as vitamin A, E and K and therefore can be stored in the body for long periods. Nevertheless, many obese persons are vitamin D deficient because the vitamin is kept in the large body fat pool and therefore is not available for metabolic activity. Patients suffering from conditions which reduce absorption of fat usually also have deficiencies of the fat-soluble vitamins. Such patients are best treated by one of the many multivitamin preparations available. The conclusion which must be drawn from this brief review of calcium and vitamin D is that everybody in the framework of osteoporosis prevention and therapy must receive 1000 mg calcium and 1000 IU vitamin D either in food or in supplements every day throughout the year. In the elderly with poor nutritional status, there may be some additional benefit from protein and multivitamin supplementation, taking into consideration that vitamin D_3 is more potent than vitamin D_2.

Recently upper limits for both calcium and vitamin D have been recommended for children of 1 year and older: calcium 2500 mg/day and vitamin D 2000 IU (50 µg)/day. When consumed in very high quantities, both calcium and vitamin D can cause health risks. High-calcium intake may decrease absorption of other minerals such as iron and zinc. The risk of kidney stones however is a complex issue because there are many possible causes of renal stones. In general, dietary calcium does not increase the risk of calcium oxalate stones by binding to oxalate in the intestine. The potential risk of excessive vitamin D intake (in some reported cases more than 20,000 IU/day) is unpredictable and may include damage to the central nervous system, which in turn can result in depression, nausea and anorexia. With increasing availability of supplements and fortified foods, it will be important to monitor intake of these substances. The dose of a calcium supplement should be adjusted, based on dietary intake, age, sex, physical condition, lifestyle and disorders and co-morbidities if present.

> Adequate calcium and vitamin D intake throughout life is essential for the maintenance of muscle and bone health. An additional advantage to increase one's vitamin D intake is to reduce the risk for autoimmune diseases, cancers, cardiovascular disease, infectious diseases and cognitive disorders.

Vitamin D metabolism is inhibited in patients with chronic renal and hepatic disorders, so that they require the activated form of vitamin D to stabilise and perhaps even to increase bone mass. *Activated vitamin D metabolites* are physiological and therefore nontoxic substances, but they are metabolically highly active so that levels of calcium in blood and urine must be checked regularly to exclude hypo- or hypercalcaemia and/or the hypercalciuria conducive to stone formation. No more than 500 mg calcium per day should be given to the patients with chronic renal or hepatic disorders. Recommended dosages are:

- Alfacalcidola 0.5–1.0 μg/day orally
- Calcitriol 0.5 μg/day orally

Several studies have shown decreases in vertebral fractures, but others have not. A few reports have suggested that alfacalcidol and calcitriol have a direct action on muscle strength and decrease the rate of falling in elderly patients. The major problem with the use of active vitamin D derivates is the narrow therapeutic window with the risk of hypercalcaemia and hypercalciuria, impairment of renal function and nephrocalcinosis. However, recommendations are fairly frequently published in the literature by recognised authorities, taking into consideration sex and age, race, ethnicity, geographic location, climate, economic and social factors, the individual medical history and family history, medical examination and results of relevant tests.

25.4 Other Vitamins Involved in Skeletal Health

Vitamin K is also important in normal bone formation. A higher-vitamin K intake helps prevent hip fractures. Vitamin K appears to be essential for conversion of osteocalcin to its active form in bone. There are three major forms of vitamin K:

K1 (phylloquinone) is the natural form found in plants, especially in leafy dark-green vegetables.
K2 (menaquinone) is produced by bacteria in the gut.
K3 (menadione) is a synthetic form.

The recommended dose for vitamin K is 100–300 IU daily. Vitamin K is particularly important for management of bone loss in patients with hepatic cirrhosis.

Vitamin A in excess may be detrimental to bone; in some studies, intake of more than 1500 μg RE/d were related to a twofold increase in the risk of hip fractures.

Recent research also suggests that low *vitamin* B_{12} status and elevated homocysteine levels interfere with the activity and number of osteoblasts and may increase the risk of bone fractures. A meta-analysis found that raising vitamin B_{12} levels in older individuals lead to a reduction in fracture risk.

26 Hormone Replacement Therapy (HRT)

26.1 Oestrogen and Progesterone

Decrease in oestrogen production starts well before menopause and initiates a continuous loss of bone.

> Oestrogen preserves bone and has an anti-resorptive effect.

After menopause, and in the absence of therapy, 1–4 % of the bone mass may be lost annually. In general, the indications for HRT are:

- Relief of postmenopausal symptoms and signs attributable to oestrogen deficiency.
- Reduction of risk of diseases associated with oestrogen deficiency (osteoporosis, cardiovascular and cerebrovascular disorders).
- HRT was thought to delay cognitive decline, but this has not been substantiated.

Long-term use (5–10 years) of oestrogen results in reduction of fractures of the hip, vertebrae and arm by about 50 %. The greatest effect is seen in the vertebral column: within 2 years of HRT, increases of up to 10 % in bone density of the lumbar vertebrae and up to 4 % in the femoral neck have been reported. The effect of HRT is more pronounced in skeletal sites with mainly trabecular bone. On cessation of HRT, bone loss resumes at the postmenopausal rate.

> Oestrogen either with or without progestin has been proven to be effective in protecting bone mass at all skeletal sites and reducing the incidence of fractures in postmenopausal women.

A significant reduction in the incidence of fractures had occurred in the years during which HRT was widely taken, confirmed by many studies, for example, from Norway.

> Hormone replacement therapy for women is now recommended for symptoms only!

Although oestrogen is considered to be the gold standard for osteoporosis prevention, not all patients experience an increase in bone mass. Because of this, the National Osteoporosis Foundation recommends BMD testing for all women on long-term hormone replacement to assure that the patients have responded to this treatment. In patients who have not responded

R. Bartl, C. Bartl, *Bone Disorders*, DOI 10.1007/978-3-319-29182-6_26

adequately to oestrogen therapy (also referred to as ERT when only oestrogen is used) or in those found to have a low bone mass, a combination of HRT and alendronate has additive benefits on bone and could be considered, as well as anabolic therapy with PTH. Every woman who reaches menopause is therefore confronted with the far-reaching decision as to whether or not to begin HRT. It is advisable to reach a decision concerning HRT and ERT only after consultation with the patient and with a gynaecologist. A BMD measurement and evaluation of the patient's risk profile, including family history, also contribute to the decision. But today, the indications are far more limited, and the operative principles are:

- Who should get HRT? – As few women as possible
- How much HRT? – As little as possible
- For how long? – As short as possible

The *mechanisms of action* of oestrogens on bone and tissues related to maintenance of bone are complex and include (Fig. 26.1):

- Increased apoptosis in pre-osteoclasts
- Inhibition of osteoclast activity
- Stimulation of collagen synthesis by osteoblasts
- Promotion of gastrointestinal absorption of calcium
- Stimulation of calcitonin secretion
- Modulation of parathyroid hormone secretion
- Improvement of central nervous functions and therefore decrease of tendency to fall
- Increased blood flow through the bones

Oestrogens increase intestinal calcium absorption and renal resorption; they facilitate vitamin D hydroxylation and decrease the age-related PTH increase.

The data from the oestrogen/progesterone arm of the *Women's Health Initiative Study* (*2003*) has influenced perceptions on the effects of HRT and its role in patient management. The study confirmed that HRT reduces the risk of vertebral, non-vertebral and hip fractures. This was a major advance in the evidence base concerning the effects of HRT on bone, but at the same time, cardiovascular and breast cancer data from the trial have had a negative effect on perceptions and as a consequence the use of HRT and ERT is now strictly limited. This is all the more so, as alternatives are readily available and do not have the potentially dangerous side effects of HRT and ERT. As a result, women, who do use HRT, limit their use to a short time after menopause. Women at high risk of osteoporosis, who wish to minimise

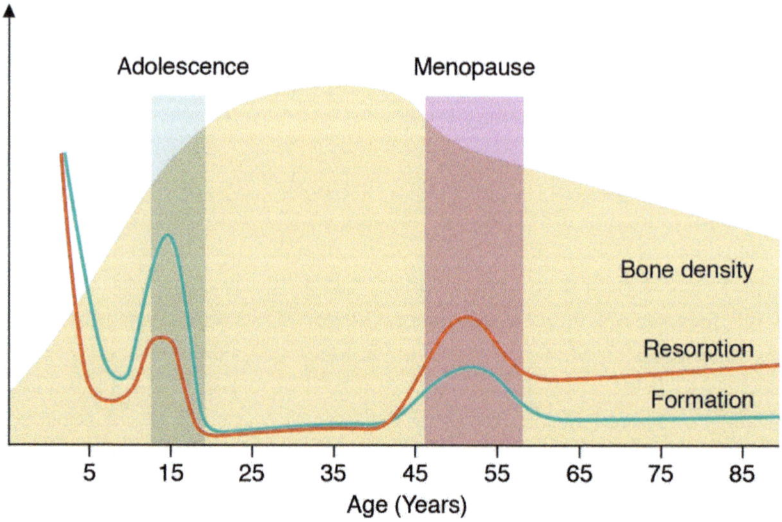

Fig. 26.1 Changes in resorption and formation and in bone mass before and at the menopause, without therapy

postmenopausal bone loss, now have the option of transferring to raloxifene or a nitrogen-containing bisphosphonate, or the combination of the two, as well as the latest anabolic therapy, if osteoporosis is already established.

HRT in women relieves vasomotor and urogenital symptoms, prevents early postmenopausal bone loss and fractures and prevents diabetes mellitus.

26.1.1 Which Oestrogens and Progestins, and How to Take Them?

The main groups of oestrogen preparations given orally or transdermally are:

- Synthetic oestrogen analogues with a steroid skeleton
- Non-human oestrogen, produced from an equine source (conjugated equine oestrogens)
- Native human oestrogens or compounds that are transformed to native oestrogens in the body

Effective daily doses of commonly used oestrogens are:

Oestradiol	Orally	2 mg
	Patch	50 μg
	Gel	1 mg
Conjugated equine oestrogens		0.625 mg
Oestradiol valerate		2 mg

For women with an intact uterus, oestrogen should be combined with *progestin* to prevent the risk of endometrial hyperplasia and cancer. Cyclic treatment is recommended for women immediately after the menopause, while continuous daily intake is suitable for older postmenopausal women when regular uterine bleeding is undesirable. Most clinical experience has been gained with the use of medroxyprogesterone acetate, norethisterone acetate and levonorgestrel. However, as pointed out previously, women should be informed about the alternatives to HRT, but if used, as little as possible, for as short a time as possible! All the above refers to the use of oral medications. However, many studies, but no clinical trials, have now demonstrated the effects of non-oral hormone therapy, in much lower doses, on bone and on the maintenance of bone mineral density.

Tibolone is a synthetic analogue of gonadal steroids with combined oestrogenic, progestogenic and androgenic properties. The endometrium is unaffected, and combination with progestin is not necessary. At a dose of 2.5 mg daily, it reduces bone turnover by 30–50 % and so increases bone mass by 2–5 % during the first 2 years. This effect on bone is similar to that of conventional HRT. The effect on fracture risk remains to be determined.

26.1.2 Which Women to Treat?

Early treatment is warranted for the following indications:

- Premature and surgically induced menopause, especially below the age of 40
- Postmenopausal women younger than 60 years and with osteopenia (T-score <-1 SD)
- Loss of bone density in excess of 1 % per year (DEXA)
- Women at high risk because of lifestyle or other factors

In postmenopausal women younger than 60 years, HRT can now be considered as one of the first-line choices of therapy for prevention and treatment of osteoporosis.

26.1.3 How Long to Treat?

Every patient must decide for herself how long to continue to take HRT. For effective prevention and management of osteoporosis, a period of

5–15 years was previously recommended, possibly even for life. The longer the therapy, the longer the bone is protected. HRT can be started even at 75 years of age, but must be continued and taken regularly, to preserve the beneficial effects on the skeleton. As soon as HRT is discontinued, bone resorption begins again, so that the bone density returns to its starting value 3–4 years after cessation of therapy. Research on the discontinuation of HRT has demonstrated that the rate of loss of bone mass is similar to the rate of loss at the menopause.

The general compliance with HRT is low and women often reject HRT:

- Only 15 % of women who would benefit from HRT actually take it.
- Only 70–50 % of the various oestrogen preparations prescribed are actually taken.
- Only 20 % of women who embarked on therapy with oestrogen take it for more than 5 years.

Since HRT is no longer recommended except in low doses for short periods and only for oestrogen deprivation symptoms such as hot flushes, but not for prevention of osteoporosis, the issue of compliance is no longer relevant. For many women, lifestyle changes, increased physical activity, proper nutrition and supplements would prevent osteoporosis and obviate the need for hormones. Should osteopenia or osteoporosis be diagnosed by routine bone density measurements, treatment with bisphosphonates or other antiresorptive and anabolic agents is now readily available.

26.1.4 How to Monitor HRT?

Oestrogen replacement therapy, with or without progestin, needs to be monitored annually for efficacy and safety:

- *Efficacy*: DEXA, alkaline phosphatase and CrossLaps in the serum, selectively oestradiol and sex hormone-binding globulin (SHBG)
- *Safety*: Annual breast examination and mammogram, vaginal ultrasound

Some patients may not respond to oral oestrogens because of gastrointestinal side effects, malabsorption or enterohepatic binding of oestrogen. Alternative routes of administration include oestrogen patches or gel.

26.1.5 What Are the Risks and Adverse Events of HRT?

Over the past few years, many studies have been designed, carried out and published on the risk and benefits of HRT, especially long term. HRT had previously been taken for many years by millions of women after cessation of the menses. Results of controlled trials did not show a protective effect of HRT on reducing risk of coronary artery disease, but there was a decreased risk of colorectal cancer and of osteoporotic fractures. Most importantly however, there was an increased risk of heart disease, stroke, invasive breast cancer and venous thromboembolism. The findings of these extensive controlled trials have seriously undermined the indications for long-term HRT which should no longer be prescribed. "Better safe than sorry" as the proverb has it!

In spite of some 50 observational studies, there is still no complete consensus on breast cancer risk with HRT. Most experts agree that oestrogen may be a promoter rather than a cause of breast cancer. The risk of breast cancer for ERT-treated women appears to be time and dose dependent and increases by 25–70 % after 10–15 years of ERT. In the *HERS study*, the use of oestrogen in women with serious cardiovascular disease did not result in protection against myocardial infarction. A further large prospective study (*Woman's Health Initiative*) designed to answer many questions related to oestrogen replacement included more than 27,000 older, generally healthy postmenopausal, women. The oestrogen-plus-progestin segment was stopped when results showed that hormone therapy caused small increases in the risk of coronary events, stroke, pulmonary embolism and breast cancer. There were also some small decreases in the risks of hip fracture and colon cancer, but the overall harm outweighed these benefits. There was also clear evidence that hormone therapy does not result in better quality of life among older women without menopausal symptoms, and does not improve cognition, depression or sexual function. At present, women with postmenopausal vasomotor symptoms must weigh the risks associated with HRT treatment against the benefits of symptom relief. They require treatment for a much shorter duration than 5 years, and therefore the risk will be smaller. Given the availability of other effective drugs, the use of hormone therapy for the prevention or treatment of osteoporosis is not appropriate for most women. Obviously the indications for HRT have changed as have the variety of choices available and alternative therapies. HRT is only recommended for climacteric symptoms, at a dose as small as possible and for a limited period of time (less than 4 years). As regards osteoporosis, comparative trials have now shown that bisphosphonates produce a similar reduction in fracture risk, without the possible adverse events of HRT. It must be unequivocally stated that HRT is no longer recommended as a first-line therapy for prevention and therapy of osteoporosis.

> There is consensus today that benefits under HRT include relief of vasomotor and urogenital symptoms, prevention of early postmenopausal bone loss and osteoporotic fractures and prevention of diabetes mellitus. Risks of HRT include venous thromboembolism, cholelithiasis and cholecystitis. Oestrogen plus progestin was associated with an increased risk of breast cancer.

26.1.6 What Are the Main Contraindications?

- Vaginal bleeding of unknown origin
- Endometrial hyperplasia
- Thrombotic tendency and pulmonary emboli in the patient's history
- Breast cancer in the family or relationship
- Hypertension
- Acute or chronic hepatic disorders
- Hypertriglyceridaemia
- Malignant melanoma

26.2 Natural Oestrogens

There is much interest among postmenopausal women in "natural" alternatives to oestrogen. *Phytoestrogens*, also known as plant oestrogens, are non-steroidal molecules (isoflavones, lignans, coumestans, stilbenes and resorcyclic lactones) and occur naturally in plants and vegetables, for example, in soy products, some types of peas and beans as well as in tea, milk and beer. The plants contain three main classes of phytoestrogens: isoflavones, lignans and coumestans, which resemble oestrogen chemically and are converted in the body into very weak forms of oestrogen. These molecules do not share the common chemical structure with oestrogens, but they have two structural features that resemble oestrogens (Fig. 26.2):

- An aromatic A ring with a hydroxyl group
- A second hydroxyl group in the same plane of the A ring

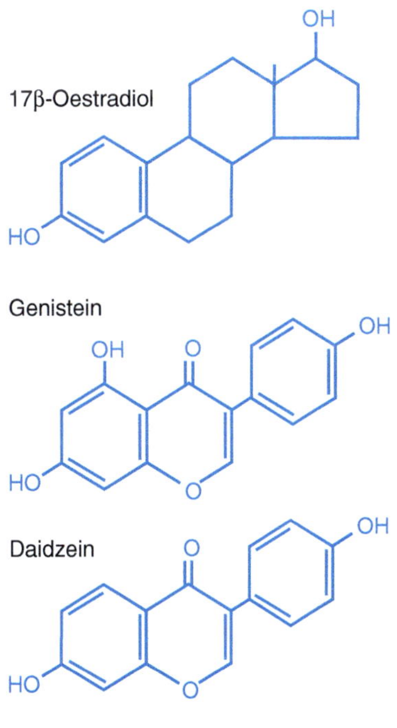

Fig. 26.2 Structures of the 17β-oestradiol and the two main natural oestrogens genistein and daidzein present in soy

These similarities allow the molecules to bind to the oestrogen receptors (ER) and thereby lead to biological activity (nuclear DNA-stimulated protein synthesis).

Though these plant oestrogens are a 1000 times weaker than animal oestrogens, they do exercise a positive effect on the vegetative manifestations of the menopause, and they also have positive effects on bone building. Some observational studies have related the lower incidence of osteoporosis in women in Eastern countries with a diet rich in phytoestrogens. *Isoflavones* are found principally in legumes and soybean products. In terms of dietary sources, most soy products contain about 2 mg/g of isoflavones, and the upper limit of isoflavone intake should be approximately 50 mg/day from diet and supplements. *Lignans* are found in fruits, vegetables and beer and *coumestans* in bean sprouts and fodder crops. Two small studies have demonstrated that they significantly reduced the fracture risk. An additional advantage is that, presumably, they have no tumour-promoting activity. The recommended dose of ipriflavone is 600 mg daily, taken in two or three separate doses. Though these results are promising, larger studies are necessary to demonstrate the value of phytoestrogens in osteoporosis, in particular in the Western countries. Phytoestrogens have the potential of significant biological effects, although the spectrum of these effects may be quite different from that of oestrogen or SERMs. However, cell and animal studies have shown that this effect is mediated, at least in part, via the classical oestrogen receptor mechanism, presumably via the osteoblasts. Stimulation of both cell proliferation and alkaline phosphatase, a marker of osteoblastic cell differentiation, suggests that *genistein* may enhance bone formation activities. Genistein also inhibits the synthesis and secretion of interleukin-6, which further indicates that this substance may decrease osteoclast differentiation and function through an osteoblast-mediated effect, as already suggested for E_2.

> Recommendations concerning the use of soy and other isoflavone supplements to help postmenopausal women with low BMD must await further randomised clinical trials, to satisfy objectively the needs for evidence-based medicine.

One must also keep in mind that herbal products are not regulated by the FDA, which means that the purity, safety and effectiveness of the herb are not necessarily assured and the amount of active drug per milligram dose may vary with different manufacturers. There may be also the possibility of contamination with other compounds, when collected, distilled and manufactured in capsules. Furthermore, the metabolism of the active drugs and consequently their action appear to be highly influenced by other factors of the diet, intestinal function, intestinal bacteria and individual variations. However, standardised plant extracts as substitutes for HRT are now available, and results of trials are awaited.

26.3 Dehydroepiandrosterone (DHEA)

This substance has gained a great deal of attention from the media and the public, and many people now take DHEA to prevent or reverse various age-related changes. DHEA is one of the major circulating adrenal androgens. Serum DHEA levels peak by the second decade of life and then steadily decline by about 10% per decade. The regulatory role of DHEA in bone metabolism has been evaluated in several studies, indicating that adrenal androgens may prevent bone loss induced by oestrogen deficiency. When using pharmacologic doses of DHEA, variable effects on blood lipids and body composition have been reported, but none of these studies investigated the effects on bones.

Consequently DHEA supplements should be deferred until the results of ongoing studies with this hormone are published.

26.4 Testosterone

Secondary osteoporosis should always be suspected if a decrease in bone density occurs in a young male. Possibilities are hypogonadism or Klinefelter syndrome, for which the therapy of choice is early institution of *testosterone replacement therapy*. Hypogonadism in the male is associated with low values of calcitriol and decreased intestinal absorption of calcium. Under therapy with testosterone, gains in BMD correlated better with serum oestrogen levels than with testosterone, indicating that conversion of testosterone to oestrogen may be an important factor. Testosterone serves as a prohormone because most oestradiol in men is derived from aromatisation of testosterone.

Testosterone administration in older patients with mildly low serum testosterone levels results in increased muscle and bone mass without main side effects.

Treatment with testosterone may also increase muscle mass and improve well-being. The use of testosterone therapy should be limited to men with low levels of free testosterone who have no contraindications such as benign prostatic hypertrophy or prostate cancer. Safety of treatment should be monitored by blood tests and by levels of glucose and prostate-specific antigen (PSA) in the serum.

Recommendations for testosterone replacement in patients with low serum levels are intramuscular injections 100–250 mg every 3–4 weeks or testosterone gel 25–50 mg daily. However, transdermal administration of testosterone seems to have lesser effects, and its impact on fracture risk has not been examined.

26.5 Anabolic Steroids: Strong Muscles for Healthy Bones!

The efficacy of these drugs in osteoporosis has long been recognised and is due to their effect on the muscles, although a direct action on bone-forming cells has also been described. These drugs are indicated in the elderly when there is reduction in muscle mass (sarcopenia), muscular weakness or even cachexia. Anabolic steroid therapy in the elderly has a significant anabolic effect on bone in addition to its anticatabolic effect. Treatment should be restricted to 3 years, and the well-known side effects (virilisation in women) and hepatic damage must be taken into consideration. Moreover, men may experience a reduction in sexual function. In addition, cancer of the prostate must be ruled out before therapy is started, because it could be stimulated by anabolics. *Nandrolone* decanoate is the preparation most frequently prescribed: 50 mg i.m. every 4 weeks.

This drug can be used as adjuvant treatment in elderly women as well as in male patients with osteoporosis.

Part VII

Treatment Strategies and Drugs in Osteoporosis

27 Management of Pain in Osteoporosis

Pain has been reported in up to 62 % of female patients with osteoporosis. There are various causes for pain in osteoporosis, including concurrent degenerative disc disease, osteoarthritis and vertebral fractures.

Osteoporotic back pain is usually acute, of sudden onset and caused by a fracture in the lower thoracic or lumbar vertebrae. On examination, there will be a painful spot in the area of the back where the vertebral fracture has occurred. The muscles next to the spine will be very tense and painful to touch. This pain can last for long periods ranging from a few weeks to months.

Start with the patient, not the disease!

In all patients, an X-ray of the affected skeletal area should be taken to demonstrate or rule out a vertebral fracture and to document the extent of destruction of bone. A bone scan may demonstrate an acute inflammation around an area of fractured bone and may show the fractured vertebrae long before a regular X-ray, because of the increased uptake in that area. It has further been suggested that covert small fractures – microfractures – due to mechanical stress can also cause pain. When the intraosseous pressure exceeds a certain level, fluid in the bone enters the subperiosteal space and exerts pressure on the nerves and induces a painful periosteal reaction. Pain during healing of a fracture may well be related to local release of cytokines, prostanoids, histamine and bradykinin into the surrounding area.

27.1 Acute Phase

Before introducing measures for pain relief, the patient's pain should be evaluated for a drug-induced cause. BPs are the agents of choice for most patients with osteoporosis, and though as many as 26 % of patients taking these agents experience some sort of bone or back pain; discontinuation is usually not required. For immediate treatment of *acute pain*, peripherally active analgesics are generally administered first, as these reduce the pain faster and better than the centrally acting analgesics. These include acetylsalicylic acid, paracetamol, metamizol and especially non-steroidal anti-inflammatory drugs (*NSAIDs*), which act by local inhibition of prostaglandins. But these should only be taken for short periods of time, because of their possible harmful effects on the gastric mucosa, the kidney, the liver and the bone marrow (gastrointestinal ulcers, renal insufficiency, hepatotoxicity and aplastic anaemia). Especially in older patients, the cardiovascular status may worsen secondarily due to overuse of these drugs. However, the latest in the series of anti-rheumatic drugs such as COX-2 inhibitors does not have these side effects.

R. Bartl, C. Bartl, *Bone Disorders*, DOI 10.1007/978-3-319-29182-6_27

Bone pain caused by bone marrow oedema can be rapidly and effectively treated with intravenous BPs, which have largely replaced calcitonin for this purpose.

When the pain is very strong as in a recent fracture, any of the medications listed above can be combined with a weak opiate. In cases when patients require large doses or a combination containing *opioids* to control osteoporotic pain, a switch to an opioid alone should be considered. Patients will still receive the analgesic effect, but without the increased risk of gastrointestinal bleeding and other adverse side effects.

Caution should be used, though, as patients using opioid analgesics may be at higher risk for vertebral fractures, secondary to falls related to the use of the opioids. Patients should regularly be assessed for risk of falls, and possibly for increased need of pain control, and for titration of maintenance medication. If the treatment outlined above is not enough, a pain expert can be consulted and the treatment adjusted according to the advice given. It is advisable to avoid muscle relaxants as they increase the risk of falling because of their sedative action.

Bed rest is recommended for the acute stage but only until the acute pain has subsided. Subsequently, short periods of careful weight-bearing alternating with exercises are incorporated into the daily schedule. In the acute stage, a wet dressing with cold water is applied to promote blood flow, while a warm-water dressing may be advantageous in the chronic phase. In selected cases, orthopaedic supports may also contribute to alleviation of pain (Fig. 27.1a, b). Acute pain caused by fracture usually resolves within 10 weeks. A different approach is required for patients with cancer-induced bone pain, as numerous factors must be taken into consideration: the age and sex of the patient, the type and stage of the cancer, the location and degree of the pain and type, extent and duration of the therapy. It is expected that a greater understanding of the neurobiological mechanisms underlying cancer-induced bone pain will shortly be translated into improved pain management.

27.2 Chronic Phase: Short Term

The pain gradually eases as the fracture heals but can also merge into *chronic pain* which is due to the development of a skeletal deformity after the fracture, as well as unbalanced and disproportionate strain on the muscles, and damage to the vertebral joints. Patients frequently complain of nocturnal pains (reminiscent of Sudeck-like pains) which respond to administration of non-steroidal anti-inflammatory agents. This chronic pain may be responsible for loss of sleep, irritability, fear and depression, which in turn highlight the pain even more. Moreover, sensitivity to pain varies greatly between patients and each must be evaluated and treated individually. Many patients with back and leg pains induced by osteoporosis have turned to complementary medicine and have been relieved by acupuncture.

The first priority in all patients is to break the circle of pain and its consequences, and this is accomplished by physiotherapy and by analgesics, calcitonin (either subcutaneously or nasally) or BP (intravenously). Other treatments to decrease pain in vertebral fractures include percutaneous injection of artificial cement into the vertebral body (vertebro- and kyphoplasty). These invasive methods should be reserved for those patients unable to achieve adequate pain control after vertebral fracture by traditional pharmacologic and nonpharmacologic therapies. Further discussion of vertebroplasty and kyphoplasty is provided in Part VIII.

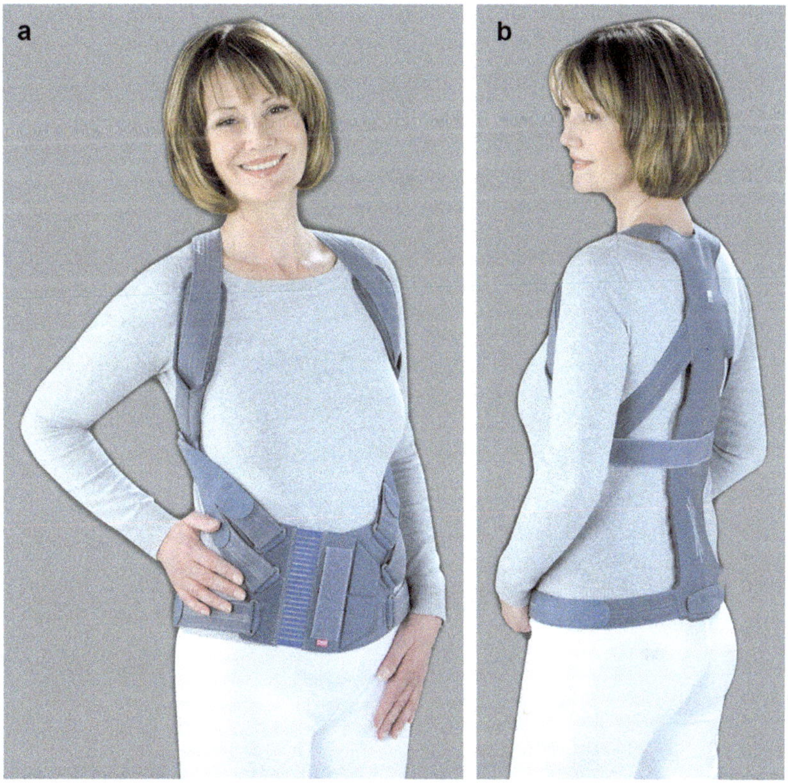

Fig. 27.1 (**a**, **b**) Orthopaedic support (Spinomed active) may also contribute to alleviation of pain

27.3 Chronic Phase: Long Term

Once the pain has become bearable, the patient must be mobilised and the muscles must be strengthened. This is best accomplished by *physiotherapy*, special exercises and the ancillary measures noted above. Every patient should have an individualised program drawn up by the responsible physician in consultation with the physiotherapist. Swimming in particular, in warm or cold water, presents the ideal combination of relieving the vertebral column of weight while strengthening the muscles. As the pain lessens and the patient's condition improves, more sport-oriented measures are introduced. Active training to strengthen bones and muscles also contributes to reduction of chronic pain. Exercises should be performed regularly and be adapted to the patient's age and general condition. The program is developed and taught under specialist guidance to begin with and later should be continued by the patient in his/her home on a regular basis. A major aim is the stabilisation and strengthening of the muscles of the back – especially those of the lower thoracic and lumbar spine. Care must be taken to avoid exercises which carry an increased risk of vertebral fractures, especially those which flex the lumbar spine, increasing thoracic kyphosis and forward flexion.

Treatment Strategies in Osteoporosis

28

28.1 Evidence-Based Strategies for Therapy of Osteoporosis

The major aim of therapy is prevention of fractures! The properties of all *ideal therapeutic agents* are:

- The medication is well tolerated and safe with minimal side effects.
- It has oral and intravenous bioavailability.
- It has been proven to increase bone mass, improve bone quality and reduce fractures at all sites including the hip.

It should be pointed out right away that there are considerable variations in both quality and credibility in results of randomised trials dealing with efficacy of different treatment schedules. When results of these clinical trials are assessed and compared, questions and problems arise with respect to the following criteria:

- Duration of the study
- Number and age of the patients
- Definition of exclusion criteria
- Primary aim of the study
- Fracture incidence versus fracture rate
- Fractures prior to start of study
- Definition of "fracture"
- Definition of "control group"
- Status of vitamin D and calcium
- Risk profiles of the participants
- Method and accuracy of bone density measurements
- Differences in statistics used for analysis

It is now possible to evaluate results of studies and reports of experiences in an objective and balanced fashion (*evidence-based medicine*) especially with reference to:

- Meta-analysis of randomised controlled studies
- Individual randomised controlled studies
- Studies based on observations
- Results of basic research
- Results and reports of clinical experience
- Results based on recommended guidelines

With the continuing worldwide acceptance of evidence-based methodology, the classification of levels of evidence and the grading of recommendations are becoming better and more widely known and are the basis of an effective and rational treatment of osteoporosis. When this rigorous approach of evidence-based medicine is adopted, the most conclusive evidence for reducing fracture risk ("*A class*" *recommendation*) has been shown for the following antiresorptive and osteoanabolic drugs (Fig. 28.1):

- Nitrogen-containing BP
- Denosumab
- PTH and teriparatide

R. Bartl, C. Bartl, *Bone Disorders*, DOI 10.1007/978-3-319-29182-6_28

- Raloxifene (SERM)
- Strontium ranelate

These A-recommended drugs/substances should have first priority in osteoporosis therapy. In contrast, no reliable or definite data are available as yet for calcitonin, etidronate, fluoride and calcitriol so that no conclusions could be drawn as to fracture risk. Thus, it has now been conclusively shown that PTH and teriparatide, the N-containing BP (e.g. alendronate, risedronate, ibandronate and zoledronate) and recently denosumab achieve the greatest reduction in fracture risk: on average 50 % reduction in vertebral and extravertebral fractures after 1 year of therapy (Table 28.1). The concept of a placebo-controlled trial has been challenged on the basis that it is no longer ethical to place osteoporotic patients on placebo now that proven effective therapies are available.

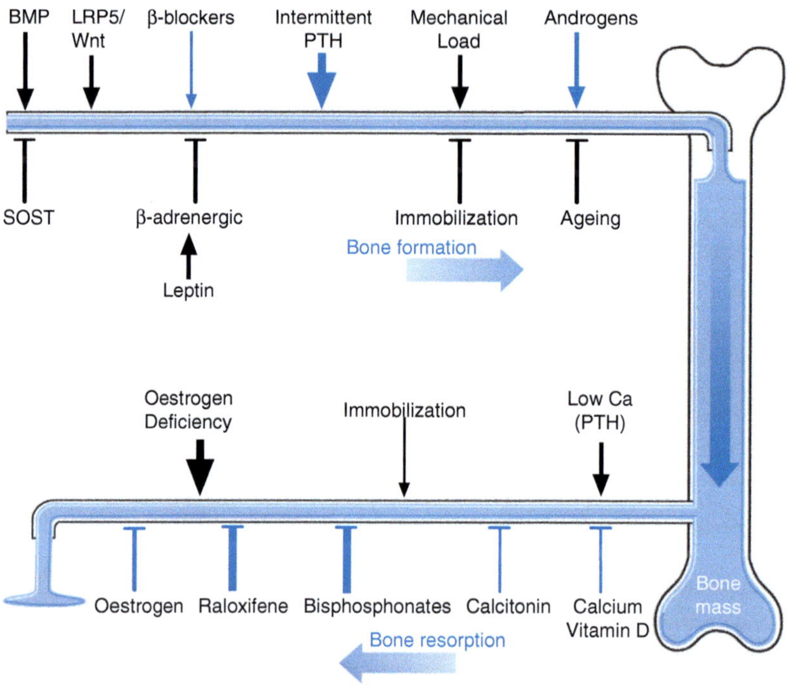

Fig. 28.1 Physiological factors, therapeutic agents and their influence on bone remodelling and on bone mass. Physiological (*black*) and pharmacological (*red*) stimulators and inhibitors of bone formation and resorption are listed. The relative impact, where known, is represented by the thickness of the *arrows*. Abbreviations: *BMP* bone morphogenetic proteins, *SOST* sclerostin, *LRP5* low-density lipoprotein (LDL)-receptor-related protein, *PTH* parathyroid hormone, *SERM* selective oestrogen-receptor modulator (Modified from Harada and Rodan (2003)), denosumab has completed the antiresorptive agents in the last years. Odanacadib, a CatK inhibitor, is a further new and promising drug in osteoporosis

Table 28.1 Drugs used and approved to treat osteoporosis

	Oral daily	Oral weekly	Oral monthly	Subcutaneous daily	Subcutaneous every 6 months	Injection quarterly	Infusion annually
Alendronate	10 mg	70 mg					
Risedronate	5 mg	35 mg	150 mg				
Ibandronate			150 mg			3 mg	
Zoledronate							5 mg
Strontium ranelate	2 g						
Teriparatide				20 μg			
Denosumab					60 mg		

28.2 Comprehensive Approach to Therapy of Osteoporosis

Successful therapy of osteoporosis includes the following aspects:

- Treatment of pain
- Initiation of physical activity and exercises
- Prevention of falls
- Adaptation of lifestyle for skeletal health
- Bone-conscious nutrition
- Vitamin D and calcium supplements
- Hormone replacement therapy (HRT) for short periods only!
- Antiresorptive therapy (BP, denosumab, raloxifene)
- Osteoanabolic therapy (PTH, teriparatide)

Based on the results of the evidence-based medicine cited above, the following *treatment strategy* is employed in our outpatient clinic, after patient examination, results of tests, medical history, family history and evaluation of personal risk profile:

- Patients are given vitamin D and calcium supplements.
- HRT or its equivalent is discussed with each female patient, but is no longer advocated for treatment of osteoporosis alone.
- Early administration of a modern (nitrogen-containing) bisphosphonate or denosumab.
- Alternatively, administration of raloxifene, strontium ranelate or PTH for a limited period and followed by a bisphosphonate.

28.3 Indication for Treatment: Combining BMD with Clinical Factors

The WHO has defined osteoporosis as a T-score below −2.5 and osteopenia when T-scores vary between −1.0 and −2.5. This is a practical definition that allows researchers to classify degrees of low bone density within populations. However, from a clinical standpoint, this definition lacks the ability to make decisions regarding fracture risk and treatment thresholds. The *NORA study of a* cohort of about 150,000 postmenopausal women showed that 82 % of those with fractures had T-scores greater than −2.5. Additionally, the *Study of Osteoporotic Fractures* showed that 54 % of postmenopausal women with hip fractures did not have an osteoporotic T-score at the hip (DXA). Therefore, relying purely on T-scores to determine future fractures is inadequate and unreliable!

There have been several attempts to combine BMD values with clinical risk factors to allow clinicians to determine when to start specific treatment. The *NOF* has developed recommendations for treatment and these *guidelines* have been adopted by many health-care organisations:

- T-score less than −2.0
- T-score less than −1.5 with at least one major risk factor (e.g. personal and family history of fractures, smoking, propensity to injurious falls, weight less than 127 pounds [58 kg])

In German-speaking countries, factors such as BMD values (only DXA method accepted), age, sex, some risk factors and presence of vertebral fractures are taken into consideration in order to determine indications for specific drug therapy. Therefore, based on currently available evidence of fracture prevention in randomised clinical trials, there are at least three groups of postmenopausal women who should receive the highest priority for osteoporosis treatment with pharmacologic agents:

- Patients with vertebral fractures
- Patients with a BMD-defining osteoporosis according to the WHO (T-score of less than −2.5 at the hip or the spine)
- Patients with a T-score between −2.5 and −2.0 and other risk factors for fracture

It is easy to decide to treat patients with

- A vertebral or hip fracture (low trauma)
- A T-score at one or both skeletal sites of below −3, irrespective of age and presence of other risk factors
- A T-score at one or both skeletal sites of below −2.5 and main risk factors using the FRAX tool (with all its limitations)

But all too often, clinicians realise that it may be difficult to determine exactly "what is evidence-based medicine". Management of the individual patient, therefore, requires a combination of clinical experience and a careful study of the available data from large trials. The development of the absolute risk assessment tool (FRAX) has significantly aided the process of identifying those patients whose fracture risk is high enough to justify the use of drugs, especially for those who have not yet fractures (asymptomatic).

"There is convincing evidence that drug therapy, in the right patient, has substantial benefit" (M. McClung, 2015).

Bisphosphonates (BP) 29

A new era in the treatment of disorders of bone began about 45 years ago with the introduction of BP into clinical practice. BP are deposited on the surface of the bones, inhibit osteoclasts and thus resorption of bone. Consequently these drugs have long been given to patients with Morbus Paget, with hypercalcaemia, with multiple myeloma and with osseous metastases. BP not only inhibit resorption of bone, they also inhibit growth of metastases in bone and marrow.

BP inhibit resorption in osteoporosis and – in particular the latest nitrogen-containing BP – have no adverse effects on bone formation and therefore lead to a long-lasting (periods of years) positive bone balance. BP have been successfully used for prevention and therapy in all forms of osteoporosis. Compact and spongy bone show equal increases in bone density. Moreover, the long-term incorporation of BP into the bones has no detectable deleterious influence on bone quality and strength.

> The concept of "frozen bone" under modern bisphosphonate therapy is simply not true. A basic level of remodelling is consistently maintained even under long-term bisphosphonate therapy. Disturbances of mineralisation have not been observed under the new BP currently in use.

The nitrogen-containing BP are today the most effective medications available for treatment of all forms of osteoporosis in both men and women and in young and old, in congenital and acquired osteoporosis, in primary and secondary, in high and low turnover and in pre-, peri- and postmenopausal and involutional osteoporoses. BP have also been given to children – even very young ones – but this should only be done in authorised paediatric centres under strictly controlled indications and conditions.

29.1 A Brief Survey of BP

These are synthetic compounds, analogues of pyrophosphate in which the oxygen atom of the central P-O-P bond has been replaced by carbon, resulting in a P-C-P group (Fig. 29.1a, b). This exchange has made the BP resistant to enzymatic hydrolysis. In addition, different BP can be synthesised by substitution of both hydrogen atoms on the carbon atom, and these BP differ in their biological properties, their activities, their pharmacodynamics and their toxicity. There are two side chains (Fig. 29.2a, b):

- One binds to bone mineral.
- One determines class and potency (nitrogen molecule).

The dynamics of these new BP manifest themselves in their potency – they are 20,000 times

R. Bartl, C. Bartl, *Bone Disorders*, DOI 10.1007/978-3-319-29182-6_29

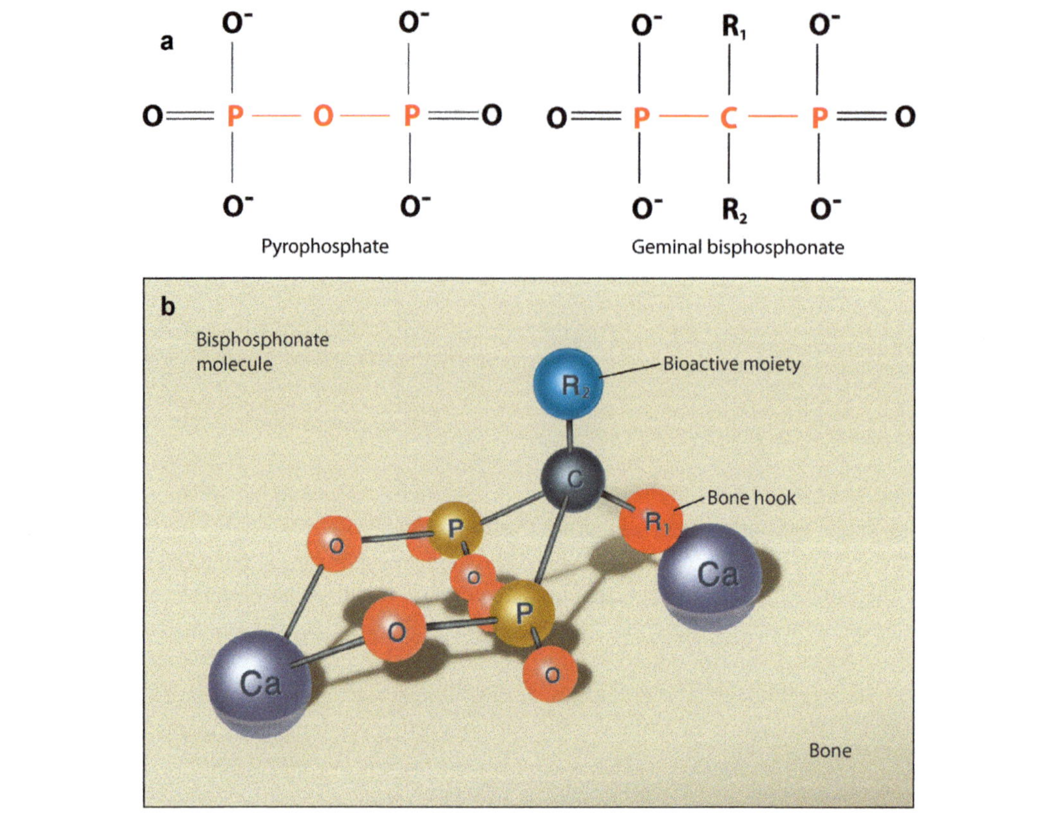

Fig. 29.1 (**a**) Chemical structure of pyrophosphate and of bisphosphonates, (**b**) spatial structure of a bisphosphonate molecule binding to the surface of bone

more potent than etidronate, the first-generation bisphosphonate (Table 29.1). BP have a high affinity for certain structures on the surface of bone. Most of the bisphosphonate absorbed in the gastrointestinal tract is deposited on bone within hours especially in resorption bays (Howship's lacunae) or in the acid environment under the osteoclasts. This causes a most effective inhibition of osteoclasts and of resorption, as well as reactivation of the suppressed osteoblasts and thereby to an overall positive "bone balance" and increase in bone mass. The BP deposited on the surface are later (weeks or months) built into the bone and may remain there for many years, until eventually they may reach the surface again in a remodelling cycle. However, due to their extremely low concentrations, these BP remain inactive, even when "recycled", which means when the bone on which they are deposited undergoes remodelling again.

The *mechanism of action* is not yet completely understood, but some aspects have been elucidated (Fig. 29.3):

- Incorporation of BP into hydroxyapatite crystals and into the bone matrix leads to decreased solubility of the bone substance and disturbances of mineralisation – physical-chemical effect.
- Reduction in recruitment and fusion of osteoclast precursors – direct influence on the monocyte-macrophage system.
- Inhibition of osteoclast activity by means of inhibition of the proton-ATPases – a direct toxic effect.
- Inhibition of enzymes of mevalonic acid metabolism – by the N-containing BP.
- Shortening of osteoclastic survival by induction of apoptosis, probably associated with a lengthening of osteoblastic survival (alterations

in the periods of the phases of the remodelling cycles).

- Indirect inhibition of osteoclastic resorption by way of factors produced by osteoblasts – interference with "coupling" in the osteoblast-osteoclast cycle.
- Increased synthesis of collagen type I by osteoblasts.
- Inhibition of production of prostaglandin E2, of proteolytic enzymes, of interleukins 1 and 6 and of many other cytokines.
- Inhibition of adherence of osteoclasts and tumour cells to the surface of bone.
- Effect on afferent nerve fibres in bone with inhibition of release of neuropeptides and neuromodulators at the nerve ends.
- BP have an anti-apoptotic effect on osteoblasts and osteocytes, for which connexin 43 is required.
- Individual BP may also exhibit particular individual activities.

From a laboratory point of view, inhibition of osteoclastic resorption results in decreased excretion of the breakdown products of collagen in the urine and a reduction in the level of calcium in the blood in patients with hypercalcaemia. In the

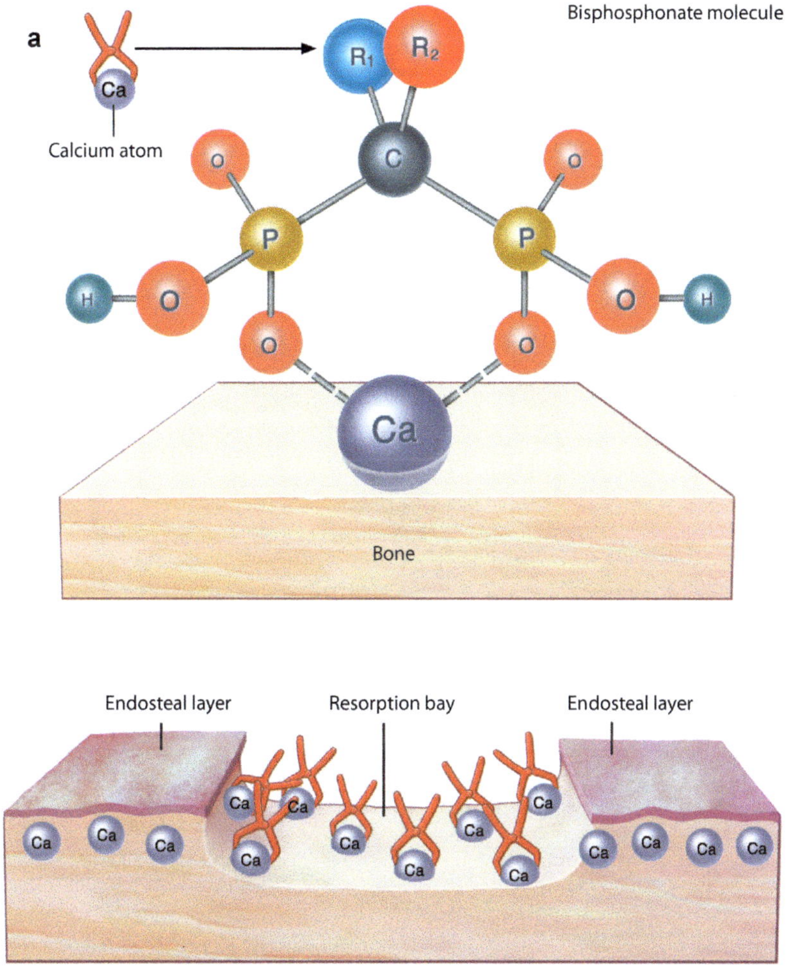

Fig. 29.2 (**a**) Molecular structure of bisphosphonates: they are stable analogues of pyrophosphate with a central P-C-P binding instead of the P-O-P. The various bisphosphonates are distinguished one from another by the ligands R1 and R2. The bisphosphonates depicted here as small tongs are deposited on the surface of the bone in the resorption lacunae. Here they are taken up by osteoclasts or incorporated into bone by osteoblasts. (**b**) Diagrammatic representation of the four compartments of bisphosphonate absorption and excretion: Gastrointestinal tract, blood, bone and kidney

Fig. 29.2 (continued)

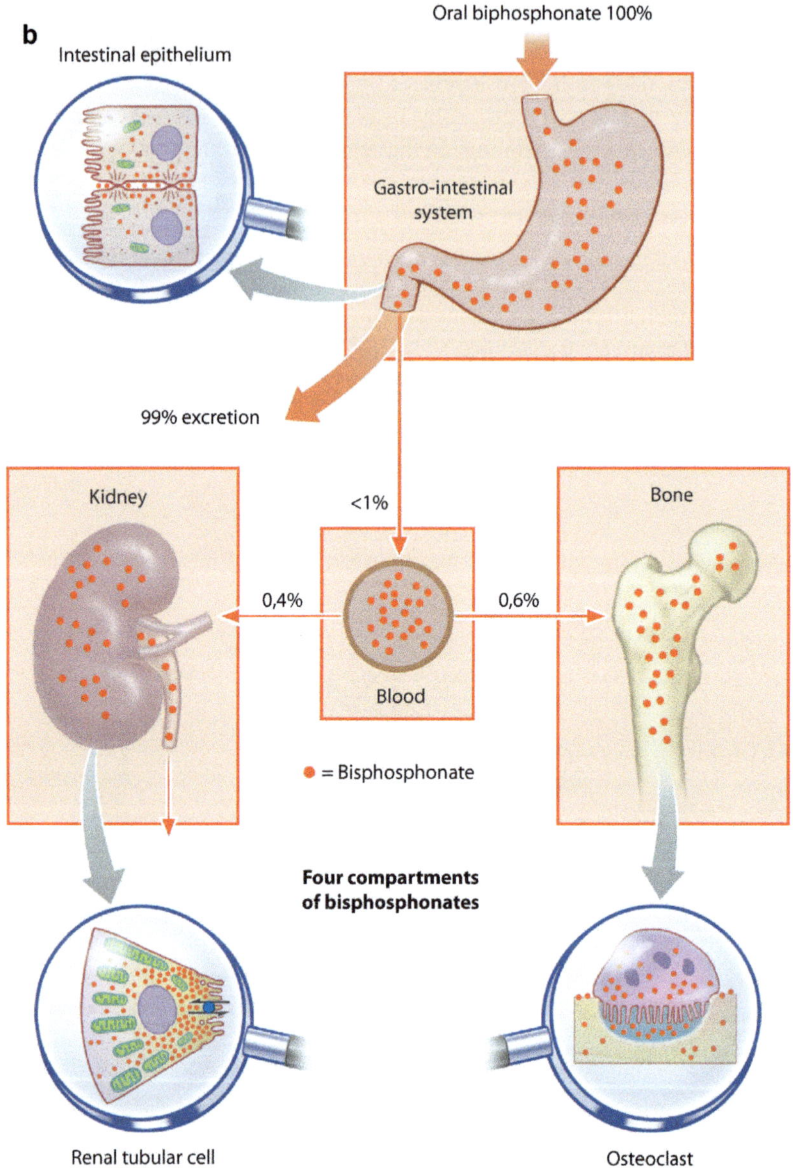

Table 29.1 List of available BP according to side chains and relative potency

Substance	Trade name	R1	R2	Relative potency
Etidronate	Didronel®	–OH	$-CH_3$	1×
Clodronate	Ostac®	–CL	–CL	10×
Pamidronate	Aredia®	–OH	$-CH_2-CH_2-NH_2$	100×
Alendronate	Fosamax®	–OH	$-CH_2-CH_2-CH_2-NH_2$	1000×
Risedronate	Actonel®	–OH	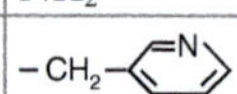	5000×
Ibandronate	Bondronat® Bon(v)iva®	–OH	$-CH_2-CH_2-NH_2-CH_3$ C_5H_{11}	10,000×
Zoledronate	Zometa® Aclasta®	–OH	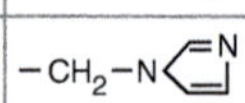	20,000×

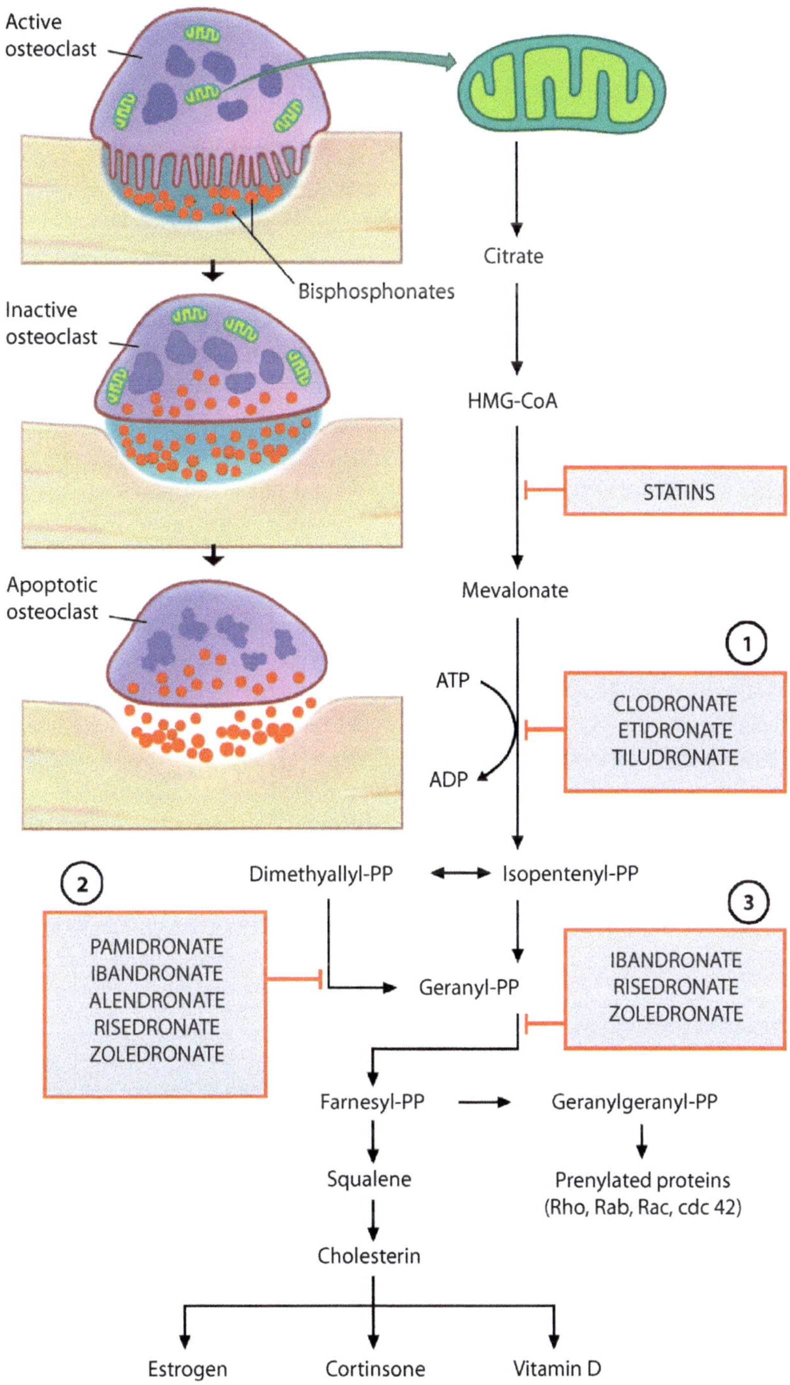

Fig. 29.3 Cellular and biochemical mechanisms of action of the nitrogen-containing bisphosphonates: *left*: layer of bisphosphonate (*red dots*) on bone beneath osteoclasts in resorption lacunae. The bisphosphonates are taken up by the osteoclasts which lead to their inactivation and retraction of the ruffled membrane. Higher doses lead to increased apoptosis of the osteoclasts. *Right*: biosynthetic pathway for sterols and isoprenoids, which takes place in the cytoplasm of the osteoclasts. Steps of inhibition by statins and bisphosphonates. *HMG Co-A* 3-hdroxy-3-methylglutaryl-Co-A, *PP* pyrophosphate. *1*, *2* and *3* show the different generations of bisphosphonates each with its own specific targets. Effects of the second and third generation lead to an accumulation of isopentenyl-PP, which in turn stimulates the acute phase reaction. However, this may be reduced by simultaneous administration of clodronate

long-term, inhibition of resorption results in a positive calcium balance with a continuous increase in bone mass, especially in trabecular bone because of its large surface area. Moreover the increase in bone mass is accompanied by an increase in mechanical resistance of the bone. BP and other antiresorptive agents improve *bone strength* by various effects:

- They reduce the size of the remodelling space and repair the resorption cavities caused by increased osteoclastic activity.
- They maintain the trabecular architecture, especially the horizontal trabeculae.
- They decrease cortical porosity.
- They increase mineralisation density by a prolongation of the bone formation period.
- They maintain osteocytic viability. Indeed, recent studies indicate that osteocytes act as mechanosensors and thereby participate in regulation of bone remodelling. There is also evidence that oestrogen, BP and raloxifene all prevent osteocytic apoptosis.
- They significantly alter maturation and properties of bone collagen suggesting a contribution of the organic matrix to the anti-fracture efficacy of these drugs. BP exert more profound changes in the organic matrix than raloxifene does, probably due to their more potent suppression of turnover (>50 % suppression).

The osteomalacia (disturbance of mineralisation) observed after long-term use of the first generation of BP has not occurred with the latest aminoBP (i.e. those with an amino group in one of the side chains) even after 8 years of therapy. Increases in mineralisation, in collagen maturity and in non-enzymatic cross-links have been observed after 3 years of therapy. Changes in lamellar structure of the trabeculae were also not observed. It has recently been reported that in dogs given a 6× greater than the normal therapeutic dose of alendronate or of risedronate, both drugs substantially decreased bone turnover, but there was an increase in histological microcracks. Moreover, there was a greater increase in bone strength in the alendronate and in the risedronate groups than in controls. To summarise, in humans none of the currently used aminoBP were found to have any deleterious effects on bone quality, estimated by preclinical mechanical testing and clinical fracture risk. Studies are available on the determination of the active ingredients in BP as well as reviews of the analytical methods applied.

However, one cautionary note: a recent investigation on the in vitro effects of pamidronate and alendronate on osteoblasts showed that these aminoBP inhibited osteoblast growth and caused osteoblast apoptosis. These inhibitory effects were observed at the same concentrations of BP that caused osteoclast inhibition. To what extent these in vitro studies reflect the in vivo situation remains to be determined.

Recent investigations have shown an antiproliferative effect of BP on growth of tumour cells. The inhibition of osteoclasts results in a reduction in the production of IL-6 and in the release of growth factors from the bone matrix. Evidence is also accumulating that BP have a negative influence on osseous and probably also on visceral metastases possibly by way of interactions with adhesion molecules on the tumour cells and/or by forming a film on the surface of the bone, which inhibits attachment of the tumour cells to the osseous surface. Data from studies on hyperlipidaemic patients with osteoporosis and on therapy with BP showed that these also have a beneficial effect on lipid metabolism. Table 29.2 summarises the main indications of BP.

Table 29.2 Disorders that benefit from BP therapy

All variants of osteoporosis
Paget's disease
Bone metastases
Primary hyperparathyroidism
CRPS I and II
Bone marrow oedema syndrome
Multiple myeloma
Fibrous dysplasia
Gorham's disease
SAPHO syndrome
Myositis ossificans progressiva
Drug-induced bone loss
Post-transplantation
Heterotopic ossification and calcification (etidronate)
Aseptic necrosis
Osteomyelosclerosis, painful

29.2 Pharmacokinetics

As mentioned above, the P-C-P bond is completely resistant to enzymatic hydrolysis. Consequently, the currently used BP are absorbed unchanged and are deposited on bone and eventually excreted. They are not metabolised in the body, and interactions with other medications do not occur. Intestinal absorption is minimal – somewhere between 1 and 10% and with the latest BP probably less than 1% (Fig. 29.4). Absorption may be further reduced if BP are taken with food or drink especially with bivalent salts such as calcium and magnesium. Consequently it is essential to ingest the BP on an empty stomach and only with water. The manufacturers recommend taking alendronate and risedronate with a full glass of tap water on an empty stomach half an hour before breakfast. The patient must remain in the upright position to ensure absorption and to avoid adverse reactions. The tablet should not be regurgitated together with gastric juices and remain in the oesophagus, because that could damage the mucus membrane. If a patient has difficulties in swallowing or there is a pre-existing reflux esophagitis, an alternative method of administration or a different therapy should be chosen.

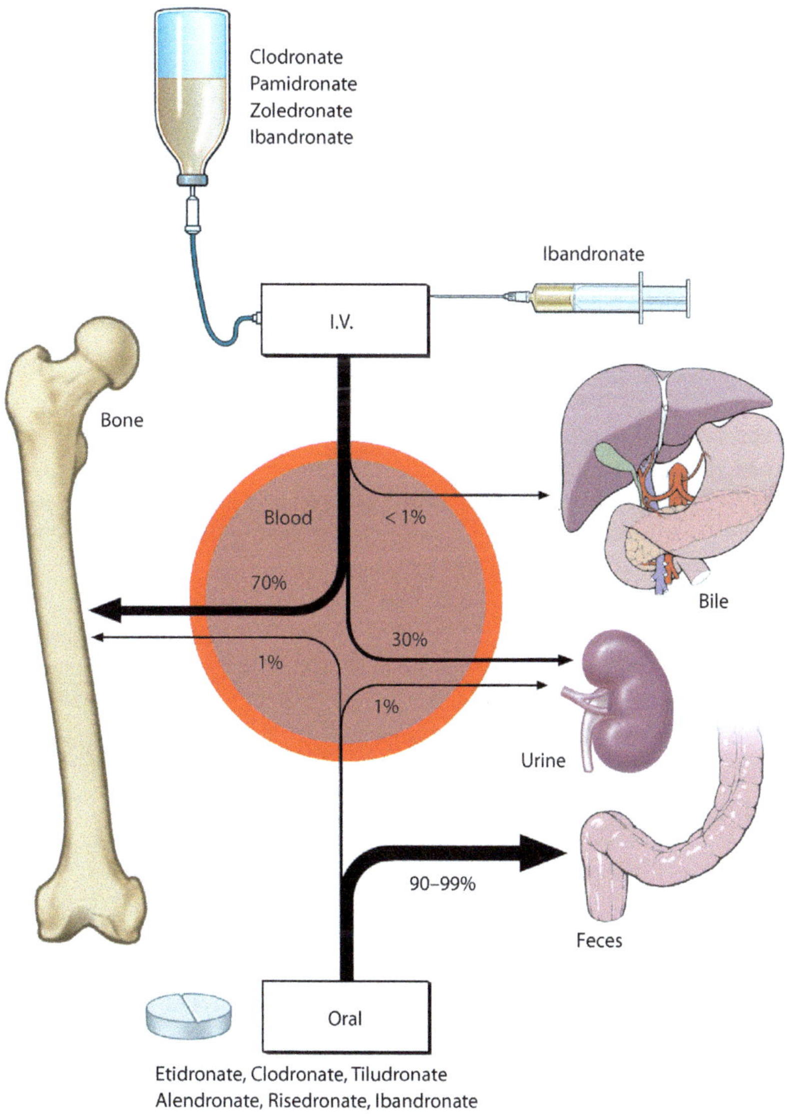

Fig. 29.4 Pharmacokinetics of bisphosphonates

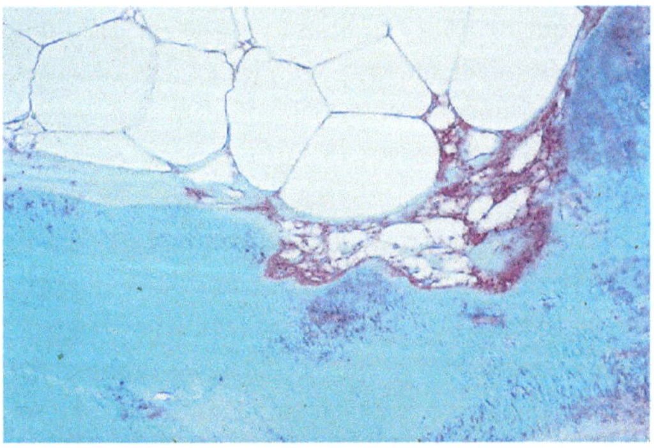

Fig. 29.5 Deposition of bisphosphonate (*red*) on bone in a resorption lacuna and in the cytoplasm of an osteoclast visualised by means of an antibody to ibandronate, in sections of a plastic embedded undecalcified iliac crest biopsy taken from a patient 2 days after 4 mg ibandronate i.v.

20–50 % of the absorbed bisphosphonate adheres to the surface of the bone (Fig. 29.5); the rest is excreted in the urine or the faeces during the day.

In contrast to its short stay in the peripheral blood (half-life of 1–15 h), the *half-life of BP in the bone* is much longer – a matter of years, as is the case for other substances such as tetracycline, which have a high affinity for bones. Individual BP may have different interactions with bone that result in differences in their pharmacologic behaviour. For example, risedronate has a lower kinetic binding affinity for the mineral substrates on the bone surface than alendronate does. These differences may contribute to the apparently shorter half-life of risedronate and to its faster clinical on- and off-responses compared to alendronate. Preliminary results suggest that ibandronate and zoledronate have higher kinetic binding affinities than alendronate and risedronate.

29.3 Toxicity

BP are very well tolerated when taken as prescribed. Side effects and adverse reactions are few and rarely severe:

- *Gastrointestinal complaints*: These have been reported in 2–10 % of the patients and include nausea, vomiting, stomach aches and diarrhoea. However, in large placebo-controlled studies, these were reported equally by both test and control groups. Inflammation and ulceration of the oesophagus, occasionally reported, can easily be avoided by strict adherence to the directions for taking the medication. Lesions of the mucus membrane occur in two stages. Regurgitation of gastric acid damages the oesophageal epithelium; aminoBP diffuse into the adjoining epithelial cells and inhibit synthesis of cholesterin (inhibition of the mevalonic acid pathway) which in turn prevents cholesterin-dependent repair of the damaged mucosal cells. Bedridden patients or patients with reflux esophagitis should not be given oral aminoBP or at best only under the strictest medical supervision.
- *Acute phase reaction*: This can occur within 24 h of the first intravenous infusion of an aminobisphosphonate. The reaction consists of a rise in temperature, joint and bone pains, myalgias, increase of IL-6 and C reactive proteins in the blood, as well as changes in lymphocyte counts.
- Very rarely an infusion or oral treatment must be stopped because of the outbreak of a *skin allergy* or photosensitivity.
- *Ocular reactions* have been observed, but very rarely (1/1,000 patients). Uveitis scleritis and episcleritis have been observed after pamidronate. With cessation of the infusion and administration of glucocorticoids, the ocular inflammation improved rapidly.
- About 3 % of patients who receive infusions of BP experience *moderate hypocalcaemia and hypomagnesaemia* which however do not require any medical treatment. AminoBP should not be given together with aminoglycosides since both medications reduce the calcium level in the blood which may last for considerable periods of time. We have not observed any clinically significant hypocalcaemia as a consequence of infusion of BP.
- *Renal function* should be checked before intravenous infusion of BP. Renal clearance of BP is accomplished by glomerular filtration and by active tubular excretion

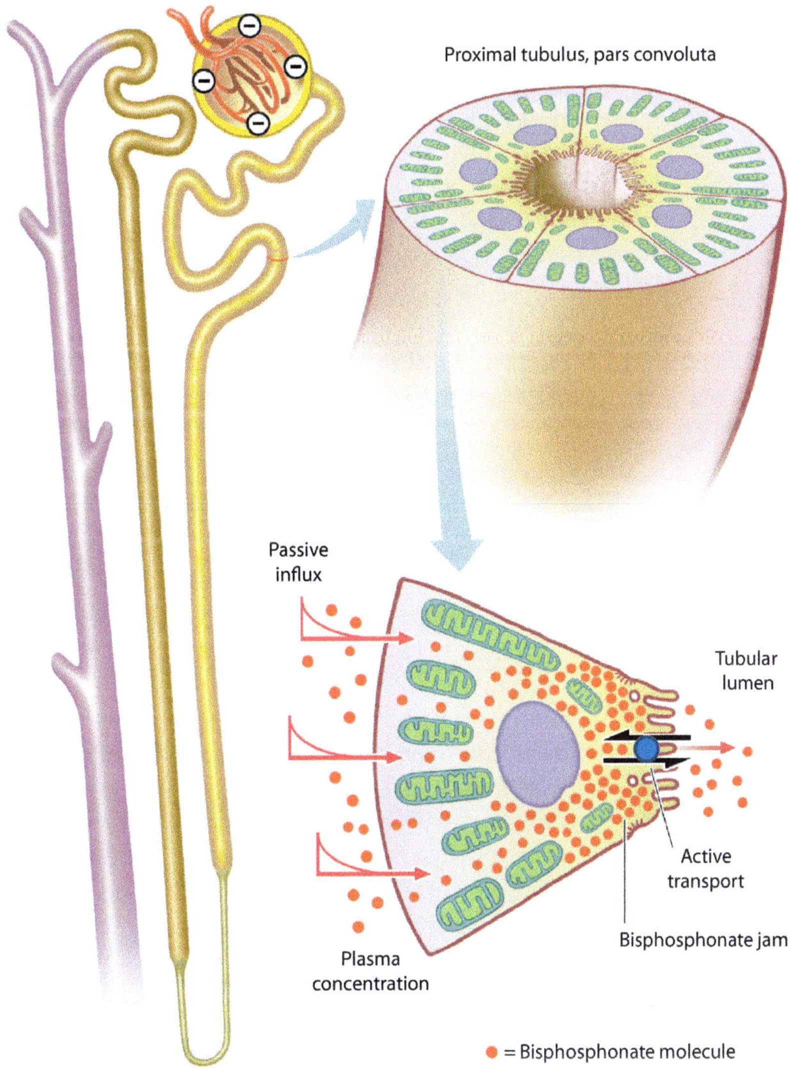

Fig. 29.6 Active elimination of bisphosphonate by renal tubular cells

(Fig. 29.6). At high dosages kidney pain may occur as well as mild, clinically non-significant albuminuria.

> Bisphosphonate should not be given to patients with GFR <30–35 ml/min and should be administered over 15–30 min. Other agents with nephrotoxic potential such as nonsteroidal anti-inflammatory drugs or diuretics and dehydration must be taken in consideration.

- No data on humans suggest that the administration of modern BP, at least in doses used for osteoporosis, interferes clinically with *fracture repair*. The amount of callus formed was either unchanged or was increased, but never decreased. The slowing of callus turnover was accompanied paradoxically by a higher mechanical strength.
- *Acute and chronic toxicity studies* using oral alendronate in female animals showed no evidence of mutagenicity, including those most relevant to human carcinogenic potential. Carcinogenicity studies in rats and mice at

maximum tolerated doses showed no increase in tumour incidence associated with alendronate treatment. There was also no effect on fertility or reproductive performance in male or female rats.

- *Low-energy fractures of the femoral shaft* (atypical subtrochanteric femoral fractures, AFF) have recently been observed in some patients on long-term therapy (> than 6 years) with alendronate. Alendronate users had a threefold higher risk of atypical fractures than women with risedronate. Cases of atypical fractures in users of intravenous BP (zoledronate or ibandronate) are very rare and only in longer-term use. The fractures had a simple transverse pattern and were presumed to result from propagation of a stress fracture presumed to be due to impaired repair of microdamage. One other previous study had identified low-energy femoral shaft fractures in some patients after an average of 4.8 years of therapy with alendronate. The speculation has been made that these atypical fractures of the femur were due to atypical skeletal fragility as a result of severely suppressed bone turnover, due to inherent conditions as well as to the prolonged antiresorptive therapy.
- *Atrial fibrillation* being possibly associated with bisphosphonate use was not confirmed in any trial and is generally discounted by most experts and by the FDA.

> There is no established causality between bisphosphonate use and atrial fibrillation or oesophageal cancer.

29.4 Osteomyelitis/Osteonecrosis of the Jaw (ONJ)

Numerous articles on the association of therapy with BP and the occurrence of osteonecrosis of the jaw (ONJ) have appeared in the international medical press since the publication of the first report of a single patient in 2003 (Fig. 29.7a–d). Many of these reports were published recently in the last few years, especially in 2008. Included are studies of related and possibly causative factors as well as retrospective investigations of large numbers of patients. The suggested associated factors include:

- Suppression of the activity of local macrophages by BP.
- Microfractures in heavily burdened jaw bones.
- Anomalies of the vascular system in the jaws. Studies have shown that the jaw bones have a greater blood supply than other bones as well as a high bone turnover rate, and therefore there is a high concentration of BP in the jaws.
- Infectious inflammatory processes during immunosuppression.
- Anti-angiogenic effects of BP leading to local necrosis.
- Inhibitory effect on local physiological processes in bone.
- Administration of BP oral or, mostly, intravenous.
- Enhancement of inflammatory/necrotising processes caused by prior or current chemotherapy and/or corticosteroids already present before administration of BP leading to an increased concentration of BP.

Many articles and position papers have been published on how to deal with the problem of ONJ (A survey in the book *Medication-Related Osteonecrosis of the Jaws* by S. Otto, Springer 2015). These include specific up-to-date practice guidelines. An excellent example is the Canadian Consensus Practice Guidelines for Bisphosphonate-Associated Osteonecrosis of the Jaw, June 2008. It should be stressed that the guidelines in this consensus were compiled with the collaboration of recognised, established authorities from all over the world. The guidelines include recommendations given by international experts as well as the results of evidence-based investigations for the avoidance, the diagnosis, the therapy as well as the management of the gums, of the jaws and especially of the patients themselves. However, relatively little attention has been given to the possible association of periodontal conditions with systemic disorders that may also be present, perhaps

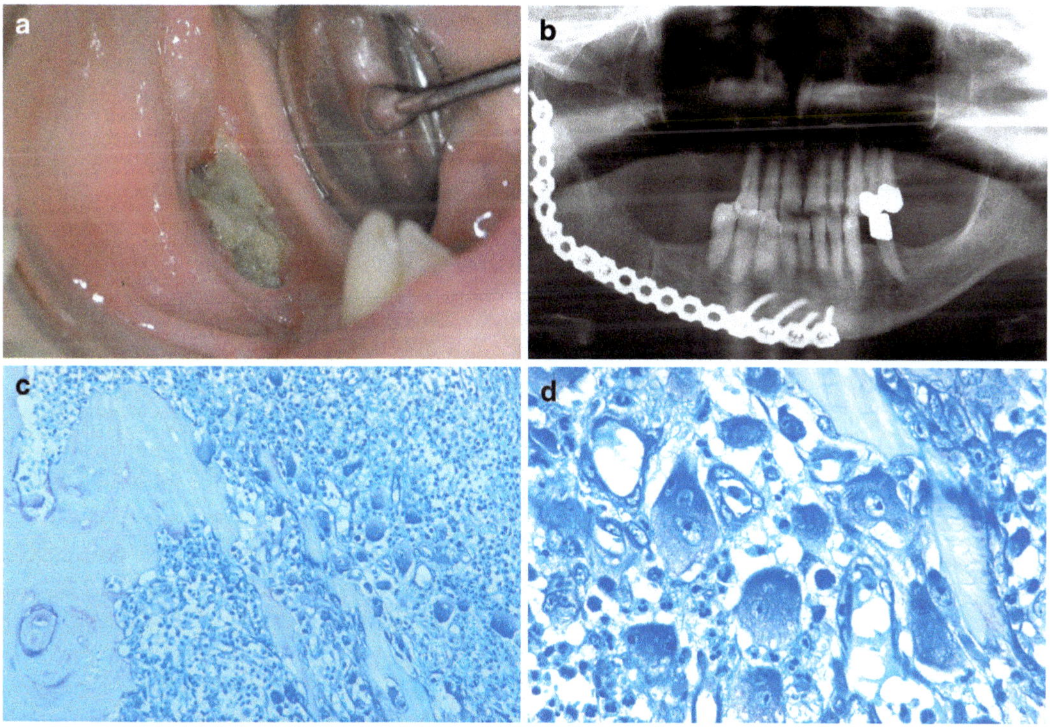

Fig. 29.7 (**a**) Osteoporosis of the jaw (ONJ) in a patient with breast cancer, 1 year after therapy with a bisphosphonate given monthly i.v., (**b**) surgical stabilisation of the necrotic area of the jaw, (**c**) histology of the necrotic jaw if the same patient showing chronic osteomyelitis with necrotic bone and osteoclastic resorption, Giemsa staining, (**d**) at higher magnification increase of large, multinucleated macrophages, lymphocytes and granulocytes in the surrounding bone marrow, Giemsa staining

even for longer periods of time and whether their management took the state of the jaws into consideration. These systemic disorders include diabetes and renal, respiratory and cardiovascular diseases. In elderly patients, such co-morbidities may have been present for quite a long time, and their presence as well as the therapy given could very well have impacted the state of the gums and the jaw bones.

As mentioned previously, the vast majority of the cases of ONJ reported so far represent only a minuscule % of the more than 20 million patients already treated with BP for many years. Many studies have confirmed that nearly all the patients who developed ONJ had malignancies. In one recent report in which the medical records of 1,086 patients were evaluated, the following percentages were calculated: 3.8 % per 100 with myeloma, 2.5 % per 100 with breast cancer and 2.9 % per 100 with prostate cancer had developed ONJ during the 5-year study. All these patients received BP i.v., which led to the hypothesis that there could be complex interactions between the BP and the chemotherapies the patients were receiving at the same time, and this possibly warrants further investigation.

In contrast, another study concentrated only on patients who were prescribed oral, not i.v. BP, and only for indications other than malignancies and who had developed ONJ. These patients were studied in order to identify potential contributing factors. The cases included 85 patients with osteoporosis, ten patients with Paget's disease and individual patients with other conditions. Most of the patients (9 % of 63 patients) who supplied dental information had undergone a dental procedure before the onset of the ONJ, and in addition 81 % of these patients had co-morbidities and were taking at least one other drug which affects bone turnover. The authors concluded that the circumstances of

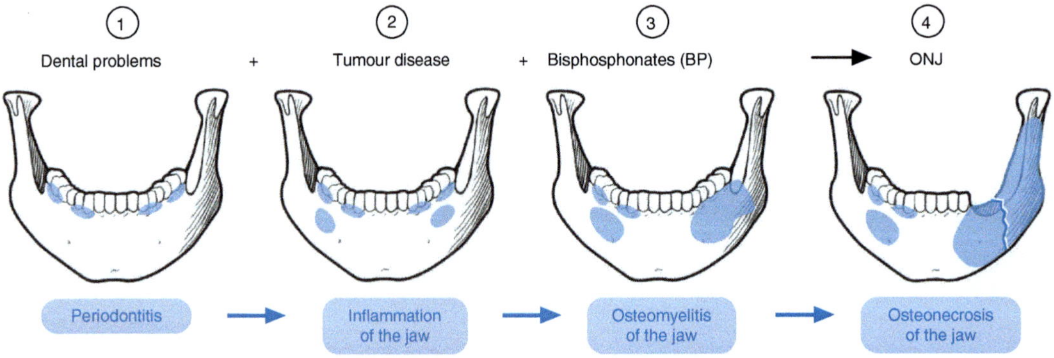

Fig. 29.8 Cascade of events and reactions in the development of ONJ in patients with neoplasias

each patient must be taken into consideration and that a multiplicity of factors may be associated with the development of ONJ (Fig. 29.8). Another study pointed out that ONJ is rare in metabolic bone disease and in Paget's disease, i.e. 1 per 100,000 person years. Interestingly, according to another study, smoking and obesity are strong risk factors for ONJ, which suggests that patients should be asked and, if necessary, advised on lifestyle factors before initiation of the bisphosphonate therapy.

To Summarise Osteonecrosis of the jaw has been reported in cancer patients receiving high doses of intravenous BP, especially pamidronate or zoledronate. The incidence of ONJ in osteoporotic patients treated with oral and/or intravenous BP is extremely low (in the order of 1/100,000 cases), and its causal relationship with bisphosphonate therapy has not been established. No causative relationship has been unequivocally demonstrated between ONJ and bisphosphonate therapy. ONJ occurred after tooth extraction. Furthermore, the underlying risk of developing ONJ may be increased in osteoporotic patients by co-morbid diseases. Finally, two studies have confirmed the hypothesis that genetic susceptibility may also participate in the host's reaction to bacteria: complex interactions between pathogenic bacteria and factors in the host's inflammatory reaction such as polymorphisms of interleukin 6 were shown to participate in the aggressivity of periodontitis, and this could represent one important genetic determinant in the individual patient's propensity to develop ONJ. On a more optimistic note, the FDA has recently approved the use of recombinant human platelet-derived growth factor (rhPDGF) for the repair of periodontal defects. PDGF is a crucial factor in the biological repair of many skeletal conditions, and it is anticipated that it will prove effective in the prevention and/or therapy of ONJ.

29.5 Contraindications

BP should be avoided during pregnancy and breast-feeding though adverse reactions in these conditions have not been reported. On the contrary, they have been used successfully in some patients both during pregnancy and lactation without any detrimental effect on mother or baby, as recently reported.

29.6 BP Currently Used in Osteoporosis

BP are now regarded as the treatment of choice for postmenopausal osteoporosis, due to proven efficacy and a good safety profile. NICE has recently recommended BP as first-line therapy in patients with established osteoporosis. The following oral BP have been approved so far:

- Alendronate 10 mg daily or 70 mg once weekly
- Risedronate 5 mg daily or 35 mg once weekly
- Etidronate 400 mg daily for 14 days every 3 months
- Ibandronate 150 mg monthly

Recommendations for intravenous therapy:

This has now gained a high degree of compliance, especially with patients who are already taking a number of other drugs orally. Additional advantages are 100 % bioavailability and no gastrointestinal side effects; moreover, the effects on bone density and fracture rate are comparable to those of oral therapy. The following dosages and time intervals are currently used:

The administration of BP at intervals of 3 months is based on the observation that a single intravenous dose inhibits resorption of bone for several weeks; zoledronate 5 mg i.v. every 12 months results in the same increase in bone density as a bisphosphonate taken orally daily, weekly or monthly.

Clodronate	600 mg infusion every 3 months
Pamidronate	30 mg infusion every 3 months
Ibandronate	3 mg infusion or injection every 3 months
Zoledronate	5 mg infusion annually

29.7 Duration of Therapy with BP and Long-Term Studies

The optimal *duration* of bisphosphonate therapy is 2–5 years, depending on the initial severity of osteoporosis and the subsequent increase in bone density. Three phases are recognised:

- *Repair* (up to 12 months)
- *Rebuilding* (6–36 months)
- *Maintenance* (24–60 months)

Bisphosphonate therapy is a matter of years – this must be explicitly explained to each patient and re-emphasised at the start of and during therapy. The highest rate of increase in bone density occurs during the first 12 months when the resorption lacunae are repaired and refilled with bone. During the rebuilding and maintenance phases, the increase is less because during these periods the trabecular structure and width are being restored. It is assumed that repair of the trabecular bone network and the increase in bone density during the first year of therapy are together responsible for the rather remarkable decrease in fracture rate which occurs during this period. An increase of more than 3 % in bone density under alendronate therapy showed about the same decrease in fracture risk as an increase of 3 % in bone density. Similar correlations were observed in patients on risedronate therapy: an additional decrease in fracture risk was not observed with bone density increases above 3 %. Annual increases in bone density of up to 10 % are possible, but do not necessarily imply a proportional decrease in fracture risk. Under risedronate therapy, markers of bone resorption show similar relationships. For example, a decrease in urinary NTX of more than 40 % did not lead to a further reduction in fracture risk.

There is relatively less increase in bone density during the phases of repair and maintenance because the increase in mineralisation is now in the foreground. On cessation of bisphosphonate therapy in postmenopausal women, there is a moderate decrease in bone density during the first year, more pronounced in the lumbar spine than in the hip; this does not occur in men. On completion of 1–3 years of treatment, results of annual measurements of BMD will determine when bisphosphonate therapy should be resumed. Some studies have already shown that the positive effect on mineral density of both cortical and trabecular bone as well as fracture reduction is maintained for 1 year after cessation of bisphosphonate therapy. This should be checked by BMD measurements in each patient.

Long-Term Follow-Up Studies Previous fears of a "frozen, poor-quality bisphosphonate bone" liable to microfractures "cracks" have not been confirmed. There is no evidence that remodelling might be turned off completely leading to frozen bone and increased bone fragility with the doses used clinically. Some studies in dogs have shown that treatment with very high doses of BP have caused increased microcracks. However, biomechanical and bone strength were preserved, so the relevance of increased microcracks is unclear, and results of long-term clinical studies of BP to date have allayed these fears. Clinical studies of alendronate and risedronate conducted for more than 7–10 years have demonstrated that bone density consistently increased by approximately 0.7 % per annum. Therefore, over a 10-year period, bone density increased by an average of 13 %. This indicates that apparently there is no time limit for therapy with BP – the one important factor is the state of the patient's skeleton, and this should be regularly monitored. The FIT Long-Term Extension study (*FLEX*) found that BMD decreases slowly on cessation of alendronate and bone remodelling gradually increases. Recent clinical studies have concluded that increased microdamage accumulation may occur in patients on prolonged alendronate therapy. These data suggest that clinicians might consider a "drug holiday" after 5 years of alendronate in lower-risk patients. Fracture healing in patients on long-term bisphosphonate therapy does not seem to be a problem, although there are only a few studies which have addressed this important issue.

> A recent publication of the FDA recommended 5 years of treatment to be followed by a "drug holiday", except for those remaining at high risk.

To *summarise*, results so far achieved:

- Over a period of approximately 1–3 years, 70 mg of alendronate is incorporated into the bones. With such a minute amount of bisphosphonate, when the skeleton contains 2,000,000 mg of hydroxyapatite, physicochemical damage is excluded for all practical purposes. The same holds true for the other modern BP. Moreover, disturbances of mineralisation do not occur with these BP.
- Under therapy with risedronate, patients have demonstrated a significant reduction of vertebral and non-vertebral fractures after a period of only 6 months. One year after discontinuation of 3 years' treatment with risedronate, the risk of new vertebral fractures remained lower in these patients compared to that in the control patients.
- After 7 years of therapy with alendronate or risedronate, the bone mass still increased by about 1 % a year, indicating that a basic positive bone balance remained unchanged. However, a "drug holiday" after 5 years of alendronate therapy is advisable to avoid any possible microdamage accumulation, at least in low-risk patients.
- Bone biopsy findings showed that after 7 years of therapy with alendronate or risedronate, the trabecular architecture and the lamellar structure of bone were both preserved and that microfractures were not found.
- The number of normal hydroxyapatite crystals increased, thereby rendering the bone more resistant to compression.
- In contrast, fluoroapatite crystals, which are incorporated into the mineral phase of bone during fluoride poisoning, though denser than hydroxyapatite crystals, are brittle and shatter easily.

> A recent large Danish cohort study (more than 60.000 patients) has shown, that long term adherent use of alendronate in excess of 10 dose years was associated with an adjusted 30 % lower risk of hip fracture and no increase in the risk of fractures of the subtrochanteric femur or femoral shaft.

The following parameters can be used to estimate *success of therapy*:

- Decrease in collagen breakdown products in urine and TRAP in serum. These biochemical markers of bone resorption provide the earliest information on the effects of therapy.
- Increase in biochemical markers of bone formation: alkaline phosphatase.
- Increase in BMD (DXA of lumbar spine and hip).
- Decrease in fracture rate (vertebral and extravertebral).
- Decrease in osteoporotic bone pain.
- Increase in quality of life and mobility.
- Decrease in duration of hospitalisation.
- Decrease in mortality (28 % under zoledronate!).

After 3–6 weeks of therapy, a decrease in markers of bone resorption should occur. If such markers have not been reduced by 30–40 % after 2–3 months of oral therapy, the patient should be questioned as to whether and in what form the drug was ingested and appropriate measures taken according to the circumstances. Subjective parameters such as pain, mobility and quality of life can only be accepted as secondary criteria.

Resistance to therapy does appear to occur in some patients when the usual parameters such as BMD remain the same as those of the control group not on bisphosphonate therapy. The patients described so far were elderly, obese and with type 2 diabetes. The lack of response was seen especially in vulnerable regions, such as the hip, femoral neck and forearm.

Bone mineral density (BMD) should be measured annually during therapy with a bisphosphonate; although, as shown in large studies of BP, the risk of fractures may be decreased even in the absence of a measurable increase in density. Should there be no increase in BMD after a year of therapy, four possibilities should be considered:

- Medication was not taken: Telopeptides (markers of bone resorption) should be checked.
- Medication was not taken according to instructions: Discussion with patient for information and clarification.
- Possible "non-responder" when therapy was indeed taken: change to intravenous administration of nitrogen-containing BP.
- Possibly the case is not that of a primary but a secondary osteoporosis: for example, an undiagnosed primary malignant disorder may be present. Investigations – including MRI and bone biopsy – must be carried out as quickly as possible.

Even when there is no direct correlation between increase in bone density and decrease in fracture risk under antiresorptive therapy, the measurement of bone density (DXA) is still the most practical and quantifiable parameter for estimation of fracture risk both within the framework of diagnostic evaluation and monitoring of therapy. In addition results of DXA measurements have worldwide acceptance which simplifies comparison of results of trials. Results of two large meta-analyses of vertebral fractures have conclusively demonstrated that the reduction of 24–54 % in risk of fractures under bisphosphonate therapy is unequivocally due to the increase in bone density. This relationship is even more pronounced with respect to non-vertebral fractures. These meta-analyses also indicate that BP increase bone density not only by inhibition of osteoclastic activity but also by their influence on osteoblasts and osteocytes (inhibition of apoptosis). BP improve the microarchitecture of bone and thereby also decrease the risk of fractures. This graphically illustrates the close corre lation between bone density, strength and microarchitecture.

Moreover, studies of bone biopsies have shown that the increase in bone density is closely connected to the improved microarchitecture of trabecular bone. This was demonstrated by Recker et al. by means of micro-CT and histomorphometry. Their results provide a convincing argument for DXA measurement in the evaluation of effects of bisphosphonate therapy on bone. These and other studies have demonstrated increases in trabecular thickness, as well as in numbers and connections, i.e. "the nodes" of the trabecular network while the porosity of cortical bone was also decreased. These micro-CT studies have clearly demonstrated improvement and preservation of the trabecular microarchitecture under bisphosphonate therapy. It should be mentioned that though increases in bone density usually occur under therapy; lower values have also been registered by DXA. This apparent paradox has been observed especially in hip measurements after 6 months of teriparatide therapy: decreases in DXA values occurred together with increases in bone surface areas. In contrast, measurements with QCT did register an increase in bone density. Under teriparatide therapy, measurements may show a decrease in density, but bone volume and strength are increased – therefore, this is only an apparent paradox, which can be explained by the fact that DXA measurements underestimate the increase in density only in the presence of an increase in bone surface.

In practice, the success of antiresorptive therapy depends on regular and consistent administration, i.e. patient compliance. However, as shown in one study, this is attained by only a small percentage of the patients. With introduction of the once weekly tablet, there was a 60 % increase in compliance; therefore, a further improvement is to be expected with the monthly tablet. The once monthly and possibly annual tablets (or i.v. administration) are expected to work wonders with compliance. Few studies have actually been carried out on compliance with long time intervals. One such study did show that a demonstrable increase in bone density contributes to better patient compliance with the therapy. The results of a comprehensive study on adherence to oral BP among 101,038 new bisphosphonate users demonstrated that age and type of fractures were two important factors in the determination of adherence. The results also showed that adherence was correlated with time, as there was a tendency for adherence to decrease from 1 to 3 years of therapy.

Other Drugs in Osteoporosis 30

30.1 Denosumab

Denosumab is a fully human monoclonal antibody, the first RANKL inhibitor to be approved by the FDA, now available for the treatment of osteoporosis, treatment-induced bone loss, bone metastases, multiple myeloma and giant cell tumour of bone. Precursors of osteoclasts, called pre-osteoclasts, express the surface receptor RANK (receptor activator of nuclear factor kappa B), a member of the tumour necrosis factor receptor (TNFR) family. RANK is activated by the ligand RANKL, which are cell surface molecules on osteoblasts. Activation of RANK by RANKL promotes the differentiation of pre-osteoclasts to active osteoclasts. Denosumab inhibits this maturation of osteoclasts by binding to and inhibiting RANKL. This reaction mimics the natural action of osteoprotegerin (OPG) and protects bone from resorption.

In June 2010, denosumab was approved by the FDA for use in postmenopausal women with risk of osteoporosis as the trade name *Prolia*™ and in November 2010 as *Xgeva*™ for the prevention of skeleton-related events in patients with bone metastases from solid tumours.

Prolia™	60 mg	s.c. injection	every 6 months
Xgeva™	120 mg	s.c. injection	given on days 1, 8 and 15 of a 4-week cycle and then once every 4 weeks

A meta-analysis in 2012 found that denosumab was more effective than placebo, zoledronate and pamidronate in reducing the risk of fractures in cancer patients. In those with osteoporosis however, it decreases the risk of fractures, but increases the risk of infections. Denosumab is a more potent inhibitor of bone resorption than are the BP. However, whether the persistent and marked inhibition of bone turnover with denosumab will have untoward skeletal consequences is not yet known ("oversuppression of bone turnover"). The rapid and complete reversal of the inhibition of bone turnover upon stopping denosumab therapy contrasts with the persistent effects of remodelling following withdrawal of nitrogen-containing BP. BP bind avidly to bone surface and may concentrate at sites of stress reaction or bone marrow oedema, denosumab

R. Bartl, C. Bartl, *Bone Disorders*, DOI 10.1007/978-3-319-29182-6_30

does not. On the other hand, unlike BP, denosumab have no sustained binding to the bone surface and are not incorporated into the bone matrix. The inhibitory effect of denosumab on bone resorption is thus more transient, and there is possible rebound effect, when the treatment is stopped.

Denosumab and BP are both antiresorptive, and their primary effect is inhibition of osteoclast recruitment (denosumab) and action (BP).

Prolia™ is administered as a single subcutaneous injection once every 6 months. No dose adjustment is required as a function of age or weight or in patients with impaired renal function. Denosumab administration resulted in a prompt and marked decrease of serum CTX, reached a nadir at about 1 month, then gradually increased during the 6 months between doses. Markers of bone formation decreased after 2–3 months of treatment and the response paralleled that which occurred under alendronate.

Adverse events occur in at least 5 % of the patients. The most common *side effects* are joint and muscle pain. There is also an increased risk of various infections (skin, abdomen, urinary tract and ear), eczema, rashes, hypocalcaemia, allergic reactions, pancreatitis, osteonecrosis of the jaw and atypical hip fractures. Probably the increase of infections under denosumab treatment might be connected to the role of RANKL in the immune system. RANKL is expressed by T helper cells and is thought to be involved in dendritic cell maturation. Because of the serious infections associated with the use of denosumab, the simultaneous use of immunosuppressants, chemotherapy and glucocorticoids can increase the risk of infections.

Denosumab is *contraindicated* in patients with hypocalcaemia, and sufficient calcium and vitamin D levels must be reached before starting denosumab therapy. Interactions with other drugs are not known. Similarly to nitrogen-containing BP, denosumab may increase the risk of osteonecrosis of the jaw (ONJ) following extraction of teeth or oral surgical procedures.

30.2 Selective Oestrogen Receptor Modulators

In the last decade, more and more oestrogen-like substances have been developed and introduced into clinical practice. These drugs bind to the oestrogen receptors (ERs alpha and beta) throughout the body. For example, *tamoxifen* had long been given to women with a history of breast cancer, after the initial chemo- and radiotherapy and surgery. It acts as an oestrogen antagonist on breast tissue but as an oestrogen on other organs and tissues in the body, namely, bone, liver and fat. Tamoxifen inhibits growth of any residual breast cancer cells remaining in the body if they still have oestrogen receptors. However, due to adverse effects, tamoxifen has been replaced by the *aromatase inhibitors*, for example, anastrozole.

30.2.1 Raloxifene

The positive effect on bone has been further developed in raloxifene, a SERM of the second generation which has no effect on breast or uterus. Raloxifene was originally investigated as a treatment for breast cancer. Uterine bleeding, breast tenderness and water retention are not observed with raloxifene. However, "hot flushes" and leg cramps occurred in about 30 % of previously asymptomatic patients, because raloxifene blocks all oestrogen receptors remaining in the body and thereby also the effects of the small amount of oestrogen that might still be produced. Leg cramps, especially nocturnal, can be treated by supplements of magnesium which is freely available; recommended amount is 300 mg daily. An international clinical trial, the *MORE* study, showed that the risk of a vertebral fracture in patients taking raloxifene is half that of a control group. After 3 years, raloxifene 60 mg daily increased the BMD by 2 3 % at the hips and spine and reduced the risk of new fractures by 30–50 %. New clinical vertebral fractures were reduced by 68 % after 1 year of therapy with raloxifene. The risk of breast cancer is significantly reduced (60–70 %) in women taking raloxifene. This effect was mainly due to a 90 % reduction of oestrogen receptor-positive breast cancer. The *RUTH* trial is evaluating this positive effect.

In summary, SERMs now constitute a new approach to therapy and have been approved for prevention and treatment of postmenopausal osteoporosis while decreasing the risks of cardiac and circulatory disorders without the unwanted side effects and risks associated with hormone replacement therapy. Raloxifene is considered to be suitable for older women, but its possible side effects must be taken into account and the patients must be informed. Recommended dosage is 60 mg raloxifene orally daily, without restrictions as to when the drug should be taken but preferably with supplements of vitamin D and calcium. Raloxifene is the treatment of choice for postmenopausal women, especially women with one or more of the following factors:

- With a high risk for breast cancer or cardiovascular diseases
- With a high risk of vertebral fractures
- With modest degrees of osteopenia in the postmenopausal period (age 55–65)
- With osteoporosis diagnosed by DXA in the postmenopausal period (age 55–65)

30.3 Peptides of the Parathyroid Hormone Family

Currently available and approved drugs for therapy of osteoporosis inhibit bone resorption. Their great clinical value lies in reducing the activity of the osteoclasts and thereby increasing BMD and reducing fracture risk. But new bone is not produced, and reduction of fracture risk, although highly significant, is rarely more than 50 % of the baseline risk level. A different therapeutic approach is osteoanabolic therapy, with stimulation of new bone formation, for which fluoride, strontium ranelate, GH, insulin-like growth factor, the statins and PTH are the main candidates in humans for short-term administration. However, it should be mentioned that continuously elevated calcium and PTH levels as in pHPT affect insulin sensitivity and result in increased insulin secretion, but the administration of rhPTH in the doses given in osteoporosis does not affect glucose homeostasis.

> Osteoanabolic action of PTH: paradoxical effects depend on type of administration

Parathormone (PTH) This hormone is a principal regulator of calcium homeostasis. It is a polypeptide with 84 amino acids. PTH stimulates release of calcium and phosphate from bone and synthesis of active vitamin D in the kidney which promotes calcium transport in the gastrointestinal tract. In addition, when given intermittently by injection, PTH stimulates osteoblastic proliferation and differentiation and new bone formation on all available osseous surfaces (Fig. 30.1) so that bone size is changed, while the number of osteoclasts and bone resorption remains unchanged. PTH has been shown to increase bone density, strength and connectivity by which it improves the microarchitecture of bone (Fig. 30.2). Indeed, it is the first treatment for osteoporosis that leads to the formation of new bone while preserving the bone's microarchitecture. However, the underlying molecular

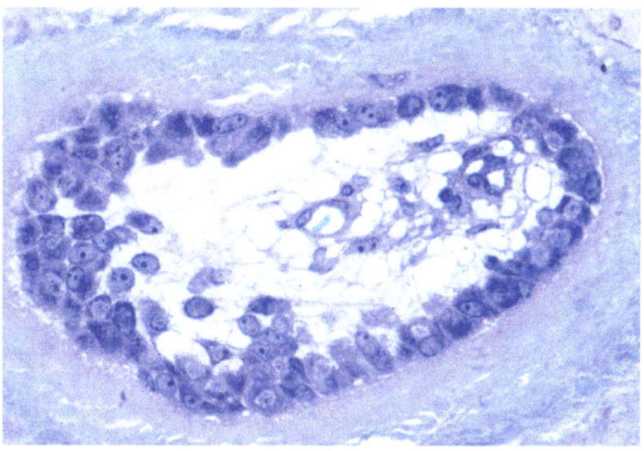

Fig. 30.1 Activation of osteoblasts and production of new bone under treatment with teriparatide

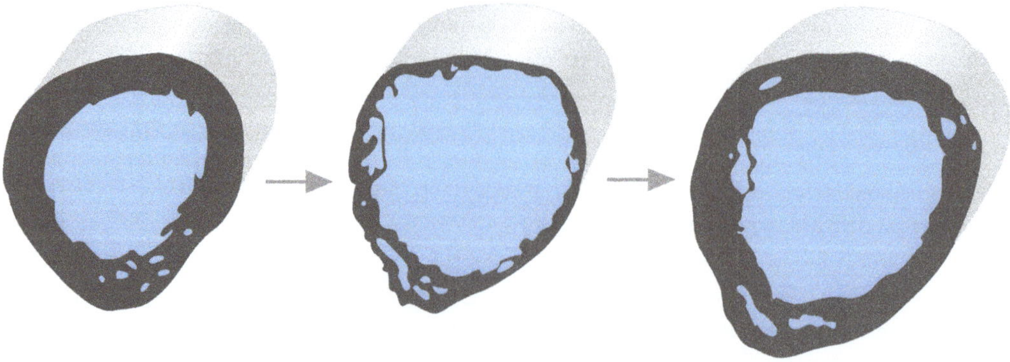

Fig. 30.2 Changes of cortical bone in osteoporosis and after treatment with teriparatide

physiology accounting for the true anabolic effect of PTH remains unknown. It is also not known why intermittent low-dose PTH administration differs so dramatically from continuous administration in its effect on bone cells. Recently, evidence has emerged that PTH reduces osteoblast apoptosis, prolonging osteoblast survival and potentiating its function of collagen synthesis. Studies on bone biopsies have confirmed these findings. Biopsies were taken before and after 18–36 months of therapy with PTH in both men and women. Results showed that PTH stimulates remodelling, resulting in an increased percentage of newly formed matrix but of lower mineral density. This would indicate that calcium and vitamin D supplements are required together with PTH.

Teriparatide (recombinant human PTH [1–34]) is the first of the bone-forming agents and has been approved in Europe and in the USA for treatment of postmenopausal osteoporosis and recently also of osteoporosis in men, with a treatment duration of 18 (Europe) and 24 months (USA). PTH stimulates bone formation and thereby induces a significant increase in BMD. Studies have already shown that age does not affect the efficacy or the safety of teriparatide. This PTH fragment is administered as a daily subcutaneous injection of 20 mcg dose. Adverse events include orthostatic hypotension, leg cramps, dizziness and injection site reactions. Metabolic changes may include hyper- and hypocalcaemia, hyperuricaemia or hypoparathyroidism. A major limiting factor with teriparatide is cost – approximately ten times the cost of bisphosphonate therapy. After completion of the 18-month course of teriparatide, it appears that fracture protection persists when followed by an antiresorptive agent (e.g. alendronate). Indeed, the administration of an inhibitor of resorption (bisphosphonate or raloxifene) after treatment with PTH potentiates its skeletal benefit. Moreover, osteoporotic patients with previous long-term exposure to antiresorptive agents also showed positive effects on BMD and markers of bone formation under therapy with PTH.

Results of many studies have now been reviewed, and these have demonstrated a significant reduction of vertebral and non-vertebral fractures in the treated patients, with or without prior antiresorptive therapy. *Full-length PTH* [1–84] is also available and provided significant protection against a first vertebral fracture in a high-risk population of postmenopausal women with osteoporosis. PTH 1–84 also provided significant protection against further fractures in women who had already experienced one osteoporotic fracture (*TOP* study). PTH 1–84 is administered as a daily subcutaneous injection of

100 mcg. The possible adverse side effects of the two formulations are similar; hypercalcaemia was observed in 14 % of the patients treated with full-length PTH. More studies are needed to determine when and if PTH monotherapy should be used and which patient population would benefit most from PTH or teriparatide. It is of interest that case reports of individual patients have shown that therapy with teriparatide can also enhance fracture healing.

Due to the high cost and need for daily injection, teriparatide is mainly indicated in patients with severe manifest osteoporosis with multiple low trauma fractures. Other candidates for teriparatide include patients with severe side effects under BP and severe osteoporosis in younger individuals.

30.4 Strontium Ranelate

Strontium is a divalent cation that is closely chemically related to calcium. Strontium ranelate contains two atoms of stable strontium and an organic moiety (ranelic acid). Strontium increases pre-osteoblast replication, osteoblast differentiation, collagen type 1 synthesis and bone matrix mineralisation. In low doses strontium increases the density of the spongy bone. It reduces resorption and stimulates formation of bone, leading to a gain in bone mass and improved bone mechanical properties (Fig. 30.3). In other words, strontium uncouples the activity of the osteoclasts and osteoblasts, in favour of bone formation.

Strontium, with a higher atomic number than calcium (38 versus 20), will absorb more X-rays and therefore results in an overestimation (up to 50 %) of the increase in bone density using DXA methods.

Strontium was well tolerated, and the most common adverse events were nausea and diarrhoea, which are usually reported at the beginning of treatment. An increase in the incidence of venous thromboembolism (VTE) has been reported.

Strontium ranelate should be used with caution in:

- Patients with severely reduced kidney function
- Patients at risk of developing a blood clot
- People at risk of heart disease, including high blood pressure, diabetes and smoking
- The original trial programme demonstrated a 60 % increase in the risk of myocardial infarction. Therefore, this finding suggests that strontium is unlikely to have a net beneficial effect in osteoporosis and its use is declining as a consequence.

30.5 Calcitonin and Fluoride

Calcitonin is a polypeptide hormone produced by the parafollicular C cells of the thyroid. It inhibits the osteoclasts by binding to specific receptors on the cell surface. Calcitonin can be given as a subcutaneous injection or in a nasal spray. However, the use of calcitonin is limited because of its side effects such as feelings of heat as well as nausea and mucosal irritation with the use of the nasal spray. However, the drawbacks of frequent injections and the high costs if nasal application preclude the long-term use of calcitonin as a first-line therapy of osteoporosis. The most valid indication for calcitonin today is the acute, intractable pain caused by a vertebral fracture, though even here its use is limited because of the superior results of intravenous BP. On the other hand, the calcitonins are physiological peptides which can be metab-

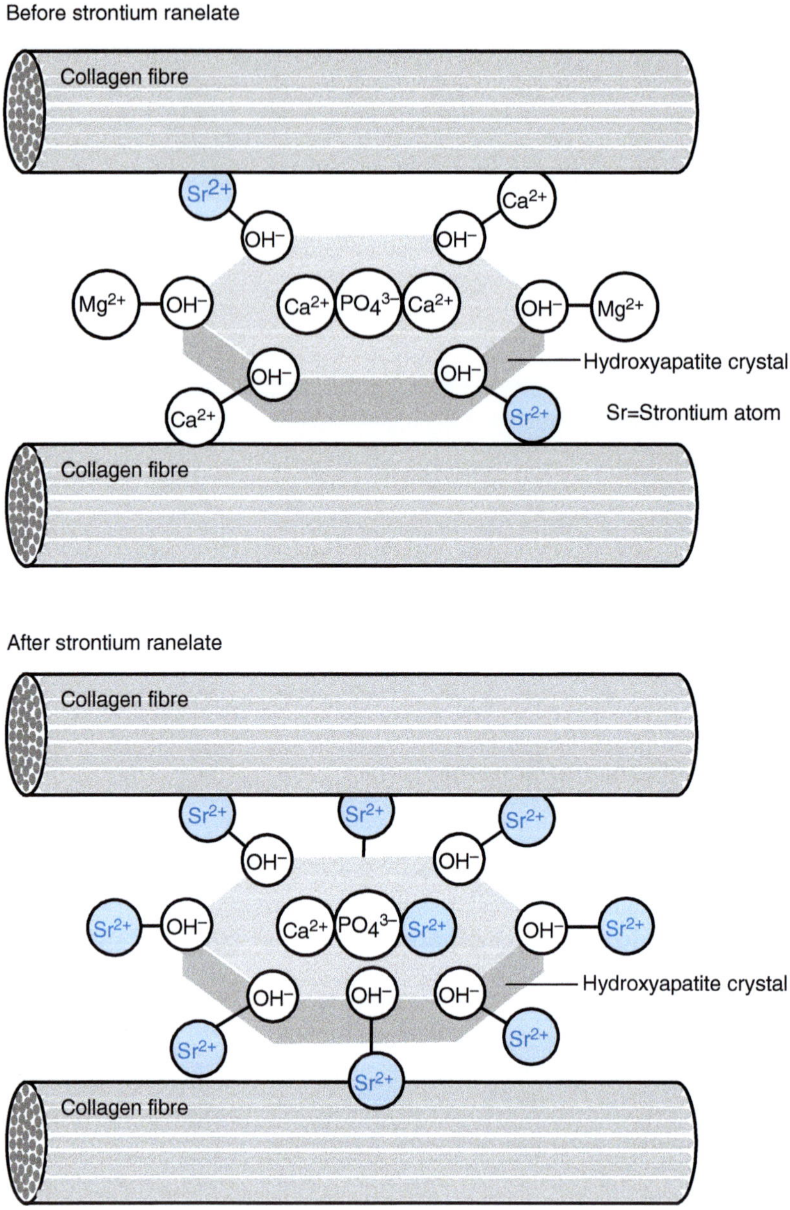

Fig. 30.3 Deposition of strontium in the hydroxyapatite crystals between the collagen fibres

olised and therefore are not retained in the body. Toxic effects have not been reported. Calcitonins are therefore suitable for children and in pregnancy and during breast-feeding. The calcitonins target the active osteoclasts and thereby reduce resorption, but have little effect on osteoblasts, so that the speculation has been made that it could lead to a continuously positive bone balance. Currently efforts are underway to produce an oral formulation to improve patient acceptance and compliance, which would enable clinical trials of its efficacy. Consequently, calcitonin may not yet be a "drug of the past".

Fluoride is still used in some countries for treatment of osteoporosis because of economic considerations, but its role in prevention of

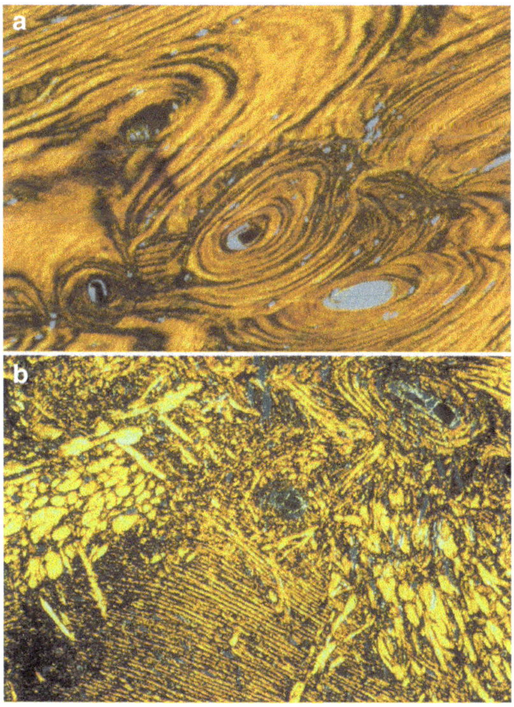

Fig. 30.4 (**a**, **b**) Bone quality under therapy: (**a**) normal lamellar bone under long-term therapy with bisphosphonates, (**b**) altered lamellar bone structure with topographic disorganisation under long-term therapy with fluoride

fractures has not been confirmed in clinical trials. The recommended dose ranges from 20 to 200 mg sodium fluoride daily (elementary fluoride constitutes half of this amount): there is general agreement that fluoride stimulates osteoblastic bone formation and thereby increases bone mass. But mechanical resistance of the newly formed bone is poor, and it is even liable to fracture easily. Fluoride is incorporated into the crystal instead of the hydroxyl group in hydroxyapatite, thereby changing crystal size and conformation, which in turn produces poor quality woven bone (Fig. 30.4a, b). A high dosage of fluoride results in increases in bone density, but vertebral fractures are not significantly reduced. Moreover, especially with high doses, there are serious adverse reactions:

- Gastrointestinal side effects: epigastric complaints, vomiting and diarrhoea.

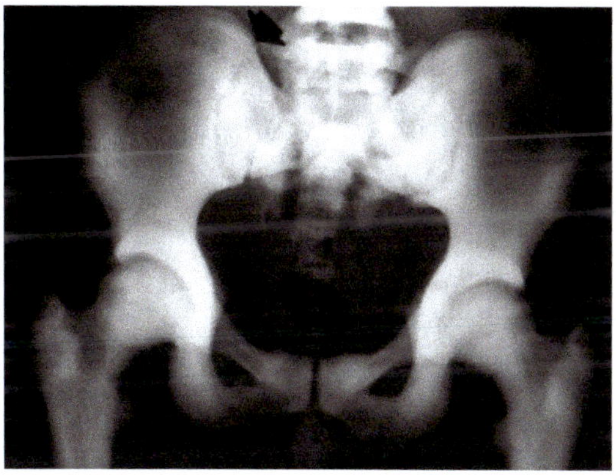

Fig. 30.5 Iatrogenic fluorosis with thickening of bone

- Lower extremity pain syndrome (LEPS): pains in the hips, knees and ankles. The cause may be delayed microcallus formation in the affected areas of these bones.
- Iatrogenic fluorosis: severe cases can be identified on X-rays as overgrowth and thickening of the bone (Figs. 30.5 and 30.6). This may be due to incorrect treatment. The patient sometimes increases the dose without medical advice because of continuing complaints and pain. However, it is not known whether there is an individual tendency to develop fluorosis.
- Exostoses and calcium deposits in the ligaments.

The latest clinical trials indicate that much lower doses (e.g. 15 mg daily) should be given over 3–4 years and always together with vitamin D and calcium. It is not known whether intermittent fluoride has any advantages over continuous administration, and the long-term effects have also not yet been clarified. Slow-release sodium fluoride at a lower dose (50 mg/day) appeared to be associated with reduction of fracture risk in one study, but confirmation of these results is not yet available. However, because of the various side effects and the availability of other efficacious agents, fluoride treatment is presently not recommended and also not approved by the FDA for treatment of osteoporosis.

Summary

When and how to intervene in osteoporosis (according to I.R. Reid 2014)?

- A 10-year hip fracture risk of 3 % or osteoporotic fracture risk of 15–20 %.
- BP are still the most widely used medications, and intravenous preparations (once a year) are most effective and convenient.
- In early postmenopausal osteoporosis, HRT may be an alternative.
- Denosumab is preferred in patients with impaired renal function and more severe disease.
- Teriparatide and PTH are, because of cost, reserved for patients at highest fracture risk and massive bone loss.
- Vitamin D supplements should be always provided for those with low-vitamin D levels in the serum.
- The use of calcium supplements is seldom justified.

30.6 Combination and Sequential Therapies

When the response to a medication is inadequate or ineffective, the doctor in charge will either change the drug or substitute another with a different mechanism of action, in order to achieve a satisfactory therapeutic result. In this context the example of the treatment of established high blood pressure is relevant. The patient usually receives several medications with different mechanisms of action in order to decrease the blood pressure to the desired level on the one hand and to minimise the side effects on the other. Although it would appear that this strategy is also applicable to the treatment of osteoporosis, some specific problems have cropped particularly with monitoring the therapy. Various studies have demonstrated that patients on therapy may definitely have a reduction in fracture risk even in the absence of a demonstrable increase in bone density. Moreover, changes in levels of markers of bone resorption under antiresorptive therapy do not always correlate with the fracture risk.

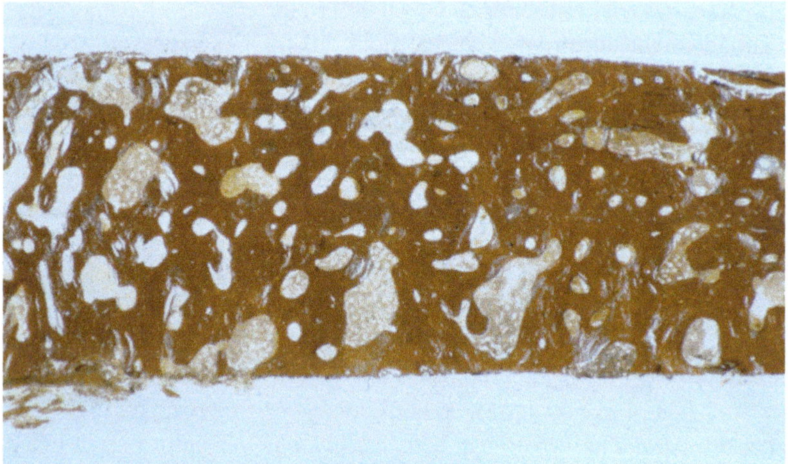

Fig. 30.6 Iliac crest biopsy of a patient with fluorosis showing marked osteosclerosis of the whole biopsy

A combination of two antiresorptive agents results in a more pronounced decrease in bone resorption which induces a greater increase in BMD than either drug alone. But studies of patients on this type of combination therapy utilised bone density measurements and bone remodelling markers as parameters, and not, unfortunately, the reduction in fracture risk – a decisive clinical criterion! The combination of SERMs and BP also provides an additive increase in BMD, but again, the use of this combination remains questionable in terms of fracture reduction and also from a pharmacoeconomic perspective.

If hormone replacement therapy (HRT) is used for a limited period of time for the management of climacteric symptoms, concomitant use of bisphosphonate may provide a further reduction in bone turnover and an additional increase in BMD. Studies have shown that such a combined treatment group had a significantly greater increase in spinal and femoral neck BMD than the increase in BMD seen by either oestrogen or alendronate alone. A greater effect on BMD also occurred with combined oestrogen and risedronate, than with either one alone.

In patients previously treated with HRT, several trials have examined the effect of adding PTH and have shown significant increases in spinal BMD, suggesting that the prior exposure to the antiresorptive HRT does not blunt a subsequent response to PTH. Therefore, patients pretreated with inhibitors of bone resorption who have not achieved a full therapeutic response are good candidates for treatment with anabolic agents.

Another important question is whether the combination of a *bisphosphonate and PTH* would provide a therapeutic advantage, but results of trials reported so far have not provided any evidence of synergy between BP and PTH, neither in postmenopausal women nor in men. Consequently, if therapy with PTH is contemplated, it should be given alone and not together with a bisphosphonate. However, treatment with alendronate immediately after the discontinuation of PTH further increased the BMD in the following year. Therefore, treatment with PTH should be followed by antiresorptive therapy to consolidate the gains made during treatment with PTH (Fig. 30.7a, b).

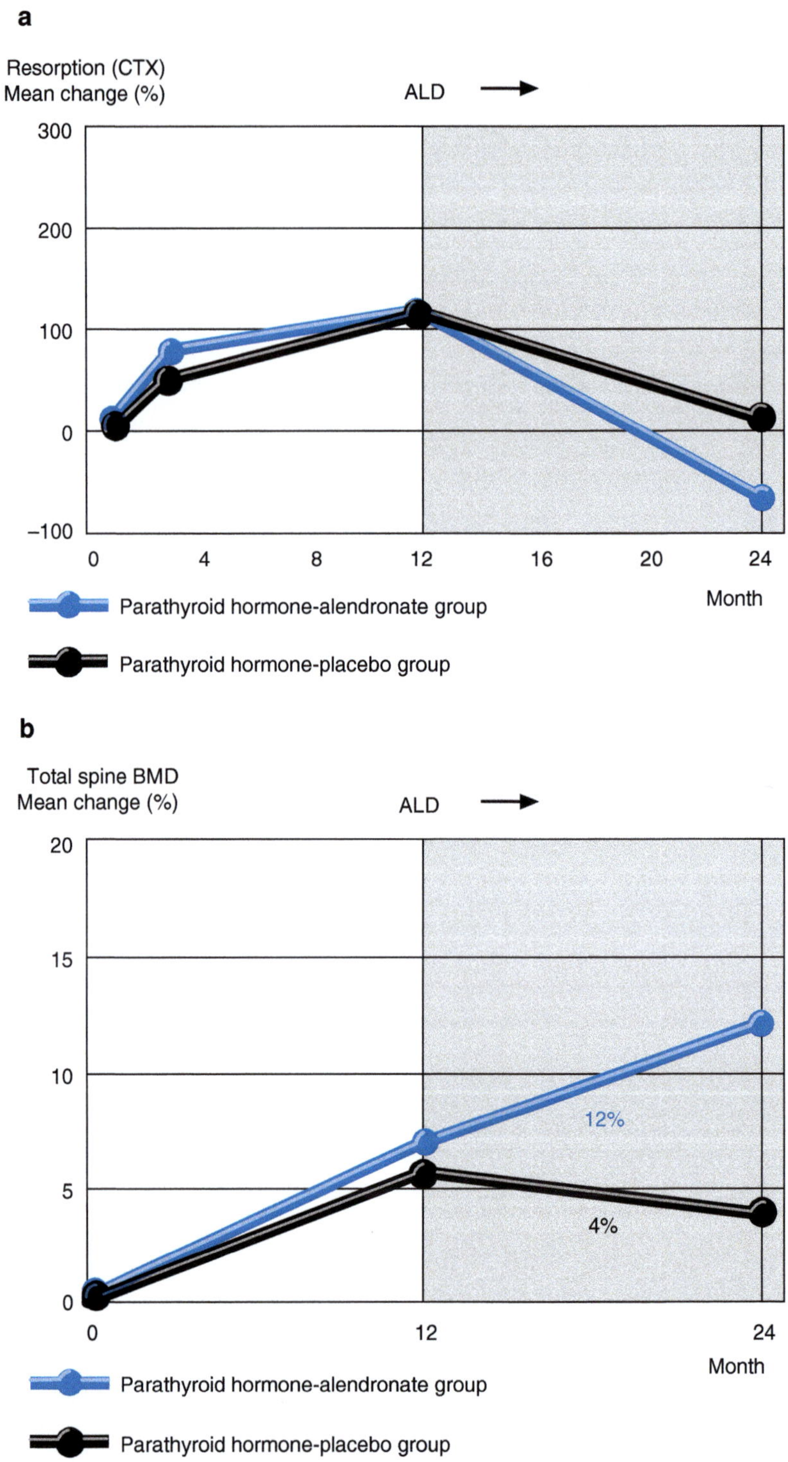

Fig. 30.7 (**a**, **b**) Treatment with alendronate (ALD) immediately after the discontinuation of PTH: (**a**) resorption marker (CTX) and (**b**) BMD of the total spine

31 Adherence and Monitoring of Osteoporosis Therapy

31.1 Adherence to Treatment

Non-adherence to medical treatment or lack of perseverance over time is a worldwide health problem in all chronic conditions, especially asymptomatic ones. It has been estimated that only half of the patients comply with long-term therapy. A large proportion of patients discontinued treatment with BP, and a majority of these did not even renew their first prescription. Adherence, although enhanced by less frequent dosing, was suboptimal in all of its aspects, i.e. acceptance, persistence and compliance (Fig. 31.1). Furthermore, risk of non-adherence increases with increased duration of treatment. In osteoporosis and osteopenia, non-adherent patients have smaller decreases in rates of bone turnover, smaller increases in BMD and a greater risk of fracture. Patients may be encouraged to adhere when presented with results of measurements of BMD or bone turnover indicating positive effects of the therapy. Compliance is also increased by utilisation of simplified and user-friendly treatment modalities such as tablets given weekly or monthly and infusions given every few months or annually. When discussing adherence or non-adherence, usually three definitions are used in the literature:

- Persistence: indicates for how long the drug is taken
- Compliance: indicates the proximity to the treatment recommendations as given in the official product information
- Primary non-adherence: when the patient has never taken the prescribed drug

Studies have shown that the regular analysis of markers of bone turnover as well as annual DXA tests to monitor bisphosphonate therapy increase persistence. Therefore, measurements of markers after a few months of therapy may provide useful information on efficacy of the therapy and improve persistence. One large study was designed to compare adherence rates between patients with one or more of seven different conditions. The results showed that adherence rates for osteoporosis medications were among the lowest (36.8 %). Younger patients (<60 years) had poorer adherence than older ones, and as co-morbidities increased, adherence among subjects with osteoporosis decreased. A population-based study carried out in Canada (Perrault, 2008) found that only 2 % of women with prior fractures were on long-term therapy with antiresorptive drugs. However, results of a recent investigation in Denmark 2008 showed that persistence has improved, both by men and

R. Bartl, C. Bartl, *Bone Disorders*, DOI 10.1007/978-3-319-29182-6_31

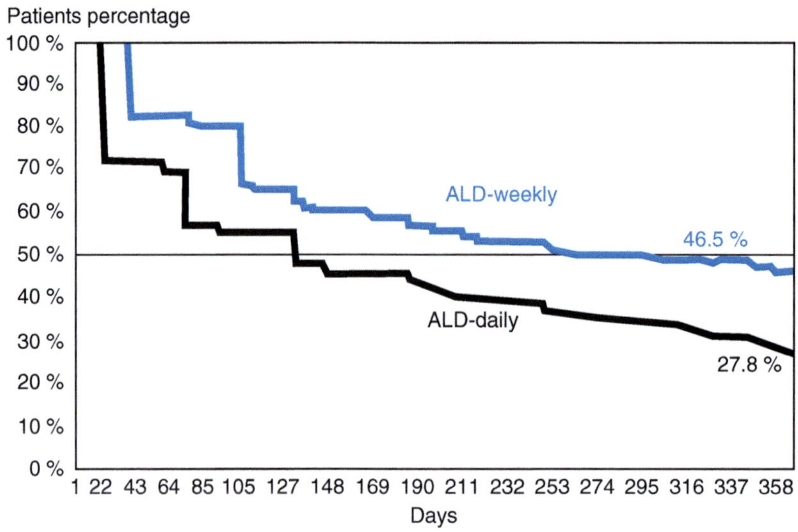

Fig. 31.1 Evidence of better compliance with alendronate (ALD) weekly versus alendronate daily

women. One large-scale study of 4,994 postmenopausal women in 33 states in the USA has been initiated to evaluate the impact of characteristics of patients and of their doctors on compliance and persistence with osteoporosis medications: the Prospective Observational Scientific Study Investigating Bone Loss Experience. This study includes 4,994 postmenopausal women, and results are awaited at the end of 2008.

31.2 Monitoring of Treatment

Patients who are not on drug therapy should be checked and evaluated at regular intervals, taking into consideration the baseline values established at diagnosis, as well as the patient's individual risk factors. Bone density (DXA) should be checked every 1 or 2 years (Fig. 31.2). A documented decrease in height of more than 2 cm or acute back pain could be symptomatic of a fracture. In such cases, immediate radiological investigation is required and further measures as indicated by the results. Since the goal of drug therapy in a patient with osteoporosis is to increase bone strength and so to decrease the fracture risk, the efficacy of osteoporosis-specific agents is monitored by means of changes in BMD and in biochemical markers (BCM) of bone turnover, although neither is a perfect indicator of response to therapeutic interventions. Patients on therapy with drugs should initially be checked every 3–6 months for the first 2 years and subsequently at 6–12 months. For evaluation of the efficacy of the therapy administered, measurements of bone density are only partially valid, but nevertheless should be checked every 2 years. A lack of increase in bone density does not necessarily imply reduction of fracture risk (Fig. 31.3). However, in some medical centres, annual DXA measurements are preferred for the following reasons:

- To encourage regular intake of the tablets
- To emphasise the necessity of long-term therapy measured in years
- To motivate the patient by demonstration of the increase in bone density

Psychology has always been an important intrinsic factor in the success of medical treatment. The patient's preferences must always be taken into consideration if at all possible especially type and frequency of administration. With long intervals, the following are advised: regular communication between patient and doctor, possibly reminders of when the next dose is due and, as indicated above, blood tests for bone turnover markers or BMD measurements of

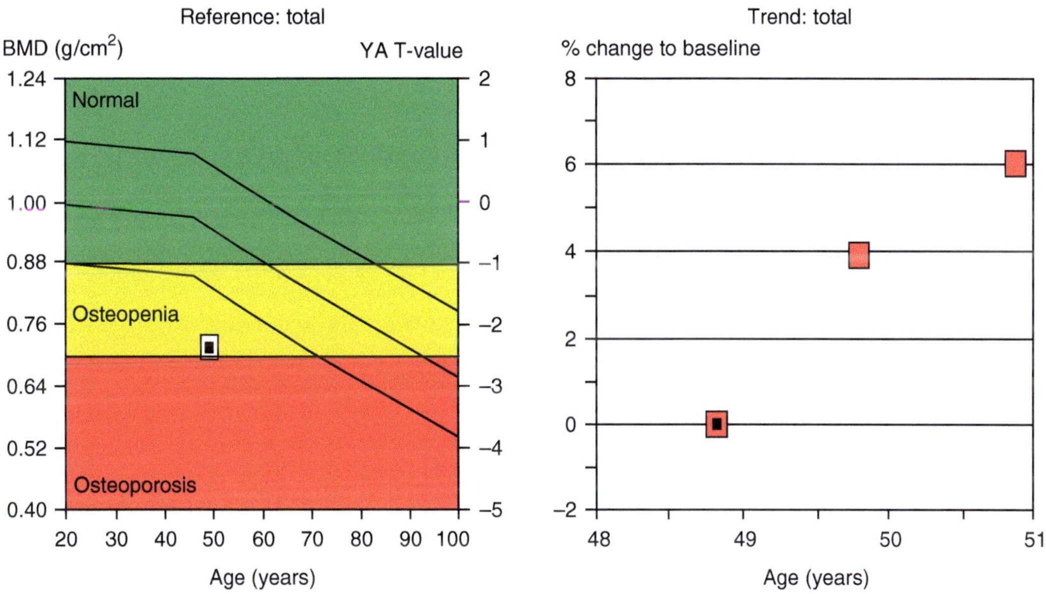

Fig. 31.2 Continuous increase of bone density (BMD) of the lumbar spine (L1–L4) under bisphosphonate therapy. Annual monitoring using DXA measurement

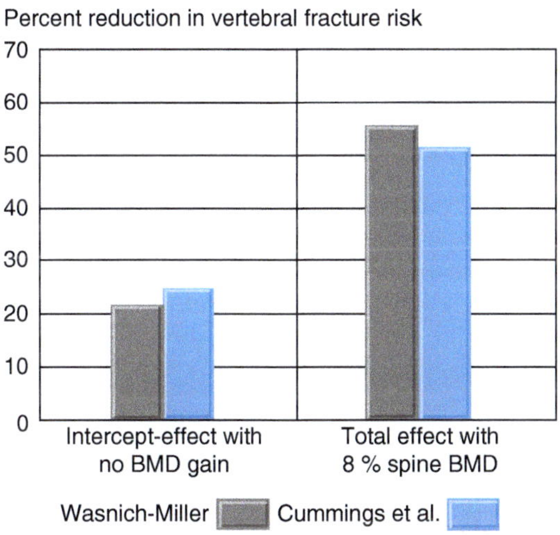

Fig. 31.3 Two meta-analyses showing the relationship between change and no change in vertebral BMD and reduction in vertebral fractures (Data from Wasnich R and Miller P 2001 Antifracture efficacy of antiresorptive agents is related to changes in bone density. *J Clin Endocrinol Metab* 87:1586–1592; Cummings S, Karpf D, Harris F et al. 2002 Improvements in spine bone density and reduction in risk of vertebral fractures during treatment with antiresorptive drugs. *Am J Med* 114:281–289)

crucial bone areas, e.g. hip or vertebra for encouragement by demonstration of progress. The details of the long-term monitoring of patients on antiresorptive and on osteoanabolic therapy are outlined below. When dealing with assessment of response to therapy, racial and ethnic differences may occasionally be observed due to the polymorphisms in the vitamin D receptor (VDR) and in the oestrogen receptor-alpha (ER-alpha) loci, which may vary in different populations.

31.3 Monitoring of Antiresorptive Therapy

It is now recognised that the increase in bone strength induced by antiresorptive treatment is only partly due to the increase in bone density. The reduction in the rate of fractures is also dependent on additional parameters, but these cannot as yet be accurately assessed by application of current methodology. These factors include:

- Increase in extent of mineralisation
- Reduction in the rate of osseous remodelling
- Repair and refill of the resorption pits
- Stabilisation of the trabecular microstructure
- Changes in cortical bone remodelling
- Changes in bone geometry

Meta-analyses of large randomised trials have retrospectively investigated the relevance of bone density and of the levels of markers of bone remodelling in the reduction of vertebral and non-vertebral fractures. Two meta-analyses concluded that 24–54 % of the reduction in vertebral fractures was due to the increase in bone density, while the reduction in non-vertebral fractures was attributed almost entirely to the increase in bone density. The observations also indicated a close correlation between the increase in bone density and the decrease in markers of bone remodelling; changes in bone turnover markers have been confirmed as reliable and significant indicators for assessment of response to therapy. Obviously, reduction in bone remodelling can also lead to changes in microarchitecture as well as in bone strength, but neither of these is necessarily manifested by changes in bone density. After treatment with alendronate, increases in BMD at both the joint and the hip were associated with reductions in the risk of non-vertebral fractures. However, for patients treated with risedronate or with raloxifene, changes in BMD did not reliably predict the degree of reduction in vertebral (raloxifene) or non-vertebral (risedronate) fractures. In these cases, the monitoring can be accomplished by utilisation of the parameters of antiresorptive therapy. Recent, up-to-date studies have demonstrated that changes in biochemical markers of bone remodelling under therapy more sensitively reflect the decrease in fracture rate as a result of the antiresorptive therapy. However, to what extent these investigations will be applicable in routine practice is still an open question. One important advantage of the application of osseous markers in monitoring is that "non-responders" can be recognised after only 1–3 months of therapy. The LSC (least significant change) is 25 % for markers of bone formation and 40–65 % for those of bone resorption. When the resorption markers decrease by about one third of the initial value (i.e. at diagnosis), the following assumptions can be made:

- The patient has taken the medication.
- The medication has been adequately resorbed.
- A biological effect on the bone has occurred.

In clinical trials the "response" rate to BP proved to be more than 90 %.

31.4 Monitoring of Osteoanabolic Therapy

When the bones to be measured have enlarged under osteoanabolic therapy, the actual increase in bone mass (bone mineral content, BMC) does not show up in the results of a DXA measurement because this is based on the following equation: bone mineral density (BMD) = BMC/area (g/cm^2). Consequently, the relatively lower density indicated by the DXA measurement is not a result of loss of bone mass, but is due to enlargement of the ossified area measured. The clinical relevance of this apparently paradoxical effect was demonstrated in a study with teriparatide. A head to head comparison of the density of the forearm was carried out using the results of DXA and pQCT measurements. While on therapy with teriparatide, the forearm is enlarged as shown by pQCT as well as by three-dimensional analyses of bone biopsies. In contrast, lower values were obtained by DXA measurements. Nevertheless, bone strength was increased, and the fracture rate of the forearm was reduced. Moreover, similar results were obtained on measurements of the hip bones. The increase in osseous remodelling stimulated by the PTH therapy first results in endosteal bone formation together with "trabecularisation" of the cortical bone. Shortly thereafter, subperiosteal bone formation leads to enlargement of the contour of the bone as well as an increase in bone mass. During the first year of therapy, this structural change is reflected in the DXA measurement as a reduction in bone density (BMC/area), while the pQCT measurements more accurately reflect the positive effects of PTH therapy. However, when correctly interpreted, DXA can still be considered the "gold standard" even for monitoring the effects of osteoanabolic therapy. Increases in BMD account for approximately one third of the vertebral fracture risk reduction with teriparatide. A larger proportion (up to 74 %) of the anti-fracture efficacy of strontium ranelate might be explained by changes in BMD of total hip. BMD monitoring of patients treated with osteoanabolic agents appears to be more informative than results of monitoring when patients were treated with antiresorptive substances.

31.5 Some Criticism of Contemporary Practice in the Literature

In recent publications, Reid (2014) and Järvinen et al. (2015) discussed the efficacy, effectiveness and side effects of contemporary drugs used to prevent and treat fractures. The WHO published diagnostic criteria for osteoporosis in 1994, and every physician was made aware that a decrease of 1 SD in BMD measured by DXA doubles the risk of fractures. Accordingly many physicians were prescribing drugs against osteoporosis to millions of otherwise asymptomatic persons on the basis of reduced BMD values alone. However, many of current beliefs and concepts in osteoporosis are debatable, and indeed, there is yet the possibility for improvement in our existing management of osteoporosis and fractures. Current prevention and treatment strategies for fragility fractures depend on the opinion that these fractures are mainly caused by osteoporosis, that the patients at high risk can be identified by DXA measurement and that the risk can be reduced by bone-targeted drugs.

However, a systematic review of all available RCTs showed no statistically significant reduction in hip or wrist fractures for women who have no prior fracture or vertebral compression at baseline. This represents the majority of women currently treated with BP and identified by BMD measurements. For secondary prevention, the incidence of hip and wrist fractures was decreased by BP, but the absolute benefit is small (1–1.3 %). Three Cochrane reviews of etidronate, alendronate and risedronate came to similar conclusions: no significant reduction in hip fractures for primary prevention and a small but statistically significant reduction in hip fractures for secondary prevention. "In secondary prevention, the small benefit of oral BP outweights the side-effects during the first 3 years of therapy, but harms outweight benefits for durations greater than 3 years".

Most fracture patients have fallen, but do not have osteoporosis, and the likelihood of falling is attributable to an ageing-related decline physical functioning and general frailty. Fractures are therefore primarily caused by falls, including the vertebral fractures. The higher incidence of fractures in women is attributable to a higher incidence of falling, not to lower BMD.

In the publication of Järvinen et al. (*Journal of Internal Medicine*, 2015, 277:662–673), the following critical questions with regard to diagnosis, prevention and treatment of low-trauma fractures have been discussed:

- To what extent do fracture patients have osteoporosis?
- Is fracture risk inherited?
- Are vertebral fractures truly osteoporotic?
- Do fractures cause excess mortality?
- Is BMD an adequate surrogate of individual bone fragility?
- Are fracture prediction tools useful for an individual risk assessment?
- Does the existing evidence justify wide-scale use of bone-targeted pharmacotherapy?
- Is bone-targeted pharmacotherapy safe?
- Is osteoporosis different from other risk diseases?

Summarising, the authors raised a final question: "Given all this, should "osteoporosis" be added to a long list of diagnoses, for which doing less, or even nothing, is better than our contemporary practice?" Perhaps new emerging therapies may give a more optimistic answer in the future. For any new class of drugs indicated to prevent fractures, it is essential that a clinically meaningful reduction in hip fractures without serious harms can be demonstrated before licensing.

32 Future Directions

None of our current therapies restore skeletal mass and strength to normal. Even the most effective drugs reduce hip fracture risk by only 40–50 % and are associated with side effects or intolerance. In all the current pharmacologic approaches to osteoporosis, whenever decreases or increases in the activity of one cell line are induced, the changes in the same direction occur in the "coupled" cell lines. Thus, whenever an antiresorptive agent reduces bone resorption by inhibiting differentiation and/or function of osteoclasts, there will also be a reduction in osteoblast function. Likewise, whenever osteoblast function is increased, there will be an increase in osteoclast function. This linkage limits the current therapies for osteoporosis. Future agents which could "uncouple" these activities, even temporarily, would enable unopposed bone formation, thus attaining greater increases in BMD, and more directed modulation of bone architecture to improve bone strength. Pharmacologic intervention in the control of osteocytes, the most abundant cell in the bone, is a further interesting and promising target in bone research.

32.1 New Forms of Established Drugs

The SERM raloxifen, now called "*estrogen agonist/antagonist*", reduces vertebral fracture risk but has not been shown to reduce the incidence of hip fractures. Three new agents in this class have been tested, but, for example, bazedoxifene and arzoxifene did not show advantages to raloxifen.

Oral formulations of *calcitonin* had a greater effect on BMD than has nasal calcitonin, but phase III fracture trials demonstrated no effects on fracture risk reduction.

A new formulation of *risedronate* is enteric coated to prevent dissolution of the tablet in the stomach and can be given after breakfast once weekly.

Oral, nasal and transdermal routes of delivering *teriparatide* are currently tested. Other PTH molecules and a PTHrP analogue are being studied.

32.2 Emerging Drugs

Shorter-Acting Antiresorptives: Cathepsin K Inhibitors, Integrin Antagonists and Prostaglandins These newer antiresorptive agents may alter osteoclast function with a much shorter biologic half-life and bone residence time than the BP. They have short duration of activity and are not stored in human tissue.

32.2.1 Cathepsin K Inhibitors

Cathepsin K (CatK) is an osteoclast-mediated product that is required to participate in the degradation of type I bone collagen, the major component (90 %) of organic bone matrix

R. Bartl, C. Bartl, *Bone Disorders*, DOI 10.1007/978-3-319-29182-6_32

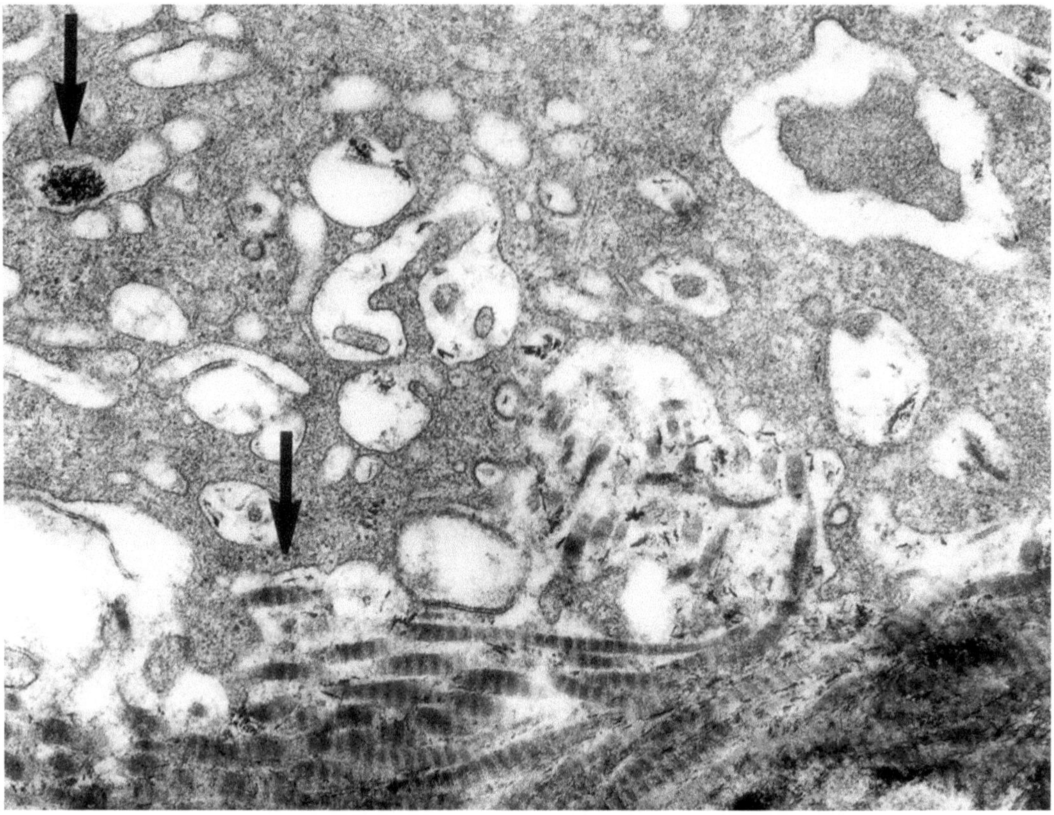

Fig. 32.1 Osteoclastic resorption of collagen fibres (*centre*) and mineralised bone matrix. Note fragments of both in osteoclastic vacuoles (*arrows*). EM

(Fig. 32.1). Inhibiting CatK suppresses the capability of osteoclasts to resorb bone matrix without reducing the number, activity or survival of osteoclasts and does not affect other osteoclastic functions such as creating a local acidic environment. Overall bone formation is not decreased; therefore CatK inhibitors may be classified as "indirect anabolic" drugs.

Four CatK inhibitors have been evaluated in preclinical and clinical studies. Anti-cathepsin K (odanacatib) is already in phase III clinical development programmes for investigation of its potential as an inhibitor of bone resorption. Results of a 12-month phase IIB study with odanacatib 50 mg once weekly demonstrated a significant increase of 3.4 % in lumbar spine BMD, an increase of osteoclasts when assessed by histomorphometry and a reduction of 57 % in sCTX and of 18 % in sBSAP (bone-specific alkaline phosphate). This modest decrease in bone formation could be used to differentiate CatK inhibitors from other antiresorptives and combinations with osteoanabolic agents. Osteoblastic activity is maintained on the endosteal surfaces. CatK inhibitors could also be used for preventing or treating osteoarthritis and metastatic bone disease.

> CatK inhibitors may be "indirect anabolic" drugs by significantly reducing bone resorption while sparing osteoblastic bone resorption. Odanacatib has a long half-life, allowing 1-weekly administration.

They can be taken orally once a week. The potential therapeutic utility of using integrin inhibitors to interfere with integrin-mediated events in osteoporosis and other metabolic and metastatic bone diseases is both exciting and promising. Osteoclast adhesion involves several integrins, and therefore integrin antagonists may be a logical mechanism-based approach to therapy of osteoclastic bone resorption in osteoporosis and bone metastases.

32.2.2 Sclerostin Antibodies

Antiresorptive drugs do not reconstruct the bone, but until recently, no therapeutic approach was available to restore bone once it had been lost. That situation has changed with the development of PTH as a highly effective anabolic therapy. Another promising way for a potent anabolic effect is the inhibition of the WNT ("wingless type and integrase") pathway, using antibodies against sclerostin. Sclerostin is produced in the bone exclusively by osteocytes and suppresses the differentiation of osteoblasts. Indeed, in preclinical studies, monoclonal antibodies against sclerostin (e.g. romosozumab and blosozumab) have been shown to promote bone formation rapidly. Inhibiting sclerostin induces a pure anabolic response, without any increase in bone resorption. Consequently, anti-sclerostin therapy can be used to treat patients with osteoporosis even until they have normal bone density and bone strength. Increases in bone formation rates and in the amounts of trabecular bone were shown in studies, without increases in resorption parameters.

> Inhibition of sclerostin induces an anabolic response not accompanied by an increase in bone resorption. Even severe osteoporosis may be reversed and "cured". First clinical data are encouraging. Inhibitors of CatK and sclerostin are interesting prospects for the next generation of osteoporosis drugs.

In 2014 the first phase II study with romosozumab has been published. The treatment was effective, generally well tolerated and safe, and severe side effects have not been reported.

Leptin This is a hormone with many diverse functions. It is produced by fat cells, acts as a "saturation hormone" and influences glucose metabolism and the production of sex hormones. It has long been known that sex hormone deficiency stimulates bone resorption while overweight inhibits it. This underlies the speculation that bone mass, body weight and sexual glands are regulated by a common mechanism in the brain. Attempts are currently underway to influence the level of leptin or its receptors and thereby develop a novel way to treat osteoporosis.

Growth Factors These are produced primarily by cells in the bone marrow, and they regulate the proliferation, function and interactions of bone cells. There are various regulators of bone formation – such as PTH, insulin, growth hormone and cortisone which all function by stimulation of growth factors in particular bone cells. In one clinical trial, bone formation was increased simply by the administration of one of these factors. It is anticipated that in the not-too-distant future, individually "tailored" growth hormones will be administered for the different types of osteoporosis. Prostaglandins also modulate metabolism of the bone. PGE2 has a distinctly anabolic effect on trabecular bone – presumably by stimulation of proliferation and differentiation of the precursors of osteoblasts.

Vitamin D_3 Analogues Novel analogues have been synthesised and examined for their action on the bone. In vitro studies showed that such analogues act on osteoblasts to suppress RANKL-dependent formation of osteoclasts, so that they could be considered as potential candidates for therapy of pathologically increased resorption.

Statins These are given for lowering concentrations of fat and cholesterol in the blood. Women who were treated with statins showed a higher bone density and a lower fracture risk than comparable women who had not been treated with statins. Animal studies have shown that statins shorten the life span of osteoclasts and thereby inhibit resorption of bone. Should this positive action of statins on the bone be confirmed, then statins could become an effective drug for the prevention of arteriosclerosis and of osteoporosis. But statins have one disadvantage: they act on the liver and therefore will never replace the bone-specific BP in the treatment of osteoporosis, though the mechanism of action of the two drugs is similar. The statins when administered orally are almost totally cleared during their first passage through the liver. It is still unclear how the statins reach the bone and how they affect bone turnover. It is also still a mystery how the statins can stimulate bone formation while the bisphosphonates, utilising the same pathway, inhibit bone resorption. Nevertheless, in the future specific statins selected for their high affinity to the bone may be useful agents for prevention or treatment of osteoporosis. The indications for such agents will be varied and numerous if they benefit both the skeleton and the cardiovascular systems.

Tetracyclines (Chemically Modified Tetracyclines, CMTs) These prevent bone resorption by inhibition of matrix metalloproteinases, as well as induction of apoptosis in osteoclasts. The possible applications and the risks of these agents are being tested in clinical trials.

ANGELs (activators of non-genomic oestrogen ligands) are another new paradigm of biology that are being investigated and may prove to be an entirely new approach to modulation of the skeletal tissue.

Oxytocin promotes osteogenesis at the expense of adipogenesis, and animal experiments have shown that administration of oxytocin to ovariectomised mice reversed bone loss and reduced marrow adiposity. Application in humans is under investigation, both as a serum marker for osteoporosis and as potential therapy.

Many other potential points of possible intervention in the complex mechanisms in control of skeletal metabolism are under investigation. A few examples would be different polymorphisms in steroid hormone receptors, delivery systems for bone morphogenetic proteins to induce the generation of new bone in special circumstances and injection of autologous mesenchymal stem cells – as osteogenic cells – to augment healing processes in the bone.

Part VIII

Osteoporotic Fractures

33 Epidemiology of Osteoporotic Fractures

Osteoporotic fragility fractures are a major public health problem around the world. The US National Osteoporosis Foundation estimates that currently more than 40 million American individuals, over the age of 50 years, are at risk of fracture, and this number will increase to 61 million by 2020. Due to the demographic change, the incidence of osteoporotic fractures will at least double until the year 2040.

Even with the emergence of highly efficacious treatment agents for osteoporosis, fractures are only reduced by about 50 %, leaving the other 50 % to suffer the consequences. Not only are osteoporotic fractures debilitating; they also have a high mortality rate. Swedish studies have concluded that more than 1 % of all deaths are related to hip fractures.

> It has been estimated that about 25 % of people over 50 years of age who suffer a hip fracture will die within 1 year.

Although a stagnation in the age-specific hip fracture incidence, for both men and women, was observed over the last decade in a Scandinavian study, there were no improvements in the survival after hip fracture, suggesting that frailty among these elderly individuals is high. The estimated lifetime risk for individuals over the age of 50 years to suffer an osteoporotic fracture is about 40 % for women and 13 % for men. These lifetime risk numbers are expected to increase in the future, as life expectancy increases in parallel.

Fractures associated with low bone mass can occur at many sites in the skeleton, but are most frequent in the proximal femur, spine, wrist, proximal humerus and pelvic ring.

> Over 75 % of these fractures occur in patients over 65 years of age. Associated clinical complications include pain, functional decline and disability, as well as loss of independent living.

These so-called *fragility fractures* result from low-level trauma that would not normally cause the bone to fracture. In the USA alone, osteoporosis is responsible for over 1.5 million fractures annually: 700,000 vertebral fractures, 300,000 hip fractures, 250,000 wrist fractures and over 200,000 proximal humerus and pelvic ring fractures. After the first fragility fracture, the future fracture risk of these individuals is clearly increased, and a meta-

R. Bartl, C. Bartl, *Bone Disorders*, DOI 10.1007/978-3-319-29182-6_33

analysis showed that there is a two- to fourfold risk increase in the following years.

The *cost to society of osteoporosis* is caused by direct care costs such as acute fracture care and rehabilitation, as well as indirect costs related to poor health. Non-vertebral fractures accounted for over 80 % of the costs, with hip fractures causing the major part.

About 25 % of fractures and a quarter of the total cost are borne by men.

By 2050 it is estimated that the direct and indirect costs worldwide alone due to hip fractures will reach about $ 130 billion per year.

34 Risk Factors of Osteoporotic Fractures

34.1 Risk Factors

The primary goal of treating osteoporosis is to reduce the risk of fractures that are associated with tremendous socioeconomic implications. Often a fragility fracture is the first manifestation of the disease osteoporosis, and a high number of patients sustaining a low-trauma fracture do not show densitometric evidence of osteoporosis. Therefore, there is a definitive need to better identify those who are at risk for fracture. Currently, tools combining bone mineral density and clinical risk fractures to assess fracture risk are under investigation.

There are two main interacting groups of factors that increase the risk of fragility fractures:

- Factors that reduce bone mass and bone strength
- Factors that increase the risk of falls

Table 34.1 gives an overview on bone factors and factors for increased risk of falling and their influence on fragility fractures. Fractures of the wrist or vertebrae are early manifestations of postmenopausal osteoporosis, while those of the proximal humerus or hip are more common in the later stages of age-related osteoporosis (Fig. 34.1). In the course of a lifetime, women lose 35–50 % of the trabecular bone and 25–30 % of the compact bone, in the absence of preventive measures (Fig. 34.2).

Generally, the lower the bone mass, the less the trauma is likely to cause a fracture, for example, coughing or rolling over in bed.

The estimated risk of fractures (for the rest of their lives) in 50-year-old women and men (percentages in brackets are for men) are:

- Proximal femur 18 % (6 %)
- Vertebral column 16 % (5 %)
- Distal radius 15 % (3 %)
- Any location 40 % (13 %)

Many, if not the majority, of "fragility fractures" occur as a result of falling, and approximately 5 % of the older people require hospitalisation, either short or longer term.

> Contemporary estimates suggest that about 50 % of vertebral fractures and all wrist and hip fractures occur as a direct result of trauma.

The most common risk factors for falls identified in 16 large studies are (see Table 34.1):

- Muscle weakness
- History of falls
- Impairment of balance and motion
- Lack of walking aids
- Visual impairment

R. Bartl, C. Bartl, *Bone Disorders*, DOI 10.1007/978-3-319-29182-6_34

- Arthritis
- Psychological factors such as depression
- Cognitive impairment
- Age >80 years

In the OFELY study, seven independent predictors of fragility fractures in postmenopausal women were identified reflecting different potential mechanisms (Fig. 34.3):

- Previous fragility fractures
- Low BMD
- Insufficient physical activity
- Decreased grip strength
- Older age groups
- Maternal history of fractures
- Patient history of falls

The following bone factors should be included in the clinical risk assessment for osteoporotic fractures (see Table 34.1):

- Reduced bone mass (density)
- Discontinuities in microarchitecture of bone
- Disturbance of mineralisation ("osteoporomalacia")

Increased fracture risk

Risk factors for decreased bone strength

Bone factors

- Bone mineral density
- Bone microarchitecture
- Bone turnover
- Bone geometry

Non-modifiable risk factors

- Gender
- Age
- Ethnicity
- Personal history of fracture
- Maternal history of fracture
- Menopause
- Loss of height

Potentially modifiable risk factors

- Vitamin D deficiency
- Low body weight
- Sedentary lifestyle
- Nicotine
- Alcoholism
- Reduced muscle strength
- Glucocorticoid therapy
- Oestrogen deficiency
- Testosterone deficiency
- Diseases (e.g. Rheumatoid arthritis, Post transplant state, Diabetes, Depression, Hyperparathyroidism and others)
- Medications (e.g. Anticonvulsants,
- Anticoagulants, and others)

Risk factors for increased falling risk

Intrinsic factors

- Dementia
- Musculoskeletal disorders
- Neurological disorders
- Cardiovascular disorders
- Frailty
- Cognitive impairment
- Poor vision
- Medications (Sedatives, Hypotensives and others)

Extrinsic factors

- Environmental hazards
- Lacking walking aids
- Low-level lighting
- Slippery surfaces

Table 34.1 Risk factors for reduced bone strength and increased risk of falling

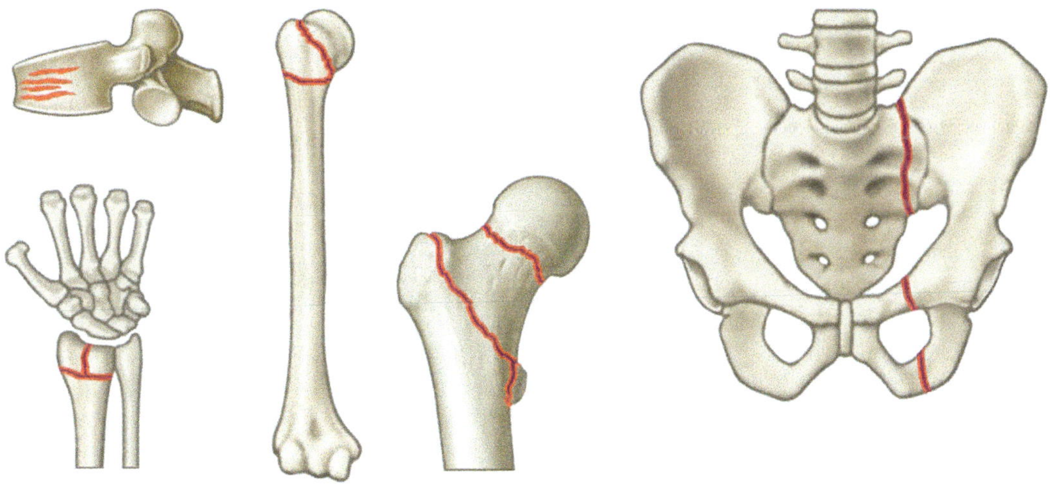

Fig. 34.1 Skeletal sites commonly involved in osteoporotic fractures

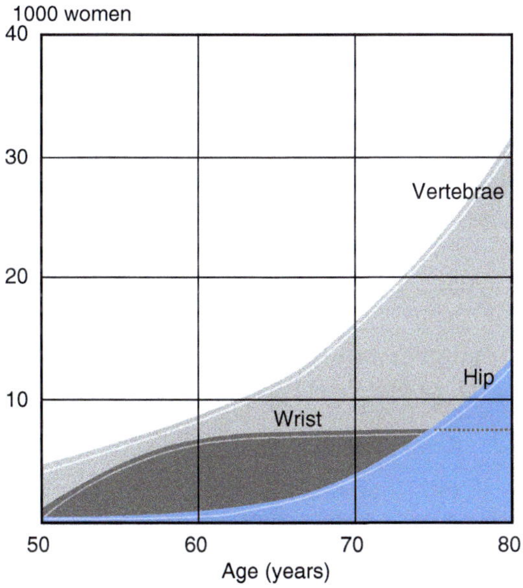

Fig. 34.2 Age-related incidence of osteoporotic fractures

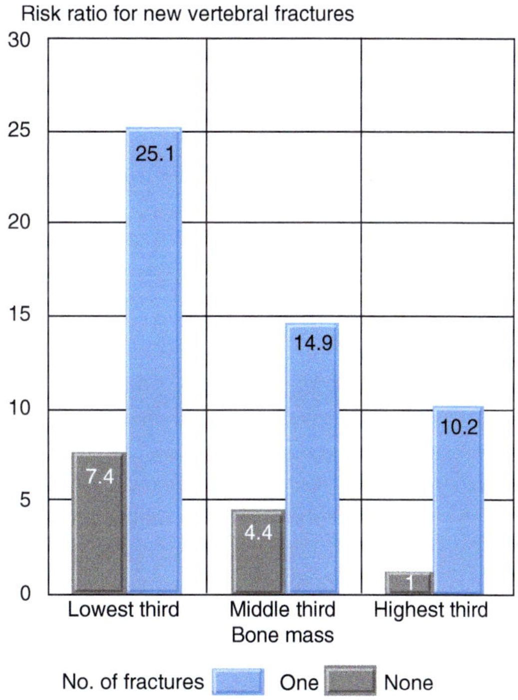

Fig. 34.3 Relationship between prevalent vertebral fractures and BMD on the risk for subsequent vertebral fractures (Modified from Ross et al. *Ann Intern Med* 1998)

- Increased bone turnover ("secondary hyperparathyroidism")
- Increased falling risk

34.2 Fracture Risk Assessment

In the current literature, BMD is described as the single most important factor influencing fracture risk. Cummings et al. showed that every decreasing standard deviation below the reference population doubles the fracture risk.

The main advantage of using BMD testing with the use of T-scores as a single surrogate parameter is to monitor the patient`s response to treatment over time. However, there are important limitations if fracture risk assessment is based only on BMD testing, as several other important factors affect fracture risk. For example, changes in BMD can only explain about one half of the fracture risk reduction induced by the antiosteoporotic treatments.

Fracture risk assessment tools were designed to calculate an individual's risk for fracture and to help in the clinical decision-making process, whether osteoporosis treatment is indicated or not. The most widely recognised is the *FRAX® tool*, introduced under the patronage of the WHO. It estimates the patient's 10-year probability to sustain a major osteoporotic fracture. Besides BMD, it takes into account clinical risk factors like age, gender, body mass index, presence of a parental hip fracture, the personal fracture history, nicotine abuse, alcohol abuse, rheumatoid arthritis, secondary osteoporosis and corticosteroid therapy.

FRAX® allows a more accurate assessment of fracture risk for an individual patient and can help to make treatment decisions. For example, a patient with osteopenia and several coexisting clinical risk fractures show an increased 10-year risk to sustain a major osteoporotic fracture and therefore should be treated.

A major limitation of FRAX® is that it cannot be used to follow-up patients, but only for patients who have not been treated for osteoporosis or osteopenia.

A further limitation is that in the risk factor analysis, all risk factors are answered in a binary fashion – only yes or no – with no graduation of each risk factor. So the number of present vertebral compression fractures (VCFs), the amount of life pack-years for smokers or the dosage of used corticosteroids is not incorporated in the risk assessment. With the lacking graduation, the tool underestimates the future fracture risk of patients with several existing VCFs compared to a patient with only one present VCF, for whom the fracture risk may be overestimated. Another drawback is that the FRAX® model only uses the BMD of the femoral neck. The BMD of the lumbar spine would be important, as it more represents the trabecular bone loss which is affected earlier in the disease process. An advantage of FRAX® is that the formula can be calculated without BMD. This allows to identify patients who might benefit to have a DXA scan.

To further improve fracture risk assessment, also other important risk factors like presence of diabetes, vitamin D level, risk of falling and presence of frailty should be included.

In the management of osteoporosis, the main task of future validated fracture risk assessment tools is to identify those individuals with a fracture risk high enough to justify treatment, especially for those who did not yet sustain a fracture and to assist the clinical decision-making process.

Fracture Healing

35

35.1 Sequence of Events in Fracture Healing

In osteoporotic patients, a minor trauma may cause extensive injury to bone with displacement, haemorrhage and clot formation; or it may affect only a small number of trabeculae without spectacular displacement or pain. Minute breaks or cracks ("microfractures") occur chiefly in weight-bearing bones, especially the vertebrae, usually after marked bone loss as in osteoporosis. Sometimes only a single trabecula is involved, as demonstrated in bone biopsies. However, in iliac crest biopsies, recognition of cracks may be difficult. It should be mentioned that these cracks are the result of the daily "wear and tear" as the body gets older, and not of a specific external trauma, or a fall. Major fractures are always accompanied by bleeding, and subsequent organisation of the clot is an integral part of the unique and highly complex healing process (Fig. 35.1). Bone, bone marrow, periosteum, surrounding muscles, nerves and blood vessels each contribute to the healing process. Fracture healing represents a repetition of the embryonic ossification process. Therefore, the bone is an exception compared to all other organs, as it does not produce scar tissue, but regenerates mature bone tissue independent of the bone turnover rate.

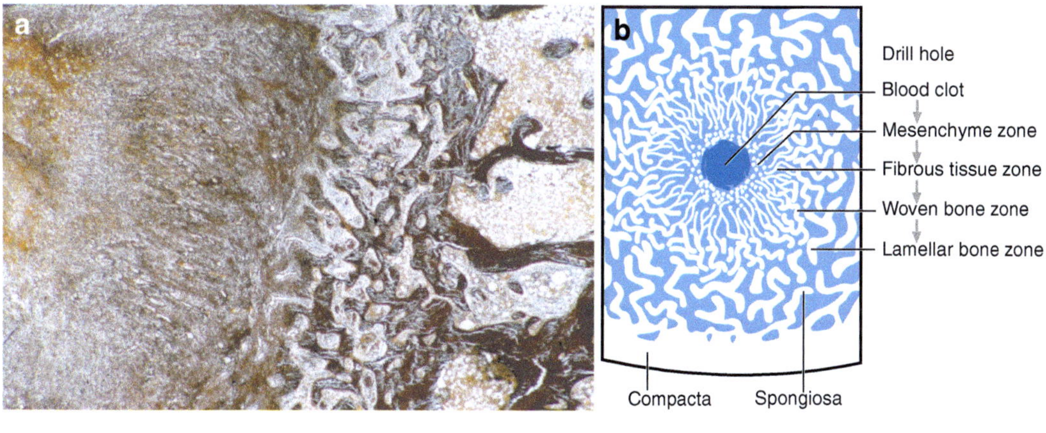

Fig. 35.1 (**a**, **b**) Sequence of repair of the hole made in the bone by taking a bone biopsy: (**a**) histology, from the blood clot (*left*) to the lamellar bone (*right*), Gomori staining; (**b**) schematic representation of the sequence

R. Bartl, C. Bartl, *Bone Disorders*, DOI 10.1007/978-3-319-29182-6_35

In brief, the following is the main sequence of events in fracture healing – both in normal and in osteoporotic bones (Fig. 35.2):

- *Inflammatory phase*: with an immediate and intense inflammatory reaction to the necrotic material: haemorrhage, vasodilatation and exudation of plasma. During the next few days, the haemorrhagic area undergoes organisation. Interestingly, it has been shown that this tissue has osteoblastic potential. The necrotic tissue is removed by phagocytosis and lysosomal breakdown.
- *Reparative phase*: this is characterised by formation of callus, a complex tissue composed of fibrous, cartilaginous and osseous elements, derived from and produced by the surrounding mesenchymal cells. This matrix, or early callus, consists of collagen and proteoglycans. At about the same time, within a week, blood vessels begin to proliferate, bringing nutrients, hormones and growth factors. The progression of soft, fibrous callus to hard, bony callus (woven bone) occurs by mineralisation of the matrix (osteoid) and by enchondral ossification. Within 3–6 weeks, the new bone has acquired a trabecular pattern, which may be observed in bone histology.
- *Remodelling phase*: this is characterised by conversion of the woven to lamellar bone. The repaired bone slowly regains its original shape and strength. Resorption of the callus is primarily due to the osteoclasts, which in turn are controlled by mechanical and electrical factors, responsible for stimulation of cellular proliferation and activity, and morphological changes.

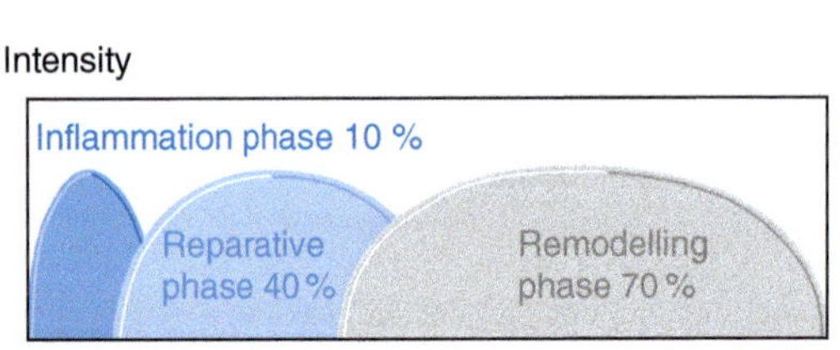

Fig. 35.2 Stages of fracture healing. Duration of the inflammatory, reparative and remodelling phases

Within these overlapping phases, the formed granulation tissue in the fracture gap that fills the fracture gap immediately is followed by chondrocytes producing cartilaginous tissue. Early in the reparative phase, the bone is formed by intramembranous ossification. Later in the reparative phase, the cartilage tissue in the fracture zone is mineralised and then will be converted to lamellar bone by enchondral ossification in the remodelling phase.

The majority of osteoporotic fractures are located in the metaphyseal region. In the metaphyseal bone with adapted fracture fragments, fracture healing with direct trabecular repair/formation takes place with minimal callus formation. In diaphyseal fractures, e.g. following intramedullary nailing or bridging plate osteosynthesis, secondary fracture healing with callus formation takes place. In animal metaphyseal fracture, healing models an increased bone formation rate, and increased bone mineral content was observed compared to diaphyseal fracture healing. Potential factors that promote direct fracture healing in the metaphyseal region are a high trabecular surface area between the fracture fragments and a high number of available osteoblasts. Future studies will investigate especially the underrecognised metaphyseal fracture healing process that is representative for most osteoporotic fractures.

Nonunion rates of the proximal femur following osteosynthesis showed an overall incidence of 20 % and a rate of 25 % in patients over the age of 70 years. In several studies, age, gender and accuracy of reduction correlated with risk of nonunion following osteosynthesis of proximal femur fractures. Studies of an osteoporotic rat model have provided evidence of an altered fracture healing in osteoporotic bone, which may have important implications in evaluating the effects of new treatments for osteoporosis on fracture healing. In the osteoporotic, ovariectomised rat, histomorphological analyses revealed a delay in healing of callus with poor development of mature bone. Experimental studies showed that both age and ovariectomy impaired the normalisation of mechanical properties and the accretion of mineral by the fracture callus, during healing of osteoporotic fractures. On the other hand, it is proven in clinical practice that also fractures with markedly reduced bone mass and bone strength can heal if fracture fixation achieved sufficient stability, suggesting that sufficient fracture healing is also present there.

35.2 Effects of Drugs on Fracture Healing

Antiresorptive agents are widely used for the treatment of osteoporosis. However, inhibition of bone resorption secondarily suppresses bone formation, which results in a substantial reduction in bone turnover, as confirmed by a 90 % reduction in activation frequency after 2 years of alendronate treatment in women. Furthermore, *bisphosphonates (BPs)* have a high affinity for mineral, and their skeletal half-life in bone is very long – about 12 years in humans. Since patients with osteoporosis are prone to fractures and because BP, oestrogen and SERMs suppress bone remodelling, animal and clinical studies are required to investigate the effects of these antiresorptive agents on the healing of fractures. Animal experiments had previously shown that high doses of etidronate interfered with the healing and mineralisation of fractures. This does not apply to the modern N-containing BP, which can be taken without increased risk by patients with osteoporotic fractures. In addition, animal experiments have shown that under therapy with modern bisphosphonates:

- The callus area as well as its calcium content were increased which could be attributed to the inhibition of bone resorption.
- The process of late callus remodelling from woven bone to the well-organised lamellar bone may be delayed under long-term therapy with BP. The consequence may be a normal radiological disappearance of the fracture line and a normal restoration of the anatomical architecture but a delayed mechanical recovery of bone strength.
- The increased callus area and increased callus mineralisation provides higher bending stiffness and callus strength compared to controls and seems to compensate for the delay in callus remodelling during the fracture healing process.

In humans the influence of BP on fracture healing is controversial. There are only five studies looking at the time to fracture healing, including a study and a control group. In distal radius studies, there was a minimal delay in time to union in the BP group, in one study more pronounced in female patients, whereas in studies dealing with femoral fracture healing, no differences between the groups could be observed. A large RCT showed that immediate initiation of BP therapy following a hip fracture showed no negative effect concerning union rate, time to fracture healing or a higher complication rate of the osteosynthesis. Currently there is no robust evidence from clinical studies to stop an ongoing BP therapy or to delay BP introduction in presence of a new fracture. Patients under antiresorptive medication with one or more new fragility fracture and no significant gain of BMD may be switched to osteoanabolic treatment to ensure a fracture protection effect. Future studies evaluating the influence of BPs on fracture healing should include higher patient numbers and a control group and should distinguish between upper and lower extremity fractures, metaphyseal and diaphyseal fractures and surgical and nonsurgical management to provide sound data.

Denosumab is another new antiresorptive drug that acts via inhibition of osteoclast formation and osteoclast recruitment. In fracture healing models, it showed similar effects as BPs, with increased callus formation and increased mineralised callus tissue compared to controls, but also remodelling and organisation of the callus was delayed. After subcutaneous injection, the antibody remains in the blood circulation for a long time compared to the short time of bone-specific BPs.

For both agents (BP and denosumab), recent clinical studies reported an increased incidence of *atypical femoral fractures*, especially in patients with long-term use. It is assumed that accumulation of microdamages due to the impaired bone remodelling rate and suppressed bone turnover with these agents leads to generation of microcracks, resulting in incomplete stress fractures or complete atypical fractures of the femoral shaft or the subtrochanteric region. Overall atypical fractures are rare, and given a correct indication for therapy, antiresorptive drugs prevent a lot more fractures than they cause.

Parathyroid hormone (PTH) is an osteoanabolic drug which is proven to enhance bone density and to reduce fracture risk in humans. In animal fracture healing models, there is a robust evidence that teriparatide greatly improves the biomechanical properties of the fracture callus. Histology showed an accelerated callus formation, intramembranous and enchondral ossification and bone remodelling rate. In humans two recent clinical studies showed only small advantages of teriparatide on fracture healing time in conservatively (cast) treated fractures of the distal radius and the pelvic ring. Currently there is no evidence that these small advantages translate into a clear clinical benefit for the patient.

Among the new anti-osteoporotic drugs, preclinical studies for a *sclerostin antibody* showed an enhancement of fracture healing, and an RCT in hip fracture patients to assess the influence on fracture healing is under investigation. The cathepsin K inhibitor, *odanacatib*, showed increased callus formation and mineralisation compared to controls in an animal fracture healing model.

Cytokines and small molecular mediators such as prostaglandins play key roles in cellular immune function, but also in the initiation of the process of fracture repair. One of the best-studied examples, showing the crucial role of these factors during repair of bone, concerns the role of *cyclooxygenase-2 (COX-2)*. In animal studies in which the effects of a nonselective *nonsteroidal anti-inflammatory drug (NSAID)* were compared to those of a COX-2 selective drug, greater impairment of fracture healing occurred under treatment with the COX-2 than with the NSAID.

Beta-blockers have also been studied in relation to skeletal health. Several studies have demonstrated that the sympathetic nervous system has a catabolic effect on bones. Indeed, functional adrenergic receptors are present in osteoblasts and osteoclasts, and sympathetic nerve fibres have been demonstrated in bone tissue. Therefore, the nervous system may well be a co-regulator of osseous metabolism and thus influence the healing of fractures.

For many drugs used in clinical practice like NSAIDs or corticosteroids as well as for external factors like nicotine or systemic diseases like diabetes, a delay in fracture healing was observed in animal studies.

Smokers as well as individuals with *chronic and heavy alcohol consumption* are not only more susceptible to falls and fractures, but also to delay in healing of fractures. Moreover, it has been reported that the maturation of the regenerating bone is abnormal and nonunion or malunion is more frequent in these patients. Smokers themselves assess their outcomes after surgery much less favourably than non-smokers. The detrimental effects of alcohol include suppression of bone formation by osteoblasts, changes in the composition of the ossifiable matrix and decrease in the ability of osteoblasts to respond to signals that normally trigger bone formation.

For impaired fracture healing with presence of a pseudarthrosis, the local application of bone morphogenetic proteins BMP-2 and BMP-7 is approved, but there is no robust data about its use in osteoporotic fractures. On the other hand, so far no study has proved that BMPs are superior to cancellous bone grafting for bone healing of nonunions. Concerning biophysical acceleration of fracture healing, low-intensity ultrasound is approved to enhance bone healing of delayed unions.

36 Management of Osteoporotic Fractures

The main goal of osteoporosis treatment is to prevent fragility fractures. Often, a low-trauma fracture of an elderly patient is the first manifestation of osteoporosis, which was an asymptomatic disease until the fracture event. Low-trauma fractures require orthopaedic trauma management including conservative management with casting or splinting, as well as surgical management with osteosynthesis or joint replacement. In elderly patients with reduced bone mass, surgical stabilisation should allow for early weight-bearing in fractures of the lower extremity, the spine and pelvic ring and for early physiotherapy in fractures of the upper extremity. For these fractures with markedly reduced bone loss, special implants are needed to provide stable fracture fixation to allow bone healing. Early fracture management, rapid mobilisation and active physiotherapy following fracture stabilisation are important to preserve joint function, to prevent joint contractures, to provide muscle strengthening for walking security and to prevent complications due to immobilisation.

General guidelines for the management of osteoporotic fractures:

- Elderly patients are best treated by rapid fracture management. Operative intervention should be minimised, in order to reduce operative time, blood loss and stress. Indeed, a delay of more than 2 days until surgical management of a hip fracture significantly increases 1-year mortality and perioperative complications.
- Surgical intervention should achieve stable fracture fixation to allow for early weight-bearing and early physiotherapy.
- For osteoporotic bone, special fracture implants are necessary to allow fracture healing. These include joint replacement, intramedullary implants, locked plating of metaphyseal fractures and locked implants for spine surgery, if necessary with cement augmentation. The primary cause of implant failure after fracture fixation is the impaired healing capacity of the osteoporotic bone.
- Rehabilitation aims at mobilisation to improve muscle function, to prevent sarcopenia due to immobility, and strategies for fall prevention. Secondary fracture prevention with specific antiresorptive or osteoanabolic drugs and vitamin D supplementation is of great importance as the future fracture risk is increased up to fourfold.

R. Bartl, C. Bartl, *Bone Disorders*, DOI 10.1007/978-3-319-29182-6_36

36.1 Fracture Sites and Their Clinical Significance

Osteoporosis causes symptoms when a bone fractures. It is important to realise that bone loss itself does not cause pain or disability. Fractures of the hip, spine, wrist and proximal humerus are the most common, although they also occur in other parts of the skeleton, particularly in the pelvic ring, ankle, ribs and increasingly in periprosthetic regions. Although any fracture can have a devastating impact on the affected individual, hip fractures are by far the most important from the perspective of public health.

36.2 Hip Fractures

Hip fractures account for most of the medical costs, as they are responsible for about 65 % of the total costs for osteoporotic fractures. More than 300,000 patients annually in the USA alone sustain a fracture of the proximal femur; 25 % are men with an average age of 80 years. One out of every six Caucasian women (15 %) will suffer a hip fracture in her lifetime. All fractures are caused by a fall. The type of fracture depends on several factors including the angle and manner of falling, bone strength of the femoral neck as well as the patient's neuromuscular and protective responses to the fall and its impact.

The two important types of fractures of the proximal femur are pertrochanteric fractures (50 %) and fractures of the femoral neck (50 % subcapital and transcervical) (Fig. 36.1). Intertrochanteric fractures are treated with joint-preserving osteosynthesis like proximal femoral nails or dynamic hip screws. Multifragmentary trochanteric and subtrochanteric fractures are best treated with intramedullary nails due to improved biomechanics and allow for early weight-bearing (Fig. 36.2). In cases of very low bone strength, the spiral blade located in the femoral head can be augmented with bone cement (Fig. 36.3).

Subcapital femoral neck fractures are mainly treated by hemialloarthroplasty or total hip replacement, as screw osteosynthesis in osteoporotic bone

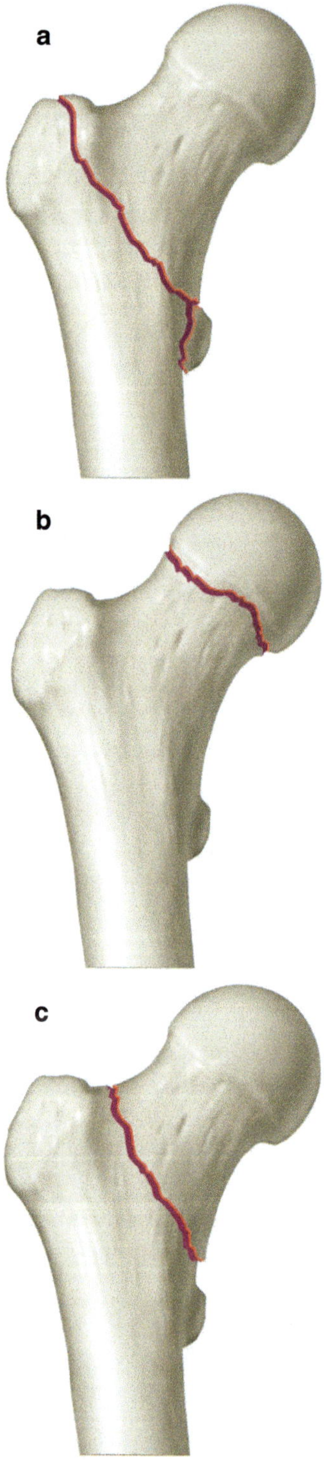

Fig. 36.1 Types of proximal femur fractures: (**a**) pertrochanteric, (**b**) medial femoral neck, (**c**) lateral femoral neck

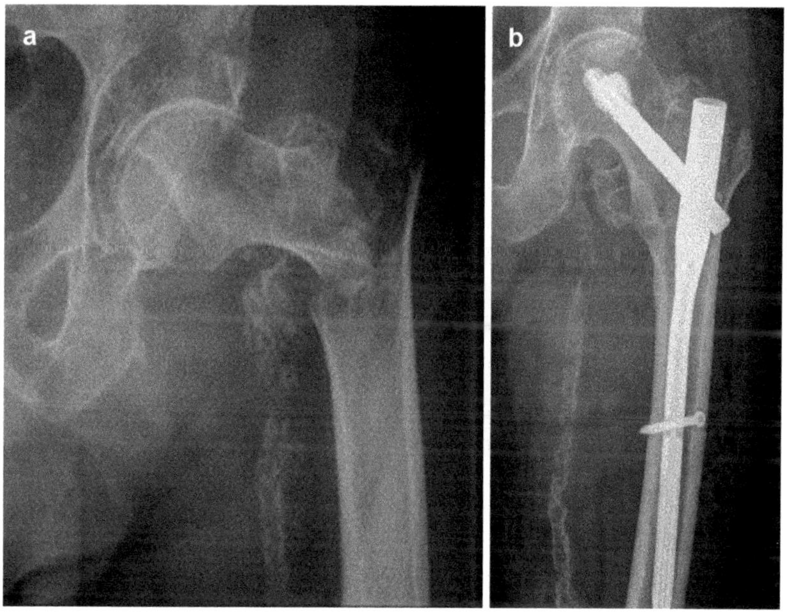

Fig. 36.2 (**a**) Dislocated pertrochanteric fracture (a). (**b**) Osteosynthesis with a proximal femoral nail (PFN)

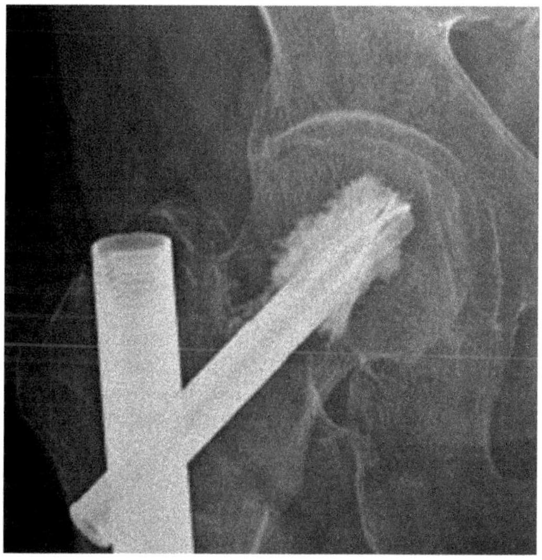

Fig. 36.3 Cement augmentation of the PFN blade in a case of severe osteoporosis of the proximal femur

showed a high implant failure rate, e.g. screw cutting out. Cemented arthroplasty provides high initial fixation stability in cases of very osteoporotic bone and allows for immediate weight-bearing (Figs. 36.4 and 36.5)

Hip fractures have very serious consequences and the majority of patients are frequently left with a disability:

- 20–25 % will die within the first year.
- Nearly 25 % require a long-term nursing facility or in-home care.
- About 40 % never fully recover their mobility and independence.

Risk factors for the first hip fracture include:

- Previous fracture at any site
- Advanced age
- Low body weight
- Low bone mineral density
- Increased risk of falling

The results of a prospective randomised hip fracture trial (Lyles et al. 2008) showed a reduction of 35 % in new clinical fractures and a reduction of 28 % in mortality in the 2 years after the fracture, achieved by a single infusion of zoledronic acid given within 3 months of the

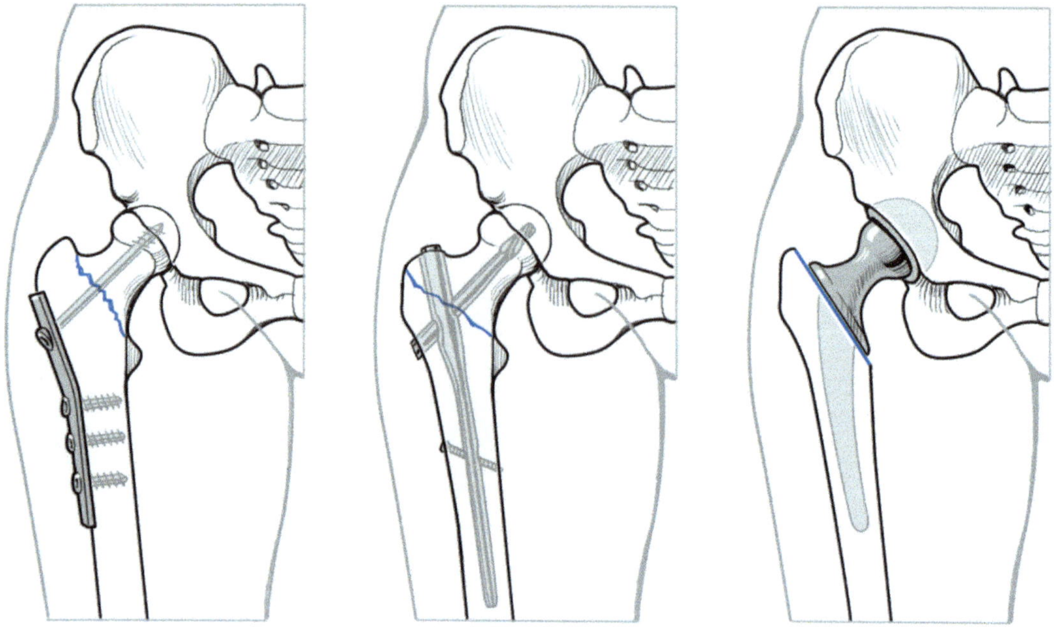

Fig. 36.4 Common surgical procedures for the treatment of proximal femur fractures

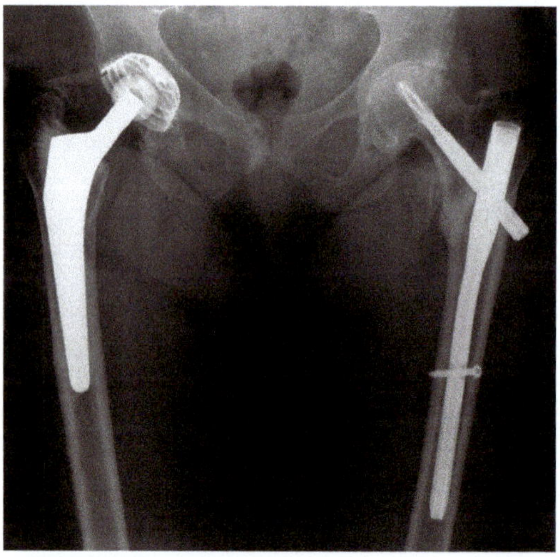

Fig. 36.5 Hip arthroplasty for the treatment of a medial femoral neck fracture. Osteosynthesis of a pertrochanteric fracture with a proximal femoral nail 3 years later

first fracture. In addition, the fracture union was not delayed by the bisphosphonate, and also the osteosynthesis complication rate was not increased.

Despite an observed stagnation in the age-specific hip fracture incidence for both genders over the last decade in several studies, no improvements in the survival after hip fracture were noted despite suggested improved osteoporosis treatment strategies and improved implant technology. The definitive need for treatment arises, as 12 % of the patients will suffer a second hip fracture in the future, with a particular high risk in the first 6 months following the first fracture. A recent European study showed that hip fractures account for about 17 % of all osteoporotic fractures but cause over 50 % of the direct costs among all fractures.

An alarming sign is the downward trend in the number of patients being treated after a hip fracture over the last decade, in a recent US study by Salomon et al. The study showed that the osteoporosis medication initiation rate following a hip fracture dropped from 40 % in 2002 to 20 % in 2011.

36.3 Atypical Femoral Fractures

Several trials showed an association for occurrence of atypical femoral fractures under antiresorptive treatment with BP and denosumab. Most patients had long-term use of antiresorp-

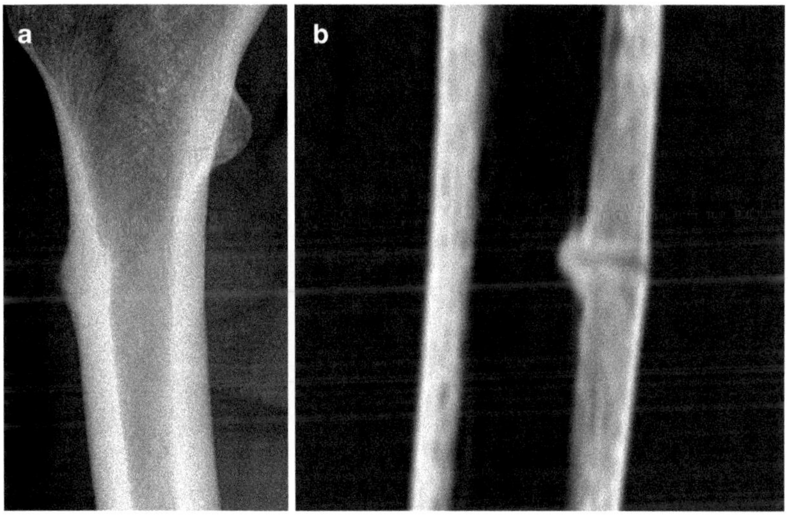

Fig. 36.6 (**a**) Atypical incomplete femur fracture with buckling of lateral cortex. (**b**) Fracture line in the lateral cortex with surrounding cortex hypertrophy (CT)

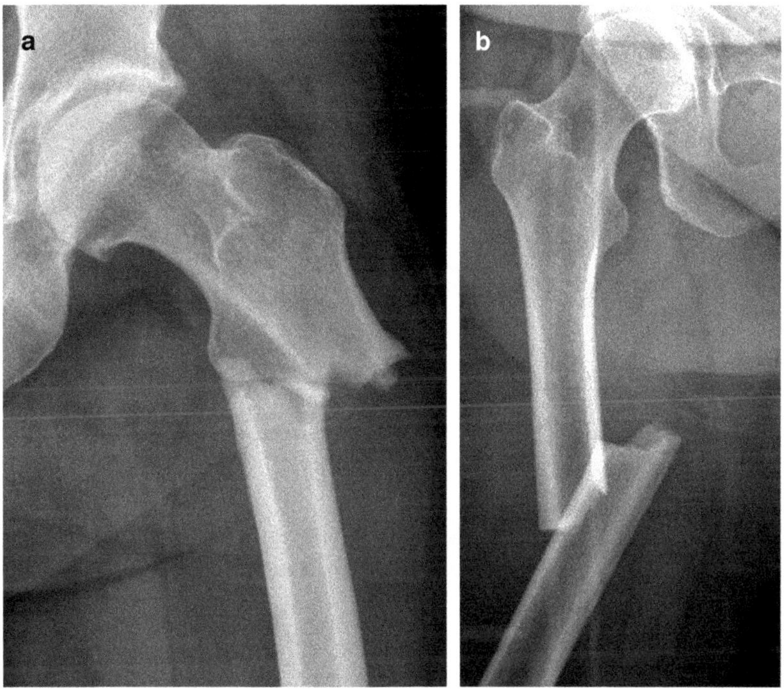

Fig. 36.7 (**a**) Complete atypical transverse subtrochanteric fracture. (**b**) Atypical transverse femur shaft fracture with cortical spike in a patient on long-term bisphosphonate use

tives for at least 3–5 years. It is assumed that accumulation of microdamages due to suppression of targeted remodelling of these drug leads to initiation of microcracks, resulting in incomplete stress fractures or complete atypical fractures of the femoral shaft or the subtrochanteric region. Patients often present with prodromal thigh pain that also can occur bilaterally. Radiographs show periosteal reaction with cortical thickening of the lateral femur cortex (Fig. 36.6a, b) in incomplete fractures and can also present with stress fracture lines in the lateral cortex. Most often complete fractures occur without an adequate trauma and present mainly as uncomminuted transverse fractures of the subtrochanteric region or the femoral shaft (Fig. 36.7a, b). Bone geometry may also influence fracture location as a more pronounced femoral bowing in the frontal plane might predispose to femoral shaft fractures.

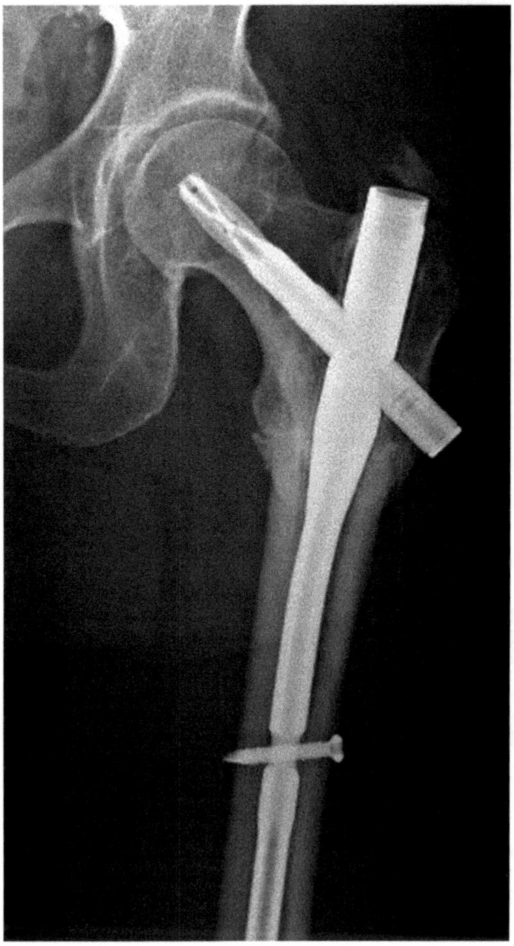

Fig. 36.8 Osteosynthesis of the atypical femoral fracture from Fig. 36.7a with a proximal femoral nail

Histology of bone biopsies showed increased remodelling and presence of woven bone around the fracture line of incomplete fractures and callus at the lateral border trying to stabilise the fracture. Another factor is the strain on the incomplete fracture on the lateral distraction side of the femur that does not allow for healing of the fracture. With early diagnosis of incomplete stress fractures with only cortical thickening, nonsurgical treatment with cessation of BP treatment and vitamin D supplementation is a possible strategy, but needs careful monitoring. There are case reports that teriparatide treatment might be an option for healing of incomplete atypical femoral stress fractures of the lateral cortex. Complete fractures are treated with a proximal femoral nail including intramedullary reaming (internal spongiosaplasty) (Fig. 36.8). The ASBMR "task force" also recommends prophylactic nailing of painful incomplete fractures with stress fracture lines in the thickened cortex after unsuccessful conservative therapy, in view of the increased complication rate of osteosynthesis for complete fractures. New studies show that women may have a higher risk of atypical femoral fractures and that in BP the risk decreases rapidly after cessation of therapy. On the basis of these studies, the authors recommend that patients who have sustained a fracture should stop taking these antiresorptive agents and that patients receiving long-term treatment should be carefully monitored as the anti-fracture effect of these drugs must be balanced against the serious adverse event to suffer an atypical fracture. After 3–5 years of treatment, the decision about continuation or a temporary discontinuation of antiresorptives can be addressed by an individual risk assessment of the patient. Studies showed that the overall incidence of atypical femoral fractures is low, ranging from about 1 in 100,000 to 5 in 10,000 in bisphosphonate users. Metaanalysis and reviews suggest a clearly favorable benefit-to-risk ratio of treatment in the first 5 years [63]. Future studies will show if once-yearly BP has a lower risk than BP with weekly dosing and if the potent antiresorptive effect of denosumab shows a potential higher rate of atypical fractures. Overall atypical femoral fractures are rare, and given a carefully selected indication, these antiresorptive drugs prevent a lot more fractures than they potentially cause.

36.4 Vertebral Fractures

Vertebral compression fractures (VCFs) are often asymptomatic and therefore not diagnosed. Indeed, only about one third of radiographic vertebral deformations come to clinical attention. Most vertebral fractures occur due to axial loading under activities of daily living, e.g. lifting, landing and bending, or are diagnosed incidentally. The greatest risk factor for compression fractures is an underlying osteoporosis, with multiple myeloma and metastatic cancer, especially of the breast, high up in the differential diagnosis of painful vertebral compression fractures. The correct diagnosis requires lateral radiographs of both the thoracic and the lumbar spine. Vertebral fractures are very common in older women; they

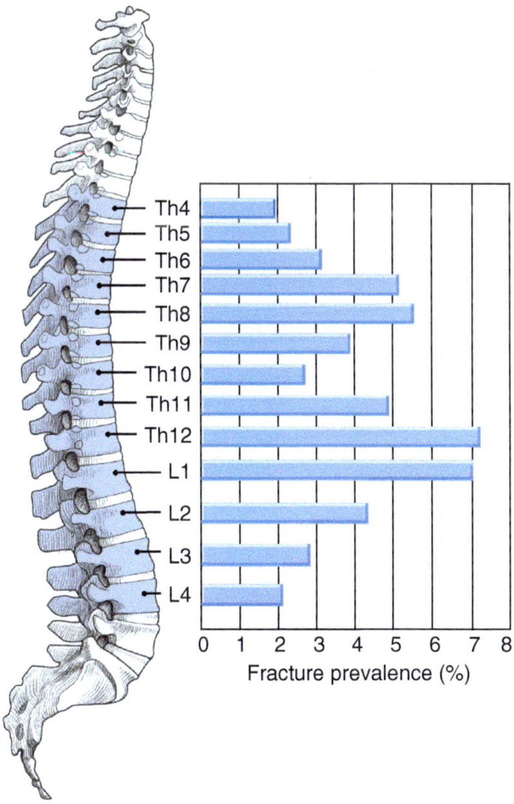

Fig. 36.9 Frequency of vertebral fractures according to their location in the spine

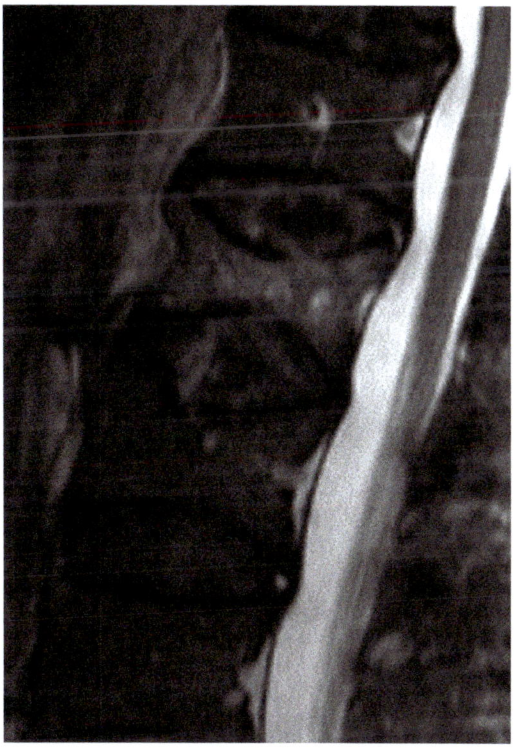

Fig. 36.10 MRI of the spine with bone marrow oedema of the vertebral body indicating a fresh compression fracture

are found in radiographs in 5–10 % of women at 55 years, rising to 30–40 % by 80 years. It is assumed that vertebral fractures occur in approximately 20 % of older persons over 70 years of age worldwide, with an estimated 1.4 million new fractures every year. The cortical shell of a vertebral body contributes only about 10 % of the resistance to compressive loads. Thinning and microcracks in trabecular bone occur with age. Although these heal with callus formation, excess accumulation of microcracks results in critical weakening which in turn leads to vertebral compression and to fracture. Vertebral fractures occur in many different circumstances, and approximately 50 % cannot be attributed to an identified loading effect. Vertebral fractures most commonly involve the mid-thoracic region and the thoracolumbar junction (Fig. 36.9). In contrast, fractures of the upper thoracic spine (T2–T6) are more likely to be due to metastatic disease or multiple myeloma. MRI can help to distinguish benign from malignant disease. Also MRI can help to identify fresh vertebral compression fractures that appear with a trabecular bone marrow oedema on fat-suppressed T2/STIR sequences (Fig. 36.10).

There is great variability in the symptoms caused by vertebral fractures. Some patients experience very little or no pain when the fracture occurs, whereas others feel severe pain. Although some affected individuals become pain-free after a few months, others may be left with long-lasting pain or discomfort. Patients with vertebral fractures experience aggravation of pain during physical activities such as bending and rising up and even standing up straight. Spinal fractures do not usually cause back pain radiating down the legs, which is more typical of radiculopathy due to disc problems. As a result of changes in body shape (expansion of the waistline and prominence of the abdomen), many patients have trouble finding clothes that fit. The long-term effects of vertebral fractures are still underestimated: many result in chronic back pain, immobility, deformity, reduced pulmonary function, increased mortality, compromised quality of life and functional decline.

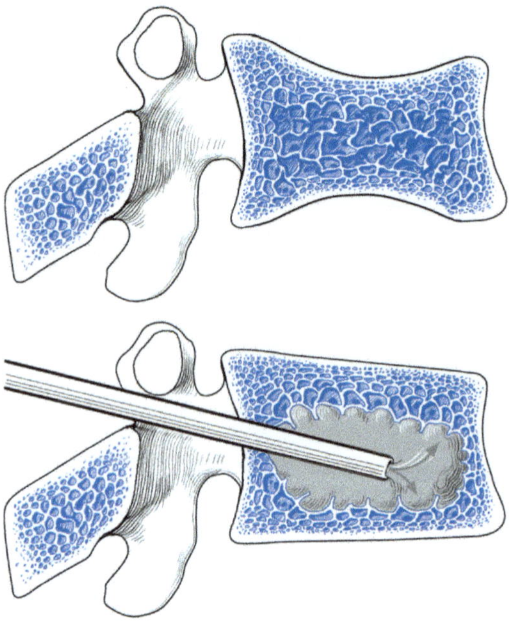

Fig. 36.11 Vertebroplasty: vertebral body fracture restoration by cement injection

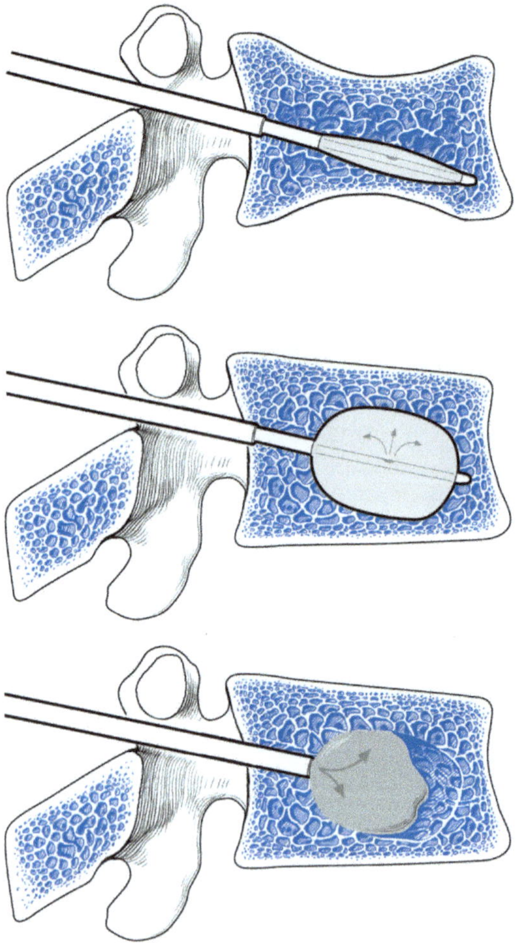

Fig. 36.12 Kyphoplasty: vertebral body height restoration with balloon kyphoplasty

The *repair phase* lasts 2–4 months during which the use of orthopaedic appliances and corsets should be limited to as short a time as possible. Their purpose is alleviation of pain, avoidance of kyphosis and preservation of pulmonary function. Sufficient analgesic treatment is necessary to allow for mobilisation therapy. Rehabilitation strategies which increase the strength of spinal muscles will reduce the load on vertebral bodies and thereby decrease the risk of fracture in the mechanically incompetent bone. Research into the risk of vertebral fractures found a four- to sixfold increase with a 2-SD decrease in the BMD of the lumbar spine. One symptomatic vertebral fracture causes a twofold increase in hip fractures, while 2 or more vertebral fractures result in an eightfold increase in new vertebral fractures.

The indication for surgical management of new vertebral compression fractures (VCFs) are persistent pain and immobility under conservative management. Painful VCF can be treated with *vertebroplasty* (*VP*), by transpedicular percutaneous injection of polymethylmethacrylate (PMMA), by means of bone biopsy needles, into the fractured vertebra to stabilise the sintered vertebra (Fig. 36.11). *Kyphoplasty* (*KP*) involves inserting an inflatable balloon or a wired expandable cage into the vertebral body under fluoroscopic guidance (Fig. 36.12). After the balloon is expanded in the vertebra, the PMMA is inserted to fill the trabecular void. Fresh wedge-shaped VCF can be corrected with this technique. Both techniques have a high rate of use and acceptance, but can be applied only for stable VCF with an intact dorsal wall. There is 95 % reduction in pain and significant improvement in function following treatment by either of these percutaneous techniques. Kyphoplasty improves height of the fractured vertebra and reduces kyphosis by over 50 %, if performed within 2–3 months of the fracture, but later on, there is less improvement in height. The achieved fracture stability and recovery of vertebral height after the procedures have been considered to be the major causes of pain relief and functional improvement. Complications occur with both

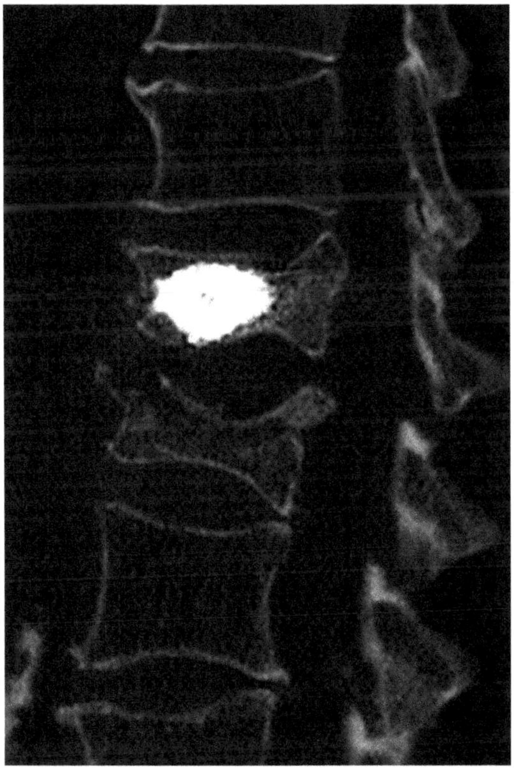

Fig. 36.13 Postoperative CT after 4 month showing a compression fracture in the adjacent level following kyphoplasty

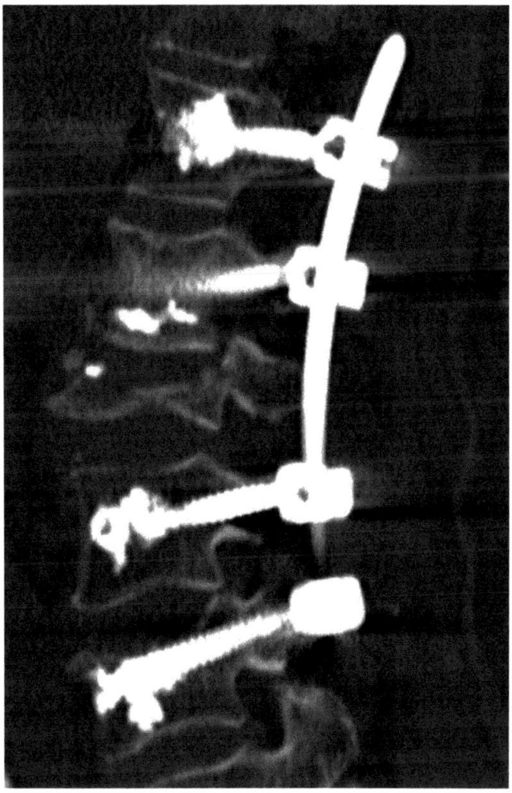

Fig. 36.14 Dorsal multilevel instrumentation of an unstable vertebral fracture with screw cement augmentation in a case of severe osteoporosis

methods mainly due to leakage of cement, less in kyphoplasty because the cement is confined within the balloon, and potential cement microemboli via the venous spinal plexus. In some cases, collapse because of new compression fractures has been observed in adjacent vertebral bodies, especially following multisegmental cement injection, in the vertebral levels above and below the vertebroplasty due to the increased stiffness of the cement-augmented vertebral body (Fig. 36.13). Two recent RCTs showed similar outcome results for the treatment of VCFs with vertebroplasty compared to sham injection, and therefore the efficacy of vertebroplasty was doubted. A large meta-analysis to analyse the results of vertebroplasty for VCFs revealed that VP was more effective in improving health-related quality of life scores and in relieving pain compared to nonoperative therapy. Also VP did not lead to an increased number of new vertebral fractures compared to all control groups. For unstable VCF or burst fractures with involvement of the dorsal wall, *transpedicular dorsal instrumentation with an internal fixator and additional cement augmentation* can be performed (Fig. 36.14). In cases with marked bone loss, a multilevel instrumentation is necessary for optimal stress distribution and to reduce bending forces on each instrumented vertebral body.

36.5 Distal Radius Fractures

Fractures of the distal radius (DRF) in elderly patients are often associated with reduced bone mass and often occur as the first fracture event in postmenopausal women. The lifetime risk of women over the age of 50 years to sustain a distal radius fracture (wrist fracture) is about 15%, whereas the risk in men is only 2.5%. It is the most frequent fracture before the age of 75 years, occurring mainly in women around the time of the menopause. Wrist fractures are usually sustained outdoors and especially during the winter season. Most of these wrist fractures occur after a fall on the outstretched arm. Wrist fractures are

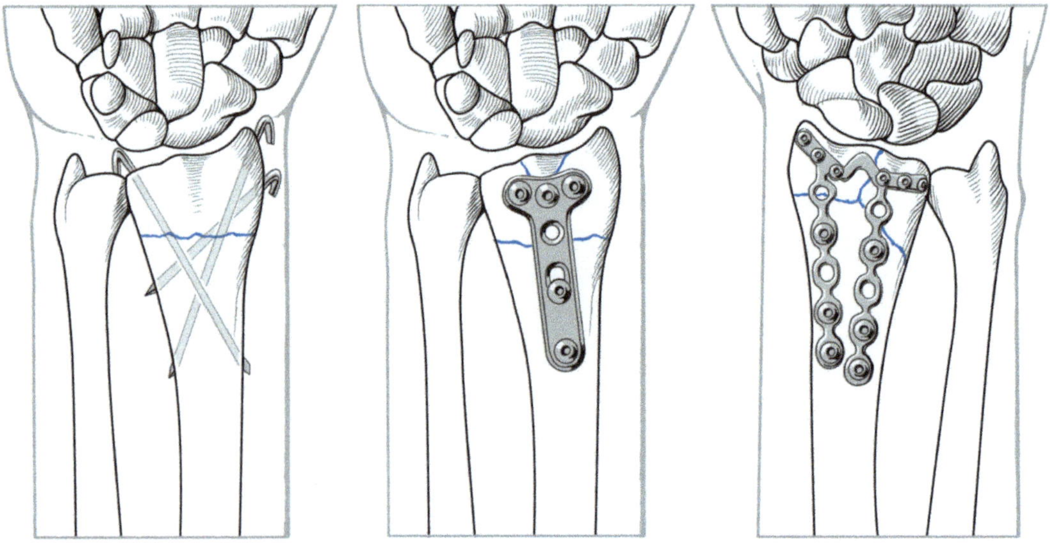

Fig. 36.15 Common surgical procedures for the treatment of unstable displaced distal radius fractures

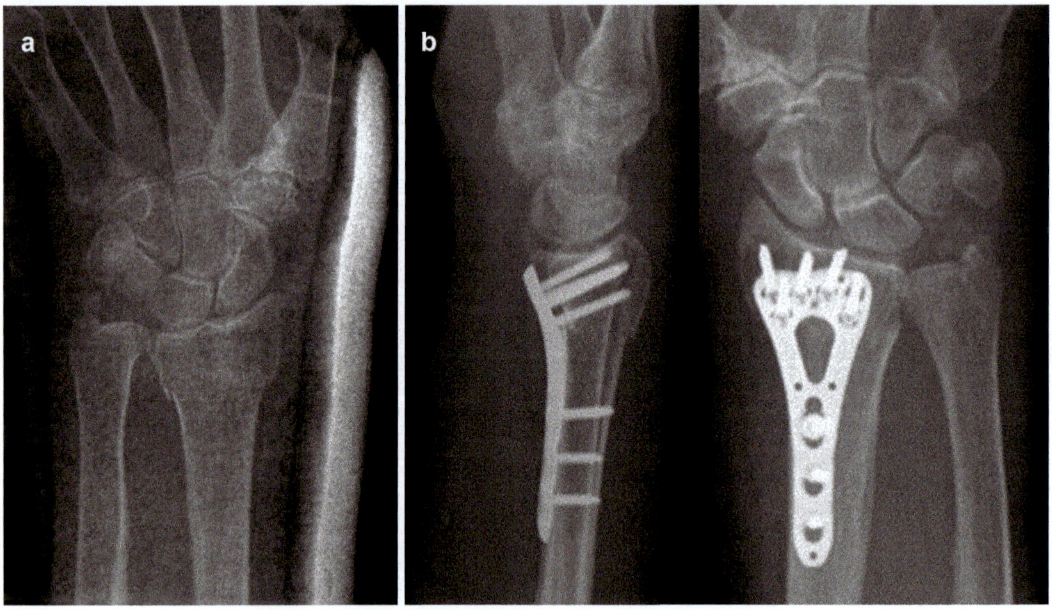

Fig. 36.16 (**a**) Cast immobilisation of a DRF. (**b**) Volar locking plate fixation of a DRF

painful and require outpatient treatment in the emergency department, though elderly patients may need to be hospitalised. The majority of non-displaced fractures can be treated by closed reduction and cast immobilisation. If fracture reduction can be maintained grossly with the cast in displaced or intraarticular wrist fractures for 2 weeks, the majority of these fractures can be managed without operation. Cast treatment with a closed cast is continued for 6 weeks. Comminuted fractures, fractures with an intraarticular step-off or fractures with redisplacement after cast treatment are best treated with a volar locking plate, which emerged as the standard for complicated fractures over the last decade (Figs. 36.15 and 36.16a, b). Plating osteosynthesis allows for earlier recovery of range of motion and wrist function, especially for an elderly high-demand population, e.g. persons who live alone or who care for their partners.

RCTs showed that wrist anatomy is better restored with locking plates compared to cast immobilisation [62]. But after 1 year, there was no difference between both groups regarding wrist function, health-related quality of life and overall activity status. Both procedures were safe and showed a low complication rate. In elderly patients the treatment strategy must consider the fracture pattern, but also the individual functional demands of the patient, the comorbidities and the activity status.

A fracture of the radius in patients between 50 and 60 years of age is always a sign of osteoporosis and calls for immediate measurement of bone density. A significant complication, after either conservative or surgical treatment, may arise in the form of algodystrophy (chronic regional pain syndrome, CRPS I). In these patients, there is often persistent pain, tenderness, swelling, stiffness and significant bone loss of the hand that may last for years after the injury. As previously outlined, osteoporotic patients are also at a higher risk to sustain additional fractures at any site. Studies have shown that mortality after a distal radial fracture is not increased, but there is a significant impairment of health-related quality of life in the following years.

36.6 Proximal Humerus Fractures

The second most common osteoporotic fracture of the upper extremity is that of the proximal humerus. Most of the proximal humerus fractures occur after a fall onto the shoulder with the arm adducted. The majority are non-displaced or minimally displaced fractures of the surgical neck and can be treated conservatively with a sling and permit early functional rehabilitation. Displaced fractures or multipart fractures require surgery with open reduction and locked plating or antegrade nailing (Fig. 36.17). In cases of marked bone loss (eggshell configuration of the humeral head), plating with cement augmentation can be performed. In displaced four-part fractures and in low-demand and frail elderly patients, hemiar-

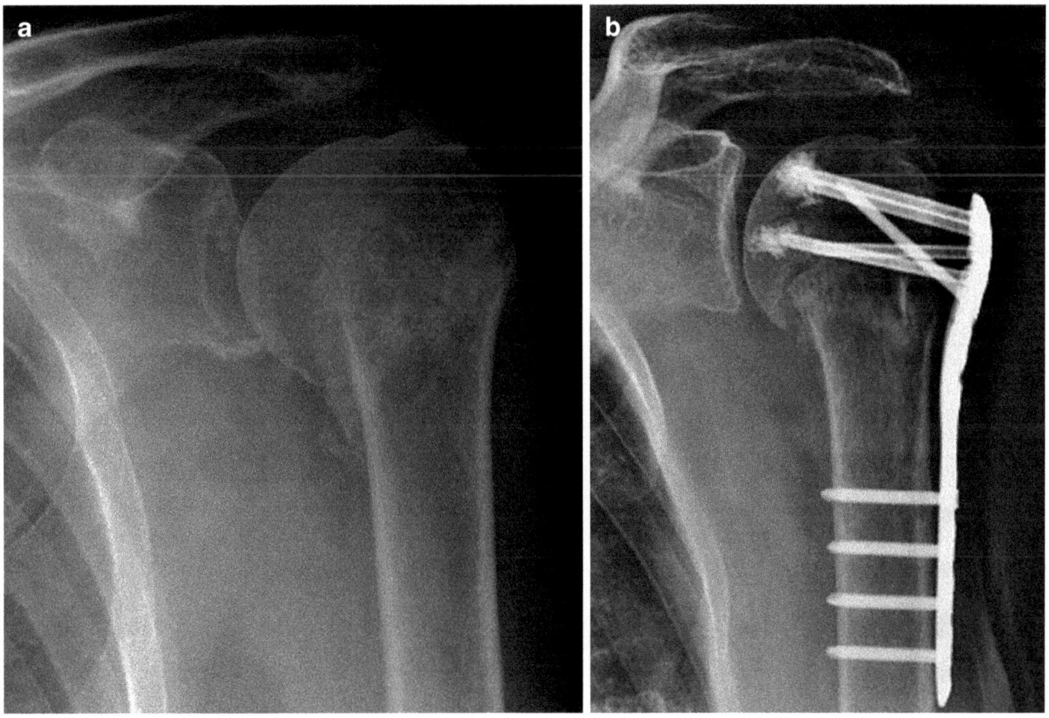

Fig. 36.17 (**a**) Conservative treatment of a simple proximal humerus fracture with a sling. (**b**) Locking plate fixation with cement augmentation of a complex proximal humerus fracture with advanced local bone loss

throplasty/reversed arthroplasty may be also considered, as complication rates of all types of osteosynthesis are high in these cases.

Elderly patients should start physiotherapy with passive motion as soon as possible to prevent capsular contracture of the shoulder joint with loss of motion in the postoperative period. Fractures of the proximal humerus are associated with an increased risk for future vertebral and hip fractures in both women and men. Conversely to the increased trend for surgical management of displaced proximal humerus fractures, a recent RCT by Rangan et al. 2015 showed no advantage of surgical (osteosynthesis and arthroplasty) versus nonsurgical (sling) management, regarding functional and health-related quality of life scores.

36.7 Other Fractures

These include fractures of the *pelvic ring*. Unilateral isolated fractures of the anterior pelvic ring (pubic rami) or the posterior pelvic ring (massa lateralis of the sacrum) can be treated with pain management and adjusted mobilisation therapy. Combined anterior and posterior pelvic ring fractures show a higher degree of instability and are associated with an increased pain level and duration of immobility. For early mobilisation, an anterior external fixator can be applied. Sacrum fractures can present as traumatic fractures or as atraumatic insufficiency fractures, sometimes also as bilateral sacrum fractures. To prevent immobility caused by the pain and potential complications with a mortality rate that is similar to hip fractures in the very elderly, a navigated sacroiliacal screw can be performed to stabilise the posterior pelvic ring (Fig. 36.18a, b).

Fractures around the *knee* (supracondylar fractures of the distal femur or fractures of the tibial plateau) carry a high risk for postoperative degenerative joint disease and arthrofibrosis. Further fractures include distal humerus fractures following low-trauma falls on the elbow and also periprosthetic fractures around hip and knee prostheses and other peri-implant fractures following osteosynthesis of a previous osteoporotic fracture. Such fractures occur due to bone stress shielding around implants, resulting in periprosthetic bone loss. Also stress risers at the tip of implants due to the increased local strain on the adjacent bone can proceed to complete fractures. These complex fractures can be managed with bridging plate osteosynthesis, but need weeks before full weight-bearing is possible (Figs. 36.19a, b and 36.20a, b).

To improve outcome assessment following fragility fractures in elderly patients, it is necessary to implement appropriate, patient-centred assessment tools, to better assess health-related quality of life activities of daily living and level of independence after the fracture (e.g. PROMIS, patient-reported outcomes measurement information system). These assessment tools need to include functional assessment (SF-36, EQ-5D, Parker mobility score), cognitive assessment (mini-mental status), frailty (level of illness, Charlson comorbidity score; nutrition status) and balance and coordina-

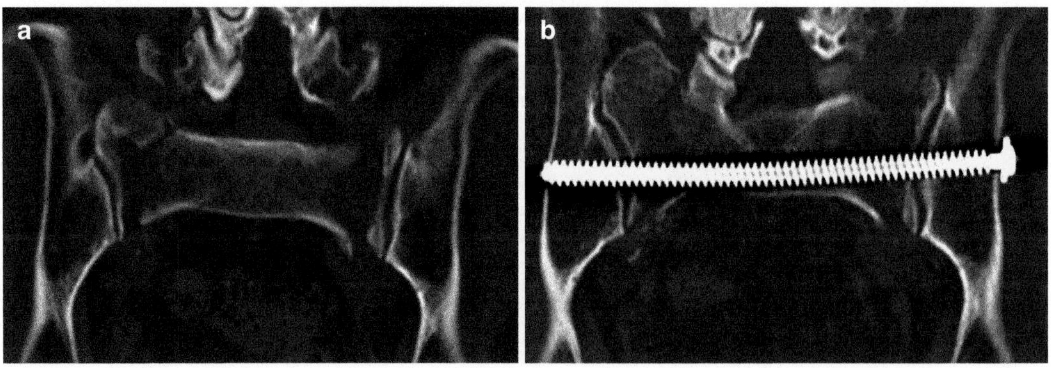

Fig. 36.18 (**a**) Bilateral osteoporotic insufficiency fracture of the sacrum. (**b**) Treatment with a navigated sacroiliacal screw

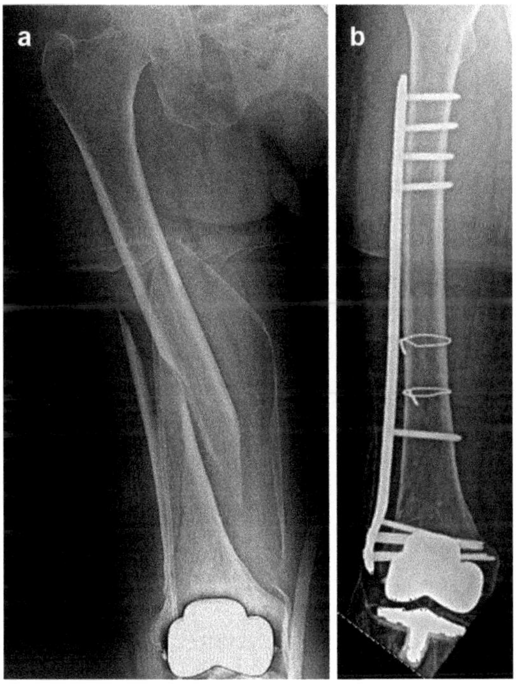

Fig. 36.19 (**a**) Periprosthetic femur spiral fracture proximal to the knee prosthesis. (**b**) Locking plate fixation

tion (timed up and go test). Implementation of such assessment tools will help to optimise in-hospital and postoperative care (mortality, perioperative complication rate, rehabilitation) and to optimise cost-effectiveness of the procedures.

36.8 Prevention of Further Fragility Fractures

As discussed above, the future fracture risk in patients with a low-trauma fracture is increased two- to fivefold in the following years. A recent meta-analysis by Bolland et al. and two other studies (RCTs by Lyles et al. and Beaupre et al.) showed that oral and intravenous administration of BP following a hip fracture is associated with a significant reduction of future fractures and with a significant reduction of mortality in the following years. The mortality reduction effect is related only in part due to the skeletal effects of BP. Study results suggest also an additional effect on cardiovascular events and pneumonia that still have to

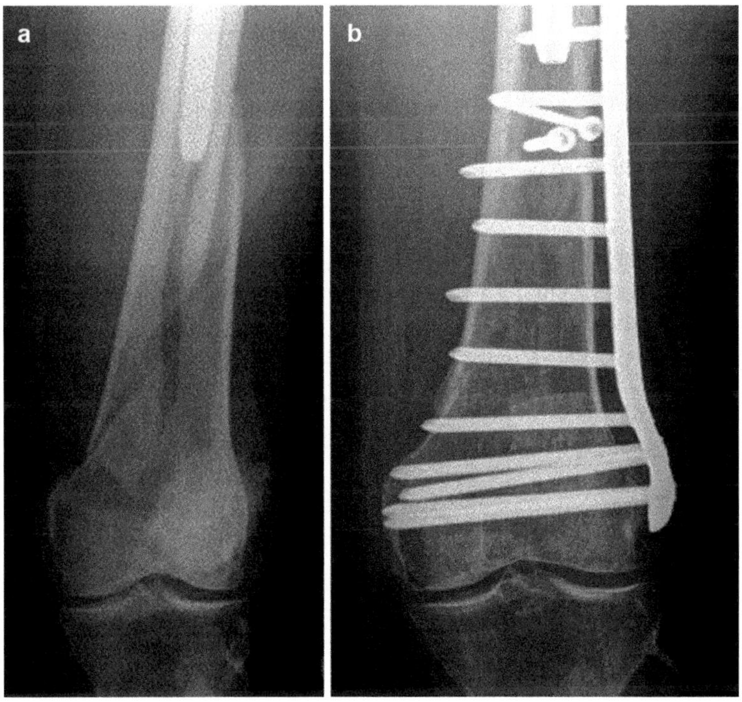

Fig. 36.20 (**a**) Peri-implant fracture of the distal femur at the tip of the femoral nail. (**b**) Overlapping osteosynthesis with a bridging plate

be determined. Post hoc analysis of patients with a prior fracture also showed a reduction of future low-trauma fractures in patients treated with teriparatide and denosumab. The most worrying finding in recent US and European studies is a stagnation/downward trend in the number of patients who receive osteoporosis medication following a first fragility fracture, which appears to have decreased by at least 30 % over the last decade. It is assumed that less than 30 % of patients with new fractures get adequate treatment according to the guidelines. Paradoxically the finding is most marked in the case of hip fractures, which account for the highest mortality rate and the major costs of all fractures. A lower osteoporosis medication initiation rate correlates with high age, male gender and patients receiving long-term care. The underlying causes for this substantial treatment gap are unclear. Potential reasons are that many doctors are in fear of rare complications and side effects of osteoporosis medications and ignore the clear advantage of these drugs in the benefit-to-risk analysis. Also a decline in BMD testing due to unclear reimbursement policies may play a role. A chance to close the treatment gap is the creation of worldwide fracture liaison services to better identify patients with fragility fractures and to improve prevention of further osteoporotic fractures.

Principles for the treatment of patients with osteoporotic fractures:

- All patients presenting a low-energy fracture should be screened for osteoporosis.
- All patients should be placed on 1000 IU of vitamin D and 1000 mg of elemental calcium daily.
- Before discharge, all patients should be started on oral weekly BP medication. As alternative intravenous BP administration (once yearly 5 mg zoledronate or 3 mg ibandronate every 3 months) can be started 2 months after the fracture or subcutaneous administration of denosumab every 6 months.
- In severe osteoporosis with multiple osteoporotic fractures or new fractures sustained under BP treatment, osteoanabolic drugs such as teriparatide (20 μg s.c. daily) or parathormone (100 μg s.c. daily) can be used alternatively.
- Within 6 weeks after discharge, all patients should undergo a DXA scan and a metabolic workup to rule out secondary causes of osteoporosis.

37 Fractures in Rare Bone Disorders

Typical fractures rarely present diagnostic problems. However, certain special types of fractures are frequently misdiagnosed. This chapter provides background information on various forms of special fractures, pathological fractures and rare bone disorders presenting with fractures.

37.1 Stress Fractures

Stress fractures occur in normal bone subjected to high stress peaks (fatigue fracture), e.g. in runners or athletes in high-impact disciplines. On the other hand, they also occur in bone that is weakened by an underlying bone disease subjected to normal stresses (insufficiency fractures), e.g. *atraumatic insufficiency fracture* of the sacrum. Fatigue stress fractures are associated with new, strenuous activities to which the bone is not adapted and are mainly located in the lower extremity. Runners often present with the medial tibial cortex stress injury that represents a prestage of the stress fracture. Due to the repetitive strain, the bone turnover is increased and microcracks occur due to a localised increase of osteoclastic activity. If the balance between formation and resorption is disturbed, the bone weakens and becomes susceptible to injury. If further strain is applied, the cracks lengthens and results in a cortical fracture. At this stage stress fractures often show linear radiolucent lines with sclerotic borders on plain radiographs. On MRI stress reactions and complete stress fractures can be diagnosed early, as they are still inapparent on radiographs. In late stages the periosteal reactions with callus formation, now present on plain radiographs, indicate healing of the stress fracture. Fatigue fractures also typically occur at the metatarsals of military recruits *(marching fracture)* (Fig. 37.1). Typically the pain is related to the strenuous activity and is relieved after cessation. In female runners presenting with the female triad (eating disorder, amenorrhea, oestrogen

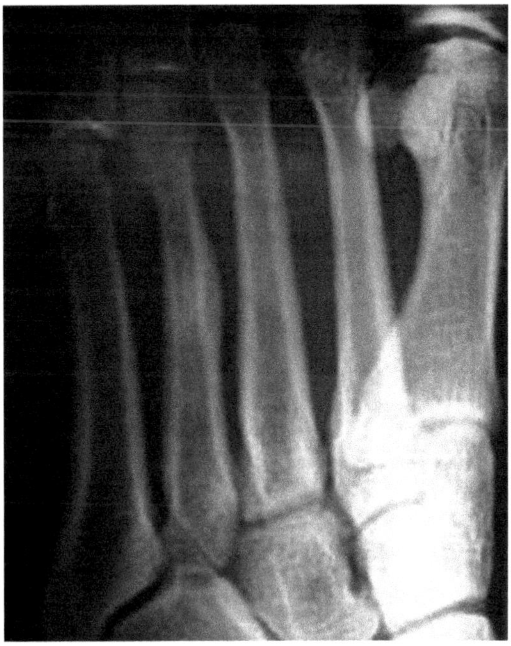

Fig. 37.1 Stress fracture of the fourth metatarsal with repair callus in a runner

R. Bartl, C. Bartl, *Bone Disorders*, DOI 10.1007/978-3-319-29182-6_37

deficiency), stress fractures are also common. Most fractures involve the weight-bearing lower extremities and typically are located in the tibia and fibula, the metatarsals, the calcaneus, the femur shaft and neck and pelvis. The vast majority of stress fractures can be managed conservatively with the REST programme, when diagnosed at an early stage. For high-risk fractures, susceptible to non-healing, that mainly are located on the distraction side of bones, e.g. the tibial shaft, femoral shaft or femoral neck, osteosynthesis in some cases is necessary to stabilise the fracture. For differential diagnosis, the repeated strenuous activity helps to differentiate stress fractures from bone infections and pathologic fractures caused by neoplasms.

37.2 Fractures in Congenital and Metabolic Disorders

Fractures are a common complication of patients with metabolic bone disease. When diagnosed on plain radiographs, these diseases already caused a substantial loss of bone strength. Therefore, fractures already occur earlier with apparently normal bone. To identify these fractures correctly, any fracture related to a minimal or no trauma should be evaluated for an underlying bone disease.

Osteogenesis imperfecta (OI) represents a group of hereditary disorders associated with abnormal collagen synthesis and composition. OI appears with genetically and clinically heterogeneous subtypes with variations within each phenotype and therefore classification is difficult (see also Chap. 40). Patients often present with osteopenia or osteoporosis, brittle bones associated with fractures and skeletal deformities, blue sclerae, hearing loss, dental deformities and abnormal skin. Figure 37.2 shows a 14-year-old osteogenesis imperfecta patient with a femur fracture sustained following a minimal trauma.

Osteomalacia presents with a poor mineralisation of bones. Patients present with skeletal deformities, bone pain, fractures and muscle

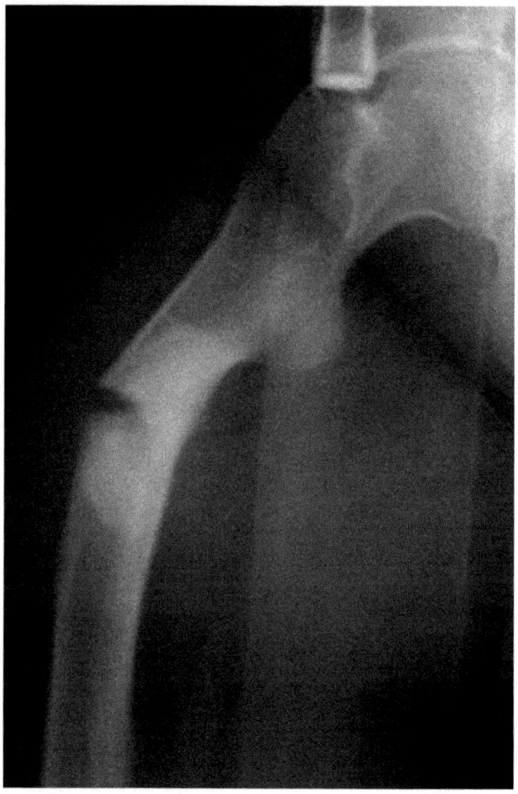

Fig. 37.2 Proximal femur fracture in a 14-year-old boy with osteogenesis imperfecta

Table 37.1 Rare bone disorders associated with fractures

Reduced bone density	Normal bone density	Increased bone density
Senile osteoporosis Postmenopausal osteoporosis Secondary osteoporoses Osteogenesis imperfecta Osteomalacia Fibrous dysplasia Homocystinuria Hypophosphatasia	Stress fractures	Osteopetrosis Metastatic bone disease (e.g. prostate, breast cancer) Renal osteodystrophy Fluorosis Paget's disease

weakness. Fractures are described as Looser zones and show up as radiolucent bands of undermineralised bone following an unhealed cortical microfracture with no present callus and in most cases perpendicular to the cortex orientation. Fractures can occur at multiple locations and typically involve the ribs, anterior pelvic ring and the medial side of the proximal femur. Pathologic fractures also occur following cortical erosions in bone cysts, in bone tumours or tumours presenting with skeletal metastasis (see also Chaps. 94 and 97). Table 37.1 gives an overview on rare bone disorders presenting with fractures.

38 Falls and Fall Prevention

About a third of older persons fall at least once a year, but less than 5 % of these falls result in a fracture. Wrist fractures usually involve a fall onto the outstretched arm. Proximal humerus fractures occur following a fall on the adducted arm. Hip fractures and fractures of the pelvic ring occur after a fall on the side. Axial loading or compression forces associated with degenerative disc alterations in elderly patients can lead to vertebral fractures.

Falling leads to increased fear of falling, resulting in reduced physical activity due to avoidance strategies. Over time immobility is also associated with increased risk of falling.

Factors associated with increased risk of falling in the frail elderly are:

- Reduced muscle mass and strength
- Slowing of reflexes
- Use of walking aids
- Loss of equilibrium
- Cognitive deficits
- Impaired vision
- Impaired coordination
- Hypnotics, sedatives and psychotropics
- Alcohol
- Environmental hazards (e.g. cables)

Studies in geriatric patients showed that 75 % of patients were mobile without walking aids before the fracture, but only 20 % of them after the fracture. Therefore, falling represents a negative "life event" in this frail patient group. Falling can be a sign of frailty, aggravation of chronic diseases and imminent loss of independence. In frail elderly patients, presence of multiple risk factors like depression, sarcopenia, weight loss and immobility further increase the risk of falling. For identification of patients at risk and also to evaluate physical function following rehabilitation after a fragility fracture, geriatric assessment scores (e.g. Charlson co-morbidity index) and fall evaluation forms should be used to assess also the psychological, cognitive and nutrition status of the patient.

Therapeutic interventions include balance programmes, strengthening exercises, reduction of unnecessary medications, optimising lifestyle and the use of walking aids and protection devices. The Cochrane Database showed that group- and home-based exercise programmes and home safety interventions reduce the rate of falls in older adults. Vitamin D supplementation in individuals with vitamin D deficiency should be given with an initial boosting dose and consequent application of 1000–2000 IU daily. In several studies vitamin D supplementation showed advantages for muscle function and reduction of falls and fracture events in elderly patients with vitamin D deficiency.

R. Bartl, C. Bartl, *Bone Disorders*, DOI 10.1007/978-3-319-29182-6_38

Part IX

Variants of Osteoporosis

39 Osteoporosis in Men

39.1 Clinical Evaluation of Osteoporosis in Men

Ageing in men is accompanied by a steady decline in levels of gonadal steroids and of growth hormones which largely determine the decrease in bone mineral density. The concept of "andropause", i.e. the natural age-related decline in testosterone levels in men, is beginning to be understood and to be accepted by health-care professionals and by the general public. Many studies have now been carried out on the effects of hypogonadism in men and its consequences, not only osteoporosis. The consequences of ageing usually also affect the bones, directly or indirectly.

However, there is insufficient awareness of the benefits of *testosterone replacement therapy*, which has already proved its value in the relatively short term, while the long-term results are awaited. Moreover, so far little attention has been paid to the direct effects of gonadal steroids and the effect their decline has on the bone and its metabolism in elderly men. Age is recognised as the most important risk factor for male osteoporosis, which occurs about 10–15 years later than in women, that is, at about 60–65 years of age, with an acceleration of bone loss after 70 years apparently due to unbalanced remodelling, which also results in deterioration of the microarchitecture of the bone.

> Men have osteoporotic fractures 10 years later than women and generally do worse.

It should be noted that a high proportion of men (approximately 60 % in some studies) no longer have optimal secretion of androgens from 60 years of age, though levels start to decrease much earlier. It should also be emphasised that the beneficial effects of testosterone therapy on bone density, on obesity, on insulin resistance and on coronary angina have already been documented in clinical trials.

Decline in other factors associated with ageing may also contribute to osteoporosis. A decrease in muscle mass (*sarcopenia*) is common even in healthy people over 60 years and increases with age and influences the status of the bones. Directed efforts to prevent the muscle loss should emphasise sustained physical activity from childhood throughout life as the years pass including appropriate exercises.

It is only in recent years that osteoporosis in men has been recognised as a major public health problem, the extent of which is increasing steadily also as a result of the increase in numbers of elderly people in the population and with a corresponding increase in cost. Moreover, men with hip fractures have a higher morbidity and mortality than women.

According to recent estimates, 20 % of all cases of osteoporosis occur in men. Osteoporosis is present in 6 % and osteopenia in 47 % of males over age 50. The clinical picture of established osteoporosis in men is comparable to that in women, with kyphosis due to wedge fractures of the thoracic column, protuberance of the abdomen and transverse skin folds over the dorsal trunk. The male/female

R. Bartl, C. Bartl, *Bone Disorders*, DOI 10.1007/978-3-319-29182-6_39

ratio of hip fractures has been calculated to be 1:3, and the vertebral fracture ratio even approaches 1:2.

Four *diagnostic steps* are recommended:

- Exclusion of other bone disorders with diminished bone mineral content (osteomalacia)
- Quantification of the degree of osteopenia (DXA of the lumbar spine and proximal femur and possibly additional sites as indicated in the individual patient)
- Evaluation of the clinical stage of osteoporosis (from preclinical and uncomplicated to advanced stage with complications)
- Exclusion of secondary osteoporosis, in addition to the primary, involutional, age-related osteoporosis

The percentage of men with secondary osteoporosis is around 50 %, higher by 10 % than that in women. Consequently men, especially the older age groups, should be carefully screened to reveal any additional underlying causes for the osteoporosis (Table 39.1). Important *risk factors* are:

- *Heavy smoking*: Smoking in men reduces BMD at the hip and the forearm and increases the fracture risk.
- *Hypogonadism*: The effects are directly related to time of onset, at about 60 years, and duration. Age-related (>73 years) decrease in measurable free testosterone levels are accompanied by clinical symptoms including erectile dysfunction, prostatism, changes in cognitive functions, in daily activities and osteoporosis.
- *High alcohol consumption*: The precise mechanism of the negative effect of alcohol on the bone has not yet been elucidated, but it appears to be on bone formation. However, other deleterious lifestyle factors undoubtedly also contribute to the reduced BMD and fractures which occur in chronic alcohol abusers.
- *Dietary factors*: Studies have shown that the consequences of eating disorders in men, i.e. the various subtypes of anorexia nervosa and binge eating, can be as bad if not worse than in women as predicted by the duration of the condition, the low BMI and severe osteoporosis. Duration of the disorder/s is also an important factor in the consequent osteoporosis. And, as pointed out previously, undernutrition in early life may also predispose accelerated ageing and its accompanying dysfunctions.
- *Weight loss*: A low BMI (body mass index) and weight loss in middle-aged men before and continuing into the andropause are strongly and negatively related to BMD of the hip.
- *Stress and anxiety*: These states could be classified as primary or secondary, for example, together with the depressive states. But there is one important difference, the age of the patients, as the patients with stress fractures are usually young and may be male military personnel. Investigation of 32 young military personnel patients and 32 healthy controls showed only that the patients had a decreased bone turnover and calcaneal stiffness, but no other pathological or biochemical cause for the fractures was found.
- *Prostate cancer*: It poses a major risk factor for osteoporosis, especially when the patient is on androgen deprivation therapy. BMD should be measured before starting therapy, which should be initiated as quickly as possible after diagnosis to prevent spread and skeletal metastases. Various non-hormonal therapies have been advocated to improve the patient's quality of life and possibly survival.

Table 39.1 Indications for DXA measurement in men

Fragility fractures
Glucocorticoid therapy (≥5 mg prednisone for ≥3 months)
Androgen deprivation therapy for prostate cancer
Hypogonadism
Height loss > inches from maximum height
Smoking
Malabsorption
Billroth surgery
Alcoholism
Medications associated with secondary osteoporosis
Recurrent calcium-containing renal stones

- *Renal disorders*: Older men with reduced renal function are at increased risk of osteoporosis and hip fractures.

The most frequent cause (about 30 %) of osteoporosis in men is *testosterone deficiency*, and it is a risk factor for hip fractures. The level of testosterone in the blood must always be determined since some patients do not suffer from sexual dysfunction and appear to have normal testes in spite of decreased levels of testosterone. Specific causes of *hypogonadism* include:

- Klinefelter syndrome
- Prolactinomas
- Kallmann syndrome
- Prader-Willi syndrome
- Male Turner syndrome (Noonan syndrome)
- Haemochromatosis
- Status post orchitis
- Castration

Androgens are crucial for peak bone mass in men and the maintenance of bone strength thereafter. The effect of androgen on the bone in men is mediated by the conversion of androgen to oestradiol via the aromatase enzyme. Hypogonadism is the major risk factor for osteoporosis in men.

Symptomatic late-onset hypogonadism (SLOH) may be particularly troublesome due to physical and mental effects, including fatigue, lethargy, reduced physical and mental activities, reduced muscle and bone mass, anaemia, increased sweating and decreased sense of well-being among other symptoms. These patients require very inclusive examinations (PSA, haemoglobin, etc.) before specific therapy, especially with androgens, is advised. Men with low testosterone levels may have a variety of physical manifestations such as increased weight and fat mass, especially abdominal. The biochemical changes include higher glucose, insulin and triglyceride levels. BMD is decreased, which is due to an increase in resorption of the bone as well as a decrease in its formation and thereby a rapid loss of bone. Moreover, it has been demonstrated in several studies that oestrogen deficiency also plays an important part in causing osteoporosis in men by the following mechanism: a high serum level of the sex hormone-binding globulin lowers the levels of both testosterone and oestrogen in the blood and reduces the availability of androgen for synthesis of oestrogen by aromatisation in peripheral tissues. It is the deficiency of oestrogen rather than androgen which is responsible for the increased bone resorption – even in men. This has been confirmed by data from the Framingham study which demonstrated that low hip BMD in elderly men is correlated with low serum oestradiol levels rather than with testosterone deficiency. Indeed, oestrogen action is clearly essential for the normal development of the bone in young males and exerts important effects on the bone in adults as well.

39.2 Special Features in Men

There are differences in frequency and in fracture site between men and women. Boys have fractures of the extremities more frequently than girls. However, this is readily explained by (a) the fact that boys are more active in sports than girls, particularly aggressive and contact sports, and by (b) the stronger physical force of young men. The diameter of the vertebral bodies and of the long bones is greater in men than in women, and this constitutes an important defence against fractures. The frequency of femoral neck fractures in men decreases during the period of 35–60 years of age and only begins to rise again after 70 years. Two main factors determine the differences in the condition of the skeleton between men and women. The first is the peak bone mass and the second is the late and slow decline in testosterone. Due to their greater physical activity and higher calcium intake, young men have a peak bone mass 25 % greater than that of young women. Moreover, the age-related bone loss that begins around 30 years of age is slower in men: 0.3 % annually compared to 0.8 % in women. Testosterone levels in men decline slowly with age so that the "andropause" as it is now called is not due to a sudden decrease in sexual hormones as in women. Women may lose up to 40 % of their trabecular bone during their lifetime but men only about 14 %. The comparatively low incidence of osteoporosis in men can be explained by:

- A higher peak bone mass at maturity
- Greater diameter of the long bones and vertebral bodies
- A low rate of bone loss in later life
- Men not undergoing sudden hormonal decline equivalent to menopause
- Andropause being characterised by a later, gradual decrease
- Men having, on average, a lower life expectancy, which is changing (fortunately)

39.3 Prevention of Osteoporosis in Men

Prevention of osteoporosis in men starts with investigation of calcium intake and blood levels of testosterone, which can be given as needed in gels, in patches, in tablets or by i.m. injections, for example, 250 mg testosterone enanthate i.m. every 3–4 weeks or testosterone patches 2.5 mg daily, though not of course to patients with carcinoma of the prostate. Isolated hypogonadotropic hypogonadism (IHH), which may occur in severely obese men, possibly because of increased oestradiol production, can be treated by an aromatase inhibitor, such as letrozole, at low dosages, 2.5 mg weekly, to begin with. However, it is important to take into account that men may be subject to fractures at higher bone densities than women and that men have higher mortality rates than women after hip fractures. Though the level of vitamin D does not automatically decline with age in healthy men, hypovitaminosis D is prevalent and therefore supplements are recommended. The following programme can be applied for prevention of osteoporosis in men:

- Daily intake of 1000 mg calcium and 1000 IU vitamin D
- Regular physical activity, adapted to each patient
- No smoking (Fig. 39.1)
- Moderate alcohol consumption only
- Monitoring of testosterone levels and treating as required
- Monitoring additional disorders and medications which possibly affect the bones
- Avoidance of falls and use of hip protection devices especially in elderly men

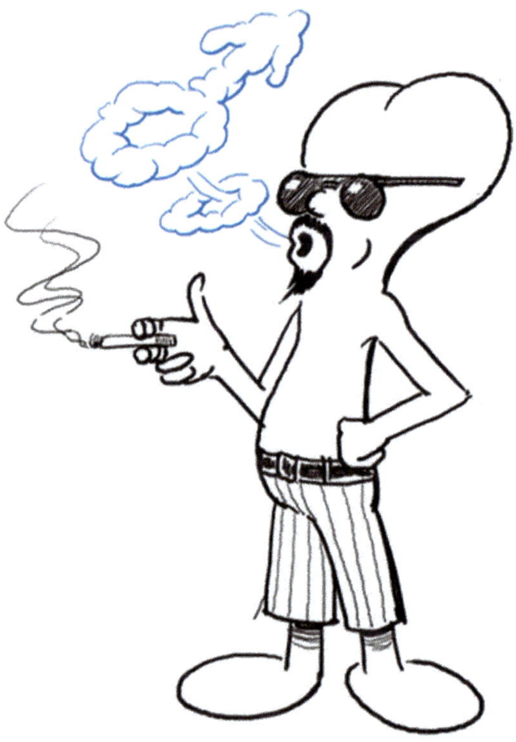

Fig. 39.1 Cigarette smoking – the bone terrorist number one and a main risk factor of osteoporosis in men!

39.4 Therapy of Osteoporosis in Men

The same guidelines apply as for women: ade encouraged. If the testosterone levels are found to be low and there are no contraindications, intramuscular, subcutaneous or transdermal testosterone will increase bone mass. As demonstrated in clinical trials, the N-containing bisphosphonates (BP) are equally effective, safe and well tolerated in men as in women.

All potent BP and also denosumab have been associated with osteonecrosis of the jaw, basically after an invasive dental procedure, but the incidence of this side effect is only about 1/10,000–1/100,000; effective recommendations for avoiding this serious complication have been published.

Alendronate, risedronate and zoledronate have been approved and are considered the BP of choice for osteoporosis in men, as already demonstrated in prospective studies.

The two most common reasons that male patients do not show an increase of bone density under therapy are:

- The patient does not take the treatment or take it correctly (about 40 % of all patients under oral treatment).
- The patient shows a deficiency of vitamin D.

However, fractures of the femoral shaft have occurred after long-term, i.e. >6 years, therapy with alendronate. Therefore, careful monitoring is required. Denosumab and teriparatide also appear to be potent but are relatively expensive.

The main reason we have to treat osteoporosis in men is that hip fracture is a fatal complication. Men older than 75 years have a 34 % chance of dying within 1 year after hip fracture.

40 Osteoporosis in Children and Adolescents

During growth, the shape, architecture and strength of the bones are modulated by three major processes: growth, modelling and remodelling. Modelling is of particular interest as it appears that bone is much more capable of responding to external loads during growth than at any other time. Remodelling also occurs during growth, but is limited, and does not participate in active growth, i.e. to accrue bone. Information on the pattern of bone mineral deposition is illustrated in Figs. 40.1 and 40.2, which show the plots and velocity curves of total body bone mineral content during growth. The authors of these longitudinal studies of boys and girls have also shown that, on average, 26 % of adult total bone mineral was accrued during the 2 years around peak bone mineral content velocity, at average ages of 12.5 years for girls and 14.1 years for boys. Furthermore, it is of interest that true bone density does not increase with size or age, and reported increases in BMD with age are a reflection of growth and an increase in size rather than an increase in bone mineral per unit volume. The crucial importance of food in childhood to achieve optimal physical and cognitive development has long been acknowledged as has the recognition that the promotion of children's health will help to reduce diet-related risks of many adult diseases, including degenerative and cardiovascular disorders, diabetes type two, cancers, obesity and osteoporosis. Consequently, nutrition guidelines for children from 2 to 11 years have just been published: the Position of the American Dietetic Association.

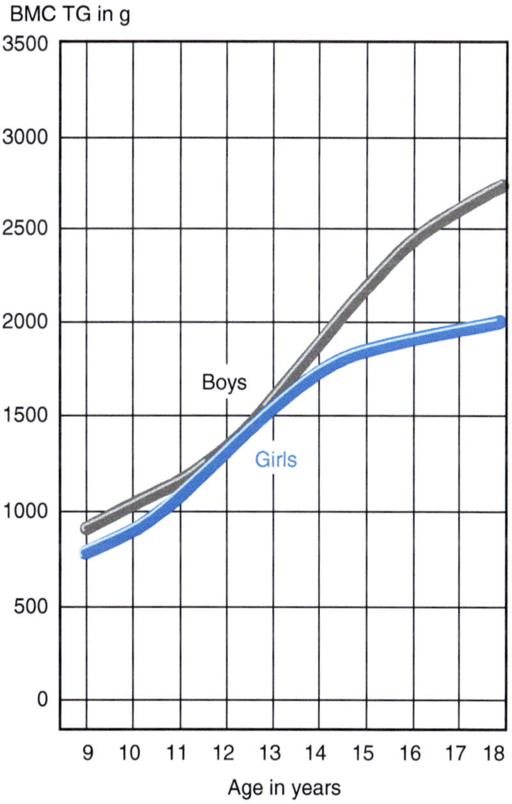

Fig. 40.1 Total body bone mineral content for boys and girls according to age (Modified from Baily 1997)

R. Bartl, C. Bartl, *Bone Disorders*, DOI 10.1007/978-3-319-29182-6_40

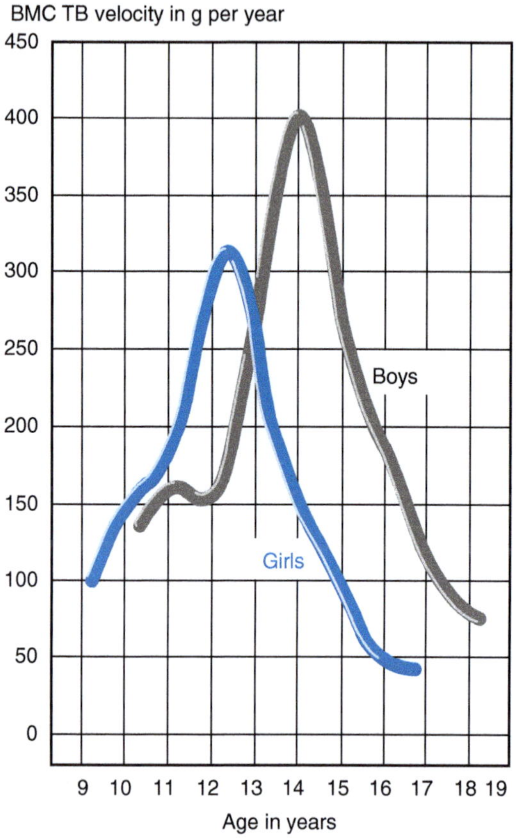

Fig. 40.2 Velocity curves depicting sex and age differences in timing and magnitude of peak bone mineral accrual (Modified from Baily 1997)

40.1 Differential Diagnosis of Osteoporosis in Children and Adolescents

Though osteoporosis rarely occurs in children, it may do so and cause severe pain, multiple fractures and lifelong limitations of movement and locomotion unless adequately treated. Osteoporosis in children is often not diagnosed until after one or two fractures have occurred or if low density is suspected on radiographs (Table 40.1). Consequently increased awareness is just as important, if not more so, than for adults, as any decrease in bone density during childhood and adolescence which remains uncorrected will have a negative impact on peak bone mass with increased risk of osteoporosis later in life.

Table 40.1 Investigation for underlying disease in childhood osteoporosis

Complete blood count and ESR
Renal and liver function (serum)
Glucose (serum, urine)
TSH (serum)
Calcium, phosphate (serum)
Alkaline phosphatase (serum)
Vitamin D and PTH (serum)
Fasting urine calcium
X-ray of the skull and lumbar spine
Bone turnover markers
Bone/bone marrow biopsy (when indicated)

Osteoporosis in children has not yet been officially defined. The *WHO definition* is based on values for adults. However, recommendations for paediatric densitometry have now been published. In practice, the diagnosis is based on a bone density measurement and an X-ray (Figs. 40.3 and 40.4):

- More than two SDs below the average value of a child of similar age with healthy bones
- Number of pathologic fractures

Musculoskeletal complaints are relatively frequent in children, accounting for about 20 % of visits to their doctors. This is not surprising taking into account that bone is a very active organ metabolically and maintains homeostasis of calcium and phosphorus, so that an imbalance may result in many osteological and other metabolic disorders.

The differential diagnosis includes rheumatic disorders, infections, metabolic bone disorders, neuropathies and specific orthopaedic conditions among others. All may be associated with osteopenia/osteoporosis. The first steps in diagnostic evaluation include family history, physical examination and elementary laboratory tests.

The major causes of osteopenia/osteoporosis in children, both congenital and acquired, are listed below in alphabetical order (this list is not exhaustive):

- Acute leukaemias, lymphatic and myeloid
- Anorexia nervosa
- Anticonvulsant therapy

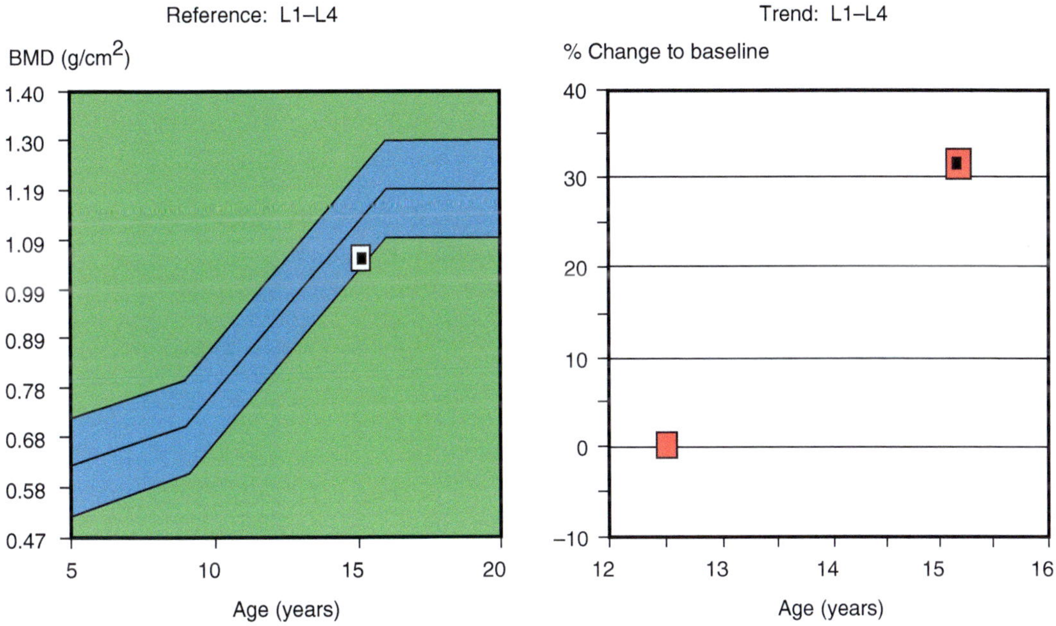

Fig. 40.3 DXA, measurement of BMD of a 15-year-old child with osteoporosis. Marked increase of BMD after therapy with a bisphosphonate for about 3 years

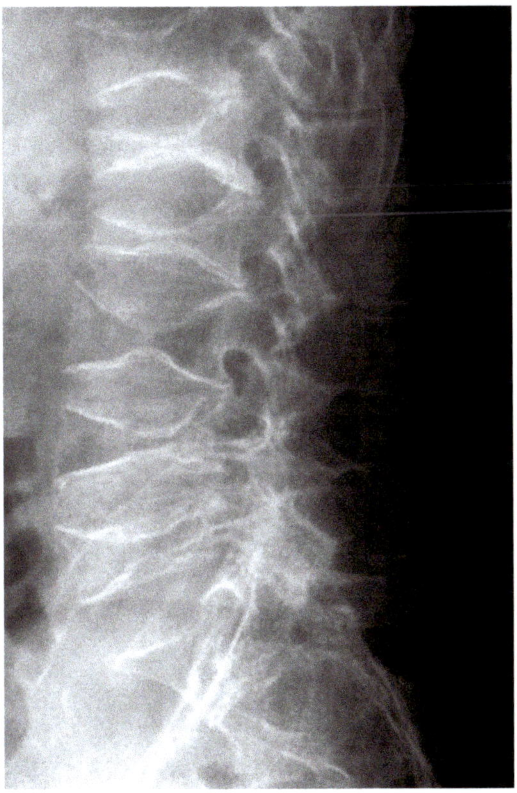

Fig. 40.4 Massive narrowing of all the vertebral bodies and ballooning of the intervertebral discs in a patient with osteogenesis imperfecta

- Asthma bronchiale
- Biliary atresia
- Cerebral palsy
- Chronic hepatic disorders
- Chronic renal insufficiency
- Crohn's and celiac diseases
- Congenital autoimmune disorders, especially those treated with glucocorticoids
- Glucocorticoid therapy
- Cushing's syndrome
- Cyanotic congenital heart disease
- Cystic fibrosis
- Diabetes mellitus
- Drugs
- Glycogen storage disorders
- Growth hormone deficiency
- Homocystinuria
- Hypogonadism
- Idiopathic hyperphosphatasia
- Hypoparathyroidism
- Infections and their consequences, if chronic, e.g. hepatitis C with metabolic risk factors
- Juvenile chronic arthritis
- Juvenile Paget's disease
- Malabsorption syndromes
- Sarcomas in children
- McCune-Albright syndrome

- Neurofibromatoses
- Obesity
- Organ transplantations
- Rheumatic
- Spinal cord injury
- Thalassaemia

Acute immobilisation decreases bone formation and increases bone resorption. Additionally bone growth is severely impaired in prolonged immobilisation, due to a lack of mechanical stimulation. Further important *mechanisms* of osteoporosis in children include:

- Inadequate production of collagen type I (congenital disorders)
- Prolonged immobilisation (fractures or neurologic disorders)
- Inflammatory cytokines (chronic rheumatic disorders)
- Deficiency of vitamin D (nutrition and gastrointestinal disorders)
- Neoplastic diseases of the bone marrow (oncologic disorders)

Glucocorticoid therapy is an integral part of the treatment of many disorders, and therefore the BMD of children should always be checked before the initiation of therapy and the relevant prevention programme initiated. The conditions include renal glomerular diseases, dermatomyositis, inflammatory bowel diseases, juvenile rheumatoid arthritis, post organ transplantation and Duchenne muscular dystrophy. Therapy with glucocorticoids and immunosuppressive drugs, e.g. given for oncologic disorders and for transplantations, but it should be stressed that the causes of osteoporosis in children with cancer are multifactorial. Several reviews have stressed that more awareness is required of the adverse effects of cancer treatment in long-term survivors, especially in view of the fact that, fortunately, increasing numbers of childhood cancer patients are surviving and require close monitoring so that timely application of preventive measures is facilitated.

Paediatric patients with *HIV infection* face a lifetime of antiviral treatment with all the attendant side effects and toxicities, which must also be treated and managed and among them osteopenia and osteoporosis with the consequences thereof. Moreover, beneficial changes in IGF-1 and lean body mass, but not in linear growth, have been noted in children under antiretroviral therapy, which has also been associated with increases in lipid measurements and in insulin resistance. These changes were presumed to be associated with immune restitution and levels of IGF1. HIV infection-associated proteinuria in children with kidney disease can be ameliorated and progression of the renal disease prevented by initiation of HAART therapy.

Insufficient physical activity, not caused by a neurologic deficit, but by the general physical condition as well as psychological aspects, could be responsible for sedentary habits which in turn account for a low BMD, for example, sedentary habits in children with haemophilia. These children may be somewhat apprehensive because of the risk of bleeding.

Adolescent athletes: According to the literature, about a quarter of teenage girls are liable to develop amenorrhoea, in spite of the increased physical activities. This hypogonadism has a negative impact on bone metabolism, which is particularly detrimental at this age, during the time of accrual of the peak bone mass, so that preventive measures are mandatory.

40.2 Therapy of Osteoporosis in Children and Adolescents

Treatment of childhood osteoporosis includes *general measures* such as:

- Adequate pain relief in children with vertebral fractures
- Orthopaedic procedures to fix fractures of the long bones
- Physiotherapy with rehabilitation to improve muscle strength
- Occupational therapy if necessary
- Protection of the spine
- Periods of bed rest in paediatric illness should be minimised to avoid immobilisation osteoporosis, for which immediate therapy should be considered if long periods of rest (matter of months) are anticipated.

Literature on the *medical treatment* of childhood osteoporosis is limited and still not evidence based, but some studies have been reported and the following recommendations made:

- *Calcium and vitamin D* supplementation is recommended though there is little evidence of benefit in the studies available. Nevertheless, a recent study from the UK emphasises the fact that the majority of teenage boys and girls fail to meet the UK government targets for calcium intakes. Most probably this applies to many other countries as well. The importance of this lies in the fact that 90 % of the peak bone mass is attained by the age of 18 years in girls and 20 years in boys. Attention has now been drawn to the fact that hypovitaminosis D is worldwide in children and youth. Studies have shown that it is even prevalent in healthy infants and toddlers! Moreover, today when obesity is considered almost a global epidemic due to its prevalence in many developed and so-called underdeveloped counties, attention must be paid to the nutritional requirements of obese children, who frequently suffer from hypovitaminosis D. These children are at increased risk of developing impaired glucose metabolism with the complications that this implies including effects on the bones. The good news is that it has been conclusively demonstrated that vitamin D can safely be given to children in high doses (14,000 IU) once a week. Moreover, as mentioned earlier, it has been confirmed that poor nutrition in early childhood may accelerate ageing and predispose to various age-related disorders. Therefore, a first priority is the provision (and of course the ingestion) of an adequate well-balanced diet from a very young age onwards.
- *Calcitriol* has been investigated in several small studies with improvement (though not significant) in symptoms, fracture risk and BMD.
- *Growth hormone* is a powerful anabolic agent, and it is well established that children with growth hormone deficiency benefit from growth hormone therapy.
- *Calcitonin* is known to inhibit bone resorption, and some small studies have shown that bone pain may disappear and radiographic signs of osteoporosis may improve under intranasal administration of calcitonin.
- *Bisphosphonates* have also been investigated in childhood osteoporosis, and there have been several encouraging studies in idiopathic juvenile osteoporosis and osteogenesis imperfecta. Concern has been expressed about potential adverse effects on the growing skeleton, though so far these have not appeared and sequential bone biopsies showed normal, lamellar bone without development of osteomalacia. There were also no adverse effects on fracture healing or growth rate. Indeed, nitrogen-containing BP are a treatment option in childhood osteoporosis, but randomised controlled studies are required. Although not yet approved by the FDA for the use in children, nitrogen-containing BP demonstrated benefits to the children treated, with no serious adverse effects. Indeed, bisphosphonates are the first agents to give paediatricians the opportunity to treat bone disorders of childhood effectively. It is important to realise that *spontaneous improvement* without any medical treatment may also occur. Thus, for some children with osteoporosis, it may be appropriate to monitor their progress over time – "watch and wait", particularly if they appear to have stopped breaking their bones. This would also depend on the cause and the circumstances of the child's daily life.

40.3 Idiopathic Juvenile Osteoporosis (IJO), Idiopathic Juvenile Arthritis (IJA) and Other Associated Conditions

In the absence of a primary causative condition, the diagnosis of *idiopathic juvenile osteoporosis* (IJO) is made. IJO is a transient, nonhereditary, rare form of childhood osteoporosis without extraskeletal involvement. In the absence of fractures, the term "osteopenia in childhood" would be more appropriate. It is important to exclude other possible causes of vertebral collapse such as acute leukaemia.

The *aetiology* of IJO has not yet been elucidated. A decrease in osteoblastic reactivity has been reported, and consequently the skeleton no longer adequately adapts to the increased mechanical loads during growth. Spontaneous remissions are the rule and with onset before puberty (mostly between age 8 and 12 years of age).

Differential diagnosis: Osteogenesis imperfecta (OI) is the commonest congenitally determined condition with osteoporosis which must always be carefully excluded (Table 40.2). *Osteoporosis-pseudoglioma syndrome* is a very rare congenital disorder with severe osteoporosis and blindness.

The *clinical picture* presents three different manifestations:

- Fractures of the extremities, especially of the trabecular bones, occasionally with an early onset, even early postnatal, pain in the ankles and knees, with fractures of the lower extremities
- Fractures of vertebral bodies with backache, kyphosis, decrease in height and difficulties in locomotion (walking, running)
- Evidence of low bone density (DXA) without pathologic fractures

Table 40.2 Differential diagnosis between idiopathic juvenile osteoporosis (*IJO*) and osteogenesis imperfecta (*OI*)

	IJO	OI
Family history	Absent	Often positive
Onset	Late childhood	Birth or soon after
Duration	1–4 years	Lifelong
Clinical findings	Abnormal gait	Abnormal dentition
	Metaphyseal fractures	Blue sclerae
	Kyphosis, back pain	Long bone fractures
Growth rate	Normal	Normal or decreased
Radiologic findings	Vertebral fractures	Thin cortex of long bones
	"Neo-osseous osteoporosis"	Wormian bones in skull
Bone biopsy	Decreased bone turnover	Increased bone turnover
Connective tissue defect	No	Collagen abnormalities

Diagnosis of IJO is made by exclusion of OI and of diseases causing secondary osteoporosis. It should be emphasised that IJO is strictly a diagnosis of exclusion and that malignancies in the marrow must be considered. Diagnosis requires X-rays of the lumbar spine in two planes. When OI is suspected, X-rays of the long bones are also required to check for the characteristic metaphyseal compression fractures. The long bones are usually of normal width in IJO, the cortex might be thinned, and metaphyseal fractures are common. On X-rays, the new bone formed in metaphyseal areas appears as a radiolucent band ("neo-osseous osteoporosis"). The onset of OI is usually much earlier in life. The children often have blue sclerae and abnormalities of collagen. Bone density should preferably be measured by DXA of the lumbar vertebrae and if possible a whole-body measurement. For children weighing less than 30 kg, a special paediatric software program is required. The modern bone marker NTX is useful for differentiating OI and IJO.

There are no known biochemical characteristics, and alterations of bone markers are nonspecific. With the introduction of *BP*, therapy of osteoporosis in children is now simple and effective. Several clinical trials have already provided evidence for an increase in bone density and a reduction in fracture risk in children treated with BP. Previous fears that such therapy might interfere with growth of the long bones have not been substantiated. In addition, the osteomalacia seen under therapy with the earlier BP is no longer observed with the newer more potent N-containing BP, which can be given orally or as infusions at 3–6 month intervals. Since randomised clinical trials in children have not yet been carried out, treatment should only be undertaken in paediatric centres, after consultation with the Ethics Committee and signed consent by the parents or guardians has been obtained. Calcium 500–1000 mg daily and vitamin D 500–1000 IU daily should also be given as basic therapy. Calcitriol – the active metabolite of vitamin D – could also be considered.

Patients with IJO can experience a complete recovery within a few years. Growth may be somewhat impaired during the active phase of the disease, but normal growth resumes thereafter. However, in some cases IJO may result in permanent disability such as kyphoscoliosis or even collapse of the ribcage. Since children undergo spontaneous remissions especially when there is osteopenia without fractures, in these cases a policy of watch and wait is recommended to begin with.

Children with IJA often have quite considerable physical impairment. Some do not respond to medications and are then treated with immunosuppression followed by autologous haematopoietic stem cell transplantation, which can induce long-term remissions. However, they have long-term (9 years in one study) impaired exercise tolerance; functional ability and joint status were also decreased. These children require special attention and management to prevent long-term complications including osteoporosis.

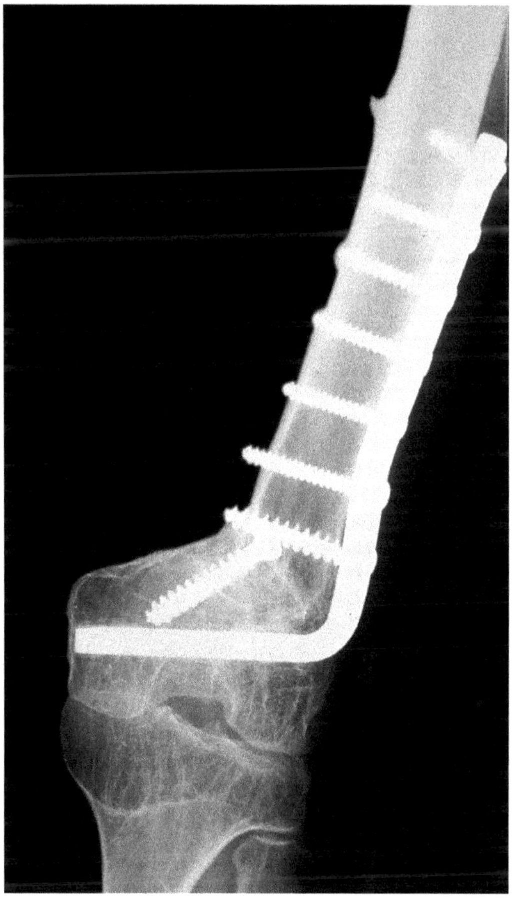

Fig. 40.5 X-ray of girl with osteogenesis imperfecta showing thin cortices and poorly mineralised bone. Note old, healed and new fractures with surgical stabilisation

40.4 Osteogenesis Imperfecta (OI)

This congenital condition should be considered in every case of severe osteoporosis occurring in infancy and childhood. A thorough family history and physical examination are important diagnostic aids. The spine frequently shows severe changes, but fractures occur primarily in the extremities (Figs. 40.4 and 40.5). Attempts to explain the pathophysiology of OI are being made by application of the still-evolving Utah paradigm of skeletal physiology; however, results have not yet been widely published and accepted.

Various genetic mutations have now been related to different types of OI showing differences in clinical features. Different mutations of the genes for collagen type I occur. When even one of the amino acids is incorrectly incorporated into the collagen molecule, a defective molecular structure may result. As a consequence, the helical structure of collagen is altered which in turn leads to a fault in the quality of the bone as evidenced by lack of lamellar structure and susceptibility to breakdown by collagenases. In addition to bone, *other organs* that incorporate collagen type I are also affected, as shown by the following manifestations:

- Thin blue sclerae (Fig. 40.6), rupture of sclerae and keratoconus
- Anomalies of the teeth which appear brown and transparent and are liable to rapid shedding
- Anomalies of the heart valves and of the aorta, prolapse of the mitral valve and aortic insufficiency
- Deafness due to damage to the stapes in the middle ear

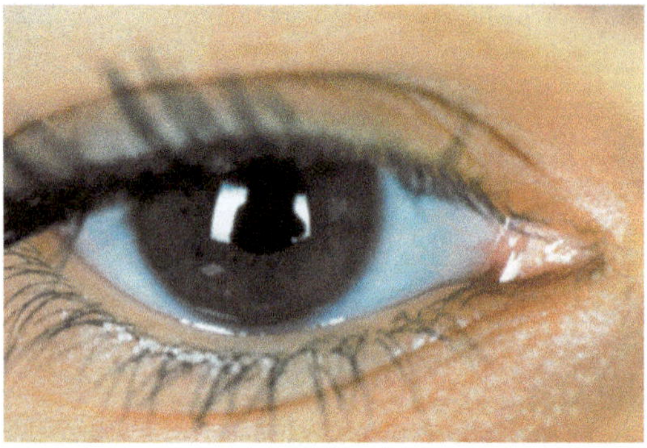

Fig. 40.6 Blue sclerae in patient with osteogenesis imperfecta

- Kidney stones and hypercalciuria
- Hyperplastic callus formation

OI occurs in one of every 20,000 live births. There are approximately 15,000 patients with OI in the USA. The condition varies from apparently typical osteoporosis to severe skeletal anomalies in childhood. Four *types* of OI are distinguished:

- Mild form with blue sclerae (type I)
- Lethal perinatal form (type II)
- Progressive deforming form (type III)
- Mild form without blue sclerae (type IV)

Previous attempts at *therapy* with fluorides were unsuccessful, as were bone marrow transplants including replacement of stromal cells. Today early administration of BP is the therapy of choice and in severe cases by infusions every 3 months otherwise orally. Recent studies have shown that oral alendronate therapy is safe and effective in children with OI, even very young ones.

During the past 3 years, we have treated 50 patients with modern BP, both orally and intravenously. All showed impressive improvements in their conditions:

- Increase in bone density.
- Increase in bone quality demonstrated in sequential biopsies.
- Decrease in symptoms especially bone pain.
- Striking decrease in fracture rate (before therapy up to 12 fractures annually!).
- Bone healing was not impaired.
- Despite decreasing bone turnover, N-containing bisphosphonates did not impair growth.

Calcium and vitamin D are given together with the BP to improve the mineralisation of the newly formed bone. Results of several clinical trials of bisphosphonates (pamidronate, zoledronate, neridronate) in children and adults with OI have now been published. BMD and physical activity increased markedly under treatment with BP, and the fracture rate decreased by 65 %. After 4 years of treatment with pamidronate, bone mineral content, bone volume and volumetric bone mineral density were 54 %, 44 % and 65 % higher, respectively, in treated than in untreated patients who were matched for age and type of OI. Patients with larger deficits in bone mass at baseline had a more marked gain of bone mass during therapy. An interesting effect of BP therapy in young children is delayed eruption of teeth, previously described in animals. A study has confirmed that under bisphosphonate therapy, tooth eruption in children with OI was delayed for a mean period of 1.67 years.

It is noteworthy that long-term adverse side effects have not been reported. On the contrary, it has been claimed that, until the advent of realistic gene therapy, BP appear to be the most efficient way of arresting the progression of OI and improving the quality of life of the patients, irrespective of type of collagen mutation, clinical severity and age at start of therapy. A recent review and update on the diagnosis, classification, pathophysiological mechanisms and current therapy have been published (Glorieux 2008). The potential for direct replacement of collagen-producing cells in the bone marrow (stem cell therapy) has led to a limited number of studies in severely affected infants, with variable results.

In *summary:* Treatment of childhood osteoporotic syndromes requires an *interdisciplinary approach* including orthopaedic surgeons, physiotherapists, occupational therapists, dentists, paediatricians and psychologists for immediate therapy, for further information and support and to prevent and care for recurrent fractures. Appropriate organisations and support groups (e.g. Osteogenesis Imperfecta Foundation) are very important for patients and their families.

40.5 Turner Syndrome and Charge Syndrome

Two other congenital disorders with very complex and distinctive features including retarded growth and development are the Turner syndrome and the Charge syndrome. They both require a multidisciplinary approach to therapy. The Turner syndrome affects only female infants, girls and women who all have a lifelong risk of osteoporosis which must be managed according to the age-related requirements, including the appropriate dietary factors, e.g. calcium and vitamins, as well as hormones at the menarche, modified HRT after the menopause and appropriate anti-osteoporotic therapy thereafter to prevent involutional osteoporosis.

40.6 X-linked Hypophosphataemic Rickets

These children also require early growth hormone treatment, which improves serum levels of phosphate and of vitamin D and normalises parathyroid function. However, the degree of improvement in rickets should be checked, by investigation of the mineralisation of bone. If there is evidence of early skeletal deformities, these must be carefully followed.

40.7 Gaucher's Disease

Gaucher's disease is the most common lysosomal storage disorder. It is due to deficiency of the enzyme glucocerebrosidase. The disease is divided into subtypes of which the non-neuropathic is the most common and has the greatest variability. Prominent clinical manifestations are hepatosplenomegaly, cytopaenias and skeletal disorders. Early recognition, diagnosis and therapy are essential to prevent disease progression which includes irreversible skeletal deformities and other severe co-morbidities. Safe and efficient enzyme substitution therapy has been available for nearly two decades. The essential factor is early diagnosis, and it has been shown that over 50 % of the effected children present symptoms well before the age of 10 years.

References

1. Baily D (1997) Int J Sports Med 18 (Suppl 3):191–194
2. Glorieux F (2008) Best Pract Res Clin Rheumatol 22:85–100

41 Premenopausal Osteoporosis

41.1 Pathogenesis

Osteoporosis in premenopausal women results from low peak bone mass, progressive bone loss or a combination of both. Low bone mineral density in this age group is associated with an increased risk of fractures and stress fractures. Studies have shown that fractures before menopause predict postmenopausal fractures. These findings suggest that certain lifelong traits such as fall frequency, neuromuscular protective response to falls, bone mass and aspects of bone quality and mineralisation affect lifelong fracture risk. In premenopausal women, the relationship between BMD and fracture risk is not so clear compared with the data and correlations in postmenopausal women. Therefore, according to current guidelines, the diagnosis of "osteoporosis" should not be based solely upon BMD measurements in premenopausal women. However, premenopausal women with Colles fractures have been found to have significantly lower BMD at the non-fractured radius, lumbar spine and femoral neck than controls without fractures. So, the International Osteoporosis Foundation (IOF) has recommended maintaining the T-score cut-off of −2.5 at the spine ort hip for diagnosis of osteoporosis in those young adults who have completed growth and who suffer from a chronic disorder known to affect bone mass. Before menopause, the absolute fracture risk is generally low, even at low levels of BMD.

41.2 Secondary Causes

Most premenopausal women with low-trauma fractures or low BMD have an underlying disorder or medication exposure that has interfered with bone mass during adolescence. In a population study, 90 % of men and women aged 20–44 with osteoporotic fractures were found to have a secondary cause (Table 41.1). Genetic factors account for up to 80 % of the variance in peak bone mass and are definitely non-modifiable. A low growth rate between the ages of 7 and 15 years was associated with a significantly greater risk of hip fractures in the following years. Modifiable factors may influence whether optimal peak bone mass is reached or maintained. These include:

Table 41.1 Secondary causes of osteoporosis in premenopausal women

Premenopausal amenorrhoea
Anorexia nervosa
Cushing's syndrome
Hyperthyroidism
Primary hyperparathyroidism
Vitamin D, calcium and other nutrient deficiency
Gastrointestinal malabsorption
Rheumatoid arthritis, SLE
Renal disorders
Liver disorders
Chronic alcoholism
Connective tissue disorders
Drugs

R. Bartl, C. Bartl, *Bone Disorders*, DOI 10.1007/978-3-319-29182-6_41

- *Diseases predisposing to bone loss*: For example, rheumatoid arthritis, thyrotoxicosis, coeliac disease, malabsorption and anorexia nervosa. Glucocorticoids, anticonvulsants and heparin are the most important drugs for early bone loss.
- *Menstrual factors:* Delayed menarche, amenorrhoea or prolonged oligomenorrhoea due to oestrogen deficiency may result in low peak mass or bone loss. Similarly, the use of the contraceptive agent depot medroxyprogesterone acetate leads to reduced oestrogen levels. Bone loss is probably partially reversible on cessation and restoration of normal oestrogen levels. Hypothalamic hypogonadism as seen in conditions including anorexia nervosa and exercise-induced amenorrhoea also causes marked bone loss.
- *Lifestyle factors*: Adequate physical activity and calcium and vitamin D intake are necessary to achieve and maintain optimal peak bone mass. Smoking and weight loss, particularly if it occurs in cycles of gain and loss, are also associated with a reduction of BMD.

41.3 Investigation

Premenopausal women with low BMD (Z score below −2.0) and/or with low-trauma fracture should undergo a thorough investigation. Evaluation for an underlying cause is important in premenopausal osteoporosis, as approximately 50 % of cases may be secondary. In a history suggestive of vertebral fracture, a spin radiograph is indicated, as fractures independently increase the risk of subsequent fractures. Vertebral deformities should be carefully evaluated to exclude other disorders such as Scheuermann's disease, which are not associated with increased fracture risk. A bone biopsy may occasionally identify unsuspected causes such as systemic mastocytosis or storage disease.

41.4 Management and Treatment

For all patients, general measures that benefit bone health should be recommended:

- Weight-bearing exercise
- Nutrition (calcium, protein, vitamin D)
- Lifestyle modifications (smoking cessation and avoidance of excess alcohol)
- Administration of oestrogen in women with oestrogen deficiency (unless contraindicated)

Pharmacologic treatment however should be evaluated on an individual basis. Currently there are no licenced treatments for use in premenopausal osteoporosis other than in glucocorticoid-induced osteoporosis. Because bisphosphonates accumulate in the maternal skeleton, they may cross the placenta and may accumulate in the foetal skeleton; they should be used with caution in women that may become pregnant. In general, bisphosphonates should be reserved for those with low-trauma fractures or ongoing massive bone loss. Other agents such as rhPTH, raloxifene or strontium ranelate are unlicensed and cannot be recommended. Contraceptive precautions are advisable in all women of child-bearing potential embarking on treatment. Follow-up should be continued until it is established that BMD is stable without treatment or that treatment response has been demonstrated by serial BMD measurements. Biochemical markers of bone turnover may be helpful to demonstrate response to antiresorptive treatment.

Pregnancy-Associated Osteoporosis

42

42.1 The Skeleton Under Pregnancy and Lactation

An increasing drain of maternal reserves mineralises the foetal skeleton. In total, the developing foetal skeleton gains up to 33 g of calcium, and about 80 % of this is deposited during the third trimester when the foetal skeleton grows rapidly. This high demand for calcium is largely met by a doubling of maternal intestinal calcium absorption, mediated by calcitriol and other hormones, which is usually enough to meet the daily calcium needs of the foetus without long-term consequences to the maternal skeleton. The increased calcium absorption early in pregnancy may stimulate the maternal skeleton to prepare for the peak foetal demands that occur later in pregnancy. Subsequently during lactation, sufficient calcium must be supplied in the breast milk to enable skeletal growth of the infant. Calcium homeostasis in human pregnancy and lactation is illustrated in Fig. 42.1.

The female body has several compensatory mechanisms to supply the increased demand for calcium during pregnancy and lactation so that problems only arise if the calcium depots (in the bones) are not full to begin with. Indeed, fragility fractures in pregnancy may be a consequence of pre-existing low BMD and increased bone resorption. Therefore, supplements of calcium and vitamins are recommended and should be taken from the beginning of pregnancy.

However, pregnancy per se is not a risk factor for osteoporosis. But risk factors are incurred if the pregnant woman is subjected to bed rest and/or is treated with muscle relaxants and/or sedatives. In some cases even corticosteroids are given.

In these situations a massive withdrawal of calcium from the bones is unavoidable and should be compensated at the very least with adequate supplements of calcium and vitamin D. During pregnancy, there is normally a slight decrease in bone density, but this loss is soon replaced after birth. However, it should be remembered that during lactation, about 500 mg calcium is excreted daily into the milk, which should be balanced on a daily basis by increased ingestion of appropriate foods and supplements. In reality, very few women suffer from osteoporotic fractures during (and because of) the pregnancy itself. The vast majority of women can be assured that the changes in bone and calcium metabolism during pregnancy and lactation are normal and without adverse consequences in the long term.

Results of a study comparing the bone status in young *primiparas* (young women immediately after the birth of the first child) with that of young "nulliparas" (young women who had not yet been pregnant and given birth) showed that the values of QUS measurements were significantly lower and

R. Bartl, C. Bartl, *Bone Disorders*, DOI 10.1007/978-3-319-29182-6_42

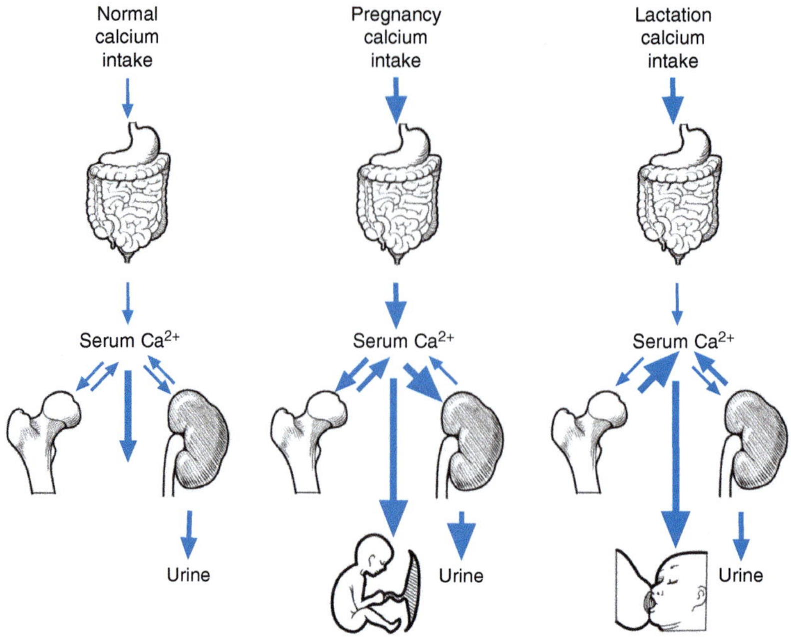

Fig. 42.1 Calcium homeostasis in normal women compared to that in pregnancy and lactation (Modified from Kovacs C, Kronenberg H.: Maternal-fetal calcium and bone metabolism during pregnancy, puerperium and lactation. *Endocr. Rev.* **18**, 832–872 (1997))

the bone markers higher in the primiparas in the early postpartum than in the nulliparas. Since later measurements were not given, definitive conclusions cannot be drawn. Possibly such early examinations were not previously recorded and the deficiency very quickly rectified, with no lasting adverse effects.

The maternal status of vitamin D during pregnancy has lately attracted some attention, and the suggestion put forward that this may affect intrauterine skeletal mineralisation, growth and development of muscles and possibly even a more sustained influence in childhood and later.

> Lower maternal vitamin D levels during late pregnancy have been associated with reduced bone mass in offspring during the neonatal period and mid-childhood. This is partly mediated by umbilical venous calcium concentration.

These possibilities raise the question of early determination of the pregnant woman's vitamin D level and administration of supplements as required. However, few investigations of possible benefits and adverse reactions of such supplements in pregnant women and on the foetus have been published. One such study from the UK was carried out on a group of pregnant women whose vitamin D concentrations were measured in late pregnancy. A total of 466 (78 %) children were examined at birth, 440 (74 %) at 9 months and 178 (30 %) at 9 years of age. The results showed that maternal concentrations of vitamin D >75 nmol/l did not influence the new born child's body size, psychological health or cardiovascular system. A low incidence of atopic disorders was observed, which requires confirmation. However, results of another study from Australia showed that maternal vitamin D deficiency increased the risk of lower birth weight and neonatal vitamin D deficiency. Low maternal levels of vitamin D may increase the risk of pre-eclampsia, a cogent reason for determination of the level of vitamin D at the beginning of pregnancy. Longitudinal studies of women have found a relationship between a history of pre-eclampsia in pregnancy and insulin sensitivity and vasodilatory functions as well as impaired insulin sensitivity later in life.

The pregnant woman is also subject to many general musculoskeletal disorders and injuries as well as specific conditions that may affect non-pregnant women at that age. A crucial factor in the determination of therapy for these conditions is the protection and preservation of the pregnancy itself. As pointed out in various reviews, most orthopaedic issues in pregnancy can be controlled conservatively, and operative interventions postponed till after delivery.

If a fracture has occurred in a pregnant woman, it is advisable not to breast-feed or at least to shorten the nursing period as much as possible. Though bisphosphonates are not yet authorised for premenopausal women, they should be considered when confronted by a manifest, severe premenopausal osteoporosis, together with the ancillary measures already outlined. In addition, the patient must be fully informed about the use of bisphosphonates, the beneficial effects and the possible, though rare, adverse side effects, the indications and contraindications and how and when they should be taken. In these patients questions concerning residual bisphosphonates within the bones and subsequent pregnancy and lactation are still open. It is quite possible that osteoporosis in pregnancy and lactation is more frequent than recognised simply because it is only recognised when an unexpected fracture occurs. Nevertheless, a few studies of osteoporosis during pregnancy and lactation have been reported including one in which three cases of severe vertebral fractures were described. The patients were treated with bisphosphonates. So far, adverse effects on the infants have not been reported. Only one patient with painful lumbar and thoracic vertebral fractures was treated with osteoanabolic therapy and had a good response. Intravenous bisphosphonate therapy during lactation has also been used in cases of severe osteoporosis with vertebral fractures which had developed during pregnancy. In another somewhat unusual case, a 30-year-old woman developed moderate back pain during the last month of her first pregnancy. The pain worsened after delivery and eight vertebral fractures were seen on radiology. The total T score of the lumbar vertebrae 2–4 was −4.7. Therefore, when back pain occurs during pregnancy and/or lactation, osteoporosis should be considered in the differential diagnosis.

42.2 Transient Osteoporosis of the Hip

This subtype of the "bone marrow oedema syndrome" is a rare, self-limited form of local pregnancy-associated osteoporosis. Some hypotheses to explain this painful condition include femoral venous stasis due to the gravid uterus, reflex sympathetic dystrophy, ischaemia, trauma, viral infection and immobilisation. These women present unilateral or bilateral hip pain and/or hip fracture in the third trimester, together with bone marrow oedema demonstrable by MRI. The symptoms and the MRI findings usually resolve within 2–6 months postpartum.

42.3 Pathogenesis of Pregnancy-Associated Osteoporosis

During pregnancy, the higher levels of sex hormones increase calcium absorption and thereby balance the loss of calcium due to the pregnancy itself. The female body has compensatory mechanisms to supply the increased demand for calcium during pregnancy and lactation so that problems only arise if the calcium depots (in the bones) are not full to begin with. Therefore, supplements of calcium and vitamins are recommended and should be taken from the beginning of pregnancy. However, pregnancy per se is not a risk factor for osteoporosis. But risk factors for osteoporosis are incurred if the pregnant woman is subjected to bed rest and/or is treated with muscle relaxants and/or sedatives. In some cases even corticosteroids are given. In these situations a massive withdrawal of calcium from the bones is unavoidable and should be compensated at the very least with adequate supplements of calcium and vitamin D.

Factors of bone loss in normal pregnancies and under lactation are:

- Pre-existing vitamin D deficiency
- Low dietary intake of calcium and protein
- Increased parathyroid hormone-related protein (PTHrP)
- Heparins for thromboembolic disorders
- Insufficient physical movement

During pregnancy, there is normally a slight decrease in bone density, but this loss is soon replaced after birth. However, it should be remembered that during lactation, about 500 mg calcium is excreted daily into the milk, which should be compensated for on a daily basis by increased ingestion of appropriate foods and supplements. In reality, very few women suffer from osteoporotic fractures during (and because of) the pregnancy itself.

42.4 Prevention and Therapy

If a fracture has occurred in a pregnant woman, it is advisable not to breast-feed or at least to shorten the nursing period as much as possible. Though bisphosphonates are not yet authorised for premenopausal women, they should be considered when confronted by a manifest, severe premenopausal osteoporosis, together with the ancillary measures already outlined. In addition, the patient must be fully informed about the use of bisphosphonates including the indications and contraindications. In these patients questions concerning residual bisphosphonates within the bones and subsequent pregnancy and lactation are still open.

43 Immobilisation Osteoporosis (Disuse Osteoporosis, Disuse Atrophy)

43.1 Causes of Bone Loss

Possible causes are spinal cord injuries, strokes, hospitalisation (prolonged), post-fracture conditions and others. Insufficient physical activity is one of the most important overall risk factors for osteoporosis. This is especially true for young bedridden patients who can lose up to 30 % of their bone density within a few months while years are required for its replacement – that is for restoration of density as it was before, i.e. "restitutio ad integrum" (Figs. 43.1 and 43.2) (see also Bartl and Frisch: Atlas of Bone Biopsy in Internal Medicine). For example, when an arm is enclosed in plaster for 3 weeks after a fracture, the immobilised bones may lose up to 6 % of their bone mass during this short period. A study of patients confined to bed has shown that, on average, trabecular bone decreases by about 1 % a week. When physical activity is resumed, bone density increases by 1 % a month, considerably slower than its loss.

> Mechanical forces deform bone and induce electric potentials and piezoelectric effects, which activate bone remodelling. As a result, osteoblasts produce enough new bone equal to the amount resorbed before. Cortical bone is more severely affected.

Examples of causes of immobilisation bone loss are:

- Damage to the vertebral bone marrow with deleterious effects on the bone
- Hemiplegia after cerebrovascular incidents
- Paraplegia of the lower half of the body
- Immobilisation after fracture of the lower extremities (rapid bone loss especially in children)
- Immobilisation after operations on the legs or feet with subsequent reduced mobility for prolonged periods
- Immobilisation due to muscular diseases or neurological disorders, e.g. multiple sclerosis

In a recent study, 20 paediatric patients (age 1–16 years, bedridden because of cerebral palsy) were successfully treated with risedronate to prevent secondary osteoporosis. It has recently also been demonstrated that there is a significantly increased prevalence of osteoporosis in both men and women with *multiple sclerosis*. Consequently bone density screening and appropriate measures including bisphosphonates need to be undertaken to avoid fractures in these patients. Shortly after the occurrence of a paraplegia, bone loss can be so rapid and extensive that relatively minimal efforts can cause fractures (e.g. transfer from bed to wheelchair or the effort of pulling up tight supportive stockings and socks). After 1 year, 42 % of paraplegic patients have osteoporosis of the femoral neck. The muscular spasms some patients

R. Bartl, C. Bartl, *Bone Disorders*, DOI 10.1007/978-3-319-29182-6_43

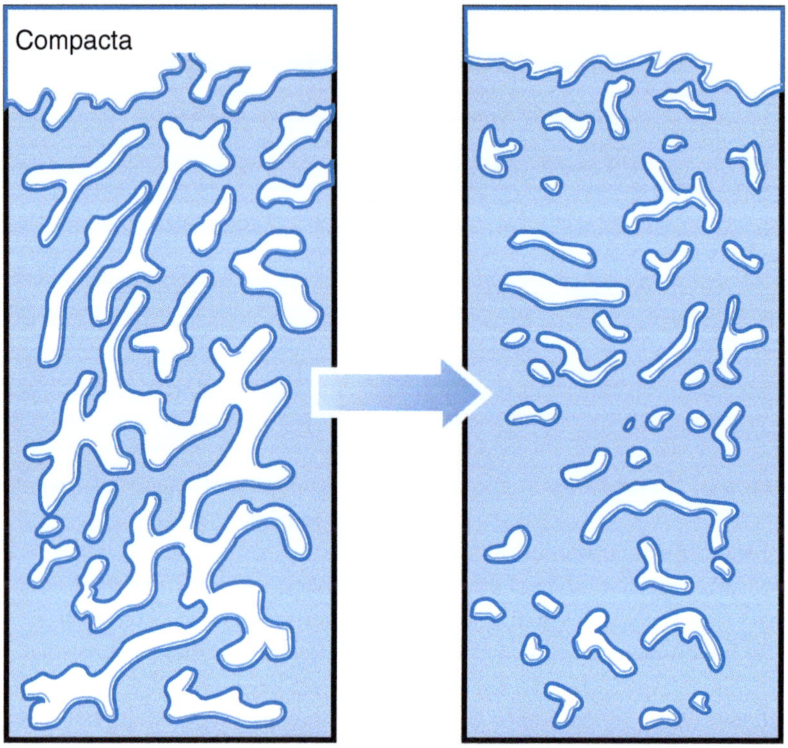

Fig. 43.1 Immobilisation osteoporosis in a child after 17 weeks of bed rest: marked reduction in volume of trabecular and cortical bone, documented in sequential iliac crest biopsies (From Bartl and Frisch 1993)

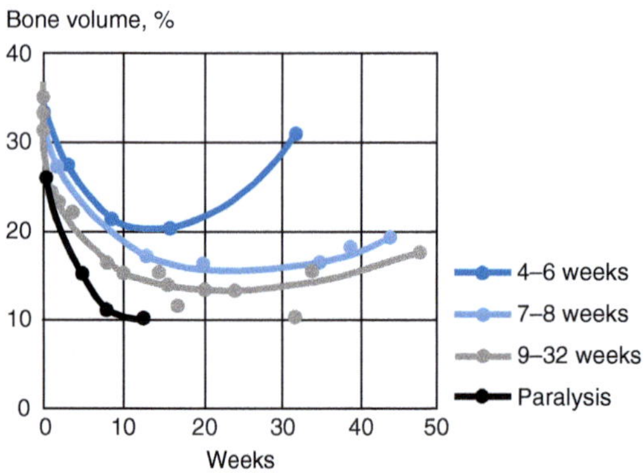

Fig. 43.2 Periods of immobilisation and recovery of bone mass in children. Note lack of recovery after paralysis (From Bartl and Frisch 1993)

undergo may have a positive effect on bone density, but such cramps are painful and patients prefer to avoid them by appropriate therapy. It is essential to emphasise that early initiation of physical training and activity is mandatory for all patients. Prophylactic initiation of bisphosphonate therapy does avert and reduce bone loss, but therapy must be continued to maintain bone in the long term.

Patients who already have osteoporosis and are immobilised for several weeks because of a fracture are likely to incur another one during the remobilisation period, unless preventive measures are taken as early as possible. The period of postoperative bed rest should be kept as short as possible and the bones protected by effective medication, e.g. bisphosphonates to prevent further loss of bone mass, by physiotherapy if at all possible and by attention to proper nutrition and supplements.

43.2 Space Travel and Force of Gravity

43.2.1 Weightlessness in Space due to Lack of Gravitational Force

Astronauts undergo specialised and regular musculoskeletal training before and during the space flight to counteract the absence of the force of gravity in outer space. In spite of this, they lose about 1 % of their bone density every month. A study of the bones of rhesus monkeys before and after a 14-day space flight revealed that they had sustained a 35 % reduction in bone volume. In the conditions prevailing in outer space, astronauts are subject to a tenfold higher bone loss than earthbound osteoporotic patients. This demonstrates unequivocally that the earth's gravitational force is nature's way of preserving the bone. The mechanisms of bone loss in astronauts have been thoroughly investigated and are used today as models for immobilisation osteoporosis. Three main factors are recognised:

- Demineralisation of bone
- Inhibition of osteoblastic activity
- Activation of osteoclasts

Timely preventive measures, i.e. before and during the flight, are mandatory. Recommendations made so far include the following: supplements of calcium, vitamins D and K, a bone anabolic agent and a long-acting bisphosphonate well before the flight, in addition to a specialised exercise training.

43.3 Therapy of Immobilisation Osteoporosis

The emphasis is on physical activity as early and as varied as possible, adapted to each patient's condition and ability. Adequate calcium and vitamin D intake is also essential for the maintenance of muscle and bone health.

Bone mass is heavily dependent on muscle mass and muscle loading of the skeleton.

The primary aim of medication is prevention; therefore, BP therapy should be started as early as possible and in accordance with the results of bone density measurements. This is especially important as the massive decrease in bone density which occurs immediately after the onset of paralysis (immobilisation) should and can be prevented. The following are recommended: the first two only if the patient is able to sit up straight for at least 30 min after ingestion, and there are cogent reasons for oral administration. Intravenous administration, as indicated below, is definitely preferable!

- Alendronate: 70 mg weekly
- Risedronate: 35 mg weekly
- Ibandronate: 3 mg injection monthly, later every 3 months
- Zoledronate: 5 mg infusion once a year

Part X

Secondary Osteoporosis in Medical Disciplines

44 Assessment of Secondary Osteoporosis

The first step is the separation of "primary" or "idiopathic" from the "secondary" osteoporoses which have an underlying cause, i.e. a specific disease or disorder. "Primary" osteoporosis refers mainly to postmenopausal and age-related involutional osteoporoses, in spite of the fact that a number of factors contributing to their pathogenesis are already known. Secondary osteoporoses are responsible for about 20 % of all osteoporotic fractures (Table 44.1). Secondary causes of osteoporosis, i.e. as co-morbidities, are also frequent in older patients who already have primary involutional osteoporosis. Physicians should consider the possible causes of secondary osteoporosis particularly when patients present as follows with:

- Unusual fractures
- Very low bone densities for their age
- Recurrent fractures despite adherence to effective therapy
- Abnormal basic laboratory tests (anaemia, hypo- and hypercalcaemia, elevated ESR)
- Unexplained bone pain
- Undetermined bone lesions on bone scan or X-ray (metastases, myeloma, malignant lymphomas, mastocytosis)

Osteoporosis is most likely to occur in the following disciplines. Only conditions not dealt with in other chapters are included here. This list represents the major secondary disorders which may affect the bones.

Table 44.1 Diseases and surgery associated with an increased risk of osteoporosis (alphabetical list)

Diseases
Acromegaly
Addison's disease
Amyloidosis
Ankylosing spondylitis
Anorexia nervosa
Chronic obstructive pulmonary disease
Congenital porphyria
Crohn's disease
Cushing's syndrome
Diabetes mellitus
Endometriosis
Gaucher's disease
Gonadal insufficiency
Haemochromatosis
Haemophilia
Hyperparathyroidism
Hypophosphatasia
Hyperthyroidism
Idiopathic scoliosis
Immobilisation
Lactose intolerance
Lymphoma and leukaemia
Malabsorption syndrome
Mastocytosis
Metastatic disease
Multiple myeloma
Multiple sclerosis
Nutritional disorders
Osteogenesis imperfecta
Parenteral nutrition

(continued)

R. Bartl, C. Bartl, *Bone Disorders*, DOI 10.1007/978-3-319-29182-6_44

Table 44.1 (continued)

Pernicious anaemia
Primary biliary cirrhosis
Rheumatoid arthritis
Sarcoidosis
Thalassaemia
Thyrotoxicosis
Surgery
Gastrectomy
Intestinal bypass
Thyroidectomy
Transplantation

45 Cardiology

Many reports have dealt with the connection between osteoporosis and cardiological conditions. For example, a recent study investigated the presence of osteoporosis in 198 patients undergoing coronary angiography because of chest pain. The results showed that 53 (27 %) had osteoporosis, 79 (40 %) had osteopenia, and only 66 (33 %) had normal BMD values. Moreover, 76 % of the patients with osteoporosis, 78 % of those with osteopenia had obstructive coronary artery disease.

> Patients who come for angiography should be checked also for osteoporosis, especially in the older age groups.

Another study investigated the level of vitamin D in 3299 patients sent for coronary angiography. The patients were followed for a median period of 7.75 years during which 95 patients died of cancer. The authors concluded that deficiency or insufficiency of vitamin D is associated with an increased risk of cancer in patients with cardiovascular disease, which itself also has a correlation with vitamin D deficiency. This was demonstrated in an investigation of 1739 people with mean age of 55 years, the Framingham Offspring Study participants, all without cardiovascular disease. Initial levels of vitamin D were assessed, and the participants were followed up for a mean period of 5.4 years, during which 120 participants with low levels of vitamin D underwent the first cardiovascular event. The authors concluded that more studies were required for confirmation and for determination as to what influence on the cardiovascular system correction of the vitamin D deficiency might have.

Patients after *operations of the cardiac valves* and on long-term anticoagulant therapy (depending on the anticoagulant used) are particularly vulnerable to loss of bone and to osteonecrosis. Additional causes are insufficient physical activity or immobilisation due to chronic cardiac insufficiency.

> Cardiac patients who are candidates for transplantation should also be checked for osteoporosis before and after so that preventive therapy may be given and fractures avoided.

Excessive alcohol consumption has also been related to cardiomyopathy and eventually to heart failure.

Atherosclerosis and osteoporosis are both multifactorial disorders related to the ageing

R. Bartl, C. Bartl, *Bone Disorders*, DOI 10.1007/978-3-319-29182-6_45

process. There is accumulating evidence that progressive telomere shortening is involved in both cardiovascular and other cardiometabolic disorders. Vascular calcification has been linked to high levels of vitamin D and to aspects of bone remodelling. Patients with vascular calcification may also suffer from osteoporosis, which requires treatment for prevention of fractures. However, other studies have shown that high levels of vitamin D not only promote vascular calcification but also constitute a risk factor for cardiovascular disease. There appears to be only a very narrow range of vitamin D levels within which vascular function is optimal and the risk of calcification and cardiac disease is avoided. Moreover, vitamin D deficiency, as mentioned above, is also a risk factor for cardiovascular disease. Patients with chronic renal disease may also derive benefit from vitamin D given for concomitant cardiac problems.

Hypercholesterolaemia and *dyslipidaemia* are linked to arteriosclerotic vascular diseases as well as to osteoporosis. Statins are usually prescribed for the disturbed lipid metabolism, but it should be noted that atorvastatin also increases vitamin D levels, so these should also be checked. The patients are also advised to pay attention to diet, with reduction of fat intake if this is above recommended levels. BP are the therapy of choice for the osteoporosis. The type, dose and route of administration are decided according to the patient's requirements and preferences.

Some previous epidemiological studies as well as comprehensive reviews found that *beta-blockers* and *thiazide diuretics* apparently have a beneficial effect on fracture risk in older adults, but information on long-term effects was limited. Two large recent studies, from the UK and the Netherlands, did not find a causal relationship between therapy with beta-blockers and reduction in risk of fractures.

A population-based case controlled study on the relationship between *atrial fibrillation* and *flutter*, on the one hand, and bisphosphonates prescribed for and taken by women as therapy for osteoporosis, on the other hand, found no evidence for an effect of the bisphosphonates on cardiac rhythm.

46 Endocrinology

It should be clearly stated at the outset that numerous endocrine disorders are inexorably associated with the metabolism of the musculoskeletal system, and only a few can be mentioned here. Moreover, many of these disorders are also closely connected to other systems, which in turn are also correlated with the function of the bone cells.

Growth Hormone Deficiency Many studies have shown that there is considerable variability in individual patient's responses to therapy with growth hormones. Nevertheless, the long-term studies have demonstrated improvements in body composition and bone mass and density as well as increases in muscle strength. However, women may also require some degree of oestrogen therapy to maintain the BMD. Therapy with growth hormone is also effective in congenital disorders such as Turner and Prader-Willi syndromes. In addition, therapy with growth hormone has beneficial effects on the cardiovascular and other systems which themselves are risk factors for the bones. An interesting hypothesis has been suggested in connection with the GH-IGF-1 axis and longevity. Studies have shown that some patients with hormone deficiency survive to 75–78 years of age or even longer, in spite of dwarfism and marked obesity. The hypothesis is that the growth hormone deficiency is a major contributing factor in protection from cancer, a significant cause of death in older populations.

Hyperthyroidism Patients with thyrotoxicosis may have generalised osteoporosis because bone formation cannot keep up with resorption, in spite of the fact that both are increased in hyperthyroidism: a classic example of high turnover osteoporosis.

> Activation of thyroid hormone receptor on osteoblasts and osteoclasts results in both increased bone resorption and bone loss.

The hypothesis had been put forward that in hypothyroidism, the thyroid-stimulating hormone TSH caused the effects in the skeleton, but recent animal studies have shown that they are due to lack of the thyroid hormone T3.

Primary Hyperparathyroidism (pHPT) Increased secretion of parathyroid hormone due to adenomas, carcinoma, congenital disorders such as Turner syndrome or parathyroid hyperplasia produces disturbances in calcium homeostasis with release of calcium from the bones. However, though there may be no or few clinical symptoms, the increase in bone turnover leads to a loss of both cortical and trabecular bone. Many studies have reported a decrease in BMD. The changes in vitamin D metabolism as well as increases in FGF 23 also contribute to

R. Bartl, C. Bartl, *Bone Disorders*, DOI 10.1007/978-3-319-29182-6_46

the decline in BMD, which increases the fracture risk. The increase in bone turnover and bone resorption in particular is manifest in complex bone changes affecting both cortical and trabecular bone throughout the skeleton and may also affect the joints and even the vessels. But it must be pointed out that the skeletal changes in pHPT are very variable as documented in different studies. Primary HPT is another example of hormonally determined generalised osteopenia/osteoporosis. However, in one study measurements of total body calcium failed to demonstrate large overall deficits of bone mineral in pHPT. Indeed, there is a broad spectrum of histologic changes in pHPT. Indeed, experimental and in vitro studies have shown that intermittent PTH inhibits adipocytes and induces osteoblast differentiation of mesenchymal cells. In our biopsy study, 20 % of the patients, particularly those with kidney stones, had no morphologic abnormalities in the bone biopsy. In intermediate bone disease, usually characterised by vitamin D deficiency, histologic parameters such as bone resorption, osteoclasts and endosteal fibrosis were predominant ("dissecting fibro-osteoclasia"). While it has been suggested that the primary osteoclastic effect in parathyroid bone disease might result in widespread osteopenia, in our study the cortical and trabecular bone volume was maintained. Only in severe cases (10 %) are the classical skeletal manifestations of pHPT seen: osteitis fibrosa cystica with marked bone loss, osteolytic destruction of the trabecular network ("brown tumours") and presence of multiple fractures. Studies on BMD and levels of vitamin D metabolites in 246 patients, age range 19–91 years, with pHPT showed that low-vitamin D status together with high plasma 1,25 (OH) (2) D were associated with increased bone turnover and decreased BMD in the patients. The long-term beneficial results of parathyroidectomy, also in elderly patients, have been documented, including an increase in BMD and reduction in fracture risk. An N-containing bisphosphonate has been suggested for patients when curative surgery is contraindicated.

In patients with pHPT, the presence of osteoporosis is an indication for parathyroid surgery in otherwise asymptomatic patients.

Secondary hyperparathyroidism (sHPT) has been described in patients with renal disease on dialysis. A Multicentre Observational Study (*COSMOS*) was recently initiated in Europe for the diagnosis, prevention and treatment of sHPT in patients on dialysis. The study will include investigation of numerous relevant parameters, including changes in bone mineral markers. The study is planned to run for 3 years, when results will be evaluated. SHPT has also been observed in congenital disorders, such as Turner syndrome.

Cushing's Disease This endogenous form of hypercortisolism is rare, in contrast to glucocorticosteroid-induced osteoporosis, which is common, severe and progressive if not treated.

Diabetes Mellitus (DM) "Diabetic osteopathy" occurs more frequently than is generally realised and is mainly due to inhibition of collagen production by osteoblasts which occurs as a direct effect of insufficient insulin and beta cell-derived protein secretion and which impedes osteoblastic bone formation and leads to deterioration of bone quality. The risk of osteoporotic fractures is increased by 12-fold in patients with type 1 DM and by 20-fold in women with type 2 DM.

In chronic disease, diabetic complications such as retinopathy, polyneuropathy and nephropathy are major causes of bone loss and increased fracture risk.

To address the question of the occurrence of diabetic osteomyelopathy as a distinct entity, we investigated iliac crest biopsies of 120 patients with manifest diabetes mellitus.

Histomorphometry of the vascular system, bone and bone marrow was performed. In our study diabetic microangiopathy was found in 82 % of the biopsies. The marked inflammatory reaction of the bone marrow stroma correlated with serologic parameters of inflammation in these patients. This may significantly contribute to the bone marrow atrophy and the "anaemia of chronic disorders" in diabetes mellitus. Atrophic reduction of the trabecular bone was also significantly higher in the patients with diabetes mellitus, but bone remodelling was normal or only slightly decreased. Insulin-dependent patients had a lower bone loss than orally adjusted diabetics. These results demonstrate the occurrence of a more or less specific *diabetic osteomyelopathy* comprising degenerative changes of the bone marrow vasculature, degenerative reactions of the marrow stroma, marrow atrophy and osteopenia with slightly decreased bone remodelling and with changes in parameters of bone quality.

To address the question of the occurrence of *diabetic osteomyelopathy* as a distinct entity, we investigated iliac crest biopsies of 120 patients with manifest diabetes mellitus. Histomorphometry of the vascular system, bone and marrow was performed. In our study diabetic microangiopathy was found in 82 % of the biopsies as shown by degenerative changes of the vessel walls, perivascular increase in fibres (collagen type III) as well as in plasma cells and mast cells.

An interesting observation has previously been associated with bisphosphonate therapy in type 2 diabetes: significant reduction in intimal thickness, suggesting an anti-atherogenic effect of etidronate, the bisphosphonate involved. However, today only the modern BP are given to these patients, and this effect has so far not been reported. Many studies have demonstrated an increased risk of fractures in patients with type 2 diabetes, but these patients did not have a decrease in BMD. The main causes were listed as other consequences of the diabetes such as visual impairment and imbalance, peripheral neuropathy, orthostatic hypotonia, ischaemic states of various organs including the legs and other conditions that predispose to falls, which were the immediate cause of the fractures. Diabetes type 2 (DM 2) has been associated with structural brain changes and accelerated cognitive decline. In patients with symptomatic arterial disease and DM 2, the hyperglycaemia and the duration of DM 2 contribute to the brain atrophy and to the deterioration of the patients' condition, including the state of the bones. Diabetes type 2 is frequently treated by rosiglitazone or by pioglitazone which belong to the thiazolidinediones (TZDs). Studies have now demonstrated that these drugs increase bone loss and decrease bone formation, thereby increasing risk of fractures, so preventive measures must be taken or the patient advised to take other drugs.

47 Gastroenterology

Chronic disorders of the liver or the gastrointestinal tract (GI) (e.g. malabsorption syndromes, lactose intolerance, Crohn's disease, colitis ulcerosa, pancreatic insufficiency and primary biliary cirrhosis) frequently cause a combination of osteoporosis and osteomalacia ("osteoporomalacia") due to deficiencies of the vitamins D, K and C. It should be mentioned that patients with Crohn's disease, even young adults, are subject to sarcopenia frequently related to osteopenia/osteoporosis. The changes which occur in patients with chronic disorders of the GI tract, as listed above, tend to worsen as the patients get older, so that regular screening for osteopenia/osteoporosis is recommended. It is noteworthy that sarcopenia is high even in young patients with Crohn's disease, and this increases the risk of bone loss. Gastric and intestinal operations (e.g. Billroth I and II and small bowel resections) interfere with absorption and utilisation of calcium and vitamin D and eventually may lead to osteopathy, especially to vertebral osteoporosis. Osteoporosis after gastrectomy and in patients using proton pump inhibitors (PPI) is due to decreased calcium absorption secondary to higher gastrointestinal pH values. Variations in intestinal absorption (with no obvious cause) may lead to hypercalciuria, and this has been linked with calcium nephrolithiasis, bone loss and idiopathic osteoporosis in some patients, including postmenopausal women. These cases are examples of the interwoven connections between gastrointestinal absorption, renal function and skeletal metabolism.

In all patients regardless of cause, administration of glucocorticoids and alcohol abuse increase the loss of bone. Large-bowel disorders are rarely associated with bone loss, since the process of absorption is generally completed in the small intestine. Coeliac disease, in particular, has been associated with numerous disorders, which in turn affect the bones. Examples are autoimmune inflammatory conditions and in particular some of the associated cytokines such as TNF-alpha and Il-1, diabetes, thyroid disease, secondary HPT, hypopituitarism and others. Each patient must be carefully assessed before appropriate therapy is given. However, today the emphasis is on early diagnosis and treatment and appropriate nutritional and lifestyle interventions to prevent the development of the disorders listed above, all of which present a danger to the bones. It should be taken into consideration that bone loss in coeliac disease already begins in childhood, if preventive measures are not taken early enough. The only effective measure able to keep coeliac disease under control is lifelong adherence to a gluten-free diet.

R. Bartl, C. Bartl, *Bone Disorders*, DOI 10.1007/978-3-319-29182-6_47

Four main causes of malnutrition may be involved in the development of osteoporosis:

- Impaired dietary intake, including anorexia nervosa
- Impaired absorption
- Increased dietary loss of nutrients, and
- Hepatobiliary and pancreatic disorders associated with intestinal malabsorption

48 Genetics

Studies of twins have shown that osteoporosis may be genetically determined – up to 50 % – and many genes are involved. Peak bone mass is therefore to some extent genetically programmed, and the subsequent degree of loss of bone density applies especially to trabecular (cancellous) bone. It has also been demonstrated that genes may have different effects on bones at different skeletal sites and play a part in overall bone development as well as in degree of osteoporosis at these sites. Recently the connection between the genes for vitamin D receptors and bone density has been of particular interest and subjects of research, though the results of such studies have been somewhat contradictory. Clinically, osteogenesis imperfecta is the most important of the hereditary osteoporoses. Other congenital syndromes with an osteoporotic component are Turner, Klinefelter, Ehlers-Danlos, Marfan and Werner. Studies of the congenital premature ageing syndrome dyskeratosis congenita have identified mutations in the genes that encode the telomerase complex. Cells of these patients have very short telomeres, and they age prematurely. The patients suffer from early greying of the hair, dental loss, osteoporosis and malignancies.

Recently it has been shown that bone may be influenced by the GH-IGF-1 axis in intrauterine (genetically determined) and in postnatal life. This effect may continue into adulthood suggesting a role for the GH-IGF-1 axis in the programming of bone mass in women. Results for men are awaiting publication. With successful enzyme replacement therapy in Gaucher's disease, the infiltration decreases, but the osteoporosis increases and should be treated prophylactically after measurement of bone mineral density. Congenital syndromes with involvement of the muscles are also prone to lead to disturbances of bone remodelling and osteoporosis. It is also of interest that a polymorphism of the growth hormone receptor gene (exon-3 deletion, d3GHR) increases the response to recombinant human growth hormone (rhGH) in children, while in adults with growth hormone deficiency, it contributes to the differences in efficacy of short-term rhGH therapy only.

Numerous studies have now accumulated on genetics and disorders of bones and joints, on congenital syndromes, on genes involved in pathways of development and differentiation, on osseous phenotypes on genes associated with onset of osteoporosis and with various types of fractures and on genes associated with skeletal metabolism and race, ethnicity and age in population studies, investigations of which SNPs may be involved in differences of response to treatment as well as their association with bones and muscles in the metabolic syndrome. All these and more have made it clear that osteoporosis is related to multiple genes and many environmental factors. Some relevant studies are listed in the references.

R. Bartl, C. Bartl, *Bone Disorders*, DOI 10.1007/978-3-319-29182-6_48

49 Haematology and Storage Disorders

Diseases of the bone marrow have a direct influence on osseous remodelling and can cause severe osteoporosis. *Multiple myeloma*, by way of the osteoclast activating factors produced by the pathologic plasma cells, regularly causes osteoporosis or, more frequently, osteolytic skeletal lesions ("skeletal-related events", SRE). *Polycythaemia vera* (PV) (Fig. 49.1) and *chronic myeloid leukaemia* (CML) (Fig. 49.2) induce widespread osteoporosis by their expansive growth, but different histologic manifestations (Fig. 49.3). Changes in the bones also occur in *osteomyelosclerosis* (OMS) (Fig. 49.4) and during leukaemic transformation when increased levels of TNF-alpha and lactate dehydrogenase (LDH) are found. Not only the degree of cellularity but also the different proliferating haematopoietic cell lines influence osseous remodelling. While in PV the trabeculae are attenuated but with normal microarchitecture and connections, a coarsening of the trabecular network with fewer connections and correspondingly large marrow spaces is characteristic of ML. Similar changes are produced by congenital haemolytic conditions which cause extreme erythroid hyperplasia and osteoporosis.

Storage diseases such as *Gaucher's disease* (Fig.49.5) or *hereditary oxalosis* (Fig. 49.6) also cause osteoporosis and/or osteolytic lesions by comparable mechanisms. On the other hand, malignant lymphomas and acute leukaemias are rarely accompanied by osteoporosis in the initial stages, but it does develop later on. The mode of spread of marrow infiltrations is a major parameter determining the pattern of osseous lesions. Processes with diffuse marrow infiltrations are characterised by a systemic osteopenia in bones, while in patients with focal, nodular or patchy infiltrations, local osteopenia or even circumscribed osteolytic lesions are found.

Patients with *red cell anomalies* such as sickle cell disease commonly also have osteoporosis and osteomalacia, with decreased BMD values. Some patients also have vitamin D deficiencies, for which the patients must be appropriately treated and treated, in addition to therapy with bisphosphonates, given according to markers of bone resorption and the BMD values.

Patients with *haemophilia* may have low BMD and osteopenia/osteoporosis, which may have begun in childhood and leads to shorter height and lower weight than normal controls. Psychological factors, especially in childhood, such as apprehension and fear of bleeding, may also be involved in restriction of some physical activities in individual cases. Other factors such as overall reduced physical activity and susceptibility to infections may also stimulate bone loss during adulthood. Clearly, patients with osteopenia/osteoporosis must be evaluated and treated on an individual basis taking into account their medical history results of tests and the individual risk factor profile.

R. Bartl, C. Bartl, *Bone Disorders*, DOI 10.1007/978-3-319-29182-6_49

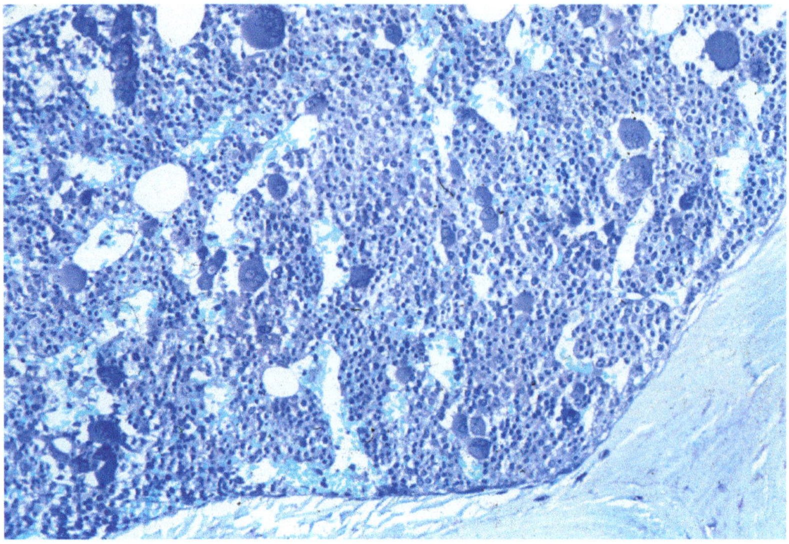

Fig. 49.1 Polycythaemia vera with massive proliferation of erythropoiesis and secondary osteoporosis. Giemsa staining

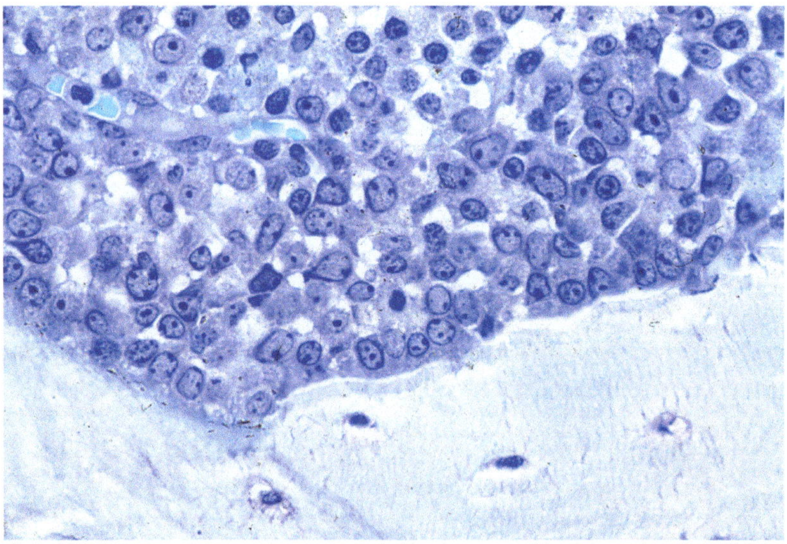

Fig. 49.2 Chronic myeloid leukaemia with a broad endosteal seam of myeloblasts and suppressed bone remodelling. Giemsa staining

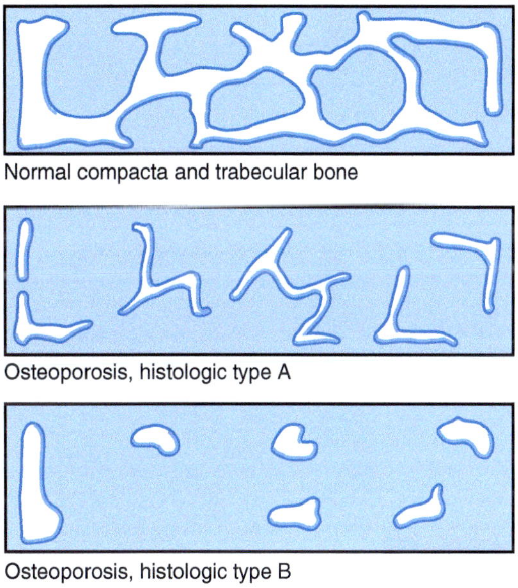

Fig. 49.3 Osteoporotic trabecular variants: *type A* in polycythaemia vera and *type B* in chronic myeloid leukaemia (From Bartl and Frisch 1993)

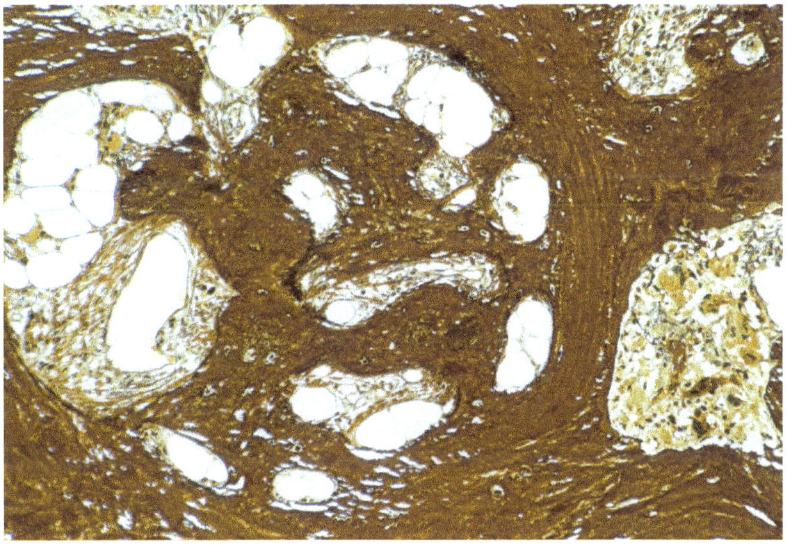

Fig. 49.4 Osteomyelosclerosis with increase in woven bone, small bone marrow cavities and decrease of haematopoiesis. Note residual cluster of atypical megakaryocytes (*right*), Gomori staining

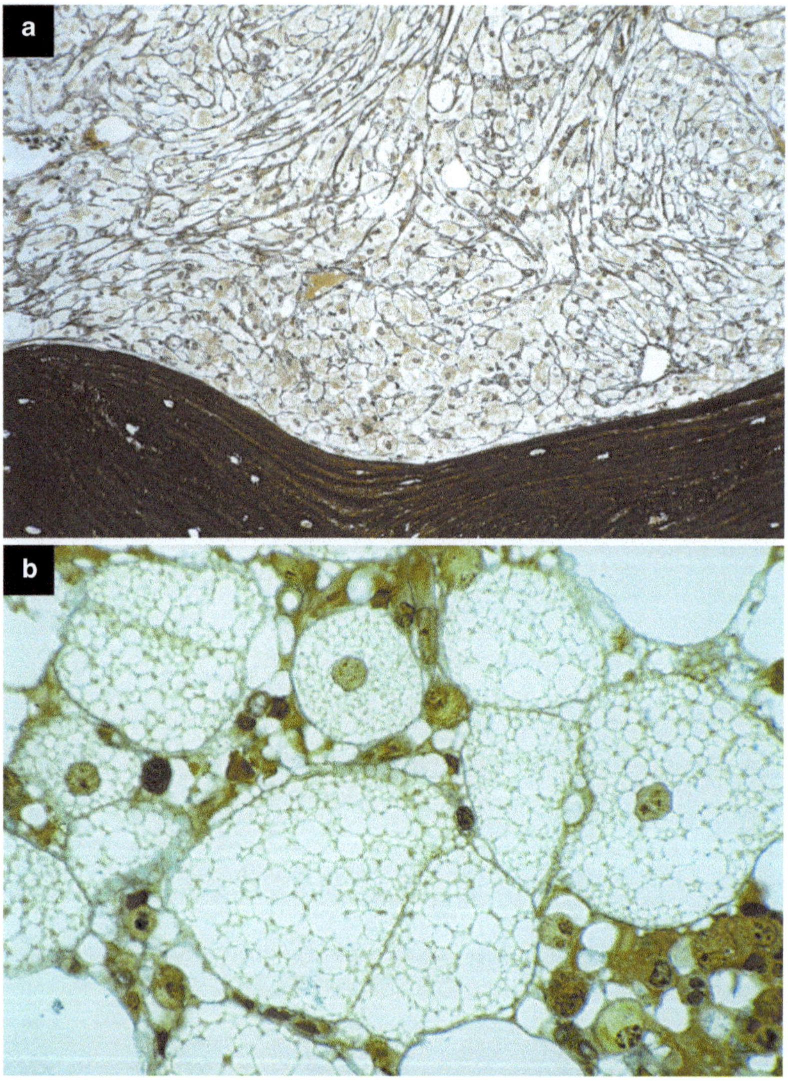

Fig. 49.5 (**a**) Iliac crest biopsy of patients with Gaucher's disease, with complete replacement of haematopoiesis and severe osteoporosis in the DXA measurement, (**b**) higher magnification showing typical Gaucher's cells of variable size, with characteristic "wrinkled tissue paper" appearance of cytoplasm, all Gomori staining

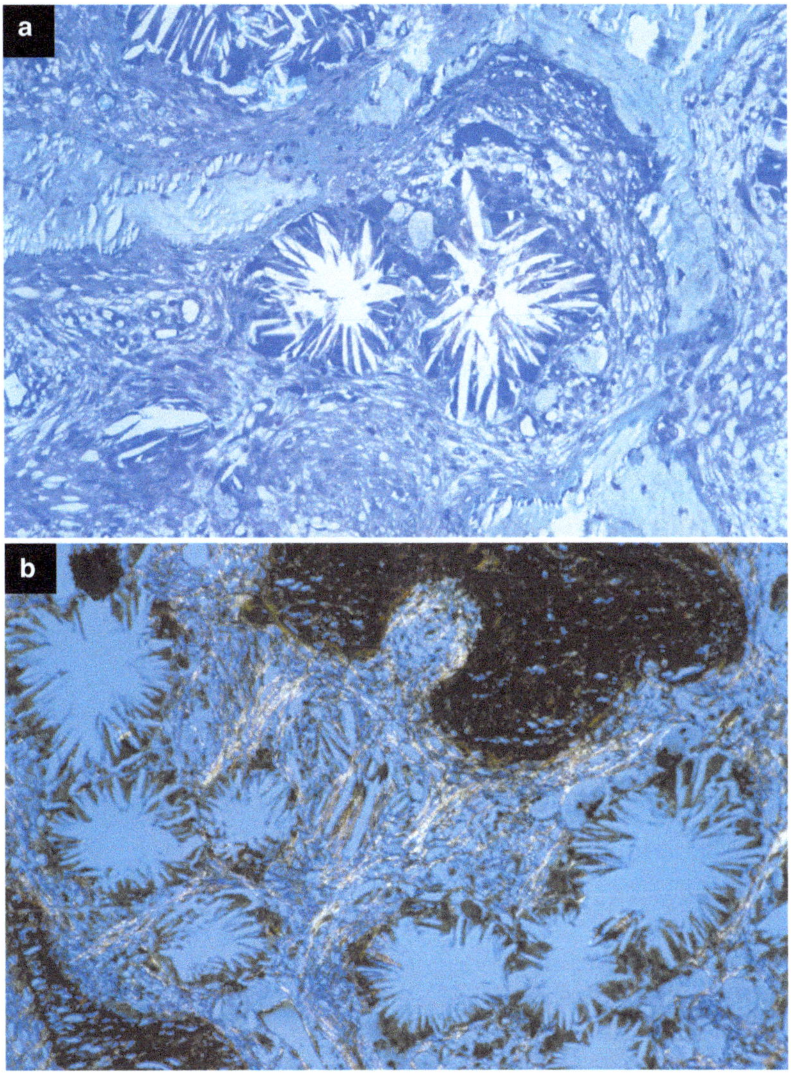

Fig. 49.6 (**a**) Iliac crest biopsy of young patient with hereditary oxalosis, complicated by chronic renal failure, aluminium intoxication under haemodialysis, renal osteopathy and pancytopenia, (**b**) multiple rosettes of calcium oxalate crystals in the intertrabecular marrow spaces surrounded by coarse fibrosis and newly formed woven bone (*above*). There is no residual haematopoiesis. Gomori staining, polarisation

50 Infectious Disorders

In view of the fact that over 33 (in some estimates 43) million people worldwide are infected with *HIV-AIDS*, this now constitutes the most important infectious disease in which osteoporosis can occur. Recent reports have shown that HIV infection is an additional risk factor for osteoporosis and pathologic fractures.

> Changes in bone mineral metabolism, bone histomorphometry and bone density document the existence of a complex *AIDS osteopathy* comprising a mixture of osteoporosis, osteomalacia and secondary hyperparathyroidism.

Immobilisation, gastrointestinal infections, lipodystrophy, hepatitis and hormone deficiencies are all further risk factors for bone loss. Highly active antiretroviral therapy (HAART) has also been shown to accelerate bone loss in HIV-infected patients and is therefore a potent inducer of osteoporosis in these patients. The hypothesis that the systemic activation of T lymphocytes leads to an osteoprotegerin ligand-mediated increase in active osteoclasts and loss of bone may in part explain the interaction of HIV infection and bone resorption. Risk factors such as nutrition, insufficient physical activity and other lifestyle influences also play a part in the skeletal changes listed above. With widespread introduction of treatment to delay progression of AIDS, early attention should be paid to these potential complications, in order to avoid them as much as possible.

Other chronic infections may also influence the bones, especially when the patient's physical ability is impaired and long-term therapy is required, which may be the case in, for example, tuberculosis. The situation is even worse if drug resistance develops. It has been suggested that adjuvant therapies, such as l-arginine and vitamin D, could stimulate mycobactericidal and immunomodulatory actions against the infection, and thereby shorten the duration of therapy. It is of note that patients with tuberculosis are reported to have deficient vitamin D levels. Studies of the effects of vitamin D therapy in these patients have not yet been reported.

R. Bartl, C. Bartl, *Bone Disorders*, DOI 10.1007/978-3-319-29182-6_50

51 Nephrology

The kidneys and the bones are both involved in calcium homeostasis; therefore, impaired renal function leads to defective calcium homeostasis and renal osteodystrophy, in the young as in the old. Chronic renal insufficiency induces osteoporosis, osteomalacia and secondary hyperparathyroidism by means of deficiencies in vitamin D metabolism. Observational studies have shown that the survival of patients with HPT may be improved by treatment with analogues of vitamin D, given while the patients are on dialysis. Chronic kidney disease (CKD) disease and end-stage kidney disease (ESKD) with the increased risk of fracture are both the subjects of growing international concern. The prevalence of both is expected to increase within the next decade together with the ageing of the populations in many parts of the world, and many studies of these patients, both completed and ongoing, deal with the therapy and prevention of osteoporosis and fractures, including treatment with bisphosphonates. Another major consideration, also from an epidemiological point of view, is the close association of CKD with risk of cardiovascular disorders, which of course are also increased in the older populations, and may be associated with osteopenia/osteoporosis. The survival of patients with CKD has benefited from therapy with calcitriol, and in recent years, the more potent analogues have shown additional advantages. These beneficial effects are also due to improvements in the cardiovascular system. It is now hoped that early therapy will benefit the kidney, slow progression of disease and postpone the necessity for haemodialysis and transplantation.

During *haemodialysis* or after *kidney transplantation*, the osteopathy is somewhat improved or it may be "set" and remain static. Interesting observations had previously been made in the early years of this decade, on mini-modelling in the iliac bone in patients on dialysis, especially after parathyroidectomy. Recent studies also of bone biopsies of patients on dialysis included young active ambulatory patients, as well as postmenopausal women. Comprehensive approach is required for the management of patients after transplantation, because of the many possible factors involved: steroid usage, hypogonadism, persistent hyperparathyroidism, poor allograft function, age-related and other chronic comorbidities and nutritional factors. Nevertheless, studies have shown that vitamin D and calcium, bisphosphonates and calcitonin may be effective. Vitamin D-based therapies have already been shown to be effective for prevention of graft rejection after renal transplantation; attention to lifestyle factors is also important. Various novel treatments are under investigation and results are awaited. Therapy-resistant osteoporosis is frequently encountered today as a consequence of chronic renal disease and haemodialysis. Patients

R. Bartl, C. Bartl, *Bone Disorders*, DOI 10.1007/978-3-319-29182-6_51

with chronic renal insufficiency and on long-term dialysis develop a complicated bone disorder called *renal osteodystrophy*. The manifestations of this disorder are severe and greatly reduce the patient's quality of life: severe bone pain, multiple fractures and extraskeletal ossifications (Fig. 51.1). Renal osteopathy is described in detail in an own chapter.

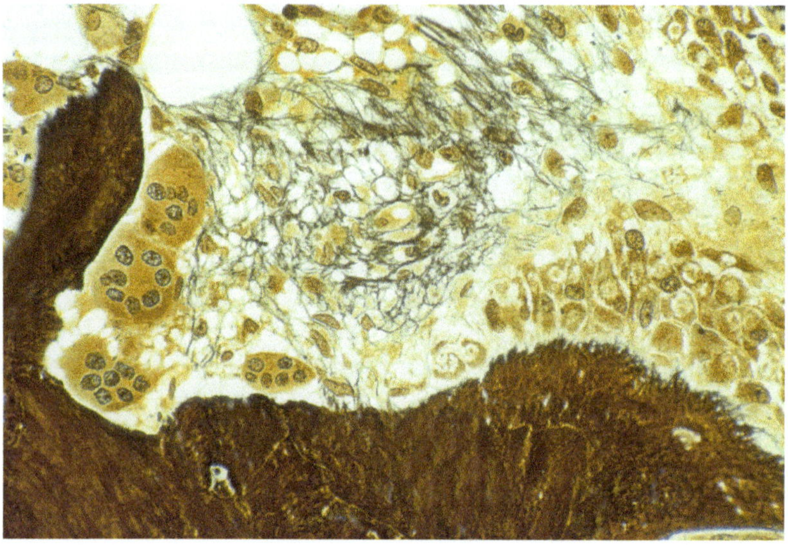

Fig. 51.1 Severe secondary hyperparathyroidism in a young patient with long-term renal insufficiency. Note multiple active osteoclasts (*left*) and a broad seam of osteoblasts (*right*). Gomori staining

52 Neurology and Psychiatry

Chronic disorders such as Parkinson's disease, transient ischaemic attacks, stroke, Alzheimer's disease, epilepsy, multiple sclerosis, amyotrophic lateral sclerosis and diabetic neuropathy increase the risk of falling and correlate with lower bone mass, caused by immobility and drugs. The same is true for depressive states in which physical activity is reduced and nutrition may be inadequate. Depression has also been associated with disorders of the cardiovascular and many other systems, with osteoporosis and with increased serum levels of various cytokines, e.g. of the TNF-alpha system, which may even contribute to the development of the depressive disorder. There also appears to be a link between depression and cognitive function which further complicates the condition. And, unfortunately, some studies have indicated that antidepressive drugs such as the tricyclic antidepressants have an increased risk of falls and fractures.

Most patients with *Parkinson's disease* have an increased risk of osteoporosis and fractures. This applies particularly to elderly females. This risk is largely due to restrictions in physical mobility as a result of the disease itself. The BMD should be monitored and appropriate measures taken, including especially adapted exercises for the individual patient. Individuals with intellectual and/or developmental disabilities are also prone to osteoporosis and fractures in the absence of preventive measures.

Many studies have found an increased risk of fractures in patients with *epilepsy* on therapy with antiepileptic drugs (AEDs), for example, carbamazepine. The increased risk is associated to some extent with length of exposure to the drug. Therefore appropriate screening and monitoring of BMD is recommended, as is attention to nutrition and supplements of calcium and vitamin D as required.

Immobilisation and Impaired Physical Activity Simple and easily applicable countermeasures developed for astronauts to reduce bone loss before and during spaceflight have also been advocated for patients who are paralysed. Changes in BMD in patients with psychiatric disorders such as schizophrenia have been described, and the causes may be related to effects and lifestyle consequences of the condition itself as well as those of the medications administered. Studies have shown that glucocorticoids represent a common factor in almost all psychiatric and somatic complex disorders, as well as in many of their therapies, and are involved in the pathophysiology of most of the organs and tissues in the body, including the skeleton. Consequently they also play a part in the effects of psychiatric disorders on the bones. Mitochondrial changes and dysfunctions with age have been documented in neurodegenerative disorders, including psychiatric conditions, which in turn affect the skeleton.

Adult and elderly patients with *multiple sclerosis* are liable to osteoporosis and to injurious falls. Out of a total of 354 patients investigated,

R. Bartl, C. Bartl, *Bone Disorders*, DOI 10.1007/978-3-319-29182-6_52

more than 50 % reported injurious falls. Management of the accompanying osteoporosis and alleviation of the fear of falling are two of the most important components of therapy, as well as of programmes for prevention of falls in these patients.

Charcot neuro-osteoarthropathy is considered to be of neurogenic origin. However, Charcot arthropathy occurs most frequently in patients with diabetes, and considering the relationship of diabetes with osteoporosis, the possibility has been put forward that Charcot arthropathy could be a late consequence of osteoporosis in diabetic patients – a most cogent reason for early diagnosis and therapy in these patients. Studies have also demonstrated that early diagnosis and conservative intervention, therapy and rehabilitation have good results and avoid surgery. In more advanced cases, surgery is necessary, for example, salvage tibiotalar arthrodesis in patients with very unstable ankles due to bimalleolar fractures complicated by the Charcot neuroarthropathy. The results were better in patients who had received antiresorptive therapy beforehand in the acute phase. Patients with vascular complications, and possibly even osteonecrosis, required more extensive surgery. It has recently been shown that the level of C-reactive protein is a reliable indicator of the presence of infections in patients with Charcot arthropathy. Increased levels were not found in patients with Charcot foot pathology, so that in these patients inflammatory cytokines were not involved in the condition.

53 Oncology

The diffuse metastatic spread of a solid tumour can mimic a primary osteoporosis, particularly in the absence of localised osteolytic and/or osteosclerotic lesions. Osteoporosis of uncertain aetiology accompanied by bone pain and pathologic fractures should always be thoroughly checked to rule out an underlying malignant condition, especially metastases of neoplasias of the breast, prostate and lungs, among others. The first induces mainly osteoporotic/osteolytic metastases and the second mainly osteosclerotic. Patients with brain tumours are particularly liable to develop osteopenia/osteoporosis due to a multiplicity of factors. These include drugs, glucocorticoids, antiepileptics, anticoagulants, chemotherapy, radiotherapy, inadequate nutrition, partial immobilisation and possible hemiplegia, and these must all be considered in the medical management. Localised osseous changes, such as vertebral compression fractures, may also occur and must be appropriately handled. Other malignant tumours such as bronchial cancers may also cause skeletal lesions, usually paraneoplastic, by means of secretion of parathormone-related proteins (PTHrPs). Various localised changes in the bone are also caused by bone tumours, such as the osteosarcomas. It has recently been demonstrated that metastatic breast cancer cells induce an inflammatory stress response in osteoblasts, with production of cytokines that attract osteoclasts, and so establish an environment in which resorption is increased and formation is reduced.

It should be borne in mind that oncologic patients of all ages are subject to the development of osteoporosis because of the antineoplastic therapy, which frequently contains glucocorticoids, and the physical restrictions imposed by the cancers and their consequences. The use of bisphosphonates in early cancer has two main objectives:

- To prevent the adverse effects of the cancer treatments on the skeleton
- To counteract the effects of the cancer itself on the bones, as it has already been established that the bisphosphonates reduce the frequency and severity of skeletal complications in patients with osteotropic cancers

It has already been demonstrated that patients with bone metastases from solid tumours together with increased resorption showed normalisation of the bone resorption markers within 3 months of treatment with zoledronate. This is a major justification for early administration of bisphosphonates in patients with metastases of breast cancer, prostate cancer, lung cancer and other solid tumours. Moreover, postmenopausal women with early breast cancer who are on therapy with an aromatase inhibitor, such as arimidex or letrozole, inevitably suffer extra bone loss which can effectively be prevented by immediate administration of a bisphosphonate such as alendronate or zoledronate, as shown in the results of the *ZO-FAST* Study (2008).

R. Bartl, C. Bartl, *Bone Disorders*, DOI 10.1007/978-3-319-29182-6_53

In addition, in patients who already have osseous complications, the bisphosphonates relieve bone pain; and in some cases, they also improve survival of the patients. It is also pertinent to emphasise the probable part played by vitamin D, its receptor's genetic variants and analogues in the prevention and the treatment of malignancies. This has been indicated by some prospective trials, for example, in patients with renal cell carcinoma, and ongoing investigations of vitamin D analogues for prostate cancer. The extraskeletal actions of vitamin D include pro-apoptotic, anti-metastatic, anti-angiogenic, anti-inflammatory, pro-differentiating and immunomodulating activities. Clearly, careful attention to vitamin D status is essential in both the prevention and treatment of malignancies.

54 Pulmonology

Patients with long-standing cortisone-dependent *asthma bronchiale* should be regularly monitored for prevention of osteoporosis. Patients with cystic fibrosis may have osteoporosis even before lung transplantation and this should be treated in advance. One of the systemic manifestations of *chronic obstructive pulmonary disease* (COPD) is skeletal muscle dysfunction, which is one factor in the development of osteopenia/osteoporosis in these patients.

Hypertrophic osteoarthropathy occurs in patients with chronic lung diseases and bronchogenic carcinoma and consists of clubbing of the digits of the hands and feet, enlargement of the extremities secondary to periosteal bone deposition and painful, swollen joints.

R. Bartl, C. Bartl, *Bone Disorders*, DOI 10.1007/978-3-319-29182-6_54

55 Rheumatology and Immunology

Skeletal damage is a hallmark of many chronic rheumatic diseases such as rheumatic arthritis (RA), ankylosing spondylitis (AS) and systemic lupus erythematosus (SLE) and is known as *inflammation-induced bone loss in the rheumatic diseases.* Vitamin D exercises a regulatory function in the maintenance of immune homeostasis, and it has been demonstrated that the net effect of vitamin D is an enhancement of innate immunity. A role has been ascribed to vitamin D in autoimmune disorders such as multiple sclerosis and rheumatoid arthritis.

Additional bone loss in the rheumatic disorders due to long-term steroid therapy and immobilisation aggravate the osteoporotic state. Various forms of skeletal destruction are recognised: local bone erosion, periarticular bone loss and generalised osteoporosis. Local bone erosion is the most typical example of inflammation-induced bone loss. The lesion affects the subchondral bone at the margins of the joints, and it emerges at the interphase between the articular cartilage and the underlying bone, first described as "caries of the joint ends". Generalised bone loss is another important and frequent feature of RA. About one third of RA patients are osteoporotic, and 10 % suffer from vertebral fractures. These patients suffer a decrease of 2.5 % in vertebral BMD and 5 % in the BMD of the hip within the first year of disease, and bone loss is doubled a year later, if the disease is not adequately treated. Severity of disease, as indicated by a high inflammatory activity, is an independent risk factor for accelerated bone loss and increased fracture risk. In patients on long-term therapy with corticosteroids, this may be the determining factor, with a relatively minor effect of the corticosteroids on the BMD. Formation of osteoclasts is facilitated by the inflammation-induced expression of cytokines such as TNF, IL-6 and RANKL. Furthermore, monocytes and macrophages accumulate in the synovial inflammatory tissues and express receptors such as RANK in response to the cytokines, and these in turn stimulate the development of active osteoclasts. Studies have shown that the replicative capacity of osteoblasts decreases with ageing and contributes to periarticular osteopenia in rheumatoid arthritis; more so than in patients with osteoarthritis.

To *summarise*, in the rheumatic disorders, the combination of joint pain, immobilisation and glucocorticoid therapy inevitably leads to a further loss of bone. Early correction of vitamin D deficiency and initiation of bisphosphonate therapy is strongly advised. In patients with chronic polyarthritis, measurement of the density of the phalanges by ultrasound has proved a useful method to monitor the state of the bones.

Ankylosing spondylitis (AS) is a chronic rheumatic disorder primarily affecting the vertebral column and the sacroiliac joints. It induces extensive damage to the vertebral column conductive to fractures and to spinal cord injury. Primary

R. Bartl, C. Bartl, *Bone Disorders*, DOI 10.1007/978-3-319-29182-6_55

preventive measures are absolutely essential in order to prevent such injuries. Management of the patients once such an injury has occurred is complex and involves extensive rehabilitation. Any patient presenting with nonspecific symptomatology should be carefully investigated for a possible specific aetiology before institution of therapy, with the possible exception of pain relief.

Part XI

Other Systemic Bone Disorders

The Patient with "Hypocalcaemia" 56

56.1 Definition and Pathogenesis

Hypocalcaemia is defined as a plasma or serum concentration of total calcium <2.20 mmol/l (<8.8 mg/dl) with normal plasma or serum protein concentration or a plasma or serum concentration of ionised calcium <1.17 mmol/l (4.7 mg/dl). In healthy people only 48 % of calcium, in the ionised form, is metabolically active. The acid-base balance is also important, because an acidosis is associated with a higher level of ionised calcium, while an alkalosis with lower level of ionised calcium shows a higher probability of hypocalcaemia symptoms.

> Only changes of the ionised calcium level in the serum are associated with clinical symptoms. The significance of normally measured total calcium in serum is therefore limited. Acidosis and alkalosis can in addition cause a shift in the relationship between ionised and total calcium.

The causes of hypocalcaemia can be divided according to whether serum PTH levels are low (hypoparathyroidism) or high (secondary hyperparathyroidism). Impaired production of PTH or vitamin D is the most common aetiology. Hypocalcaemia may have many causes. Today they are divided into three groups according to the behaviour of the parathyroid hormone (PTH).

Hypocalcaemia Due to Reduced or Absent Secretion of PTH

Various congenital and acquired diseases can lead to a failure in the development or destruction of the parathyroid gland or to a functional failure of PTH production.

- Destruction of the parathyroid gland: The most common cause of hypoparathyroidism is the surgical removal during thyroid operations or in the context of extended operations of head and neck tumours. Infiltrative processes, granulomatous diseases, metastases, irradiation or heavy metal deposits can also lead to failure of the parathyroid glands.
- Hypomagnesaemia: Magnesium is an important cofactor for PTH secretion. Hypocalcaemia associated with hypomagnesaemia is observed in severe cases of magnesium deficiency in the case of chronic gastrointestinal disease, eating disorders, alcoholism or cisplatin therapy. Administration of magnesium immediately normalises the secretion of PTH.
- Idiopathic hypoparathyroidism: An isolated failure in the development of the parathyroid gland is a rare genetic disorder. Molecular abnormalities of PTH biosynthesis in morphologically normal parathyroid glands can also lead to hypocalcaemia. A rare autoimmune illness ("autoimmune polyglandular syndrome

R. Bartl, C. Bartl, *Bone Disorders*, DOI 10.1007/978-3-319-29182-6_56

type1") is associated with Morbus Addison, diabetes mellitus and candidiasis and manifests itself in childhood.

Hypocalcaemia Due to Resistance to the Effects of PTH (PTH Receptor Defects)

The peripheral tissue resistance to PTH is referred to as pseudohypoparathyroidism (PHP) and manifests itself with hypocalcaemia and hyperphosphataemia with increased PTH levels. PHP is divided further into subgroups, where type1a is the hereditary osteodystrophy Albright and goes hand in hand with short stature and skeletal deformities.

Hypocalcaemia in Normal or Raised PTH Levels and Normal PTH Receptors

Despite normal function of PTH and normal PTH receptors, malfunction of calcium homeostasis, of vitamin D metabolism and other illnesses can lead to hypocalcaemia. Common *causes* are:

- Hypoproteinaemia: The most common cause of low levels of calcium in the plasma is low protein levels (especially albumin). In these patients the concentration of ionised calcium, however, is normal so that symptoms of hypocalcaemia are missing. Low albumin levels can be found with nephrotic syndrome, cirrhosis, malabsorption syndrome and with a too high circulation volume. The determination of ionised calcium clarifies this situation.
- Hyperphosphataemia: It occurs in serum levels of >1.46 mmol/l (>4, 5 mg/dl) and is mainly due to a decrease in the renal excretion of PO_4 in renal deficiency. A hyperphosphataemia also occurs with excessive oral or parenteral administration of PO_4. Other causes include alkalosis, tumour lysis syndrome and rhabdomyolysis. The clinical symptoms are caused by the accompanying hypocalcaemia and may lead to tetany.
- Severe tissue injuries, burns, rhabdomyolysis and tumour lysis.
- Pancreatitis: Hypocalcaemia and tetany were diagnosed for the first time in the 1940s in patients with pancreatitis. Released lipases from the damaged pancreas release fatty acids, which bind calcium. Hypocalcaemia with pancreatitis is associated with a poor prognosis.
- Chronic kidney deficiency: See separate chapter in this book.
- Sepsis: Approximately 20 % of patients with sepsis have reduced serum levels of ionised calcium combined with a poor prognosis.

Table 56.1 shows the main causes of hypocalcaemia.

Table 56.1 Causes of hypocalcaemia

Hypoparathyroid
Renal
Acute and chronic renal failure
Nephrotic syndrome
Gastrointestinal
Vitamin D deficiency
Malnutrition
Malabsorption
Acute pancreatitis
Hepatic disease
Metabolic
Alkalosis
Magnesium deficiency
Phosphate administration
Neoplastic
Osteoblastic metastases
Infectious
Measles
Drugs
Calcitonin
Bisphosphonates
Chelating agents
Aminoglycosides
Anticonvulsant drugs
Antineoplastic drugs
Postsurgical
Acute tissue necrosis
Massive blood transfusions
Toxic shock syndrome
Pregnancy

56.2 Symptoms

Patients with hypocalcaemia may be asymptomatic or they may present with life-threatening complications. The symptoms of hypocalcaemia are mainly caused by increased neuromuscular irritability (Table 56.2). Muscle spasms of the legs and back are typical. Further signs are paraesthesia of the lips, tongue, fingers and feet (laryngospasm in children). A creeping hypocalcaemia can also lead to a diffuse encephalopathy with depression, psychosis or even dementia or it is completely asymptomatic. In contrast, a sharp drop of the calcium level can trigger a prolonged Q-T interval in ECG, up to heart failure.

Table 56.2 Signs and symptoms of hypocalcaemia

Symptoms
Paraesthesias
Tetany
Muscle cramping and weakness
Abdominal cramping
Laryngospasm
Bronchospasm
Seizures
Papilloedema
Cataracts
Congestive heart failure
Depression
Coma
Signs
Chvostek sign
Trousseau sign
Prolongation of the QTc interval
Intracerebral calcifications

56.3 Diagnosis

For diagnosis, some laboratory values of the serum are necessary such as calcium (total and ionised), phosphate, magnesium, creatinine and protein (albumin) and in certain cases also vitamin D and PTH. The Chvostek and Trousseau signs are easily trigged under latent tetany. With severe hypocalcaemia, typical changes can be found in the ECG and EEG.

56.4 Therapy

The approach to treatment depends on:

- Severity of hypocalcaemia
- Rapidity with which it develops
- Accompanying complications (e.g. seizures, laryngospasm)

Therapy of symptomatic hypocalcaemia is based on oral or parenteral administration of calcium (e.g. 10 ml of a 10 % calcium gluconate solution over ten min i.v. or 1 l of a 5 % dextrose solution, to which 20–30 ml of 10 % calcium gluconate solution are added, over 24 h). Further possible treatment such as vitamin D and magnesium supplementation depends on the underlying disease. The treatment goal is to bring serum calcium into the normal range and to avoid hypercalciuria, which may cause renal stones.

Symptomatic hypocalcaemia occurs in many organs: central nervous system, muscles, cardiovascular system, abdomen, eyes, upper respiratory tract, teeth and skin. The symptoms are often general and nonspecific and frequently lead to unnecessary diagnostic measurements (e.g. laparotomy).

Osteomalacia and Rickets

57

57.1 Histology

Osteomalacia, translated "soft bones", was first recognised by the pathologist Pommer in 1885 as a specific illness and separate from osteoporosis. It is characterised by a mineralisation malfunction of the normal structured organic bone matrix in adults and histologically by a high proportion of non-mineralised osteoid ("wide seams of osteoid") (Fig. 57.1a–d). Paradoxically, the total mass of the bone matrix is raised. Nevertheless, there is an increased risk of fracture. Mineralisation malfunctions of the growing skeleton, in addition, are accompanied by changes of the epiphysis and stronger deformities of the skeleton and are referred to as *rickets*.

57.2 Pathogenesis

Many *reasons* can lead to a disrupted mineralisation (Table 57.1). First and foremost, mineral concentrations, vitamin D metabolites, acid-base balance and genetic defects of bone cells and matrix are all known causes. Six main groups can be distinguished:

- *Vitamin D deficiencies*: They occur with insufficient UV radiation of the skin (with children and older persons with disabilities), inadequate vitamin D intake through diet, in the context of malabsorption and maldigestion syndromes, celiac disease and rarely with conditions after gastric resection.
- *Vitamin D metabolism:* Dysfunctions in vitamin D metabolism can be found most commonly in chronic renal deficiency ("renal osteodystrophy"), which are described in detail in the following chapter. Osteopathies, caused by antiepileptic drugs, are also clinically significant. Osteomalacia in chronic liver parenchymal damage is rare, because 25 % functioning liver parenchyma is sufficient, to ensure an adequate 25-hydroxylation of vitamin D. In hereditary pseudodeficiency rickets, there is a genetic disorder with occurrence of a rachitic appearance in infant and toddler age. Underlying there is a defect of the 1a-hydroxylase (type I) or a deficiency of the vitamin D receptor (type II).
- *Renal tubular dysfunction (vitamin D-resistant rickets):* Less common causes for osteomalacia or rickets are genetic defects of hydroxylation in the kidney and defects of the vitamin D receptor. Onset of rickets is usually at the age of two. With the exception of renal tubular acidosis, all cases share reduced phosphate reabsorption in the proximal renal tubules ("*phosphate diabetes*"). Because of the malfunctioning hydroxylation, hypophosphataemia is accompanied additionally by a reduced intestinal absorption of calcium and phosphate.
- *Phosphatase deficiency (hypophosphatasia):* In this autosomal recessive inherited disorder,

R. Bartl, C. Bartl, *Bone Disorders*, DOI 10.1007/978-3-319-29182-6_57

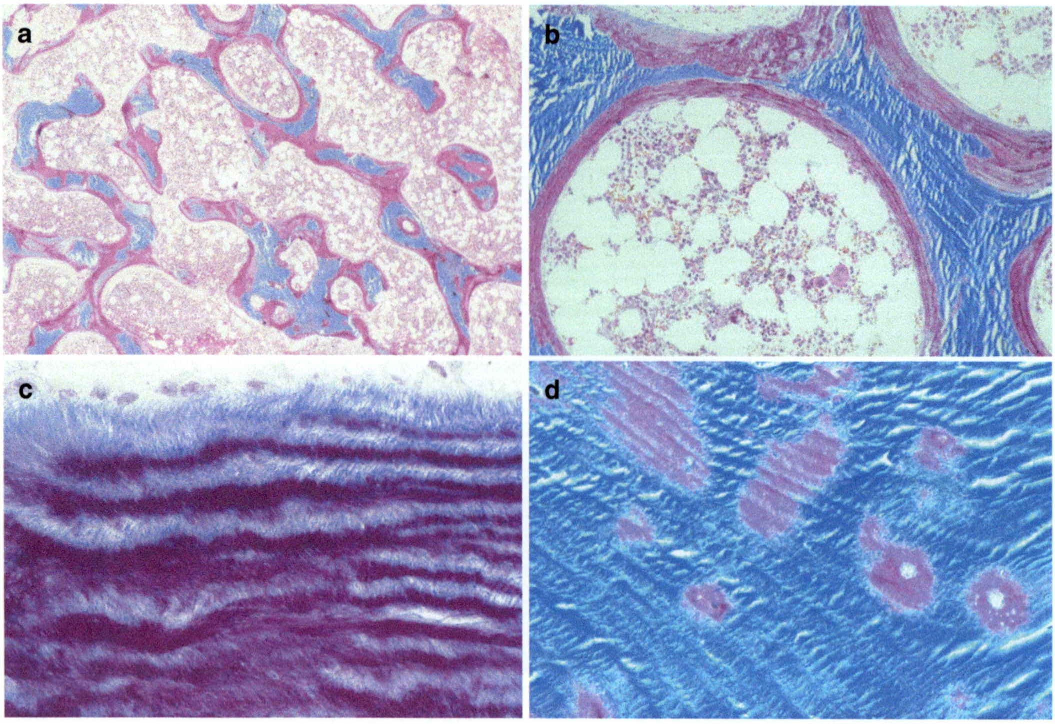

Fig. 57.1 (**a**) Dense trabecular network and increased extent of osteoid surfaces on the trabecular bone (*red*); (**b**) higher magnification with layer of osteoid as well as patchy, irregular demineralisation of the trabecular bone; (**c**) higher magnification of non-mineralised osteoid lamellae lined by a layer of osteoblasts; (**d**) isolated foci of demineralisation within the trabecula – pathognomonic for osteomalacia. All Ladewig stainings

a chondrocalcinosis frequently occurs in addition to the osteomalacia. Affected children show hypercalcaemia, hypercalciuria as well as various anomalies and deformities of the skeleton with a tendency to fracture.

- *Tumour-associated osteomalacia:* Osteomalacia images have been reported, especially in mesenchymal tumours, caused by the production of humoural factors ("phosphatonine") in the tumour tissue. These influence above all multiple functions of the proximal tubule of the kidney, especially the reabsorption of phosphate with resulting hypophosphataemia. After surgical removal of the tumour, the osteomalacia is also completely cured. Tumour-associated osteomalacia has also been reported with multiple myeloma, caused by the accompanying light-chain nephropathy and the reduced phosphate reabsorption in the kidney.
- *Drugs/toxic causes:* Although major studies have shown that fluoride stimulates new bone formation, higher doses and absence of calcium supplementation stimulate a malfunction of the mineralisation of the newly formed bone matrix, compatible with the appearance of osteomalacia. The mechanism is not known. The administration of *etidronate* in high doses leads to a suppression of the osteoblast function and above all the calcium phosphate crystallisation so that today only modern BP are used in much lower doses for the treatment of osteoporosis. Large deposits of aluminium in the bone disrupt the mineralisation and, in the case of chronic kidney disease, lead to severe osteomalacia.

57.3 Clinical Signs

The clinical picture of osteomalacia depending on the underlying condition is characterised by generalised severe and load-dependent bone pain, bone bending and muscle weakness and atrophy.

Table 57.1 Main causes of osteomalacia and rickets

Congenital
Hypophosphataemic rickets
Hypophosphatasia
Vitamin D-dependent rickets, types I and II
Primary renal tubular defects
Axial osteomalacia
Nutritional
Low dietary intake
Lack of exposure to the sun
Parenteral alimentation
Gastrointestinal
Postgastrectomy
Malabsorption
Hepatobiliary diseases
Chronic pancreatic insufficiency
Renal
Chronic renal failure
Dialysis bone disease
Renal tubular acidosis
Nephrotic syndrome
Tumour associated
Mesenchymal tumours
Metastatic carcinomas
Acute leukaemias
Malignant lymphomas
Multiple myeloma
Drugs/toxins
Fluoride
Bisphosphonates, first generation
Anticonvulsants
Barbiturates
Cholestyramine
Aluminium
Lead

The most common clinical features of osteomalacia are generalised bone pain and tenderness and marked muscle weakness. Bone tenderness can be shown by percussion of the spine, the sternum or the ribs.

These problems may be so pronounced that in individual cases they result in confinement to bed and immobility. The bone pain is interpreted as periosteum stretching pain, as a result of the soft, malleable bone. With 5–10 % of patients, pseudofractures ("Looser lines") occur in characteristic places of the skeleton that present themselves in the X-ray image as band-shaped light zones with edge sclerosis (Fig. 57.2a, b). Looser zones are the radiological hallmark of severe osteomalacia and are found mainly in bones responsible for bearing the major mechanical stresses. They are often multiple and bilateral and can be related anatomically to the arterial supply of the bone (sites of entrance of nutrient arteries). They may progress to complete fractures and may heal very slowly even under therapy. Figure 57.3 shows the predilection sites of these lesions. These pseudofractures are shown in the skeletal bone scan as "hot spots".

Muscle weakness is often misinterpreted as polyneuropathy and affects especially the abdomen and the proximal extremities. This results in the typical "waddle". Psychological symptoms such as depression and reduced performance levels are observed.

The fracture tendency results, on the one hand, from less resilient bones and, on the other hand, from muscle weakness.

Rickets in infants and children comes with typical findings such as enlargement of the costal cartilage ("rachitic rosary"), bending of the limbs, bell-shaped chest, chicken breast, enamel defects of teeth and characteristic dorsal kyphosis ("rachitic catback").

Radiographically, the disease is characterised by three changes:

- Dysfunction of bone formation in the metaphyses
- Low mineral content of bones (not to be confused with osteoporosis!)
- Periosteal apposition (osteophytes)

The earliest specific radiological change is widening of the growth plate resulting from an increase of cartilage, followed by bone loss in the metaphyseal side of the growth plate (Fig. 57.4). Soft tissue

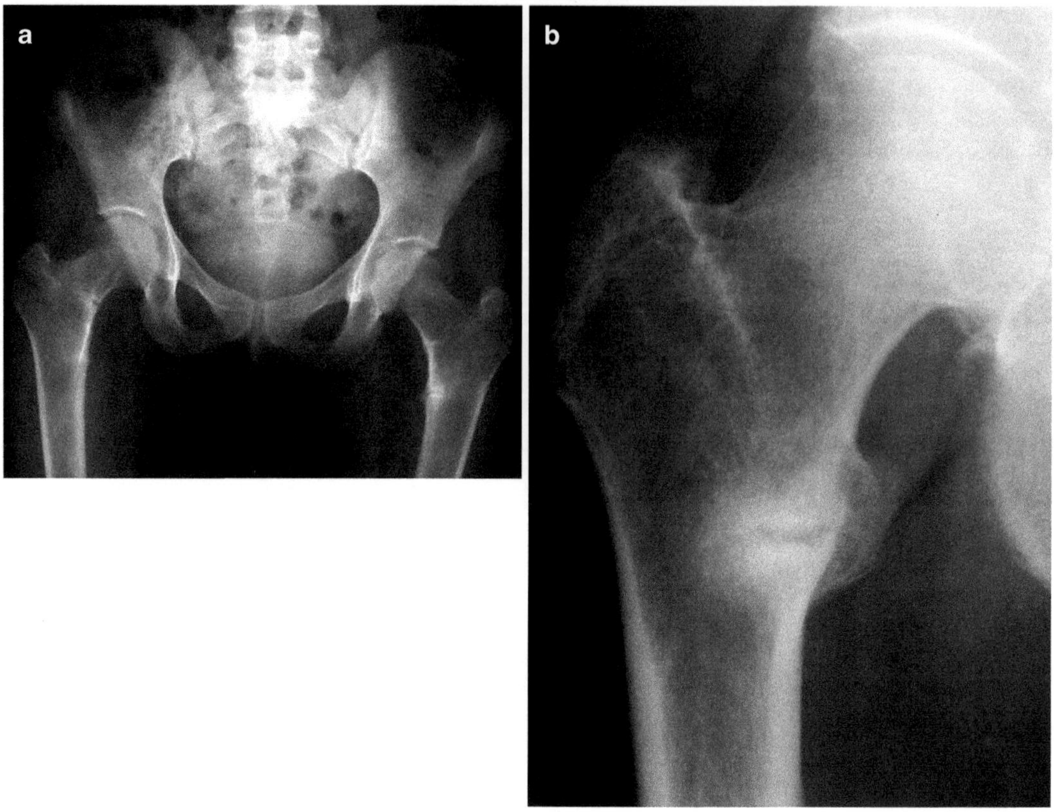

Fig. 57.2 (**a**) Bilateral Looser zones of the proximal femora; (**b**) at higher magnification, Looser zone of the proximal femur: a transverse band at right angle to the cortex and involving mainly the cortex with slight periosteal reaction

swellings around the involved joints are typical, explaining the "rachitic rosary" appearance along the middle ribs. Bowing of the forearms and the long bones of the legs as well as deformities in the pelvis with coxa vara may occur. Looser zones in rachitic children, however, are uncommon.

Rickets in premature babies of low birth weight may also occur. Predisposing factors besides prematurity include prolonged illness in the newborn and maternal pre-eclampsia, inadequate nutrition and medications that may be given to control infections.

Hypophosphatasia (HPP) is the rare genetically determined rickets or osteomalacia characterised by abnormal mineralisation and subnormal activity of tissue-nonspecific isoenzyme of alkaline phosphatase (TNSALP). HPP mainly disturbs the skeleton, the teeth and muscles. Perinatal, infantile, childhood and adult HPP are differentiated. HPP osteomalacia is remarkable, because serum levels of calcium and phosphate are not reduced and ALP activity is low. Approximately 50 % of the patients are hyperphosphataemic, and hypercalcaemia occurs frequently in infantile HPP. Serum PTH and $1.25(OH)_2$ concentrations are suppressed in hypercalcaemic variants. There is no established treatment in HPP. Only enzyme-replacement therapy will be promising in the future. In childhood HPP, dietary restriction and binders to correct hyperphosphataemia can be useful. Continuous expert dental care is important.

57.4 Diagnosis

The diagnosis of osteomalacia or rickets is established on the basis of the symptoms, as well the laboratory and radiological results. In a few cases, to ensure the correct diagnosis, histologic

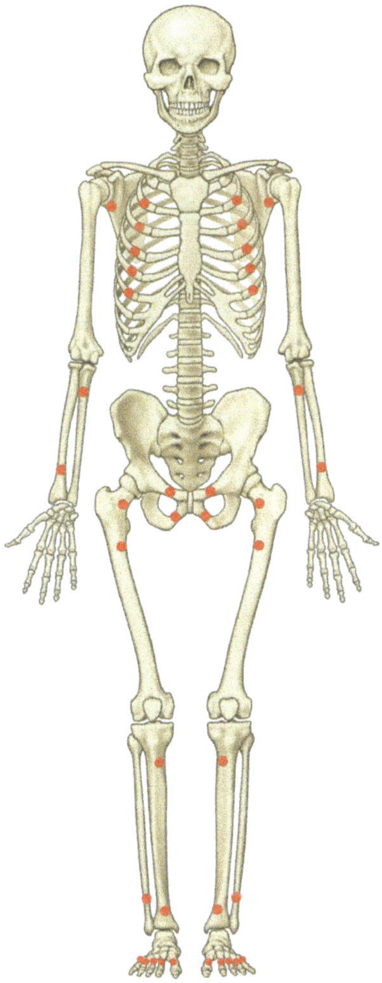

Fig. 57.3 Main localisations of Looser zones

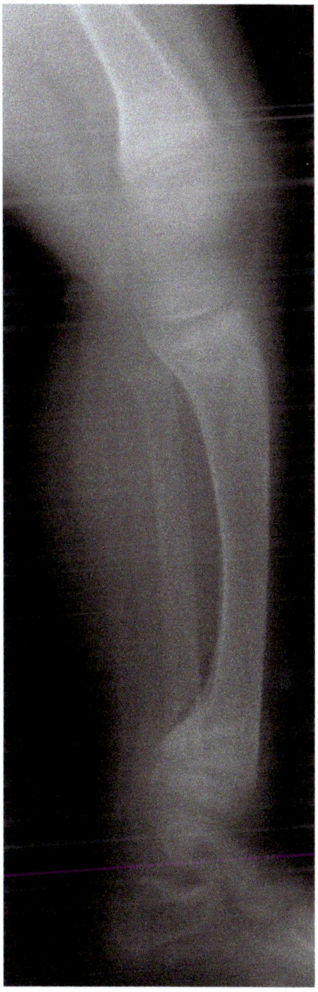

Fig. 57.4 X-ray of the knee and tibia from a child with rickets. The epiphyseal plates are widened with bending of the tibia

findings are additionally required. The evidence of a decreased serum level of 25(OH) vitamin D and an increased alkaline phosphatase (exception: hypophosphatasia) are well-known indicators (Table 57.2).

According to estimates, less than 50 % of the world's population have a normal vitamin D status (>50 mmol/l or >20 ng/ml)! In Europe, higher serum levels were found, apparently paradoxically, in Scandinavia than in southern or eastern European countries.

The Looser zones are characteristic ("Milkman's fractures"). These lines, present in 20 % of patients with osteomalacia, represent stress fractures and are most prominent on the concave side of long bones. The DXA bone density measurement gives significantly low values that should not be interpreted as "osteoporosis". They correspond to a "reduction of calcium carbonate". As the mass of non-mineralised bone tissue (matrix) with osteomalacia is even increased, an effective therapy with vitamin D results in a rapid and strong growth of bone mineral density (BMD) (up to 50 % within a few months).

A low value in the DXA measurement may not automatically be interpreted as "osteoporosis". Rather, osteomalacia must be taken into consideration with determination of alkaline phosphatase and calcium in the serum. Furthermore, with the symptom "systemic bone pain", osteomalacia can always be suspected or a malignant process and requires further laboratory chemical and – if necessary – a bone histological investigation.

Table 57.2 Differential diagnosis between osteoporosis and osteomalacia

	Osteoporosis	Osteomalacia
Clinical features	Bone pain only when fractures occur	Bone pain and muscle weakness
Biochemistry		
Calcium	Normal	Low
Phosphate	Normal	Low
Alkaline phosphatase	Normal	High
Histology	Thin trabeculae and cortex	Wide seams of osteoid, normal bone matrix
Radiology		
Bone density	Reduced	Reduced
Bone architecture	Thin, sharp cortex and slim trabeculae	Broad and coarse cortex, coarse and woolly trabeculae
Looser zones	No	Present
Bone softening	No	Present
Fractures	Present	Present
Association with HPT	No	Common in renal disorders

57.5 Treatment

The treatment of osteomalacia and rickets is directed towards the normalisation of mineralisation and treatment of the basic disease – as far as it can be influenced. Vitamin D_3, calcium, phosphate and vitamin D metabolites as well as alkalising substances are worth considering. Duration and dose of vitamin D therapy can be very different and must be adjusted according to regular serum control. As an initial weekly dose, 20,000–40,000 IE has proved its worth (1000 IE corresponds to 25 μg vitamin D_3). Later, 2000–3000 IE daily vitamin D_3 taken as small pills or tablets are usually sufficient. With malabsorption syndrome, higher doses are usually necessary. The alkaline phosphatase may rise initially, but it falls within weeks or months into the normal ranges. Radiological changes of rickets also heal rapidly. However, Looser lines take more than a year to disappear. Calcium (e.g. daily 800–1000 mg calcium carbonate as a tablet) is a necessary complement to vitamin D. With renal osteopathy, active vitamin D metabolites can be employed. With tubular dysfunction administration of oral phosphate and alkalising substances can be administered if necessary. The observation that some forms of rickets do not respond to vitamin D administration led to the detection of rare congenital anomalies of vitamin D metabolism or of vitamin D receptor.

Treatment of osteomalacia with high-dose vitamin D_3 should be combined with the simultaneous administration of calcium in order to avoid a symptomatic hypocalcaemia in the context of rapid onset of mineralisation ("*hungry bone*"). A meta-analysis has also shown that the combination of vitamin D and calcium is essential for its preventive effect on fractures.

58 AIDS Osteopathy

58.1 Pathogenesis

It is important to emphasise that there are well over 40 million people worldwide who are infected with the AIDS virus (acquired immune deficiency syndrome), and about five million more people are still infected annually. A high proportion of these are women and children. Many AIDS patients live in circumstances which do not enable them to receive the care and treatment outlined below, though greater international efforts in this direction are now being made. Put very briefly, the progression of HIV infection to the full-blown picture of AIDS is associated with loss of immunocompetence and its consequences, the occurrence of opportunistic infections and malignancies, while the immune dysregulation may lead to autoimmune phenomena such as vasculitis. Poor antibody responses have also been associated with premature exhaustion of B lymphocytes in HIV-infected patients. Fungal infections in particular increase the risk for disease progression. Co-infection with hepatitis C virus also has a deleterious effect and contributes to hepatic fibrosis. DNA microarray analysis has been used to predict hepatic fibrosis, thereby sparing the patients a liver biopsy. These patients also have reduced BMD and possibly osteopenia/osteoporosis.

Much knowledge has accumulated over the years from the work that has been done on the pathogenesis of AIDS (Table 58.1) and on the mechanisms of disease progression from infection with the virus to the full-blown clinical picture of AIDS, and these insights are being used to assist in the development of a vaccine against AIDS that has widespread applicability. However, all attempts to accomplish this goal have so far not been successful, but concentrated efforts are ongoing and results expected.

The introduction of *HAART* (highly active antiviral therapy) in 1995/1996 has changed the future and fate of the people with AIDS, at least those who are able to receive and adhere to therapy with HAART. Since its introduction, some modifications and variations have been made and are available, and these contribute to the differences in both the beneficial effects and the

Table 58.1 Aetiology of AIDS osteopathy

Basic disorder
Haemopoietic cell defect?
T-cell activation
Bone marrow inflammation
Malnutrition
Gastrointestinal infections
Immobilisation
Lipodystrophy
Testosterone deficiency
Vitamin D deficiency
Infections
Hyperparathyroidism
Glucocorticosteroids
Antibiotics
Protease inhibitors

R. Bartl, C. Bartl, *Bone Disorders*, DOI 10.1007/978-3-319-29182-6_58

adverse reactions reported during the past 10 years or so. Racial/ethnic differences, due to many different factors, have also been shown to play a part, as seen in the reactions of patients to therapies given for some of the disorders associated with AIDS, such as metabolic syndromes and malignancies, which in turn influence their consequences, such as osteopenia/osteoporosis. Studies have shown that renal dysfunction, frequent in advanced HIV-AIDS, was improved after 2-year therapy with HAART. However, neurocognitive disturbances associated with HIV/AIDS were not affected by therapy with HAART. In contrast, therapy with HAART has resulted in a dramatic reduction in morbidity and mortality among HIV-AIDS patients.

It has been estimated that >40 % of HIV/AIDS patients develop a malignancy during the course of their lives. Since the introduction of HAART and the increased survival, it is estimated that malignancies, mainly lymphomas and sarcomas, still occur in more than 40 % of patients at some time in their lives. Possibly the incidence is so high due to the increased survival. The patients suffer from the so-called AIDS-related malignancies but also from others such as lung cancer. The malignancies, their therapies and the consequences of both all have deleterious effects on the skeleton which greatly increased the prevalence of osteopenia/osteoporosis among patients with AIDS. The manifestations of rheumatic disorders in AIDS patients has changed with the introduction of HAART, but complications such as metabolic abnormalities, cardiovascular disorders and osteoporosis still occur. It should be clearly stated that rheumatic disease is also still prevalent even after therapy with HAART. Some studies have indicated that alendronate is the bisphosphonate of choice for the osteopenia/osteoporosis of the patients on HAART therapy, though few comparative studies have been published. Since over 10 years have now passed since the introduction and use of HAART, reports of cases of resistance to therapy have increased and national authorities as well as the WHO have developed monitoring, assessment and prevention strategies to facilitate evidence-based decision-making concerning the various aspects of AIDS therapy.

58.2 Manifestations of AIDS Osteopathy

Many of the problems experienced by patients with AIDS (acquired immune deficiency syndrome) require haematologic, immunologic and osteologic investigations. These problems include cytopaenias, lymphomas, infections, fever of unknown origin (FUO), haemorrhages, bone pain and pathologic fractures. It is essential to emphasise that osteopathy in AIDS is an important, highly complex complication which has so far received too little attention. Haematologic disorders and neoplasias have been extensively described and are well recognised, but not osteological problems. Since the latest treatments for AIDS now achieve longer survival times, it is all the more important to pay attention to the quality of life for which mobility and therefore skeletal integrity are crucial, particularly for the millions of children involved, because many of the more than 40 million people with AIDS are young.

Drugs used to treat AIDS may also be harmful to the bones, as is the decreased physical activity of many patients. HIV therapy-induced changes in immune factors which also participate in bone remodelling have been implicated in the increased bone resorption in HIV-infected children and adolescents. In one study, evaluation of aspirates and bone marrow biopsies ($n = 120$) frequently demonstrated dysplastic/aplastic changes in haematopoiesis, as well as inflammatory reactions in the stroma of the bone marrow. The bone itself also regularly exhibited changes designated as *AIDS osteopathy*. These changes are summarised as follows (Fig. 58.1a, b):

- Reduced bone density (osteopenia, osteoporosis)
- Increased osteoclastic activity (secondary HPT)
- Disturbances in mineralisation (osteomalacia)

Recent studies on the interaction of the AIDS infection and bone have postulated that the constant stimulation of T cells leads to activation of osteoclasts and thereby increased resorption via

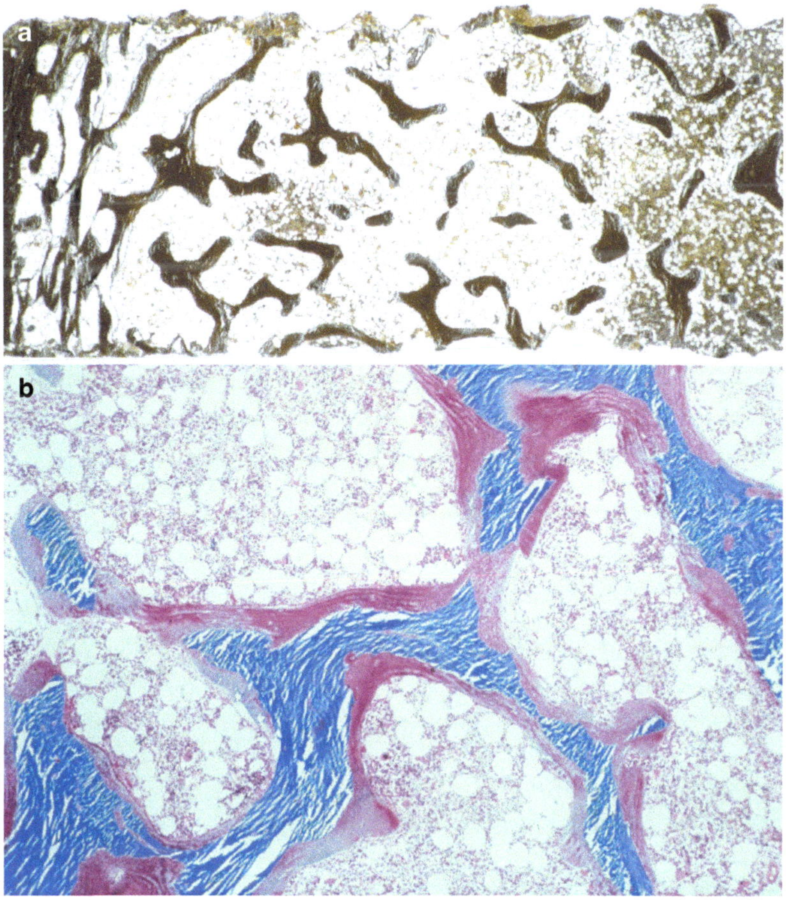

Fig. 58.1 (**a, b**) (**a**) Iliac crest biopsy of a patient with AIDS: note marked marrow atrophy and osteoporosis, Gomori staining; (**b**) at higher magnification signs of inadequate mineralisation with increased amount of osteoid (=*red*), Ladewig staining

osteoprotegerin. In adult men, the G-IGF1 axis in the control mechanism of bone remodelling is apparently also involved. In addition to the direct viral and drug-induced damage to bone cells, marrow cells and stroma, as well as the anomalies of vitamin D metabolism, many other secondary risk factors are also involved (Table 58.1). Recent international studies of bone density by DXA measurements in AIDS patients have now confirmed the frequent occurrence of osteopenia/osteoporosis and pathologic fractures and in some cases even of osteonecrosis, as shown in a large study of patients from 1999 to 2002. A recent study has demonstrated that pre- and postmenopausal women who are HIV+ are at increased risk for fragility fractures, compared with women in the general public in many cases with the same BMD as the controls. Both women and men with HIV disease are at increased risk of fracture, which is three- to fourfold increased compared with non-HIV-infected controls. The risk of having osteoporotic bone density is also increased 3.7-fold for HIV-infected persons compared with controls. Should the patients undergo additional viral infections such as hepatitis C, they will be at risk for additional complications such as diabetes, steatohepatitis, subsequent advanced fibrosis and increased BMI.

Prospective studies have shown that HAART initiating reduces BMD by 1–5 % over 1–2 years. Therapy with tenofovir has been associated with a greater reduction in BMD than with stavudine or abacavir.

The causes of the osteopathies in AIDS are very complex (as noted above) and are also influenced by the various therapies the patients have received. These in turn affect the clinical, biochemical and radiological manifestations. Moreover, fractures in AIDS patients have a very strong adverse influence on quality of life, by the additional suffering and incapacity, the added requirements for care and nursing and the effect on morbidity and mortality, as well as contributing greatly to the cost of treatment, which is still a very important factor in many developing countries with a high prevalence of AIDS infection in the population. This also accounts for geographic differences in availability of HAART.

58.3 Diagnosis

Consequently all AIDS patients should undergo an osteological evaluation at the time of diagnosis, including the following if at all possible:

- X-ray of the lumbar spine in two planes
- DXA of the lumbar spine and hip (annual monitoring)
- Examination of peripheral blood for calcium, phosphate, alkaline phosphatase, crosslaps, PTH, vitamin D, TSH and testosterone/oestrogen
- Complete blood count (CBC)

When appropriate indications are present (cytopaenias, atypical cells in blood films, etc.), and possibly (unclarified) osteopathies, a bone biopsy and aspirate should be obtained for clarification and diagnosis. It should be stressed that in AIDS the disorders of the bones of young people and adults begin in childhood – even in the neonatal and perinatal periods; therefore appropriate management of the paediatric patient is crucial.

58.4 Treatment Strategies

All patients with AIDS benefit from the established basic therapy of osteoporosis:

- Physical activity
- Bone-conscious lifestyle (e.g. giving up smoking!)
- 1000 mg/d calcium
- 1000–2000 IE/d vitamin D_3

However, should there already be osteoporosis at diagnosis (T <–2.5 SD) or if the density measurements decrease in spite of the basic therapy (as above), then addition of an oral nitrogen-containing bisphosphonate is indicated. If difficulties arise with the oral route, then a bisphosphonate can be given i.v. which also forestalls problems of compliance and uncertainty as to whether or not the medication has been taken. The schedule is the same as previously noted.

- Alendronate 70 mg orally weekly
- Risedronate 35 mg orally weekly
- Ibandronate 3 mg i.v. every 3 months
- Zoledronate 5 mg i.v. annually

When osteomalacia and secondary hyperparathyroidism dominate the clinical picture, the daily supplement of vitamin D_3 can be increased to 3000 IU daily. Alternatively an active metabolite of vitamin D can be substituted. Serum calcium must of course be monitored and given in patients with hypocalcaemia.

To summarise, the AIDS patients develop some form of osteopathy during the course of the disease. This can be a combination of osteoporosis, osteomalacia and secondary hyperparathyroidism and frequently entails difficult clinical situations involving pathologic fractures and bone pain.

Studies are in progress to clarify to what extent the viral infection itself and/or the antiviral therapy are/is responsible for the loss of bone mass. Secondary infections and lipodystrophy also add to the *osteoporomalacia*. If the diagnostic investigations (as described above) are applied and the basic therapy implemented, then AIDS osteopathy can be diagnosed and prevented in its early stages and even successfully treated in the later ones. Studies have already been published on the efficacy of alendronate plus calcium and vitamin D on bone mineral density – however, most of the patients were male with an average length of 8 years HIV infection. Results of additional studies are pending.

59 The Patient with "Hypercalcaemia"

59.1 Pathogenesis

Hypercalcaemia means a plasma or serum concentration of total calcium >2.60 mmol/l (>10.4 mg/dl) or a concentration of ionised calcium in the plasma/serum >1.3 mmol/l (>5.2 mg/dl). Hypercalcaemia usually arises through an increased absorption of calcium from the bone and is based mainly on a combination of several mechanisms:

- *Increased protein binding due to dysproteinaemia.* Since the ionised calcium is normal, this form is meaningless.
- *PTH-induced hypercalcaemia.* This is nearly always due to primary hyperparathyroidism (pHPT). In 90 % of the cases, the underlying cause is a parathyroid adenoma, in 7 % hyperplasia and in only 3 % a carcinoma.
- *Tumour-associated hypercalcaemia.* This occurs as part of a paraneoplastic syndrome or because of tumour-induced osteolytic bone disease. It occurs acutely and must be treated as a life-threatening emergency.
- *Hypercalcaemia associated with granulomatous disease or lymphomas.* This variant is caused by enhanced conversion of 25(OH)D to the active $1,25(OH)_2D$.
- *Hypercalcaemia in hyperthyroidism*, in combination with suppressed PTH secretion.

Hypercalcaemia is found in hospital patients at a frequency of approximately 1 %, caused by a tumour in 46 % and by pHPT in 35 %. In the remaining 19 %, there is a correlation with sarcoidosis, immobilisation and taking thiazides or active vitamin D.

> The four most common causes of hypercalcaemia to keep in mind and to clarify:
>
> - Incorrect values
> - Bone metastases
> - Multiple myeloma
> - Primary hyperparathyroidism

Less common causes should be examined from existing relevant information and clarified further by differential diagnosis:

- Sarcoidosis
- Hyperthyroidism
- Immobilisation
- Malignant illnesses with PTH production (PTHrP)
- Vitamin D and A intoxication
- Total parenteral nourishment
- Tertiary hyperparathyroidism
- Morbus Addison
- Milk-alkali syndrome
- Lithium poisoning
- Thiazide diuretics (hydrochlorothiazide and chlorthalidone)

R. Bartl, C. Bartl, *Bone Disorders*, DOI 10.1007/978-3-319-29182-6_59

- Hypereosinophilic syndrome
- Tuberculosis
- Familial hypocalciuric hypercalcaemia (FHH, autosomally inherited)

Once the diagnosis of hypercalcaemia is confirmed by control measurements, a distinction must be made between the pHPT, tumour hypercalcaemia and the rare hypocalciuric familial forms.

The determination of intact parathyroid hormone (iPTH) and calcium excretion in 24 h urine is also required. The following differentiation is possible:

- In pHPT, the iPTH value is usually >60 ng/l. A lower value indicates that the hypercalcaemia is not triggered by the parathyroid gland.
- In tumour-induced hypercalcaemia, the iPTH level in plasma is low (<40 ng/l) while phosphate is high.
- In typical familial hypocalciuric hypercalcaemia, calcium excretion in the urine is usually <100 mg/24 h.

In sarcoidosis and tuberculosis, hypercalcaemia is based on an uncontrolled production of 1,25$(OH)_2D$ by the monocytes of granulomas as a result of increased activity of 1-α hydroxylase.

59.2 Symptoms

Patients with mild hypercalcaemia have no symptoms. The term "hypercalcaemic syndrome" refers to a constellation of symptoms independent of the aetiology including renal (renal stones), gastrointestinal (peptic ulcer disease, pancreatitis, nausea, constipation) and neuropsychiatric changes (trouble concentrating, personality changes, depression). This syndrome has a wide clinical spectrum from asymptomatic to lethal. It is characterised by severe dehydration which is caused by the following sequence of events: hypercalcaemia, hypercalciuria, polyuria, polydipsia and polyuria. Nausea and vomiting further increase the fluid and electrolyte loss. The result is hypopotassaemia together with disturbances of cardiac rhythm. Moreover, fatigue, depression and a general deceleration of cognitive function indicate additional neuropsychiatric involvement. In severe cases the condition may progress to a hypercalcaemic crisis with somnolence and coma. With long-term hyperparathyroidism, the patient may present with bone pain and pathologic fractures.

59.3 Management

Mild, asymptomatic hypercalcaemia does not require immediate therapy. Symptomatic hypercalcaemia, however, requires immediate therapeutic intervention independent of the aetiology. Management is determined by the level of calcium in the serum, the clinical symptoms and the underlying disorder. But regardless of the cause, treatment always starts with adequate *rehydration*. When calcium is <2.88 mmol/L, investigation and correction of the underlying cause will suffice. When the PTH level is elevated, the parathyroid glands must be investigated and operated, if necessary and feasible. In cases of inoperable hyperparathyroidism, therapy with bisphosphonates is the second-line treatment of choice and this may be successful. If the level of iPTH is normal or low, a malignancy must be ruled out. In severe symptomatic hypercalcaemia (>3.75 mmol/L), immediate measures must be taken to ensure a rapid decrease in calcium levels. These include rehydration (physiological saline) and forced diuresis (furosemide). *Haemodialysis* may be required in the event of renal failure. In patients with sarcoidosis, with certain neoplasms and with vitamin D intoxication, corticosteroids are also indicated to decrease the calcium levels.

The main therapeutic aim in hypercalcaemia is inhibition of osteoclastic resorption of the bone, and this is most easily, effectively and reliably accomplished by intravenous administration of *BP* after rehydration. The following *protocols* are used:

Clodronate	Infusion of 300 mg daily over 7–10 days. The total number of infusions depends on the calcium level. Duration of infusion: 2 h
Ibandronate	Infusion of 6 mg, depending on the calcium level. Duration of infusion: 1–2 h
Pamidronate	Infusion of 30–90 mg, depending on the calcium level. Duration of infusion: 1–2 h
Zoledronate	Infusion of 4–5 mg, depending on the calcium level. Duration of infusion: 15–30 min, together with a 2-h infusion of saline

Generally speaking, a single infusion of one of the nitrogen-containing bisphosphonates restores the calcium level to normal. The treatment is repeated if the calcium levels rise again. The time required to stabilise the calcium level depends on the underlying condition and is usually about 2 weeks. Following infusion of zoledronate, the calcium level is usually normalised and stabilised by day 10. In patients with $1,25(OH)_2D$-mediated hypercalcaemia, glucocorticoids are the preferred therapy. Intravenous hydrocortisone (100–300 mg daily) or oral prednisone (40–60 mg daily) for 3–7 days is used most often.

Hypercalcaemia syndrome has a broad clinical spectrum, running from asymptomatic to lethal. The presence of a tumour must be considered by differential diagnosis in every patient with hypercalcaemia. The first step is sufficient intake of fluid. Modern BP have made further treatment of hypercalcaemia safe and effective.

60 Primary Hyperparathyroidism (pHPT)

60.1 Pathogenesis

Hyperfunction of the parathyroid glands can be categorised according to the aetiology in primary and secondary forms. In *primary hyperparathyroidism* (*pHPT*), the cause of overactivity of the parathyroid glands lies with the organ itself, while *secondary hyperparathyroidism* (*sHPT*) is a disorder of the calcium phosphate metabolism caused by renal or gastrointestinal disorders. People with *familial pHPT* are a small, but important group (about 5 % of all cases with pHPT). These familial syndromes include the multiple endocrine neoplasias (types 1, 2A and 4), the familial hypocalciuric hypercalcaemia (FHH) and the neonatal severe pHPT. About 2 % of all cases with pHPT are caused by MEN 1. This syndrome is defined by tumours of the parathyroid glands, the islet cells of the pancreas and the hypophysis. The tumours are removed surgically.

pHPT is a disorder of calcium metabolism caused by the overproduction of PTH in the parathyroid glands and is therefore characterised by simultaneous elevations of both circulating PTH and calcium levels. It is the third most common endocrine disease, with an incidence of approximately 1:1000, an age peak at 40–80 years and an emphasis on the female sex.

60.2 Pathologic Anatomy

In 80–85 % of cases, pHPT is caused by a solitary benign adenoma composed of the chief cells in one of the four parathyroid glands. A normal gland weighs about 30 g and adenomas can weigh up to 20 g. The inferior glands are most often involved, but in about 5–10 % of cases, the adenoma is sited abnormally in the thymus, mediastinum or retro-oesophageal space. In 10–15 % of patients, hypersecretion results from a diffuse hyperplasia of chief cells in all four parathyroid glands. Parathyroid carcinoma accounts for only 0.5 % of cases but is accompanied by a severe symptomatic hypercalcaemia.

PHPT is caused by:

- Solitary adenoma of one gland 85 %
- Hyperplasia of all four glands 15 %
- Carcinoma of one gland <0.5 %

Most congenital cases of pHPT result from one of the two MEN syndromes ("multiple endocrine neoplasia types I and II").

R. Bartl, C. Bartl, *Bone Disorders*, DOI 10.1007/978-3-319-29182-6_60

60.3 Diagnosis

Half of patients with pHPT were asymptomatic or discovered accidentally. PHPT can be diagnosed with the evidence of raised serum levels of calcium and PTH, assuming normal serum protein levels and kidney function. Often, a single value of PTH is also found in the upper normal range. Only low values for the intact PTH are arguments against a pHPT. Low serum levels of phosphate and vitamin D metabolites and a mild metabolic acidosis are also often found. This initial laboratory diagnosis is followed by a screening of the end organs: diagnosis of kidney stones with ultrasound or CT and of osteoporosis with the DXA measurement. Hyperparathyroid myopathy is diagnosed by electromyography. 24 h urine sampling further clarifies the existence of a hypercalciuria. Localisation of parathyroid adenomas is based on sonography of the neck, on MRI of the neck and on technetium-99 m-sestamibi scintigraphy. A selective venous catheterisation with PTH evaluation is only indicated before the second or third surgical intervention. Ectopic parathyroid glands can be located in the upper neck region as well as in the mediastinum. A second operation is occasionally necessary.

60.4 Clinical Findings

The clinical features of pHPT include the typical symptoms of hypercalcaemia associated with different renal and osseous complications. Approximately 20% of patients develop *kidney stones* (calcium oxalate and calcium phosphate) and less commonly a *nephrocalcinosis*. Radiologically, renal calcification is shown as lines or dots of calcium arranged in triangular tufts outlining the pyramids. This should be differentiated from other causes of nephrocalcinosis, which also occurs in normocalcaemic disorders of augmented calcium absorption through the gut (sarcoidosis, vitamin D intoxication), skeletal breakdown (tumours and multiple myeloma) or distal renal tubular acidosis. The risk factors for stone disease are hypercalciuria and alkaline urine. The pathognomonic skeletal presentation of pHPT is *osteitis fibrosa generalisata cystica*, which was first described by Recklinghausen in 1891 (Fig. 60.1a, b). This osteopathy is caused by an increased bone remodelling and defined in skeletal radiographies as a combination of:

- Subperiosteal bone resorption in the distal phalanges (Fig. 60.2) and skull
- Loss of the lamina dura of the teeth
- Bone cysts and "brown tumours" (cysts with bleeding) in the long bones
- Progressive bone loss with osteoporosis and pathologic fractures
- Osteosclerosis (very rare)

Occasionally, patients with pHPT develop muscle weakness, fatigue, listlessness, duodenal ulcer, pancreatitis, psychiatric disorders, arthritis,

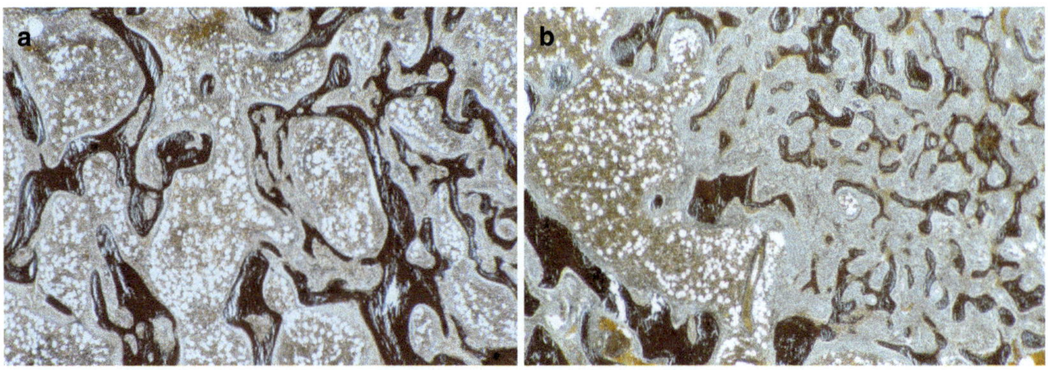

Fig. 60.1 (**a**) Bone biopsy of a patient with pHPT: dissecting osteoclasia with paratrabecular fibrosis. Gomori staining. (**b**) Small area of haematopoietic marrow (*left*) with focus of woven bone in network of fibrous connective tissue. Gomori staining

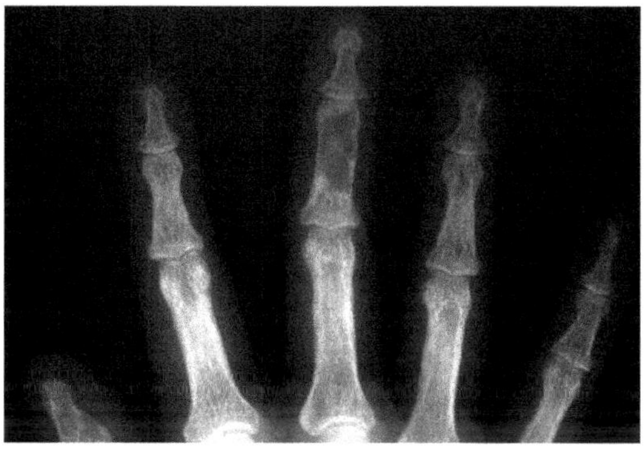

Fig. 60.2 Radiologic features of hyperparathyroid bone disease. Note the marked subperiosteal bone resorption involving the phalanges, as well as the cortical porosity

insulin-resistant diabetes mellitus and cardiovascular problems.

Twenty percent of the patients, particularly those with kidney stones and with asymptomatic hypercalcaemia, had no morphological abnormalities in the bone biopsy and histomorphometric values were within normal limits.

Our observational study in the 1970s showed that patients with pHPT and vitamin D deficiency more commonly have bone abnormalities with massive osteitis fibrosa, while patients with pHPT and normal vitamin D levels especially mobilise calcium from the gastrointestinal tract, show only minimal bone changes but mainly develop kidney stones and nephrocalcinosis (Table 60.1).

60.5 Bone Biopsy

Increased bone turnover is the most consistent feature found in iliac crest biopsies, and there is a lack of balance between formation and resorption. There is paratrabecular fibrosis in the affected areas extending inwards into the marrow spaces. Osteoclastic resorption usually outpaces osteoblastic bone production so that the trabeculae become excavated with cystic formations and

Table 60.1 Clinical and histologic data in patients with pHPT disease: bone versus stone disease

Variant of pHPT	Stone disease	Bone disease
Number of patients	43	36
Trabecular bone (vol%)	26	21
Osteoid (vol%)	2	11
Fibrosis (vol%)	0	31
Haematopoiesis (vol%)	45	21
Osteoclasts (number/mm^2)	1	11
Osteoblasts (number/mm^2)	3	19
Age of patients (years, median)	44	55
Size of adenoma(s) (mm^2)	90	143
Renal calculi	+++	0
Osteolysis (X-ray)	0	+++
Serum ALP, increased	normal	+++
Vitamin D deficiency	0	+++

wide osteoid seams. The cortical bone is likewise affected. There are areas of haemorrhage with haemosiderin-laden macrophages, also called *brown tumours* (Fig. 60.3a, b). Some degree of HPT may also contribute to osteoporotic features.

Calcification of the vessel walls also occur.

Histologic features of the bone in pHPT:

- Increased bone turnover
- Excavating and dissecting osteoclastosis in the cortex and in the trabeculae (Fig. 60.4)
- Surface erosion cavities with broad osteoid seams
- Numerous osteoclasts, most morphologically normal
- Irregular cement lines, but no mosaic pattern
- Para- and intertrabecular fibrosis, which may replace the bone marrow
- Replacement of trabecular network by connective tissue
- Aggregates of haemosiderin-laden macrophages

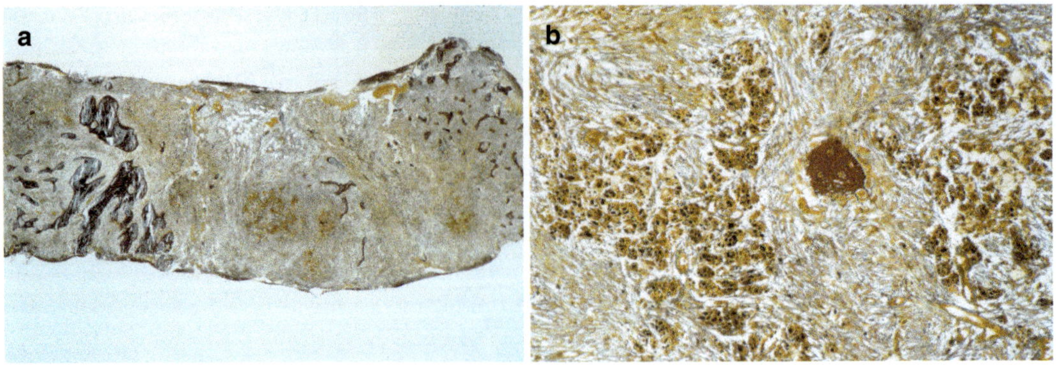

Fig. 60.3 (**a**) "Brown tumour" of pHPT bone disease with osteolytic destruction of trabecular bone. Gomori staining. (**b**) At higher magnification, residual fragments of the bone undergoing remodelling, surrounded by aggregates of haemosiderin-containing cells. Gomori staining

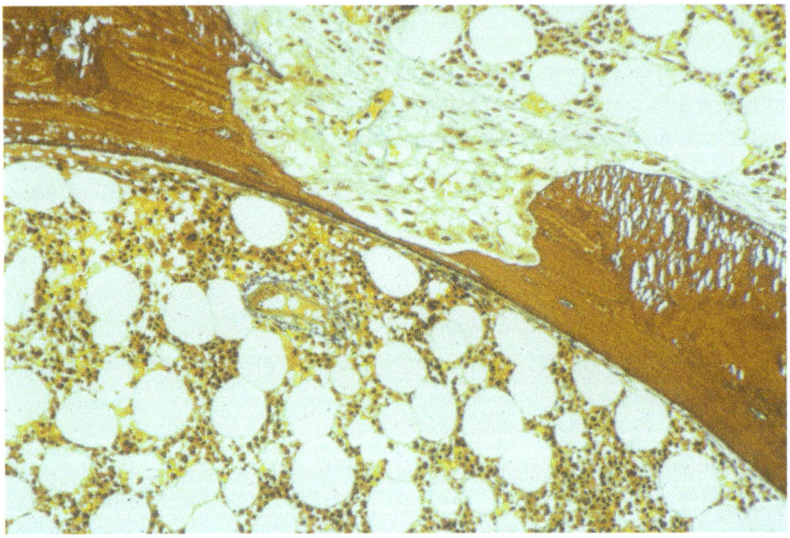

Fig. 60.4 Transsecting osteoclasia of a trabecula in a patient with HPT. Gomori staining

60.6 Therapy

About half the patients with the diagnosis of pHPT are asymptomatic, and the first decision is whether any treatment is necessary. Many patients will remain asymptomatic for many years. A *conservative therapy* is worthy of consideration in the following situations:

- Asymptomatic patients >50 years and calcium <3.0 mmol/l
- Patients with poor general condition
- Patients who refuse an intervention

The administration of modern intravenous BP such as ibandronate and zoledronate has proved to be very effective in patients with hypercalcaemia. The interval between the infusions depends on the extent and response of hypercalcaemia.

Ibandronate	6 mg every 3–6 months as an infusion
Zoledronate	5 mg every 3–6 months as an infusion

These infusions lower the increased calcium levels effectively and stop bone loss. In addition, daily 1000–2000 IE of vitamin D_3 are useful, especially in patients with vitamin D deficiency. Patients with pHPT have a high consumption of vitamin D and therefore often have early vitamin D deficiency. Active forms of vitamin D inhibit PTH secretion and reduce the growth of the involved parathyroid gland(s). Recent studies have shown that vitamin D administration in patients with pHPT does not worsen hypercalcaemia, but rather lowers the increased PTH values and bone remodelling. A systematic control of calcium, vitamin D and PTH is necessary to determine the need for further bisphosphonate infusions and vitamin D administration.

Nowadays, an asymptomatic pHPT must not necessarily be treated surgically, but can easily be well controlled with intravenous bisphosphonates and vitamin D.

The treatment of choice for symptomatic pHPT is *surgical* removal of the parathyroid adenoma or partial resection of diffuse hyperplasia (removing three or four parathyroid glands and autografting part of the tissue in the forearm). Operative and postoperative complications are less frequent when parathyroidectomy is performed by an experienced surgeon.

Guidelines for parathyroid surgery in asymptomatic pHPT (2002 NIH consensus conference), asymptomatic pHPT with one of the following criteria:

- Serum calcium >1.0 mg/dl above the upper limit
- 24 h urine calcium excretion >400 mg
- Reduction of creatinine clearance by ≥30 %
- DXA bone density T-score of <–2.5 at any site
- Age <50 years

Postoperatively, with successful surgery there is a sudden drop of the serum calcium value, which returns to normal within a few days. In case of osteitis fibrosa cystica, there is a massive influx of calcium into the damaged and undermineralised bone (*hungry bones syndrome*). Additional doses of vitamin D and calcium are therefore necessary for an effective and rapid mineralisation.

61 The Patient with "Dense Bones"

In the majority of cases, artefacts, calcifications of the damaged ligamentous apparatus or degenerative changes (spondylophytes) are causes of increased bone density values of the vertebral body in the DXA measurement. In these cases, comparison with the measurements of the hip or with an X-ray of the lumbar spine quickly brings clarification. When artefacts, calcifications, degenerative reactions and especially a measurement error are excluded, further clinical, radiological, laboratory and biopsy investigations of the diagnosis "increased bone density" are required. These may be generalised, multifocal or local, they can be painful or accidentally discovered, they can be congenital or acquired, and they may have completely different causes: inflammatory, toxic, medical, neoplastic or metabolic. Bones with increased bone density do not correlate with higher strength, and there is even an increase in fracture risk due to loss of elasticity and abnormal bone modelling. Caused by irritation of endosteal and periosteal afferent nerve fibres, there may be a dull bone pain.

For the diagnostic report, some *nomenclatural definitions* are useful and necessary:

- *Osteosclerosis* is an increase of the cancellous bone at the expense of the medullary cavity without simultaneous thickening or deformity of the bone shape so that it should better be described as a "spongiosclerosis". There is either a decreased bone loss or an increased bone formation, which in both cases result in a positive bone balance and an increase in cancellous bone mass. Developmental abnormalities or deformities of the skeleton are not present. In the case of lead poisoning, a high bone density is only simulated in the X-ray image.
- *Hyperostosis* describes a widening of the compacta with or without deformation of the bone shape. In the subtype of *endostosis*, bone tissue is formed inside the bone at the endosteal surface. There are small islands of sclerotic bone, either solitary or multiple in the vicinity of joints, known as *osteopoikilosis. Periostosis* arises from the periosteal bone surface, which lead to an outward thickening of the compacta. Reactive periostoses include the periostitis ossificans of inflammatory or traumatic origin and periosteal thickening in response to subperiosteal haemorrhage. Onion-shaped periosteal bone areas found in Ewing sarcoma are a sign of slow tumour growth. Hyperostoses are also found in inherited osteopathies, while haematological, neoplastic or metabolic osteopathies usually show osteosclerosis with replacement of the bone marrow.

With radiologic proof of osteosclerotic or hyperostotic changes, the following questions must to be answered by *differential diagnosis*:

- Does the increased bone density affect the entire skeleton as in osteopetrosis, or is it present in only one or a few bones as in melorheostosis?

R. Bartl, C. Bartl, *Bone Disorders*, DOI 10.1007/978-3-319-29182-6_61

- Is the increased bone density homogeneous and uniform as in osteopetrosis, or is it patchy and random as in osteoblastic metastasis?
- Are compacta and spongiosa equally affected as in renal osteodystrophy, or is there a mainly diaphyseal thickening of the cortex as in Morbus Camurati-Engelmann?
- Are there changes and deformations of the bone shape as in Paget's disease of bone, or are there local bone expansions as in certain bone tumours?
- Is the bone contour faded as in fluorosis or smooth and sharp as in osteomyelosclerosis?

Pronounced osteosclerosis with marked increased density of spongy bone can be found especially in haematopoietic (myelofibrosis), metabolic (hyperparathyroidism) and toxic (fluorosis, bisphosphonate overdose) diseases (Table 61.1). A major reason for this topographic preference of cancellous bone is the much higher rate of bone remodelling of cancellous bone in contrast to the cortical bone with a low bone turnover. In many cases of osteosclerosis diagnosed by DXA measurement or by X-ray, no cause can be evaluated (Fig. 61.1). Systematic osteological and haematological check-ups are useful in these cases.

> Measurement errors, artefacts or degenerative changes must first of all be excluded when increased bone density is measured by DXA. Even intensive diagnostic investigations may not detect the cause of osteosclerosis in all cases, so check-ups including bone biopsies are recommended in these cases (Fig. 61.2).

Table 61.1 Main causes of osteosclerosis

Congenital
Osteopetroses
Carbonic anhydrase II deficiency
Pycnodysostosis
Progressive diaphyseal dysplasia
Hyperphosphatasia
Pycnodysostosis[a]
Melorheostosis[a]
Chemical poisoning
Fluorosis
Hypervitaminosis D and A
Heavy metal poisoning
Bisphosphonate intoxication
Endocrine disorders
Primary HPT
Secondary HPT
Acromegaly
Hypothyroidism
Healing osteomalacia
Sarcoidosis
Inflammatory disorders
Sclerosing myelitis[a]
Sarcoidosis[a]
Radiation[a]
Osteomyelitis[a]
Hepatitis C
Haematopoietic disorders
Sickle cell disease
Osteomyelosclerosis
Malignant lymphomas[a]
Multiple myeloma (sclerotic variant)[a]
Systemic mastocytosis[a]
Osteoblastic metastases
Prostate carcinoma[a]
Breast cancer[a]
Paget's disease[a]

[a]May occur as widespread or as patchy osteosclerotic lesions

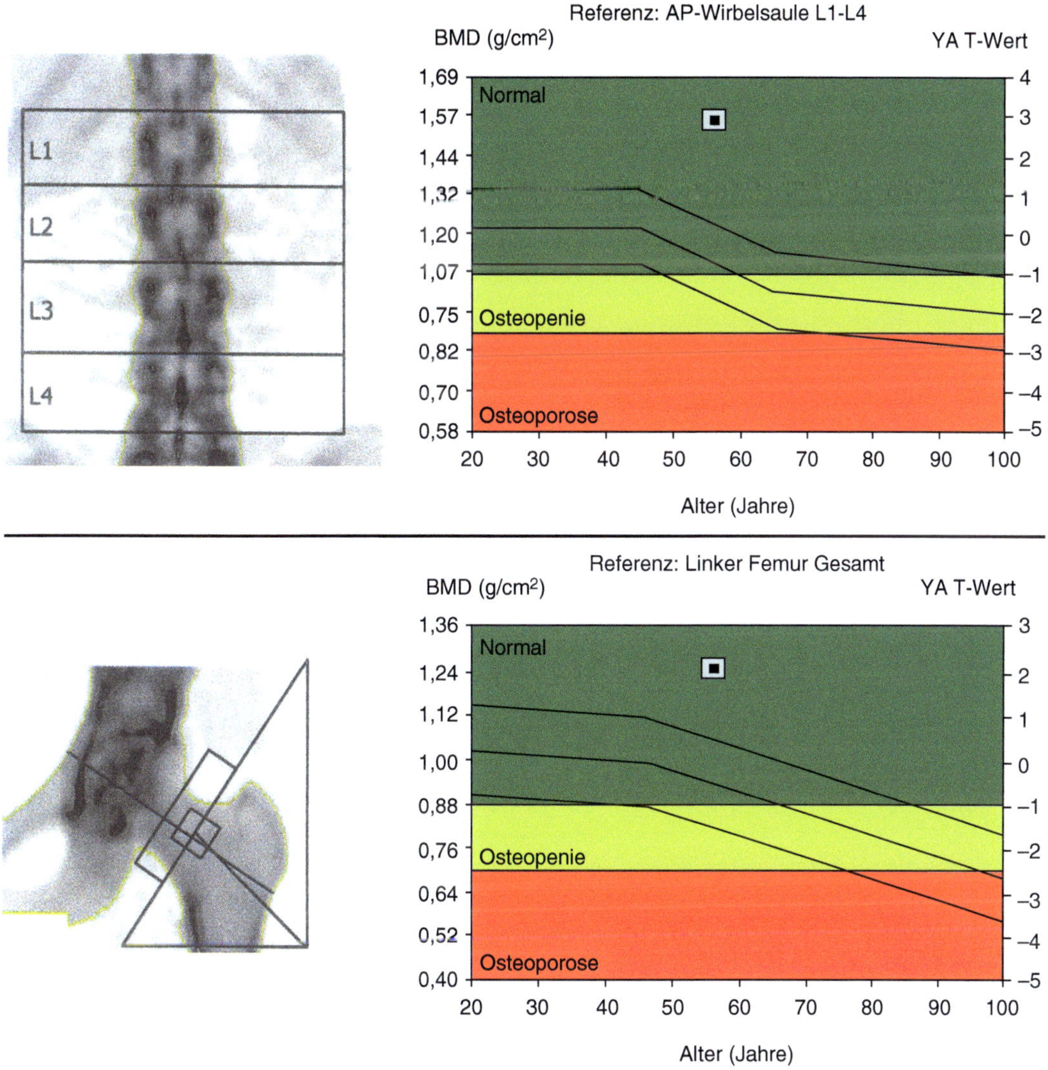

Fig. 61.1 Measurement of bone density of the lumbar spine and hip using the DXA method: marked osteosclerosis of the whole skeleton but of unclear aetiology

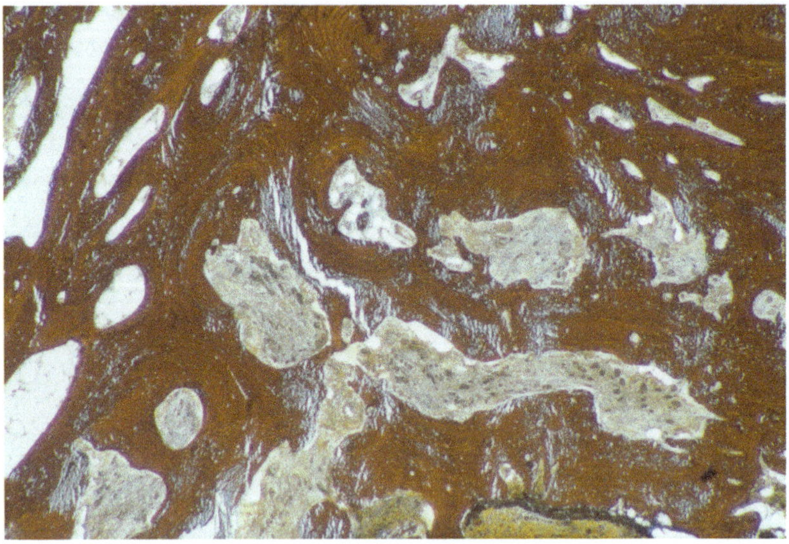

Fig. 61.2 Patient with bone pain and massive osteosclerosis of unknown significance. Iliac crest biopsy revealed metastases of a prostatic carcinoma dispersed in small marrow cavities. Gomori staining

62 Osteosclerosis and Hyperostosis

62.1 Osteopetrosis (Marble Bone Disease)

Osteopetrosis, also known as marble bone disease or *Albers-Schönberg disease*, is a rare osteopathy with high bone density. The incidence of severe osteopetrosis ranges from 1 in 200,000 to 500,000 live births. The cause is a congenital dysfunction of osteoclasts, which leads to a defective formation of bone marrow spaces and to an insufficient modelling of the structure of cancellous bone (Fig. 62.1). Osteoclast differentiation and activation are very complex and multifactorial and depend on haematopoietic cells' competence as well as signals from osteoblasts and stromal microenvironment. In some forms of osteopetrosis, osteoclasts are present, but cannot resorb bone and in other forms osteoclasts are totally absent. Consequences of defective osteoclastic modelling are a high risk of fractures as well as bone marrow failure (infections, anaemia, bleeding). Three types can be differentiated:

- *Benign type* (late onset, "Albers-Schönberg syndrome"): This form is autosomal dominant and refers to the milder, adult form of osteopetrosis. The patients are asymptomatic for a long period, but cranial nerve palsies, deafness (sclerosis at the base of the skull) and mild anaemia may occur. This type of mild osteosclerosis is often coincidentally detected by DXA measurement (Fig. 62.2a, b) or X-ray (Fig. 62.3). The long bones show diffuse symmetric sclerosis and transverse metaphyseal sclerotic bands. The vertebrae frequently have a "rugger jersey" appearance due to osteosclerosis beneath the endplates. Some patients with increasing bone marrow insufficiency later develop anaemia and bone marrow insufficiency and need transfusions or a splenectomy.
- *Malignant type* (early onset): This aggressive form is an autosomal recessive form. Patients present in infancy and usually die before age ten. Abnormal or absent osteoclasts correlate with an insufficient or absent modelling of bone marrow spaces and increased bone density ("osteosclerosis"). The progression of the disease leads to modelling deformities of long bones ("Erlenmeyer flasks") and diffuse symmetric sclerosis. Bone marrow insufficiency caused by absent medullary cavities proceeds and leads to death in the first year of life. Allogenic HLA-identical bone marrow transplantation has been successful in some children. After transplantation, the marrow contains preosteoclasts and normally functioning osteoclasts. A cure is most likely when patients are transplanted before age 54. Prednisone, calcitriol and interferon-γ are effective in only a few cases, but may stop the progressive course.
- *Renal of tubular acidosis type (RTA)*: This form is autosomal recessive and also causes osteosclerosis. In addition, a renal tubular acidosis develops, which persists even after successful bone grafting. A long-term treatment with bicarbonate and electrolytes can

R. Bartl, C. Bartl, *Bone Disorders*, DOI 10.1007/978-3-319-29182-6_62

correct the renal losses. In addition to sclerotic bones, patients with *carbonic anhydrase II deficiency* show dense cerebral calcifications, a complication that causes mental retardation.

The primary defect of osteopetrosis is deficient or absent osteoclastic bone resorption but normal osteoblastic bone formation. The reasons are different genetic defects, e.g. overexpression of OPG with blocking of RANKL or blocking of the proton pump in the osteoclasts with reduced production of acid. HLA-identical allogenic bone marrow transplantation has proved to be successful. A cure is achieved, above all, in children under 4 years of age. An improvement of the complications is reported under interferon-γ-1β, 1,25 $(OH)_2D$, methylprednisolone and calcium-/phosphate-rich diet.

62.2 Pyknodysostosis

The French impressionist painter Henri de Toulouse-Lautrec probably suffered from this autosomal recessive form of osteosclerosis. It is a congenital *defect of cathepsin K*, a lysosomal metalloproteinase in the osteoclasts, which is responsible for the resorption of the bone matrix. Osteoclasts are present, but defective. Pyknodysostosis is a form of dwarfism with short limbs and high fracture rate, but with a normal life span. Clinically it is characterised by growth retardation, a typical skull shape with a prominent forehead and occiput, small hands and hypoplastic finger nails. Radiologically, a generalised high bone density is characteristic. A normal cortical structure with reduced bone remodelling is found histologically. In contrast to osteopetrosis, medullary cavities with haematopoiesis are present. Serum chemistries are normal, and unlike osteopetrosis, there is no bone marrow failure. Fractures of long bone are typical, sometimes with delayed union and massive callus formation. Jaw fractures with osteomyelitis of the mandible may require antibiotics and surgery. There is no known effective treatment for this bone disease.

62.3 Hepatitis C-Associated Osteosclerosis (HCAO)

This complication is a rare diffuse osteosclerosis acquired in adults after hepatitis C infection. After a latent period of some years, the patients

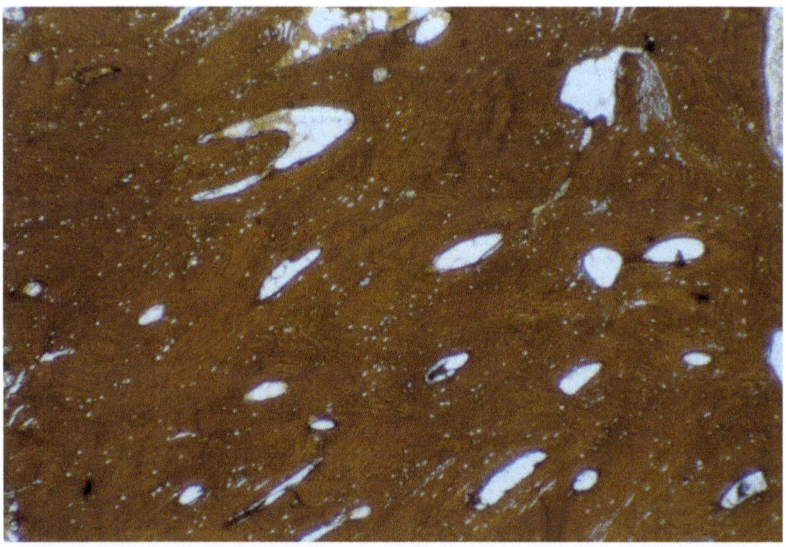

Fig. 62.1 Iliac crest biopsy of a young patient with osteopetrosis, malignant type. Note almost complete obliteration of the marrow cavities and absence of osteoclasts. Gomori staining

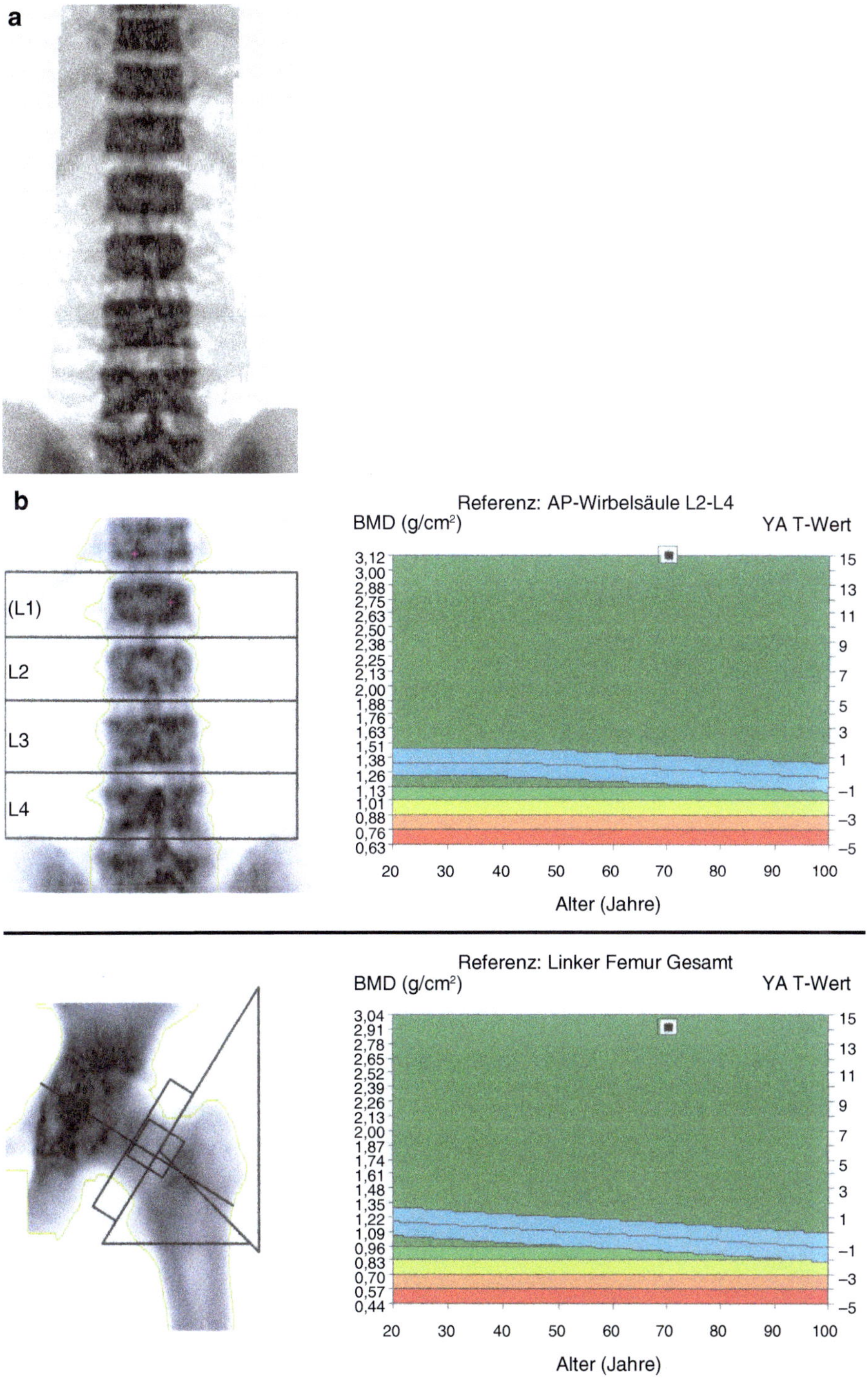

Fig. 62.2 (**a**, **b**) DXA measurement of the spine of a patient with osteopetrosis, benign type, (**a**) measurement of the whole spine using a modern DXA machine, in order to demonstrate massive homogeneous osteosclerosis of the whole spine, (**b**) massive increase of bone density of the lumbar spine and hip

develop bone pain, a generalised increase in bone density and increased serum levels of ALP. Bone biopsy shows a decrease of osteoclasts with reduced bone loss and dense lamellar bone.

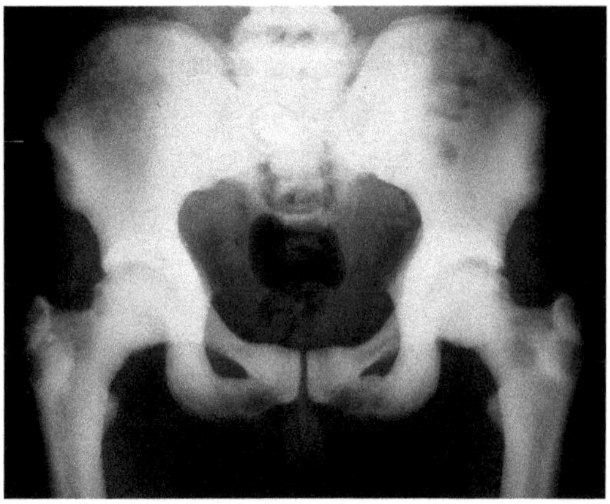

Fig. 62.3 Osteopetrosis with overall increase in bone density in the ilium and femur

62.4 Progressive Diaphyseal Dysplasia (Camurati-Engelmann)

With a frequency of one occurrence in one million births, it is a very rare autosomal dominant inherited hyperostosis. The dense bones are the result of excessive periosteal osteoblastic activity in the diaphysis (Fig. 62.4a, b). The cortical thickening of long bones, caused by both periosteal and endosteal bone deposition, narrows but does not obliterate marrow cavities. In addition, the skull is often hyperostotic. Only severe cases later also develop osteosclerosis in the axial skeleton. Gait abnormalities, muscle hypoplasia and bone pain are clinically present. Cortical thickenings of the diaphysis are shown on X-ray. A sclerosis of the skull (Fig. 62.5) and the spine is also observed in pronounced cases. The course of this condition is highly variable.

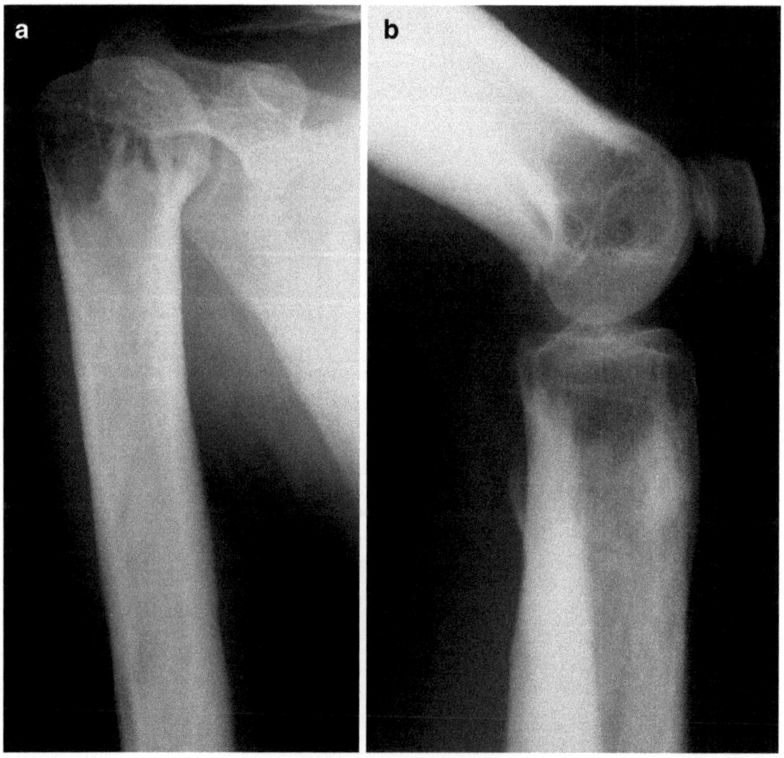

Fig. 62.4 (**a**, **b**) Camurati-Engelmann disease: Excessive osteoblastic activity and hyperostosis in the diaphysis of the humerus (**a**) and the femur/tibia (**b**). The metaphyses and epiphyses are spared

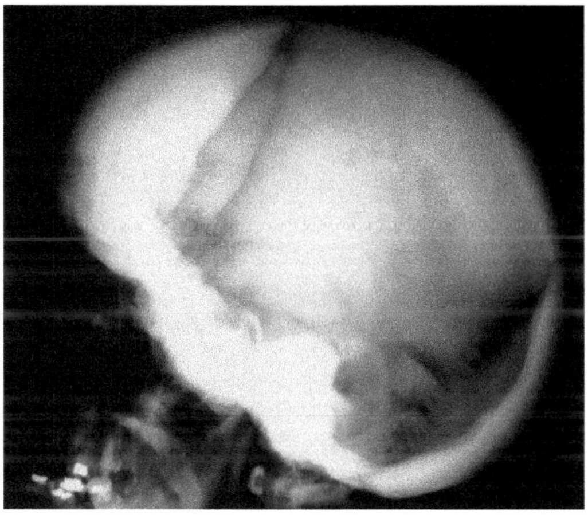

Fig. 62.5 Massive sclerosis of the skull in a patient with Camurati-Engelmann disease

Other congenital hyperostoses are the endosteal hyperostosis-type van Buchem and type Worth and *pachydermoperiostitis* with typical periosteal new bone formation and skin thickening. Descriptions of further extremely rare congenital hyperostoses can be found in the appropriate textbooks.

The genetic defect of Camurati-Engelmann disease has been localised on chromosome 19. The mutation causes a stimulation of TGF-β1 resulting in an exclusive thickening of the endosteal and periosteal surfaces of the diaphysis of long bones.

62.5 Diffuse Idiopathic Skeletal Hyperostosis (DISH)

This is not an uncommon illness; it is also referred to as "disseminated skeletal hyperostosis" and goes hand in hand with excessive ankylosing ossifications of the ligaments of at least four vertebrae. The consequences are spondylophytes with partially full bony bridging of the segments. Also in other regions of the skeleton, ossification of ligaments is found.

The cause of the formation of spondylophytes is unclear; the patients are typically HLA-B27 negative. Patients with DISH have a higher BMI, elevated uric acid values and a high risk of diabetes mellitus.

In patients with calcifications of ligaments, ankylosing spondylitis (Morbus Bechterew), spondylosis, fluorosis and acromegaly must be excluded.

63 The Patient with "Changes in the Shape of Bones"

In some local and generalised bone disorders, *changes in the shape of bones* may also occur as a result of atypical remodelling and growth (Fig. 63.1). Paralysis in childhood may also lead to deformities of the skeleton, which are often similar to those in congenital bone disorders. Four types of malformation can be distinguished:

- *Changes in the shape of the skeleton resulting from congenital disorders:* Gigantism and dwarfism (Marfan syndrome, acromegaly), chondrodystrophia foetalis (Turner syndrome), osteochondrodysplasias, dysostosis multiplex (Morbus Hurler, Morquio, Hunter, Sanfilippo), neurofibromatosis Recklinghausen and osteogenesis imperfecta (deformation of long bones).
- *Changes in the shape of the skeleton resulting from acquired disorders:* Bone tumours and tumour-like conditions, bone metastases, inflammatory processes and osteomyelitis, Paget's disease, fibrous dysplasia, Gorham disease and osteomalacia ("rachitic catback", "rachitic rosary" and "Harrison grooves").
- *Changes in the shape of the skeleton resulting from traumatic influences*: Fractures lead to axial and rotation deformations.
- *Changes in the shape of the skeleton resulting from toxic (drug) influences:* The classic example is thalidomide embryopathy occurring in the 42nd–48th days of pregnancy.

Congenital and acquired deformities of the skeleton are an important symptom of orthopaedic disorders and are associated with massive constraints of mobility and capability. Acquired deformities are due to degenerative, toxic, inflammatory and tumorous changes and especially trauma (fractures).

R. Bartl, C. Bartl, *Bone Disorders*, DOI 10.1007/978-3-319-29182-6_63

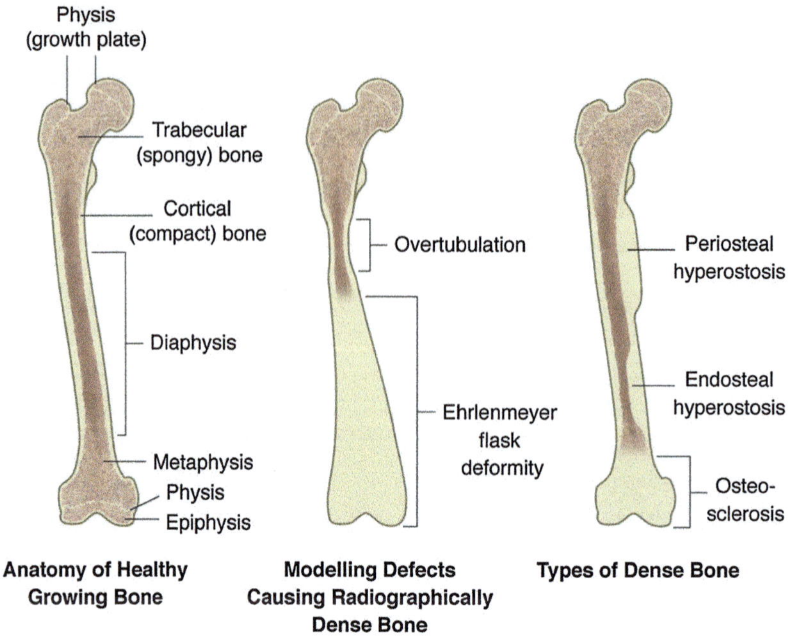

Fig. 63.1 Variants of hyperostosis and alterations in the shape of bones (Modified from M. Whyte in "*The Bone and Mineral Manual*", edited by Kleerekoper, Siris and McClung (Elsevier, 2005))

64 Genetic Disorders of Bone and Connective Tissue (Skeletal Dysplasias)

Even single gene mutations may manifest as generalised or local disorders of the skeleton known as *skeletal dysplasias* or constitutional bone disorders. Patients with these disorders usually have short stature, abnormally shaped bones and often with pathologic fracture. There exist more than 170 variants of skeletal dysplasias, and the most frequent are osteogenesis imperfecta, osteopetrosis, osteopoikilosis and achondroplasia. Recent progress has led to the identification of many gene mutations that cause skeletal dysplasia, for example, osteogenesis imperfecta, an autosomal dominant condition caused by defects in type I collagen. Subsequent biochemical and molecular studies revealed both quantitative and structural defects in either of the two chains that form the type I collagen heterotrimer. Many dysplasias once thought to be different disorders are now known to be variants of a different expression of the same gene defect. New genetic, biochemical and molecular informations will be the basis of a future classification system of constitutional skeletal dysplasias.

64.1 Mucopolysaccharidosis

Proteoglycans are ubiquitous components of the extracellular matrix and the cell surface and are among the largest and most complex molecules of the body. They consist of a protein core and various glycosaminoglycans. Genetic defects of the degrading enzymes in the lysosomes lead to storage of metabolites in cells causing various deformities and organ complications. They are summarised as mucopolysaccharides (MPSs) and mucolipidoses (MLs). The MPSs are rare, with an incidence of 1 in 100,000 births. Morbus Hurler, Morbus Sanfilippo and Morbus Morquio diseases are known. Short stature, mental retardation, corneal clouding and deafness are clinically prominent. Life expectancy is usually reduced due to damage of internal organs.

64.2 Marfan Syndrome

This syndrome belongs to diseases of the collagen metabolism. It is autosomal dominant and is based on defects of the extracellular microfibril, the large glycoprotein *fibrillin-1*. The disorder affects all connective tissue organs, in particular the eyes ("lens tremble"), skeleton (arachnodactyly, scoliosis, tall stature), heart (mitral valve prolapse), aorta (aortic dilatation), lungs (spontaneous pneumothorax) and skin (striae). Scoliosis has, above all, a rapid progression and needs an early operative stabilisation.

64.3 Ehlers-Danlos Syndrome

It is clinically variable and genetically heterogeneous. Defects of *collagen and other proteins* of the extracellular space cause structural changes of collagen with hyperelasticity and vulnerability

R. Bartl, C. Bartl, *Bone Disorders*, DOI 10.1007/978-3-319-29182-6_64

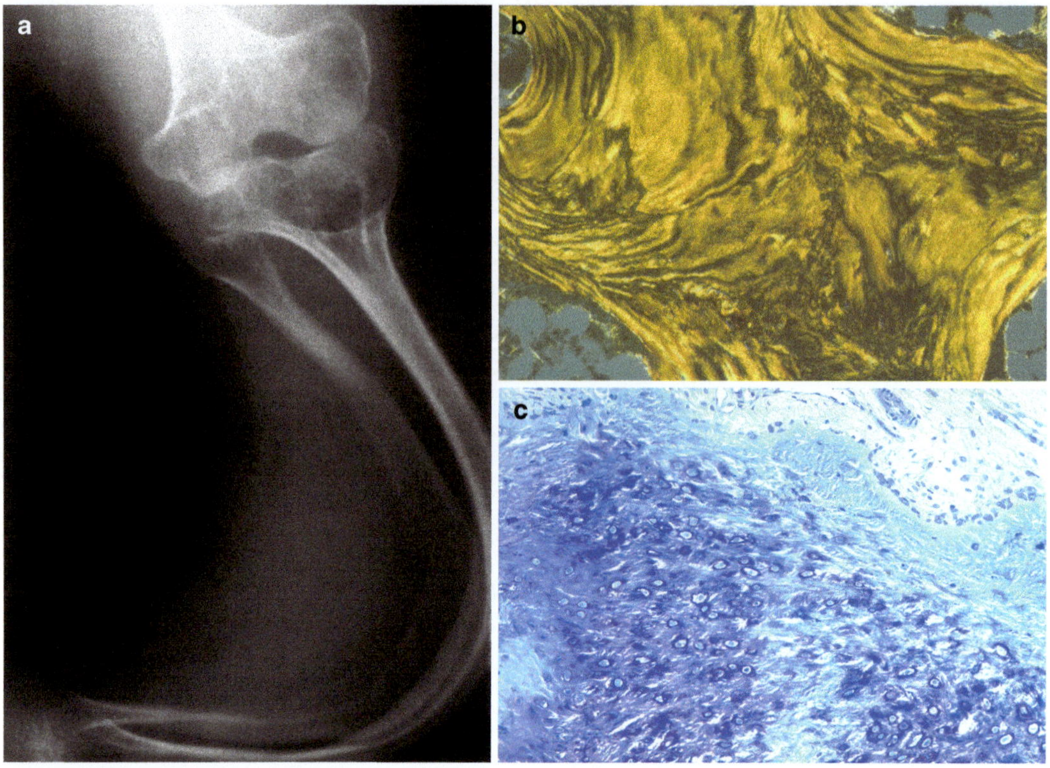

Fig. 64.1 (**a**) Osteogenesis imperfecta (OI): (**a**) Massive bowing of the right lower leg in a patient with OI, (**b**) part of cortical bone with altered lamellar structure but without woven bone pattern. Gomori, polarisation. (**c**) Overview of growth plate of young patient with OI illustrating disorganisation and irregularity of the different zones of cartilage. Thin cortex covered by a rim of osteoblasts upper right. Giemsa staining

of the skin, hypermobile joints, calcifications of soft tissues and osteoporosis. Internal, cardiac and vascular complications such as valve damage and vascular dilation are characteristic.

64.4 Osteogenesis Imperfecta (OI)

The congenital disorder type I comprises defects of both *chains α1 and α2 of the procollagen type 1* and is discussed more precisely in Chap. 40. Figure 64.1a–c shows a massive deformation of the lower leg in a patient with OI as well as some characteristic alterations of bone and cartilage.

64.5 Chondrodysplasias

While osteogenesis imperfecta and osteopetrosis are disorders of bone formation, chondrodysplasias, the largest group of skeletal dysplasias, are disorders of cartilage structure and growth. *Achondroplasia* is one of the most common chondrodysplasias and is characterised by a retarded cartilage growth, a problem most manifested at the growth plate. As a result, the long bones, the spine and the base of the skull are abnormally shaped or short: patients have a markedly short stature, also called "little people" or "dwarfs". The articular cartilage and membranous bone formation are normal, so bones have a normal width. Other syndromes of achondroplasia are *hypochondroplasia* and, at the severe end of the spectrum, *thanatophoric dysplasia*, which is incompatible with life.

64.6 Homocystinurias

These disorders are caused by an autosomal recessive inherited deficiency of *cystathionine-β-synthase*, which catalyses cystathionine formation

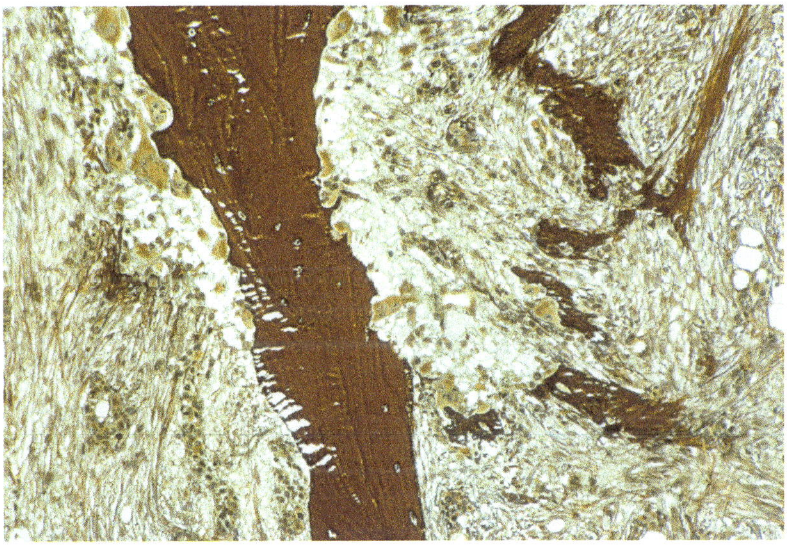

Fig. 64.2 Iliac crest biopsy of a patient with Morbus Fabry: Complete replacement of the bone marrow by storage cells and fibrosis. Note marked osseous remodelling, osteoclastic bone resorption with Howship lacunae (*centre*) and multiple foci of newly formed woven bone (*right*). Gomori staining

by homocysteine and serine. As a result, homocysteine accumulates and dimerises to homocysteine, which is excreted in the urine. The excess homocysteine has adverse side effects on connective tissue and in particular in the vessels, eyes, nervous system and skeleton. Most patients present with dislocated optic lenses and mental retardation. Some patients develop a Marfanoid habitus and radiologic evidence of osteoporosis. Life-threatening vascular complications (coronary, renal and cerebral arteries) are the major cause of morbidity and mortality.

64.7 Fabry's Disease

This is also called *angiokeratoma corporis diffusum* and is inherited in an X-linked recessive way. The clinical manifestations are mainly due to intralysosomal deposits of trihexoside in cells of the RES, in endothelial cells of vessels and in the glomeruli of the kidney. The storage cells have a foamy appearance, and in the bone marrow, they may induce a marked perivascular and paratrabecular fibrosis with osteoclastic bone resorption (Fig. 64.2).

Part XII

Local Bone Disorders

A local bone lesion can pertain to one (monostotic), several (oligoostotic) or multiple (polyostotic) sites of the skeleton. These forms of local osteopathies must be distinguished from systemic, metabolic forms and require an individual approach to diagnostic and therapeutic strategy. Various causes and mechanisms can underlie a local osteopathy:

- Dysplastic
- Circulatory
- Neural
- Immobilisation
- Traumatic
- Infectious
- Inflammatory
- Metabolic
- Haematopoietic
- Endocrinologic
- Cellular defects
- Neoplastic

Clinical evaluation of a bone lesion is always a diagnostic challenge. A quick clarification is necessary to exclude or to detect and treat a malignant process at an early stage!

65 Paget's Disease of the Bone

65.1 Definition and Pathogenesis

Paget's disease, or Morbus Paget (named after Sir James Paget who first accurately described the disease in 1877), is also called *osteodystrophia deformans* or *osteitis deformans*. It is a localised non-inflammatory disease of bone caused by uncontrolled, increased bone resorption, by pathological large multinucleated osteoclasts (Fig. 65.1), which in turn induces disorganised bone formation. This disease illustrates graphically what happens when there is complete local deregulation of osteoclasts together with partial abrogation of "coupling" in the osteological meaning of the term. Osteoblasts are stimulated to replace the resorbed bone, but the osteoid is randomly produced and not laid down as lamellae, so that the resulting bone is dense but mechanically inadequate. The focally greatly increased bone turnover is accompanied by hypervascularisation and increased blood flow. Deformities of the effected bones are the rule. Mono- and polyostotic forms of Paget's disease are recognised.

About 1–3 % of people over 40 years of age have Paget's disease of bone (more men than women 3:2), but initially only 5 % are symptomatic or require therapy. More recent estimates put the number of affected people (55 years or older) at 2–7 % in the USA and Western Europe. The cause of Paget's disease is presumed to be a viral infection of osteoclasts and/or an abnormality on chromosome 18, resulting in multinucleated, hyperactive and unregulated giant osteoclasts. Mutations in SQSTMI have been associated in up to 40 % of familial and sporadic cases. Other genetic anomalies have been found, but the aetiology of Paget's disease has not yet been determined. Moreover, why all osteoclasts are not involved is still a complete mystery!

65.2 Symptoms

The following symptoms are indicative of Paget's disease: the variability of the symptoms that characterise Paget's disease is caused by the variability of the locations:

- Pain and warmth of the affected area (pelvis, spine, extremities, skull).
- Bone pain that is stabbing and deep and often stronger at night. Pain could also be due to compression of nerves or associated arthrosis.
- Bending and deformities of the affected bones with risk of spontaneous fractures ("saber tibia", "hat that became too small" appearance).
- When the base of the skull is involved, hearing loss and damage to the cranial nerves can occur.
- Compression fractures may result if the vertebrae are involved.
- Secondary arthrosis can occur due to incorrect weight-bearing.

R. Bartl, C. Bartl, *Bone Disorders*, DOI 10.1007/978-3-319-29182-6_65

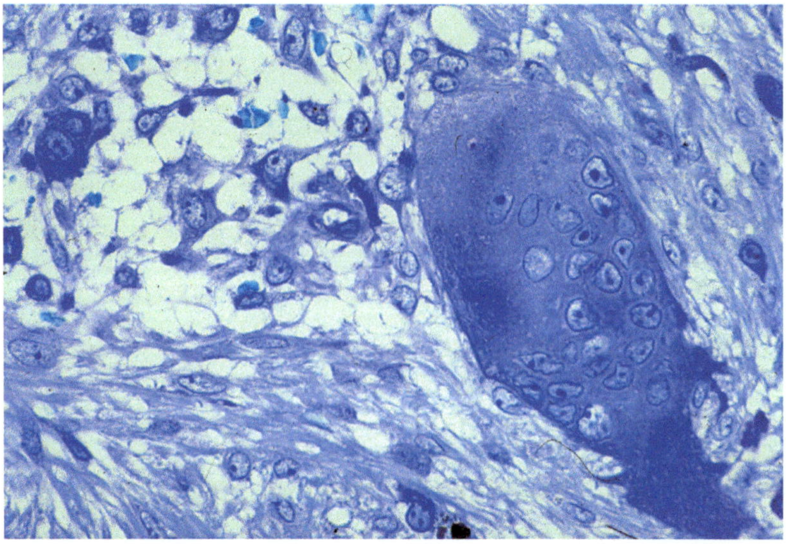

Fig. 65.1 Giant multinucleated and nucleolated osteoclast within loose connective tissue but far from any osseous surface. Note small developing osteoclast (*upper left*. Giemsa staining)

- When large areas of the skeleton are affected, the accompanying hypercirculation may cause cardiac insufficiency.
- Inner ear involvement can cause deafness. It has been assumed that Beethoven's deafness was caused by Paget's disease of bone.

65.3 Course of Disease

The course of the disease can be divided into three stages which are identified locally:

- *Lytic stage*: The osteolytic process spreads at the rate of 1 cm annually.
- *Repair stage* (also called "mixed stage"): After the period of rapid resorption, osteoblasts fill the cavities with bone, thereby producing cement lines with the mosaic patterns characteristic of Paget's disease (Fig. 65.2).
- *Sclerotic stage*: When the disease has progressed for several years, relatively large areas consist of dense bone, but this is not capable of weight-bearing or stress (Fig. 65.3).

Transition from mono- to polyostotic forms of Paget's disease must be excluded by periodic X-ray examinations and bone scans.

65.4 Diagnosis

Imaging techniques highlight a focal increase in bone remodelling and depict the extent of skeletal involvement (mono- or polyostotic) (Fig. 65.4). In addition, characteristic X-rays plus increased alkaline phosphatase levels as well as other markers of bone remodelling in the serum confirm the diagnosis. Conventional X-ray and/or CT demonstrate typical changes, and the following points are considered:

- Alterations in contours of the bone (Fig. 65.5).
- Careful evaluation is required when the vertebrae are affected.
- Thickening of the cortical bone.
- Coarsened trabecular structure with alternating lytic and sclerotic regions.
- Narrowing of the foramina of the spinal column (Fig. 65.6).
- Thickening of the skull.
- Fibrosis and hypervascularisation of the bone marrow surrounding the foci of involved bone.

Bone biopsy can be useful in the initial stages of Paget's disease for differential diagnosis and

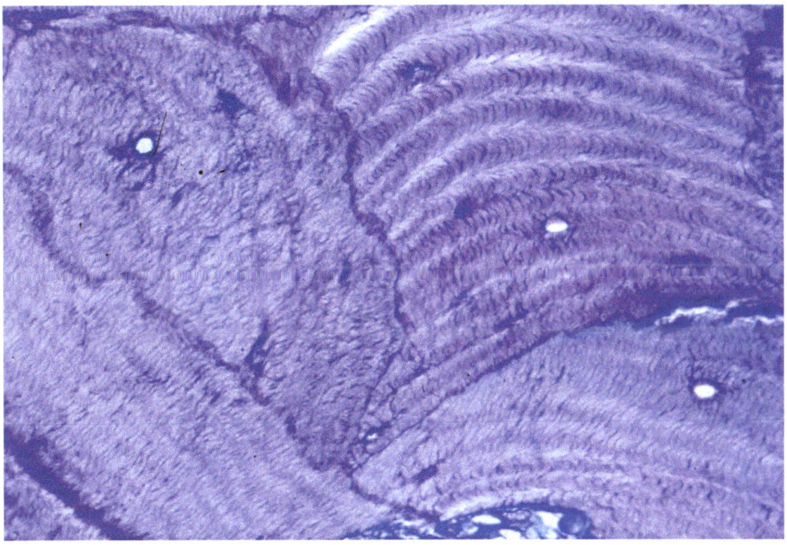

Fig. 65.2 Trabecula showing marked mosaic pattern of cement lines. Ladewig staining

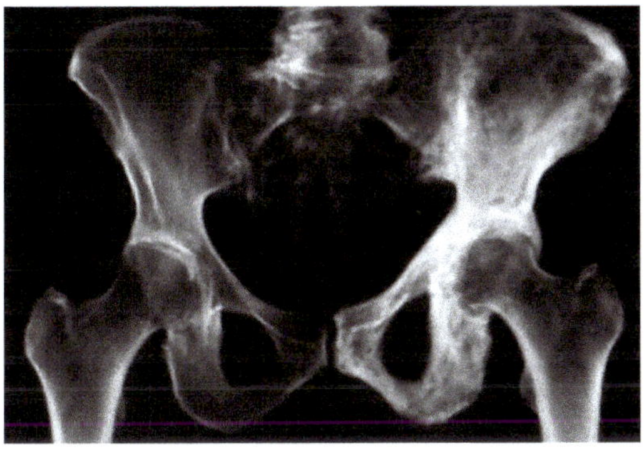

Fig. 65.3 Paget's disease of bone with widespread painful involvement of the left pelvis, sclerotic stage

for ruling out metastasis or arthrosis. The most important features (Fig. 65.7a, b) are:

- Cement lines forming mosaic structures and woven bone
- Multinucleated osteoclasts containing nucleoli and showing signs of activity: localisation in resorption bays and presence of pronounced ruffled membranes
- Striking reactive osteoblastic bone formation
- Fibrosis and hypervascularisation of the surrounding bone marrow
- Two histologically unmistakable features characterise M. Paget: the giant, multinucleated osteoclasts and the mosaic structure of the newly formed bone.

Biochemical markers of disease activity are *alkaline phosphatase* in blood and pyridinoline cross-links in urine. The level of osteocalcin in the serum is used for monitoring. Osteocalcin production by osteoblasts is dependent on vitamin K; the level reflects the degree of bone remodelling.

65.5 Differential Diagnosis

For differential diagnosis, the following must be excluded:

- Skeletal metastasis
- Primary bone tumour
- Malignant lymphoma
- Severe arthrosis
- pHPT and renal osteopathy.

The danger of later transformation to sarcoma is minimal (<1 %), particularly in the present era of bisphosphonate therapy. Tumour-associated Paget-like lesions seen on X-rays, CT or scans must be investigated by bone biopsy, but are rare.

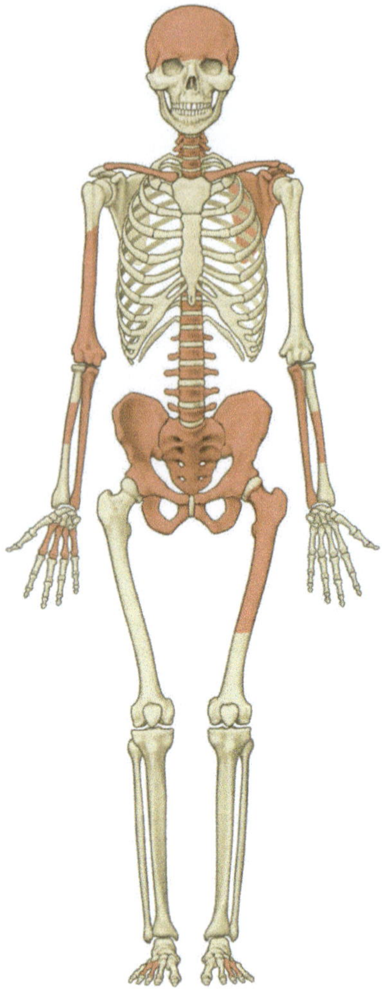

Fig. 65.4 Paget's disease locations

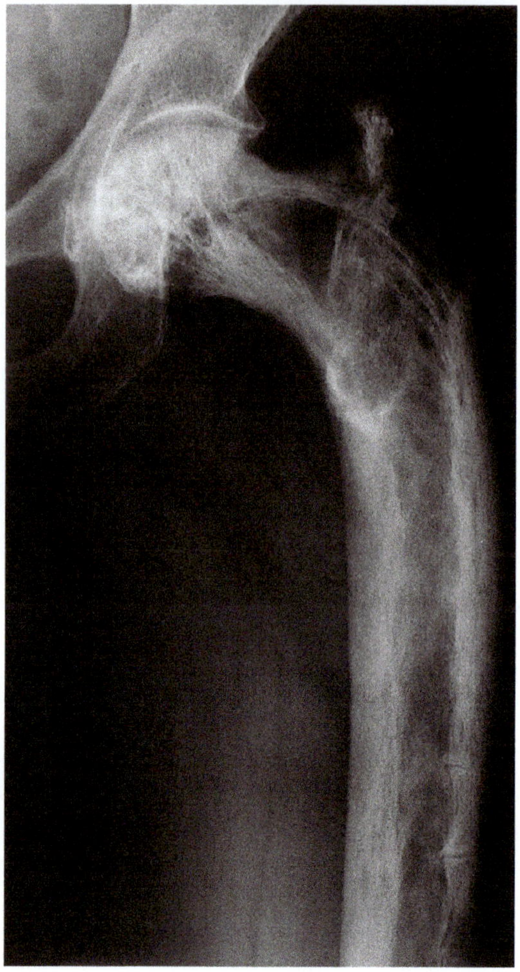

Fig. 65.5 Paget's disease of bone in the left femur. Note both deformation and thickening of the shaft, increase in width and "trabecularisation" of the compact bone and the irregular, stout cancellous bone with an especially large Ward's triangle. The trabeculae are particularly stout along lines of compression and tension. As a consequence of the completely disorganised osseous remodelling and replacement of lamellar by woven bone, numerous "fatigue fractures" have occurred. These were repaired within a year of bisphosphonate therapy. The patient became free of pain and the alkaline phosphatase in the serum returned to normal levels within 6 months

65.6 Treatment Strategies

Treatment is indicated if there are local changes, pain and risk of complications that may require neurosurgical or orthopaedic intervention and if there are high alkaline phosphatase levels (more than 5U/l). Skeletal deformities and fractures require orthopaedic interventions (Fig. 65.8). Two separate indications for therapy are derived from the clinical course of the disease:

- *Alleviation of symptoms*: severe headaches, backaches and radicular nerve pain
- *Prevention of complications:* fractures, deafness, paralyses, skeletal deformities (Fig. 65.9), and sarcomatous transformation

Bisphosphonates (BP) are the treatment of choice, and many have been authorised for use in Paget's disease of bone (see below). The latest is zoledronate, and now that this is authorised, therapy of Paget's disease is simplicity itself. For patients with extensive and/or active disease (as indicated by high levels of alkaline phosphatase in serum), intravenous administration is the

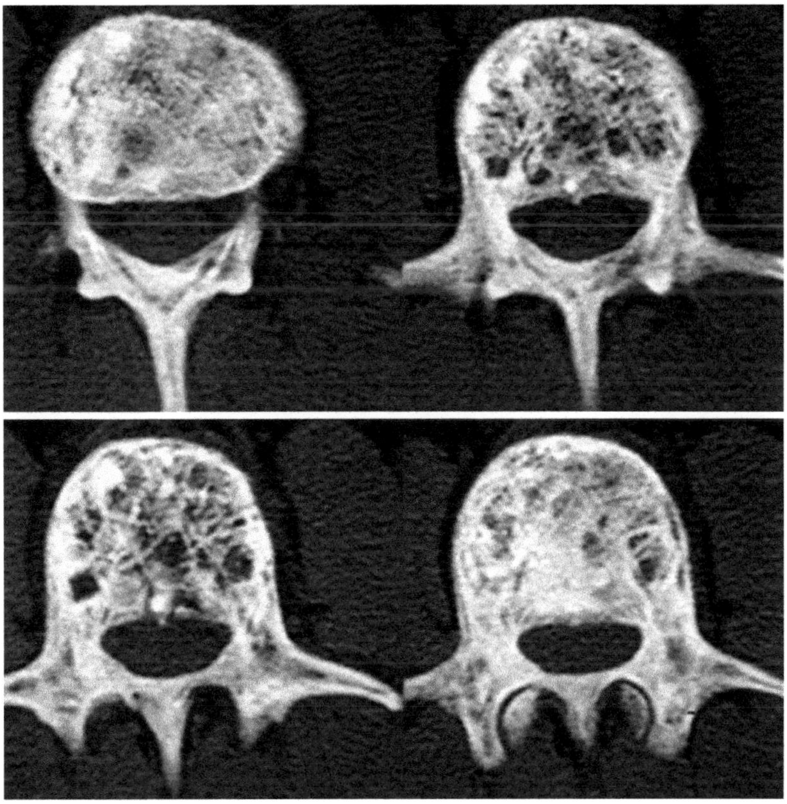

Fig. 65.6 Paget's disease of bone in area of lumbar spine (CT). Note the altered structure of the trabecular bone. Significant narrowing of the vertebral canal is evident – *lower right*

method of choice. Analgesics or non-steroidal anti-inflammatory agents are now rarely required. The following protocols for infusion can be used:

- *Pamidronate* 30 mg infusion to begin with, then 60 mg in 500 ml NaCl given slowly for 30–60 min monthly until the pain has been alleviated and the alkaline phosphatase level has returned to normal. Thereafter, only regular clinical and biochemical monitoring is required.
- *Ibandronate* Given in 250 ml NaCl infusion for 15 min monthly, 2 mg for the first and 6 mg for subsequent infusions till normalisation as above.
- *Zoledronate* 5 mg infusion for 15 min. Usually one infusion is enough to normalise the bone markers. Thereafter, monitoring as above.

Alternatively, oral therapy can be given, preferably one of the potent BP:

Tiludronate	400 mg daily for 3 months
Clodronate	800 mg daily for 3 months
Alendronate	40 mg daily for 3 months (authorised in the USA)
Risedronate	30 mg daily for 2–3 months

BP halt progression and may even induce regression of Paget's disease. This is usually accomplished within 2–6 months depending on the intensity of therapy. Histologically, therapeutic success is indicated by decrease in osteoclast number and by formation of lamellar bone. The effects of therapy can last for several years. Should symptoms such as bone pain and/or rise in markers of bone resorption recur, administration

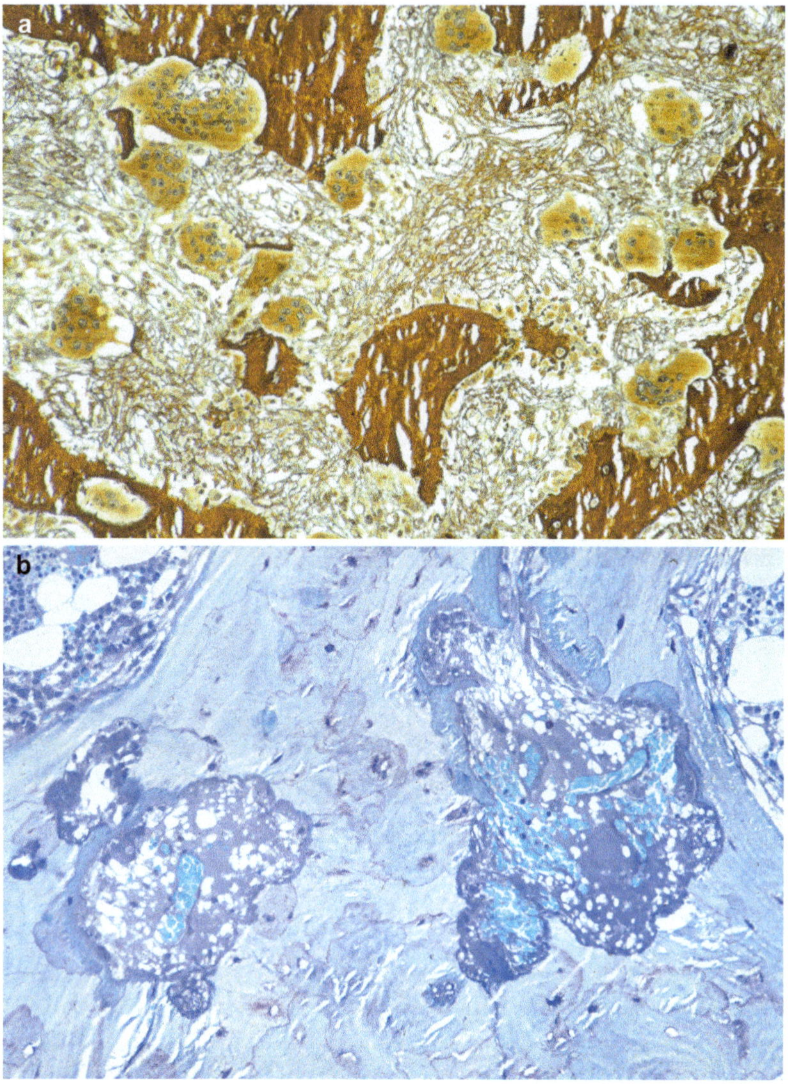

Fig. 65.7 (**a**, **b**) Typical histology of bone in Paget's disease: (**a**) Multiple multinucleated and active osteoclasts in deep resorption lacunae. Note the marked fibrosis in the marrow spaces, Gomori staining. (**b**) Marked remodelling with dissecting osteoclasia and mosaic structures in the adjacent bone, Giemsa staining

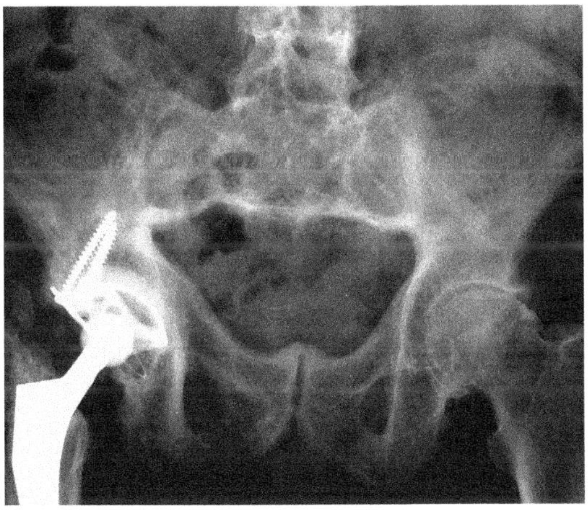

Fig. 65.8 Active phase of Paget's disease, mixed type of the pelvis und lumbar spine with coarsening of the trabecular pattern and prosthesis of the right hip

of a BP should be repeated. The following markers are generally involved: alkaline phosphatase, osteocalcin and β-CrossLaps. Therapy with a different BP is given if resistance is suspected. Bone scans and X-rays are used to check for spread and/or malignant transformation and should be carried out annually (or semi-annually as required) as part of monitoring of the disease and the efficacy of therapy. Current reviews of Paget's disease have confirmed the long-term safety and efficacy of zoledronic acid 5 mg for attainment of long-lasting remissions.

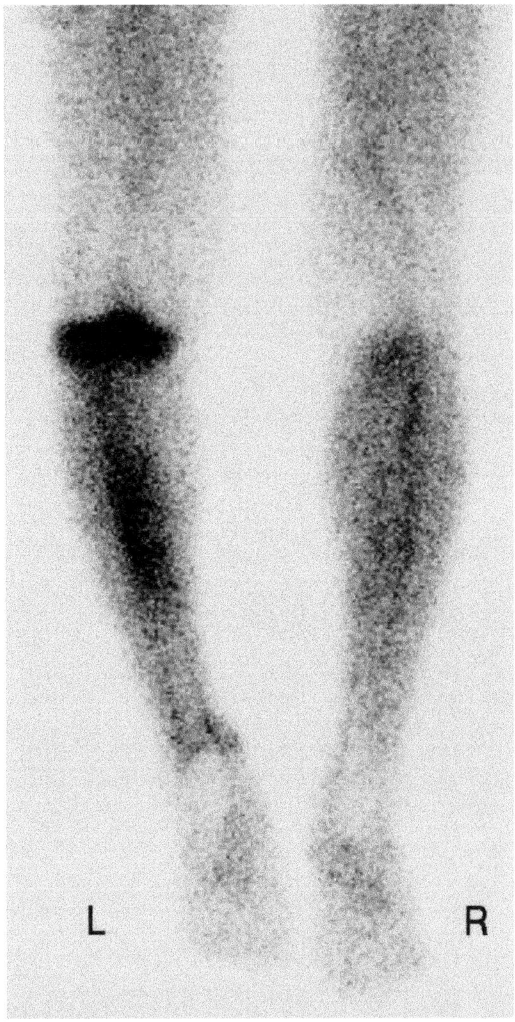

Fig. 65.9 Bone scan showing deformity of the affected tibia in a patient with Paget's disease

66 Fibrous Dysplasia

66.1 Definition

Fibrous dysplasia is a local developmental fibro-osseous aberration of the skeleton. The aetiology is not clear, but it does not appear to be hereditary. Increased production of Il-6 has been implicated as a causative factor. The disease occurs mainly in the first two decades of life, and both sexes are affected (Fig. 66.1). When there are polyostotic fibrous dysplasias of bone together with café au lait skin pigmentation and endocrine disorders, the condition is known as Albright syndrome or *McCune-Albright syndrome (MAS)* (Fig. 66.2). The underlying pathologic process is substitution of fibrous tissue for both bone marrow and bone with activation of osteoclasts. The aim of therapy is normalisation of the increased osteoclastic activity by administration of bisphosphonates.

66.2 Diagnosis

The main clinical symptoms and signs are:

- Bone pain
- Osteolysis or local osteopenia
- Deformity of bone
- Spontaneous fractures

The pelvis, long bones and skull (Fig. 66.3) are particularly prone to this disorder. Fig. 66.4a, b shows the destruction of trabecular bone by fibroblasts and causing fragility and distortion of the normal bone contours. Malignant transformation occurs in less than 1 % of cases. Both mono- and polyostotic variants are recognised. Involvement of the legs usually presents with limp, pain, fracture and deformities ranging from coxa vara to the classical shepherd's crook deformity (Fig. 66.5a, b).

66.3 Treatment

Surgical correction was the only treatment available until recently. Early administration of BP can curtail secondary osteoclastic bone destruction and thereby prevent deformity of bone. Successful treatment with BP has already been reported, although the groups of patients were small. The studies underscored the alleviation of pain, improvement in function, decrease of fracture risk and prevention of deformity. In practice intravenous BP therapy is recommended, but should be administered at an osteological clinic, after informed consent has been obtained and documented.

- *Ibandronate* Monthly infusion of 6 mg for 4–6 months
- *Pamidronate* Monthly infusion of 60 mg for 4–6 months
- *Zoledronate* 5 mg infusion annually

X-rays, CT and/or bone scans can be used for monitoring.

R. Bartl, C. Bartl, *Bone Disorders*, DOI 10.1007/978-3-319-29182-6_66

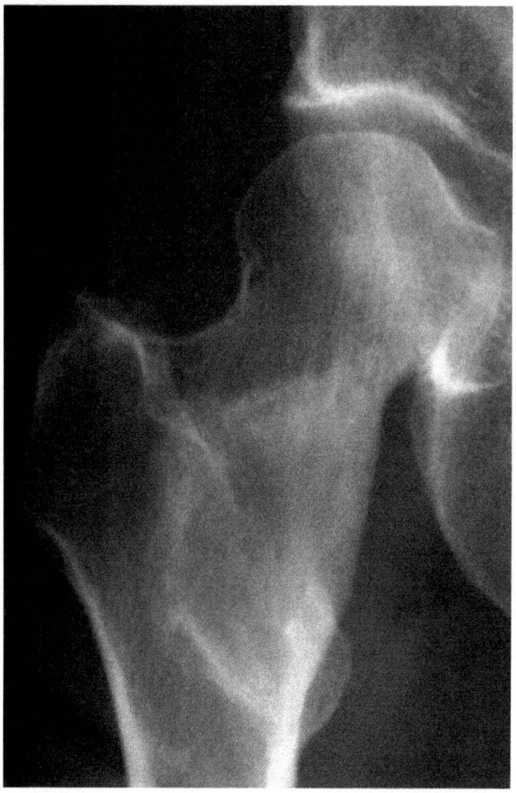

Fig. 66.1 Fibrous dysplasia of the right proximal femur

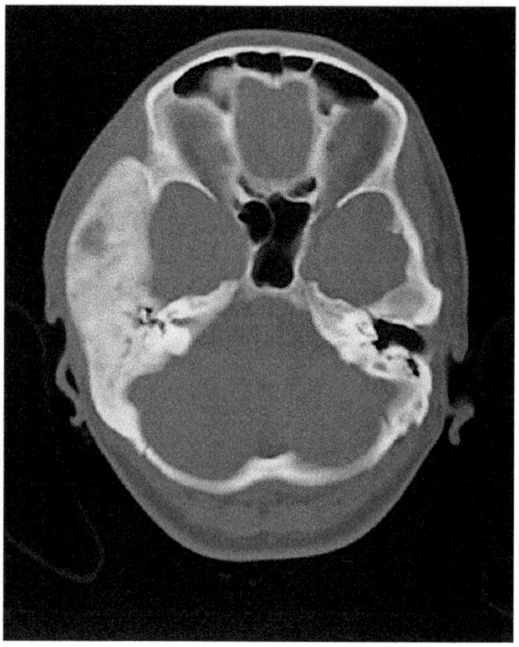

Fig. 66.3 Fibrous dysplasia. CT showing involvement of the cranial bone on the right. The diagnosis was confirmed by histology. A moderate reduction in size of the skeletal lesion and a significant decrease in bone pain were achieved by bisphosphonates, which were initially administered intravenously and later orally

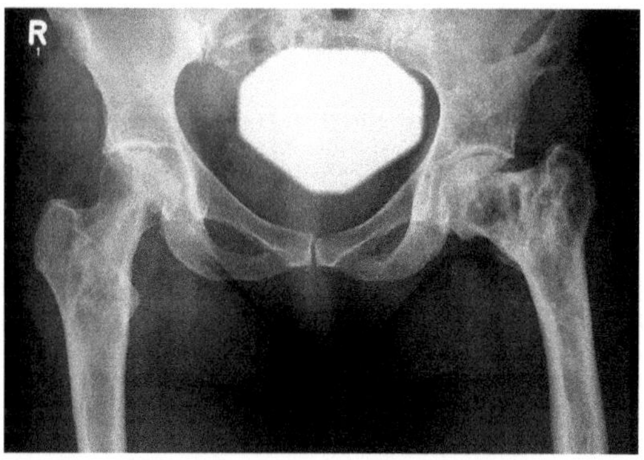

Fig. 66.2 McCune-Albright syndrome with involvement of both hips. Note the irregular and stout cancellous bone, similar to the radiological changes observed in Paget's disease of bone. There was marked bone pain in the involved areas, and the alkaline phosphatase in the serum was increased

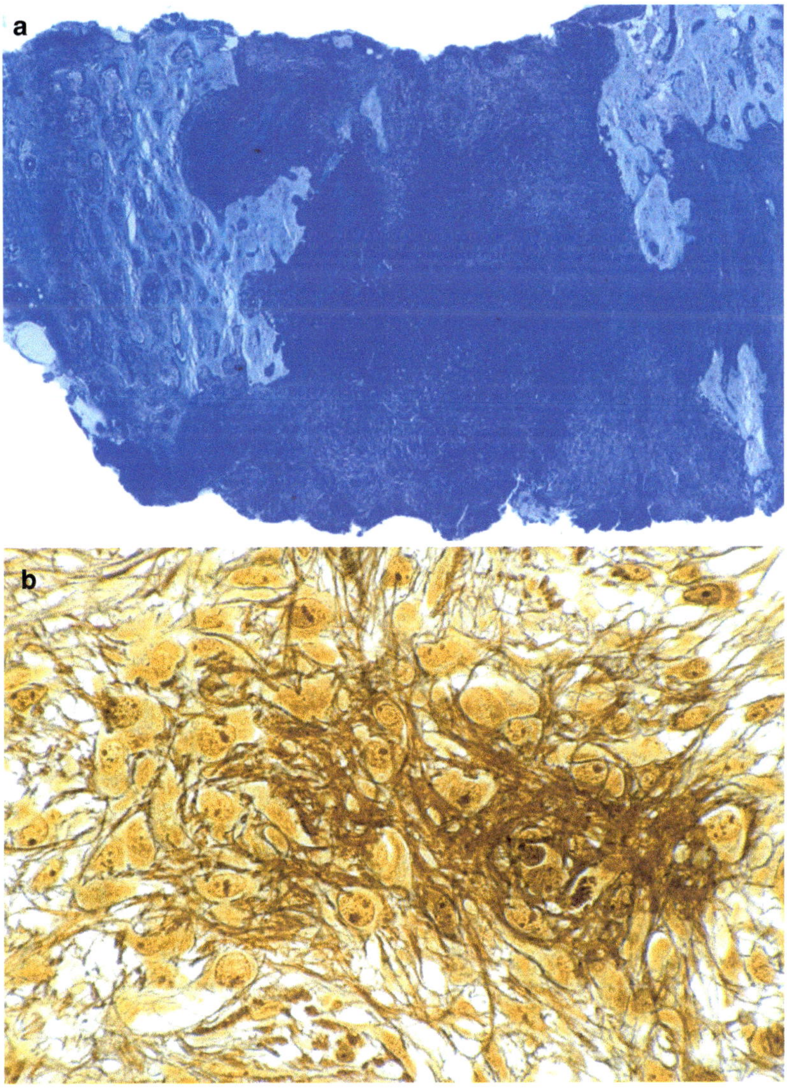

Fig. 66.4 (**a**, **b**) Fibrous dysplasia: (**a**) overview of biopsy section demonstrating complete transformation of trabecular bone and bone marrow into a mass of fibrous tissue. Note cortical bone at left. Giemsa staining. (**b**) Higher magnification with focus of fibroblasts and fibrocytes and production of fibrosis. Gomori staining

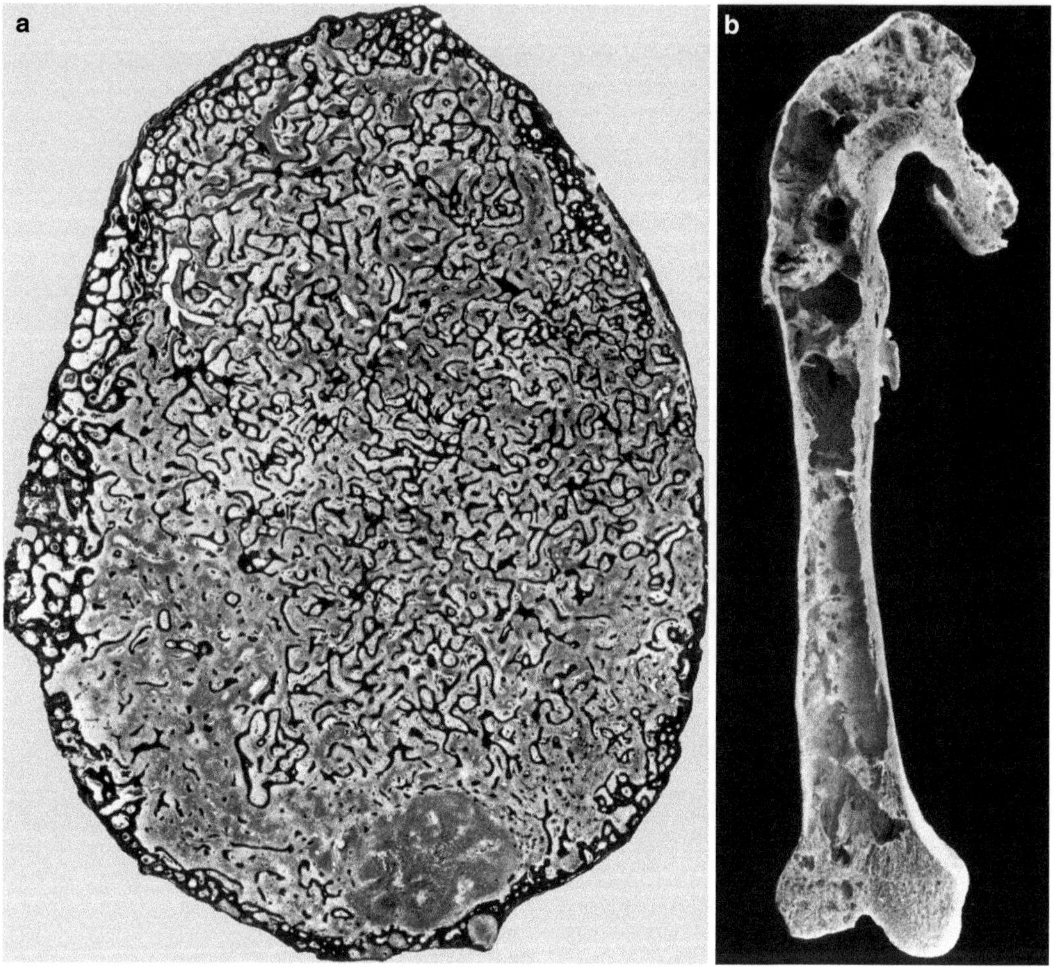

Fig. 66.5 (**a**, **b**) Polyostotic fibrous dysplasia with a cross section of the fibula, showing a fine network of small trabeculae surrounded by fibrous stroma. (**b**) Femur of a patient with advanced fibrous dysplasia showing the classical shepherd's crook deformity (With kind permission of Springer, from [38])

67 Vanishing Bone Disease (Gorham-Stout Syndrome)

67.1 Definition

This syndrome is also known as *massive osteolysis*, *disappearing bone disease* and *phantom bone*.

Gorham's vanishing bone disease is the ultimate osteoporosis showing complete disassociation of the normal coupling mechanism. The cause is unknown, though overactivity of cytokines especially Il-6 has been implicated. Gorham's disease is occasionally fatal. This disorder was first described by Jackson in 1938 as "a boneless arm" (Fig. 67.1). In 1953, Gorham and Stout published 24 cases and emphasised the angiogenic component of the disease. Subsequent surveys of the literature revealed nearly 150 documented cases (Devlin et al. 1996); more have been reported since then, up to 175 cases as of Feb. 2008. Occasionally, the disease has also been identified in children, as in a recent case in the humerus of a 14-year-old boy.

67.2 Aetiology and Pathophysiology

The cause has not yet been elucidated. Haemangiomatosis and lymphangiomatosis have been implicated, possibly due to an endothelial defect, with production of abnormally high levels of cytokines which stimulate osteoclasts. Some studies have reported the presence of numerous leaky lymphatic vessels near the osteolytic lesions as well as chylous ascites. Investigations have now revealed several lymphangiogenic pathways that could be relevant in Gorham's disease. Many investigators have described prominent osteoclasts particularly in the lytic front of the lesions. However, no reactive osteoblastic activity has ever been documented indicating that the physiological "coupling" between bone resorption and bone formation has been completely abrogated. This clearly demonstrates a communication defect between osteoclasts and osteoblasts resulting in absence of stimulation of osteoblasts, i.e. no reaction to the osteoclastic activity. In one patient interleukin-6 – a cytokine that stimulates osteoclasts and is produced by various cell types including endothelial cells, either directly or by way of VEGF – was implicated; initially high levels of Il-6 dropped after therapy with bisphosphonates and radiation.

67.3 Clinical Findings

A review of the recent literature based on findings in 46 patients revealed the following features (Fig. 67.2):

- It affects young adults without preference for male or female.
- Genetic, endocrinologic and metabolic disturbances have not been found.

R. Bartl, C. Bartl, *Bone Disorders*, DOI 10.1007/978-3-319-29182-6_67

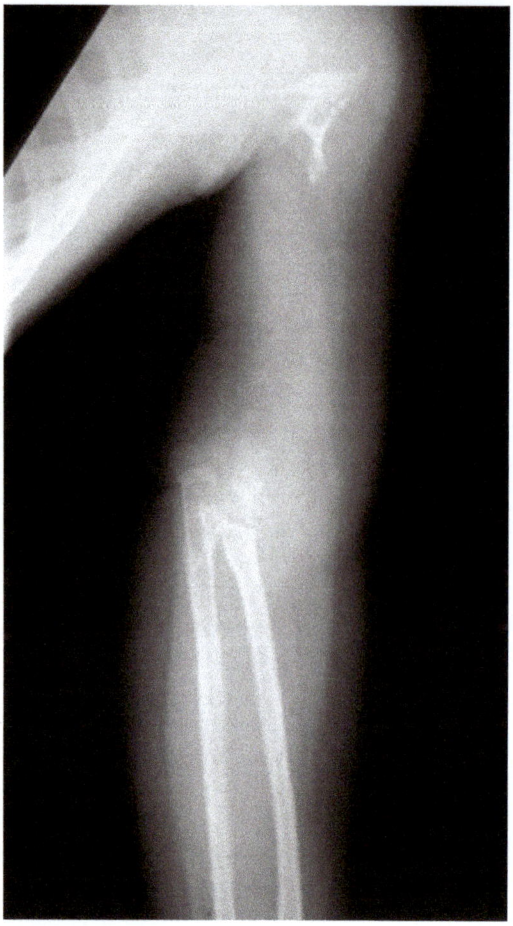

Fig. 67.1 Almost complete disappearance of the left humerus in a 14-year-old patient with Gorham-Stout syndrome

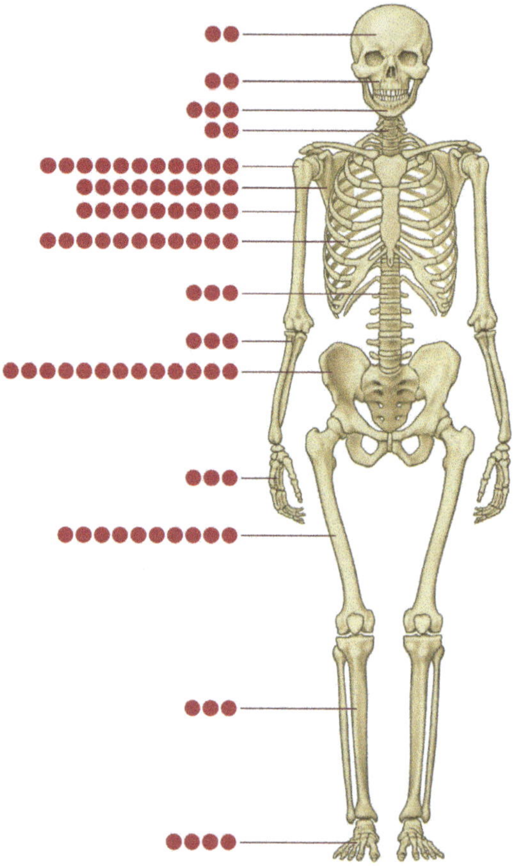

Fig. 67.2 Frequency and topography of skeletal involvement in vanishing bone disease (Gorham's syndrome). Every red dot represents one patient reported in the literature

- It starts in a single bone and spreads to adjacent bones.
- In 38 of 46 cases, the condition was already polyostotic at diagnosis.
- The pelvis, vertebrae, ribs, proximal bones of the extremities and cranial bones are frequently involved.
- Progression and spread of the disease are unpredictable.
- When the ribs are affected, pulmonary insufficiency is frequently a lethal consequence.
- Chylothorax is a common complication.

67.4 Diagnosis

The diagnosis of Gorham-Stout syndrome is established by X-rays which demonstrate the absence of bone in the affected areas. Occasionally vertebral compression fractures in severe osteoporosis must be considered in the differential diagnosis. When localised to the mandible, it must be differentiated from osteonecrosis due to other causes (Mignona et al. 2005) (see also section on periodontitis). In early phases of the disorder, osteolytic lesions due to a malignancy must be ruled out. Bone biopsies taken from an involved area show increased osteoclastic resorption by morphologically normal osteoclasts. The absence of osteoblasts is particularly striking. This indicates complete abrogation of the "coupling" mechanism. The resorption lacunae are filled with fibroblasts, blood vessels and oedematous connective tissue. Infiltration of the involved areas by plasma cells, lymphocytes and mast cells suggests an immunologic component.

67.5 Treatment

Before the introduction of bisphosphonates, progression of the Gorham-Stout syndrome was inexorable. All previous attempts to treat this condition have failed. But, as in all other states of skeletal destruction: immediate initiation of bisphosphonate therapy proved to be highly effective. Case reports have demonstrated rapid disappearance of local symptoms and pain after i.v. administration of bisphosphonates, and follow-up over the subsequent 24 months revealed a stable condition with no evidence of progression (Hammer et al. 2005).

Focal osteolysis – the unbalanced hyperactive osteoclastic resorption – can be halted immediately by intravenous BP, which stop progression of the disease. The following are recommended:

- *Ibandronate* 6 mg infusion monthly for 4–6 months
- *Zoledronate* 5 mg single infusion

X-rays should be taken every 4–6 months for follow-up. Restitution of the vanished bone has not been observed, even under therapy with bisphosphonates. Trials with anabolic agents have not yet been reported.

68 SAPHO Syndrome

68.1 Definition

SAPHO syndrome is a strange disease of the skin and bone which also occurs in children (Kerrison et al 2004). Generally SAPHO syndrome includes the following dermatologic and osteologic manifestations:

- *S*ynovitis
- *A*cne
- *P*ustulosis
- *H*yperostosis
- *O*steitis

Sternoclavicular hyperostosis, which occurs primarily in the fourth to sixth decades of life, is the most impressive; it has also been observed without dermatological changes. Characteristically this disorder involves the clavicle (Fig. 68.1a, b), sternum and the proximal sections of the adjoining upper ribs. All the effected skeletal parts are swollen, sensitive to pressure and unduly warm. Occasionally the subclavian veins are obstructed, and this results in oedema. About 30–50 % of the patients show a purulent plantar or palmar eczema which leads some experts to classify this syndrome as a particular type of psoriasis.

68.2 Diagnosis

Laboratory investigations demonstrate signs of an inflammatory reaction (high ESR, mild leucocytosis and increase in alkaline phosphatase), while rheumatoid factor and histocompatibility antigen HLA-B27 are negative. Paget's disease, osteitis and bone tumours must be excluded by imaging techniques. Chronic diffuse sclerosing osteomyelitis should also be considered. It is a local inflammatory condition accompanied by intractable pain. Therapy with a bisphosphonate resulted in alleviation of symptoms and decrease in markers of bone turnover (Wright et al 2005).

68.3 Therapy

Until recently therapy was confined to analgesics (NSAR and/or glucocorticoids). Although bacteria were isolated from some biopsies, attempts at therapy with antibiotics were unsuccessful. Other medications including colchicine, methotrexate, cyclosporine, calcitonin and vitamin D_3 were equally ineffective. The almost unbearable bone pain is quickly alleviated by therapy with bisphosphonates especially i.v. which constitutes

R. Bartl, C. Bartl, *Bone Disorders*, DOI 10.1007/978-3-319-29182-6_68

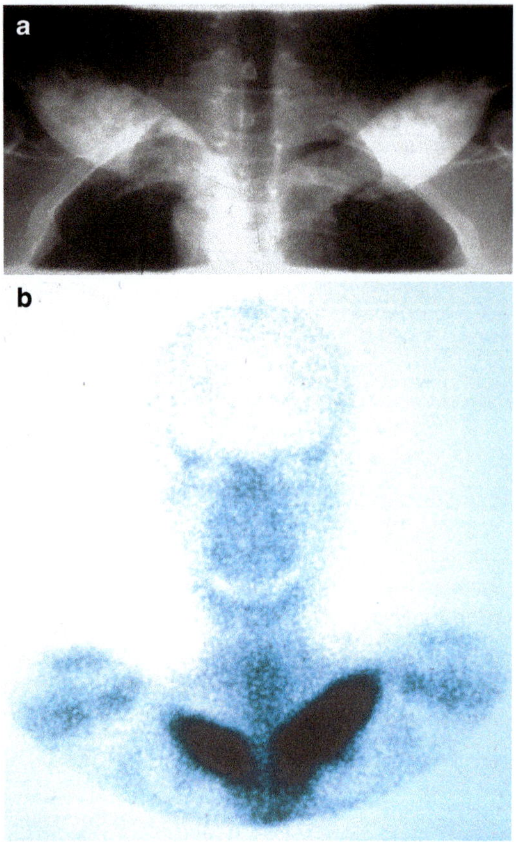

Fig. 68.1 (**a**, **b**) SAPHO syndrome: (**a**) massive enlargement of both clavicles on X-ray, (**b**) same, as seen in bone scan

a breakthrough in the treatment of this disorder. With continued therapy, the symptoms decreased, and progression of the disorder was halted. In five cases the following protocol was used successfully:

Ibandronate 6 mg, 15 min infusion monthly

Children with SAPHO syndrome have been treated with cyclic pamidronate therapy. X-rays, CT, MRI and or bone scans can be used for monitoring. Moreover, this bisphosphonate therapy has been highly successful even in patients with long-standing treatment – refractory sternoclavicular hyperostosis.

69 Bone Marrow Oedema Syndrome

69.1 Definition and Pathogenesis

Bone marrow ischaemia, osteochondral lesions and microfractures lead to an inflammatory response reaction in the epi- and metaphyseal region. Macrophages, monocytes and osteoclast precursors located in the bone marrow react with a release of cytokines and proinflammatory mediators leading to a capillary leak of the bone vessels followed by fluid outflow into the bone marrow interstitial space (Fig. 69.1). Increased blood flow, reduced venous outflow and lymphocyte invasion further aggravate the bone marrow oedema (BME). Histological findings show fibrovascular regenerates and increased bone turnover with increased osteoclast activity. The bone marrow is hypocellular with oedema in the interstitial space and present lymphocytosis, plasmacytosis and fine fibrosis. Sinusoids show dilatation and disruption of their walls (capillary leak). Osteoclast activation leads to bone resorption and microfracturing of trabeculae (Fig. 69.2a–c). Bone mineralisation rate is reduced, but without marked loss of bone mass, as in the case of osteoporosis. The presence of active, intact bone cells is responsible for the repair capacity and the reversibility of the bone marrow oedema syndrome (BMES) after correction of the activated bone turnover. Increased fluid pressure and inflammatory mediators within the bone compartment activating the afferent nerves in the bone marrow cause the typical pain. In experimental studies the normal intraosseous pressure was found to be 20–30 mmHg. The increased bone turnover with increased osteoclastic activity due to an intraosseous inflammatory reaction with a capillary leak leads to fluid accumulation in the bone marrow interstitial space.

The differentiation of BME to early stages of osteonecrosis (ON) is of decisive importance. In some classifications (e.g. ARCO), BME is listed as an early stage of osteonecrosis. Several studies have shown a high reversibility rate of BME following treatment, so that BMES is now regarded as a distinct clinical entity with varying duration apart from avascular bone necrosis. Currently the pathophysiologic mechanism of bone marrow oedemas is still under debate, but the main theories support an inflammatory response reaction following a bone microtrauma or a resulting bone marrow ischaemia following nontraumatic conditions.

69.2 Diagnosis and Clinical Findings

In general, healthy middle-aged individuals are affected. Due to unspecific clinical findings, the correct diagnosis of BMES is often delayed. An MRI is usually done after several weeks or months of persistent functional impairment. In the literature the symptomatic period is described

R. Bartl, C. Bartl, *Bone Disorders*, DOI 10.1007/978-3-319-29182-6_69

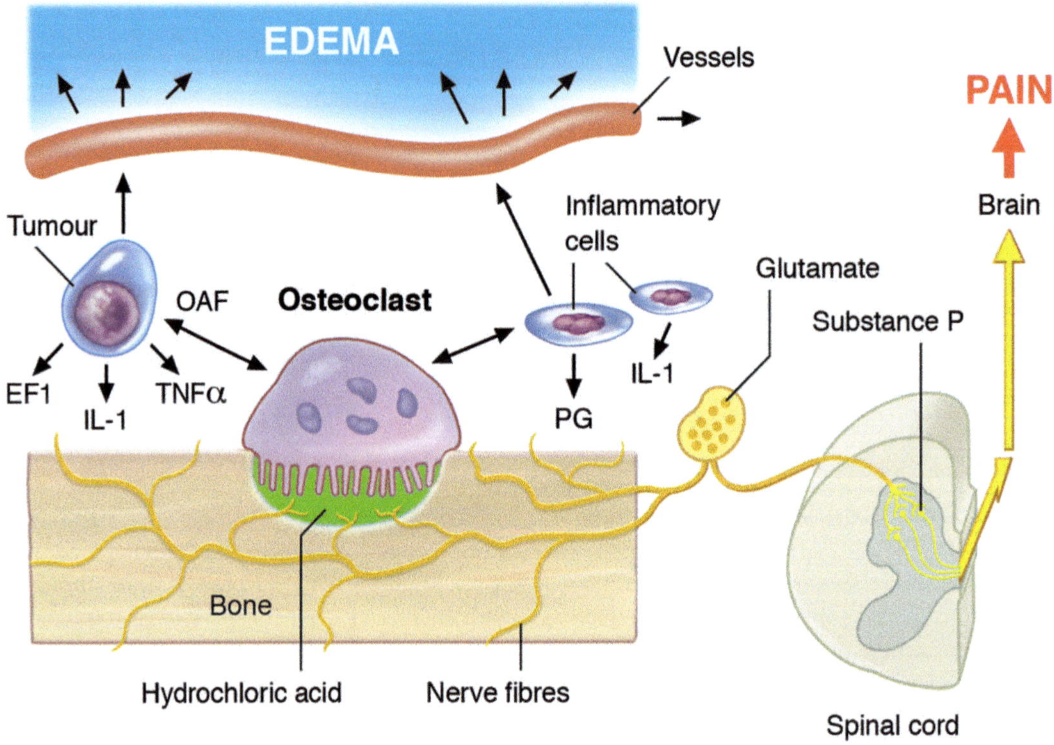

Fig. 69.1 Pathophysiology of bone marrow oedema syndrome

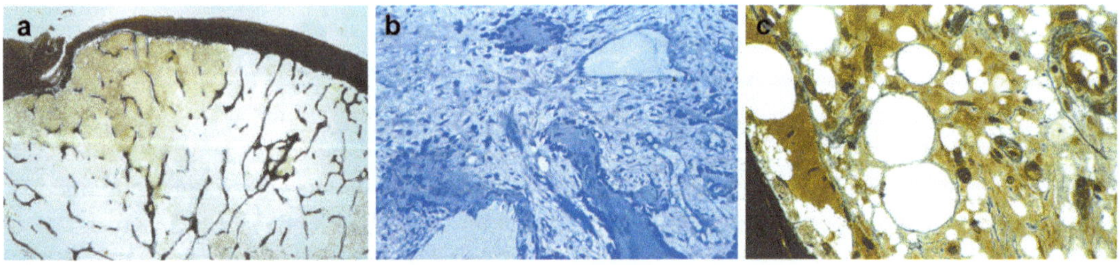

Fig. 69.2 (**a**–**c**) Histology of a BME area: (**a**) low magnification of a section of a subchondral BME region (*light brown*). (**b**) Microfracture with production of new woven bone in the subchondral region (*Giemsa staining*) and (**c**) massive bone marrow oedema in the surrounding bone marrow area (*Gomori staining*)

with a duration of up to 24 months with especially long disease courses following conservative treatment. BMEs mainly occurs around joints in the epiphyseal and metaphyseal region. In most cases the symptomatic onset cannot be linked to a special traumatic event. Bone marrow oedemas can be diagnosed accidentally, or following bone drilling, after intensive physical activity (e.g. marathon running, jumping) or as reactive BMEs with underlying chondral lesions, osteoarthritis or rheumatoid arthritis (Table 69.1). Over time BMEs show changes in size, location and intensity. A typical dull pain is present at rest, due to the increased fluid pressure within the bone compartment, and is aggravated under activity. Patients report about pain and a functional deficit of the affected joint. Studies have shown that pain levels do not correlate with the extent of the BME on MRI.

A special subtype is the pregnancy-related BMES, formerly called *transient osteoporosis* with a painful osteopenia and undermineralisa-

Table 69.1 Classification of bone marrow oedema syndrome (BMES)

Traumatic, mechanic	Fracture
	Stress fracture, insufficiency fracture
	Bone bruise
	Osteochondral lesion
Ischaemic	Bone necrosis
	Osteochondritis dissecans (OD)
	CRPS
	Pregnancy related
	Coagulopathies (e.g. sickle cell anaemia)
Reactive	Degenerative/inflammatory (osteoarthritis)
	Neoplastic
	Osteomyelitis
	Metabolic
	Iatrogenic (e.g. bone drilling, OATS)
	Toxic, medication associated

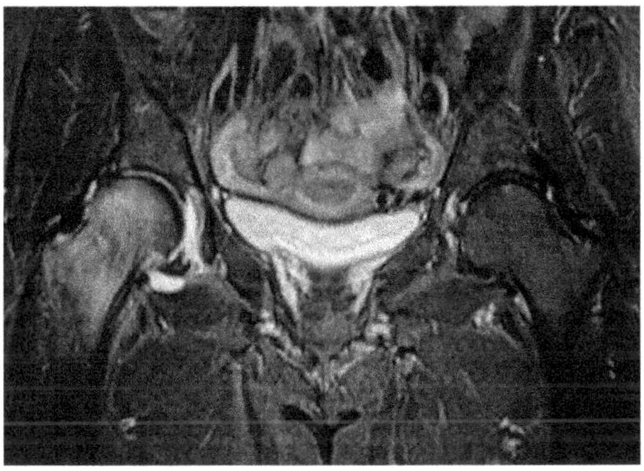

Fig. 69.3 BME of the femoral head and the metaphyseal region postpartum

tion that occurs in the third trimester of pregnancy or in the postpartum period. BME mainly affects the hip (Fig. 69.3).

Another special subtype is the migratory BMES that can affect various joints of the lower extremity. BME can migrate from one femoral condyle to the other or can jump over the joint line to the proximal tibia (Fig. 69.4a–c).

69.3 Imaging

In the early stage, radiographs do not show abnormalities, whereas in chronic stages, local osteopenia can be seen. MRI can detect bone marrow oedemas with high sensitivity and specificity already in the early stages. Also differential diagnosis like osteonecrosis ("double-line sign"), osteochondral lesions, bone bruises and stress fractures can be distinguished with MRI. The oedema region appears hyperintense in T2-weighted, STIR, proton-weighted sequences and fat-suppression techniques and hypointense in T1-weighted images. Bone scans can indicate regions of high bone turnover but have no accurate specificity.

69.4 Treatment Strategies

Treatment is related to the BME subtype and underlying diseases. Given the intact repair capacity, a conservative approach with pain med-

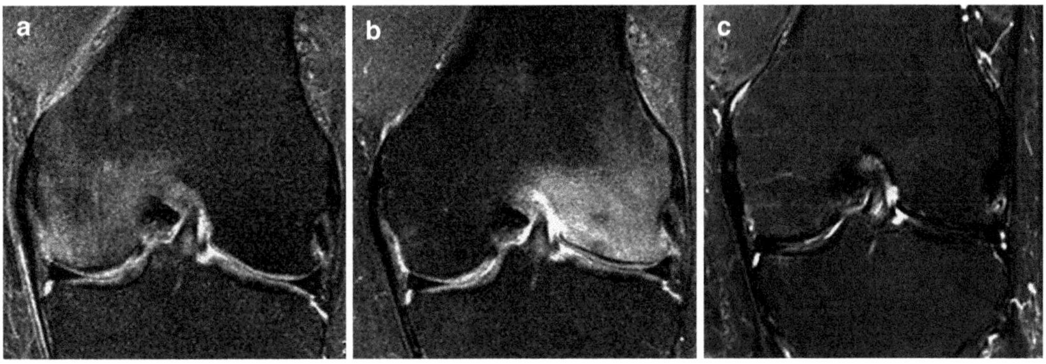

Fig. 69.4 (**a**) Migratory BME of the medial femoral condyle, (**b**) the lateral femoral condyle 4 months later, and (**c**) complete regression of the BME after BP infusion therapy

ication and unloading of the affected joint is justified. Additional *vitamin D supplementation, pain medication* and *anti-inflammatory drugs* should be given. In chronic cases without functional improvement, an infusion therapy with an *N-containing BP* should be applied. Infusion therapy is strongly recommended in cases of functional decline correlated with BME progression and risk factors for osteonecrosis.

The following *infusion protocols* can be applied:

- Ibandronate 3 infusions with 6 mg every 3 weeks; infusion time 30 min.
- Zoledronate Single infusion of 5 mg; infusion time 30 min.

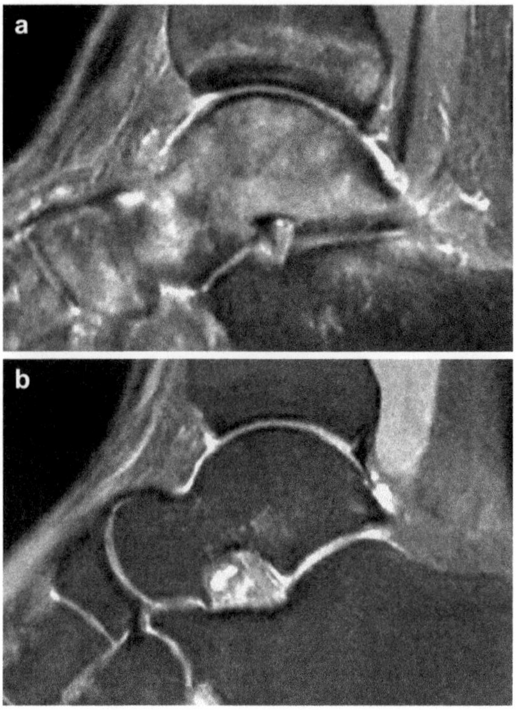

Fig. 69.5 (**a**) Marked BME of the ankle and foot following an ankle supination trauma with CRPS-like symptoms for more than 6 months. (**b**) Complete regression of the BME following BP infusion therapy and functional recovery with full return to sports activity after 3 months

Intravenous BP act via osteoclast inhibition and reduce the increased bone turnover in the bone compartment. The intravenous therapy shows a rapid therapeutic effect and therefore should be preferred over oral medication. Infusion therapy can be applied in an ambulatory setting and comprises a low rate of potential side effects. It represents an off-label use and should be discussed with the patient. Contraindications are pregnancy, lactation and current surgery on jaw bones. In most cases there is already a significant functional improvement and pain reduction after application of the first infusion. In the author's experience in over 1000 BMES cases treated with BP infusion therapy, no cases of kidney dysfunction and no case of osteonecrosis of the jaw was observed. In about 10 % of the cases, there is a mainly mild, first-dose-dependent, acute-phase reaction with flu-like symptoms. In a case-control study, BP infusion therapy showed a significant faster functional improvement and pain reduction compared to a control group treated with pain medication and partial weight-bearing. Control MRI showed a complete regression of BME in 70 % and a significant BME reduction in 25 % of the cases within 6 months (Figs. 69.5a, b, 69.6a, b, and 69.7a, b). A clear advantage is the fast regain of activity in the active population and in athletes compared to conservative therapy.

An alternative option is the infusion therapy with prostacyclin analogues (Iloprost, Ilomedin®) that act via an increased blood flow and also represent an off-label use. Due to the potential severe side effects, the infusion therapy must be done in an in-hospital stay. Iloprost is applied at a dose of 25 and 50 μg (1.5ng/kg/min over 6 h) over 5 days.

Other therapeutical options are the application of *denosumab* (60 mg every 6 months), a potent osteoclast inhibitor or an osteoanabolic therapy with PTH (20 μg daily dose) tested in case reports. For all therapy regimens, additional vitamin D supplementation, pain medication and pain-adapted partial weight-bearing should be applied. Given the fact that BMES represents a distinct clinical entity apart from bone osteone-

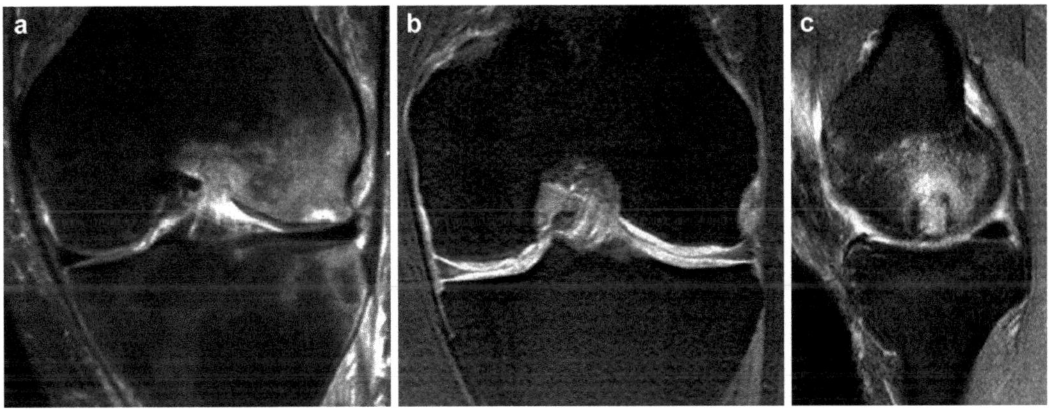

Fig. 69.6 (**a**) BMES of the lateral femoral condyle in a 58-year-old patient showing a focal subchondral area of initial bone necrosis (M. Ahlbäck) following arthroscopy. (**b**) Complete regression of the BME and restitution of the subchondral bone necrosis area following BP infusion therapy. (**c**) Reactive BME of the femoral condyle in a 27-year-old patient following osteochondral transplantation

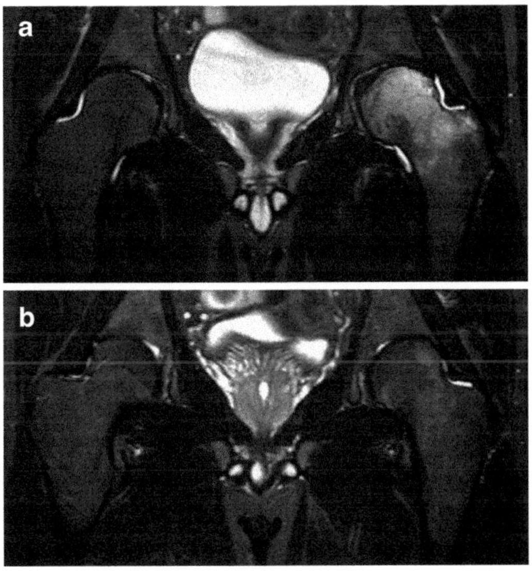

Fig. 69.7 (**a**) BME of the femoral head including the metaphyseal zone. (**b**) BME regression after BP infusion therapy

crosis, pain medication and partial weight-bearing with additional drug therapy were established as treatment standards.

Surgical procedures can be applied in cases of ischaemic BMEs of the femoral head, refractory to conservative treatment or infusion therapy. A core decompression of the epi- and metaphyseal BME is done to lower the intraosseous pressure and to initiate bone revascularisation and to prevent the progression to osteonecrosis. Surgical decompression can also be combined with infusion therapy to further improve revascularisation.

Depending on the BME subtype, other surgical procedures like *chondrocyte and mesenchymal stem cell transplantation*, *osteochondral transplantation* (*OATS*), *microfracturing* or *osteotomy* with limb alignment correction can be done in cases of osteochondral lesions and reactive BMEs.

70 Complex Regional Pain Syndrome (CRPS, Sudeck's Disease)

70.1 Definition and Pathogenesis

Also known as *algodystrophy*, *Sudeck's disease* or *sympathetic reflex dystrophy*, this disorder is a highly unpleasant, unpredictable and painful complication of injuries and trauma, especially fractures. The cause, development and effective treatment of CRPS are largely unknown. It has not been observed in children. Putative causes range from disorders of vegetative innervation to endocrine and psychosomatic disorders. Triggers of CRPS include fractures, repeated reduction maneuvres following fractures, operations, infections and nerve injuries. The severity of the underlying injury bears no apparent relationship to the severity of the symptoms of Sudeck's disease, which can be triggered even by trivial trauma. Most frequently affected are distal parts of the extremities, like the wrist and hand, mainly following conservative or surgical management of distal radius fractures (90 %) and the ankle/foot region. Women are affected twice as much compared to men. A psychosomatic component is discussed. Unlike in BMES several bones and small joint regions are affected. The initial phase with a sympathetic dysregulation with swelling and hyperthermia of the affected area is followed by a neurogenic-dystrophic process. Following the inflammatory stage, there is a hypoperfusion due to the sympathetic dysregulation, leading to acidosis and dystrophic changes with neuropathic pain, joint stiffness, muscle dysfunction and local osteopenia.

Two types are recognised:

- *CRPS type I* develops after a trauma.
- *CRPS type II* is triggered by a peripheral nerve injury.

70.2 Diagnosis and Clinical Findings

The diagnosis of CRPS type I is based on clinical findings. The following criteria have to be fulfilled:

- Disproportionately strong pain, neuropathic pain, hyperalgesia (Fig. 70.1).
- Asymmetric swelling and hyperthermia.
- Asymmetric skin discoloration and sweating.
- Increased hair growth on the area involved.
- Reduced range of motion, muscle weakness and joint stiffness.
- The symptoms cannot be explained by another disease.

The following investigations contribute to the diagnosis:

- Thermography (area of overheating)
- Bone scan (area of increased uptake)
- Radiographs (patchy rarefaction of the bone)
- MRI (oedematous areas around the joints and muscles involved)
- Quantitative sensoric measurements (pain characteristic)

R. Bartl, C. Bartl, *Bone Disorders*, DOI 10.1007/978-3-319-29182-6_70

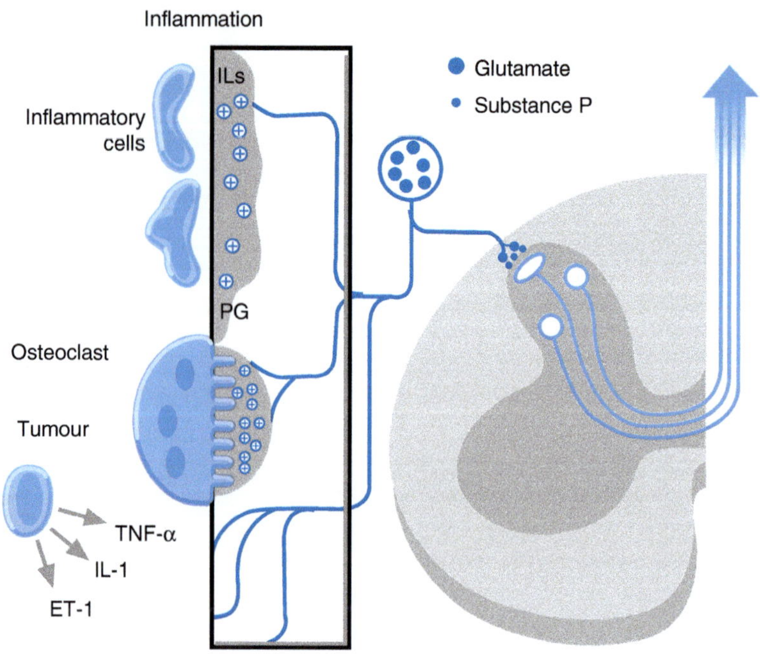

Fig. 70.1 Mechanisms of bone pain in inflammatory and neoplastic disorders

70.3 Course of Disease

The course of the disease is divided into three main stages:

Stage of inflammation (up to 3 months): Typical symptoms include localised pain, discolouration and hyperthermia of the skin, doughlike oedema and functional limitations of the joint. MRI shows presence of bone marrow oedema.

Stage of dystrophy (3–6 months): The dermatologic symptoms regress, leaving a trophic disorder of the skin. There is an increase in restriction of joint movement and spotty areas of demineralisation are seen on radiographs.

Stage of atrophy (6–12 months): This end stage is characterised by generalised atrophy of the skin, muscles and bone (Fig. 70.2a). Stiffness of the joint is further increased as massive rarefaction of the bone occurs.

70.4 Treatment Strategies

A relationship of confidence and trust must be established between patient and doctor, to ease the fear, tension and anxiety which always accompany this chronic condition. First, it is essential to break the vicious circle of pain and dystrophy to get pain control by rest and physiotherapy. Frequently the diagnosis is established delayed, usually following cast management or osteosynthesis of a fracture. All procedures leading to pain aggravation are contraindicated.

Immobilisation and passive physiotherapy, analgesics, anti-inflammatory drugs and cold dressings to counteract overheating are useful measures in stage I. Corticosteroids are used due to their anti-inflammatory and anti-oedematous effect. *BP* reduce osteoclast activity and are given to treat bone loss and decalcification, and also due to their analgesic effect (Fig. 70.2b), BP are first-line therapy in CRPS I following fractures. Medications to treat neuropathic pain (e.g. gabapentin) are also useful. Invasive interventions like blockade of the sympathetic nerve supply (stellate) or calcitonin therapy can also be considered. Physiotherapy, ergotherapy and exercises ("motor learning") are strongly recommended in stages II and III.

70.5 Bisphosphonates

Since 1988, 4 RCTs with BP to treat CRPS I showed alleviation of pain and regain of function in most cases.

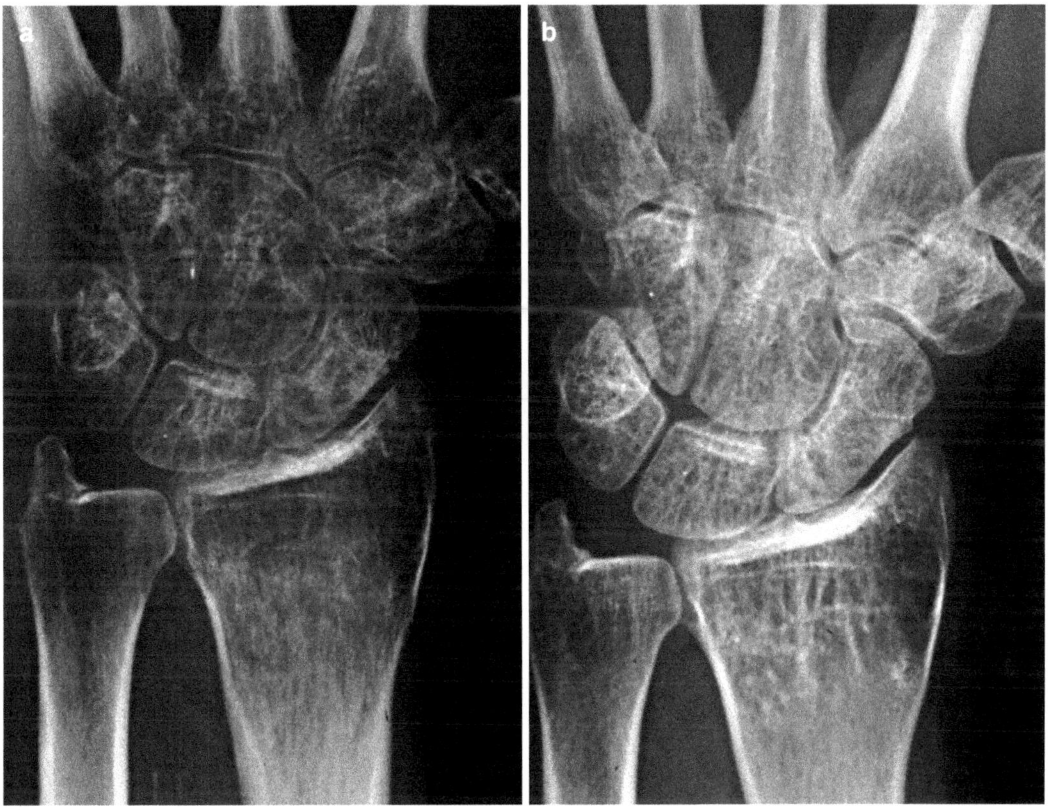

Fig. 70.2 (**a**) CRPS I with massive bone loss and decalcification of the wrist and carpus following a distal radius fracture. (**b**) Control radiograph with regain of bone mass and normalisation of mineral content following intravenous BP therapy

In CRPS I cases caused by fractures, BP are now first-line therapy.

Currently one of the following N-containing BP is given for 4–6 months:

- *Ibandronate* Infusion of 6 mg monthly, four times
- *Pamidronate* Infusion of 60 mg monthly, 4–6 times
- *Zoledronate* Infusion of 5 mg as a single dose

Initially a half dose of 3 mg ibandronate or 30 mg pamidronate can be given to avoid potential acute-phase reactions (previously described), which could be much more pronounced in patients with CRPS I, than in other patients.

BP became more and more important in the treatment of CRPS I as the complex pathomechanism has been studied in detail.

The sympathetic dysregulation in the inflammation stage leads to hypoperfusion and hypoxia of the affected limb area finally resulting in local acidosis. Acidosis leads to osteoclast activation and bone resorption and reduced bone mineralisation (Fig. 70.3). Osteoblast growth and collagen production are further inhibited, resulting in reduced bone formation. BP are potent specific osteoclast inhibitors and play a key role in reversing bone resorption and regulating bone homeostasis in cases of CRPS I. Acidosis also activates the BP.

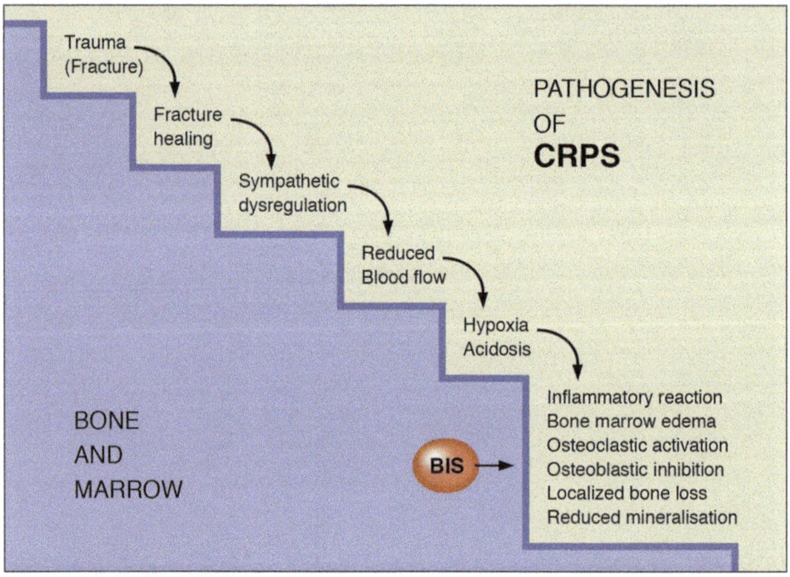

Fig. 70.3 Mechanisms of local bone loss in complex regional pain syndrome

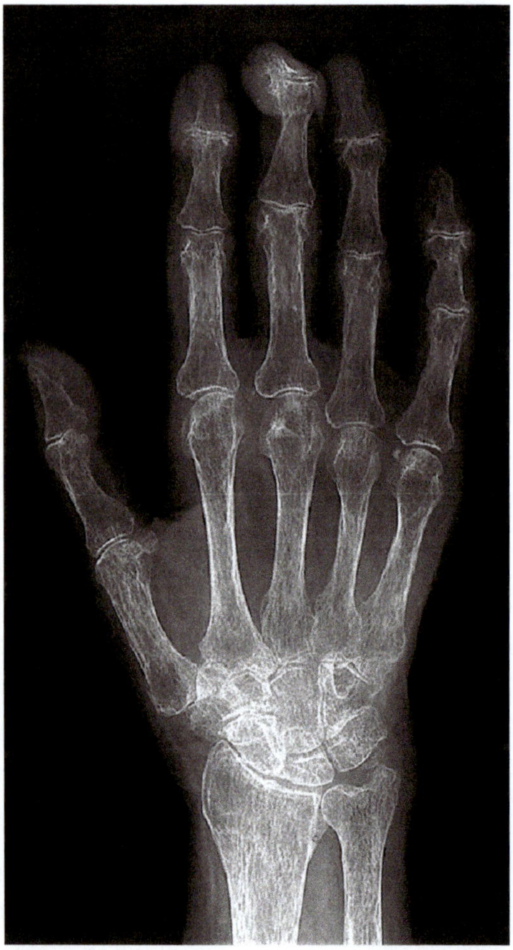

Fig. 70.4 Massive and spotty decalcification of the hand in CRPS (Sudeck's disease), Stage III (stage of atrophy). Even this late stage is curable with intravenous BP

Osteoclasts are the main causative cells in the pathogenesis of bone marrow oedema and CRPS. BP are potent specific osteoclast inhibitors and play a key role in reducing bone marrow oedema, reversing bone resorption and regulating bone homeostasis in all cases of CRPS (Fig. 70.4).

71 Ischaemic Bone Disease

71.1 Definition and Pathogenesis

Bone dies just like other tissues, when interrupted from blood supply. This dead bone is also called *skeletal infarction*, *osteonecrosis*, *avascular necrosis*, *bone infarction* or *medullary infarct*. The disease occurs more frequently in males than in females (8:1), and the patients are usually less than 50 years of age.

> Ischaemic bone disease is a focal bone infarction, which may be idiopathic or secondary to various conditions. Severe joint destruction may result. Early diagnosis is best made by MRI.

Bone infarcts may be asymptomatic or may cause painful collapse of subarticular bone that leads to joint destruction and fracture. The disease may affect only one bone, more than one bone at the same time or more than one bone at different times. In 30–70 % of cases with non-traumatic AVN, the disease is bilateral. Medullary infarcts mostly occur in the metaphyseal and diaphyseal regions of the femur and tibia (Figs. 71.1a, b and 71.2a, b). Usually they are asymptomatic and are discovered incidentally. Calcification of the dead marrow and reparative new bone assume a "smoke ring" shape, a well-demarcated zone with serpiginous borders, together with cystic alterations. T_2-weighted images of MRI show the "double line" sign, highly characteristic of bone necrosis.

> Characteristic radiologic signs of medullary infarcts are the "smoke ring" shape, serpiginous, well-demarcated borders, the "double line" sign, calcifications and cystic changes.

The femoral head is the most common location for osteonecrosis, but it may also occur at other sites including the distal femur, proximal tibia, humeral head, waist of scaphoid, talus, wrist and foot. In the early stage of the disease, radiographs will be normal. MRI demonstrating bone marrow oedema is especially sensitive for detecting early osteonecrosis. Relatively late in the pathologic process, X-rays show patchy areas of osteopenia or osteosclerosis that reflect skeletal repair.

> Radiologic signs of *osteonecrosis of the femoral head*, late stage are:
>
> - "Crescent sign" beneath the subchondral plate
> - "Double line sign"
> - Collapse or flattening of the articular surface

R. Bartl, C. Bartl, *Bone Disorders*, DOI 10.1007/978-3-319-29182-6_71

- Mottled osteosclerosis, subchondral cysts and osteophytes
- Extensive fragmentation of the necrotic segment

In avascular necrosis, laboratory evaluation will be normal, but may reveal causal factors such as connective tissue disease, diabetes mellitus, hyperlipidaemia, coagulopathies or gout.

71.2 Histology

Necrosis of bone and bone marrow due to interruption of blood flow starts by disruption of sinusoids and small blood vessels, followed by extravasation of erythrocytes, bone marrow oedema, degeneration of haematopoietic and fat cells and death of bone cells, including osteocytes, osteoblasts and chondrocytes. Especially for nontraumatic ischaemic necrosis, the predisposed sites seem to reflect the conversion of red marrow to fatty marrow with ageing. Furthermore, a genetic basis to idiopathic osteonecrosis of the femoral head is suggested by the occurrence of disease in twins and a clustering of cases in families. Repair begins with ingrowth from adjacent healthy tissue of blood vessels, fibroblasts and macrophages which remove the necrotic debris and reconstitute the marrow stroma with formation of woven bone. Necrotic bone is partially removed by osteoclasts.

71.3 Pathophysiology

Skeletal infarction may result from destruction, obstruction or compression of blood vessels. Haematopoietic cells are most sensitive to hypoxia and acidosis and die usually within 12 h after removal of blood supply. Bone cells die within 2 days and adipocytes within 5 days. After reperfusion, repair of ischaemic bone occurs in three phases:

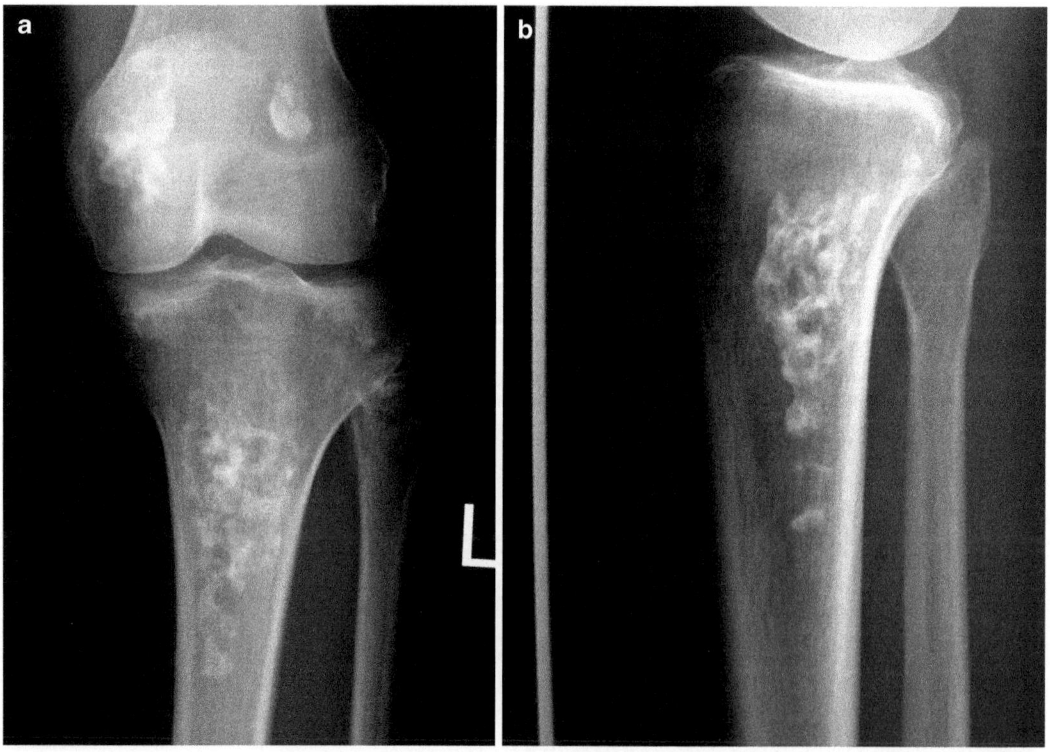

Fig. 71.1 (**a**, **b**) Medullary infarcts of the femur and tibia. (**a**, **b**) Calcification of the necrotic fatty tissue results in serpiginous, well-demarcated smoke ring patterns

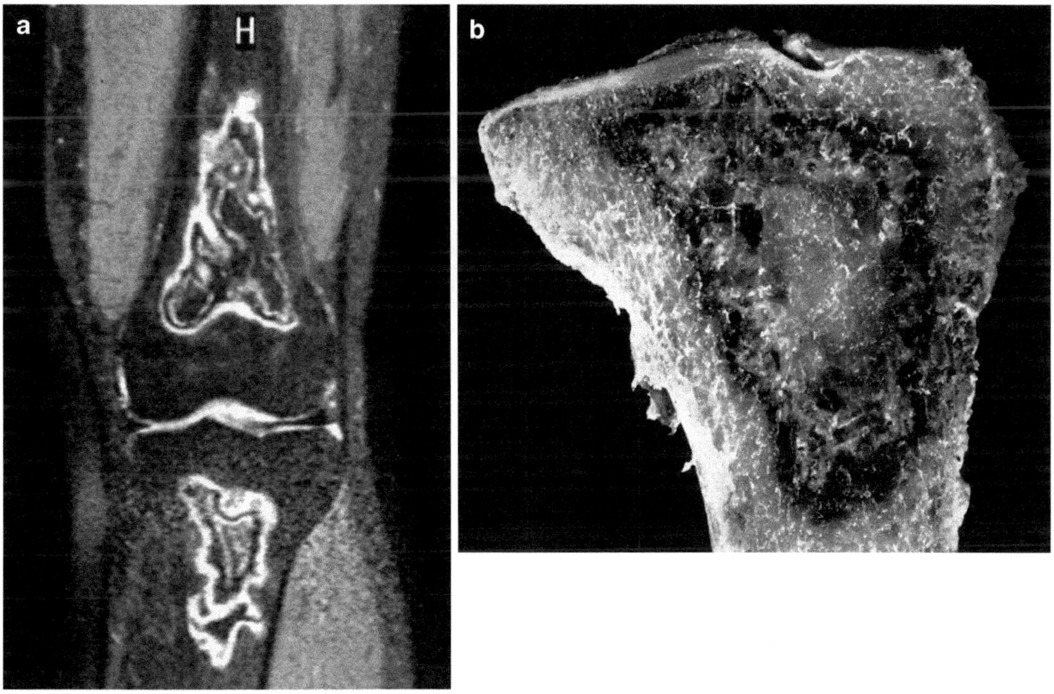

Fig. 71.2 (**a**, **b**) Acute medullary infarct of the knee: (**a**) MRI (T_2 weighted) of an acute medullary infarct of the distal femur and proximal tibia. (**b**) Acute medullary infarct of the epi- and metaphysis of the tibia under systemic corticosteroid therapy. With kind permission of Springer, from [28].

- Movement of undifferentiated mesenchymal cells, macrophages (osteoclasts) and monocytes into the dead marrow tissue
- Angiogenesis with production of small vessels and fibres
- Cellular differentiation to bone cells and fibroblasts

Arteries of the bone may be interrupted by various mechanisms:

- Trauma, fracture and joint dislocation
- Infiltrative processes
- Vascular occlusion
- Diabetes mellitus
- Associated diseases
- Osteochondroses
- Radiation osteonecrosis

Many conditions are associated with osteonecrosis, and a summary of related conditions is given in Table 71.1.

Table 71.1 Causes of osteonecrosis

Endocrine and metabolic
Ethanol abuse
Cushing's disease
Diabetes mellitus
Hyperuricaemia
Hyperlipidaemia
Drugs
Storage disorders
Haemoglobinopathies
Trauma
HIV
Dysbaric conditions
Collagen vascular disorders
Irradiation
Pancreatitis
Organ transplantation
Haemodialysis
Burns
Intravascular coagulation
Idiopathic

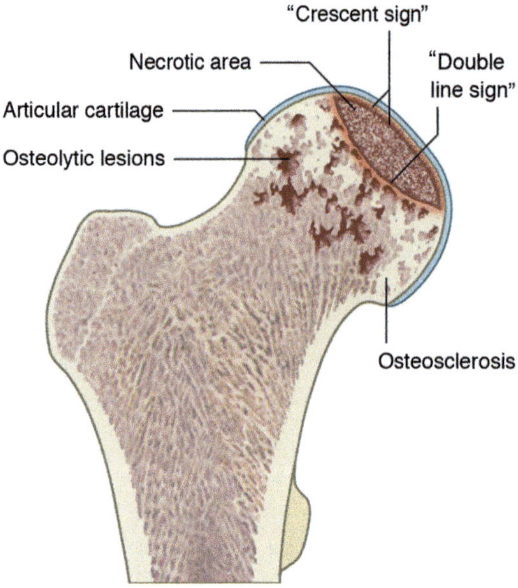

Fig. 71.3 Osteonecrosis of the femoral head

Table 71.2 Staging of osteonecrosis

Stage	Findings	Diagnostic methods
0	All methods non-diagnostic, necrosis on biopsy	Biopsy
1	Radiographs and CT normal, positive results from at least one method listed opposite	Bone scan, MRI, biopsy
2	Radiographic abnormalities without collapse (sclerosis, cysts, osteopenia)	Bone scan, MRI, bone biopsy, radiographs
3	"Crescent sign"	Radiographs, CT
4	Flattening or evident collapse	Radiographs, CT
5	As for stage 4, with narrowing of joint space	Radiographs
6	As for stage 5, with destruction of joint	Radiographs

Trauma may interrupt the blood supply and cause skeletal infarction. Two important situations are typical for this type of bone infarction:

- *Necrosis of the femoral head* is usually caused by intracapsular femoral neck fracture (Fig. 71.3). It is the most important clinical syndrome of bone infarction and often leads to significant disability. Lateral epiphyseal vessels, branches of the arteria profunda femoris, are lacerated following displaced femoral neck fracture. The amount of necrosis varies, depending on the degree of displacement, and in some cases the entire femoral head dies and collapse within some months. The clinical evolution of osteonecrosis of the hip may be divided into various stages (Table 71.2). Other bones prone to develop osteonecrosis after fracture are the talus and the carpal navicular.
- *Osteochondrosis dissecans* usually affects adolescents. Joint trauma with damage to the cartilage and subchondral bone and hypoperfusion of the bone tissue are discussed as main mechanisms. The medial femoral condyle and the medial dome of the talus are the most common sites of osteochondrosis dissecans (OD) (Figs.71.4a, b and 71.5a, b). The radiologic features of osteochondrosis dissecans are diagnostic: a cup-shaped radiolucent defect with a sclerotic rim, adjacent to the articular surface. This defect may enlarge owing to cystic changes in the adjacent trabecular bone.

Infiltrative processes in bone such as infections or tumours (primary as well as metastatic) destroy or compress the blood vessels, and the bone area supplied by these vessels then dies and becomes necrotic ("sequestrum").

Vascular occlusion also causes ischaemic bone disease called "skeletal infarction", until some years ago also called "idiopathic necrosis", "aseptic necrosis" or "avascular necrosis". Unlike infarcts in other organs such as the heart or brain, which are caused by arteriosclerotic occlusion, osteonecrosis of bone results from intravascular coagulation in small arteries or venules. This type of osteonecrosis can occur anywhere in any bone. However, the subchondral regions of the femoral head, distal femur, proximal humerus, talus and scaphoid are frequently involved. In addition to the subchondral regions, the medullary canal in the shafts of long bones may also become infarcted. Aseptic necrosis rarely occurs in healthy patients, and usually an underlying medical problem is present:

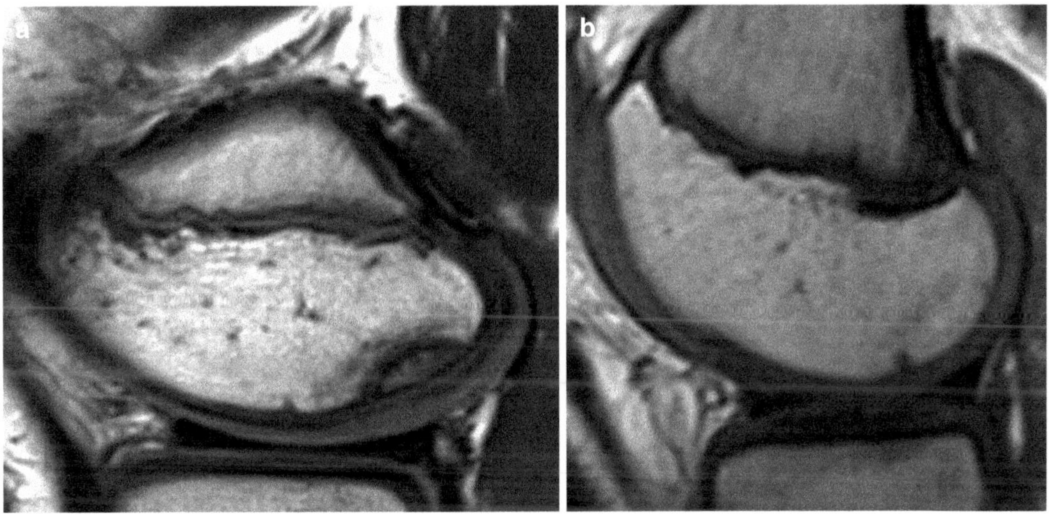

Fig. 71.4 (**a**, **b**) Osteochondrosis dissecans of the femoral condyle: (**a**) before treatment, (**b**) after surgical treatment with drilling

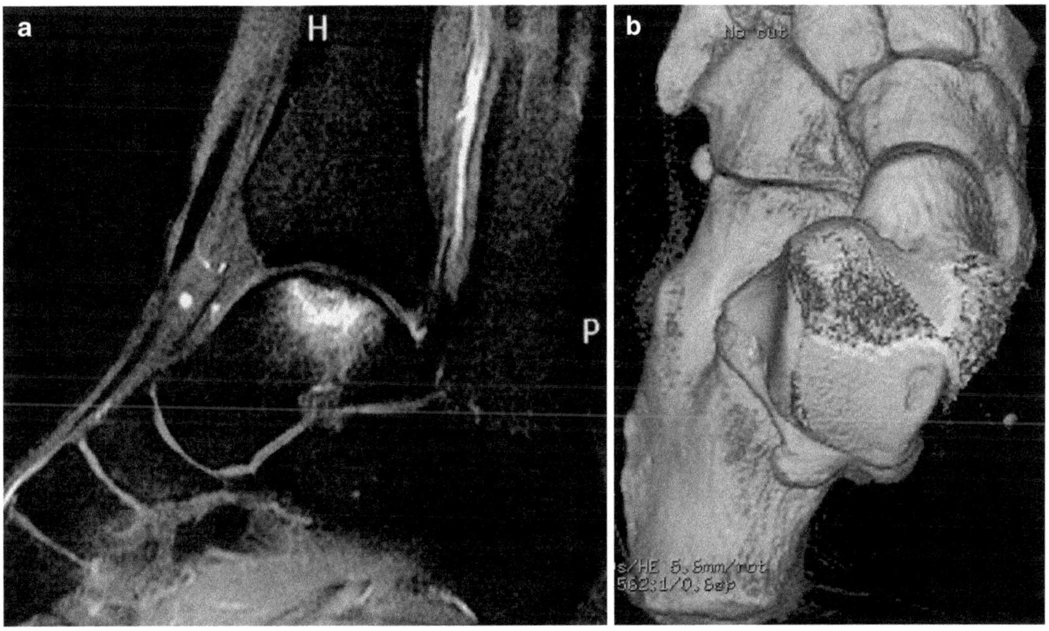

Fig. 71.5 (**a**, **b**) Osteochondrosis dissecans of the talus

- Intravascular coagulation (DIC)
- Vascular stasis
- Fat embolisation (hyperlipidaemia)
- Increased intraosseous pressure (bone marrow oedema or haemorrhage)
- Hypercoagulability of blood (hypofibrinolysis)

A wide range of *associated diseases* predispose patients to osteonecrosis:

- Alcoholism
- Excessive steroid therapy
- Chemotherapy

- Decompression sickness (Caisson disease)
- Vascular compression
- Haemoglobinopathies (e.g. sickle cell anaemia)
- Storage diseases (e.g. Gaucher's disease)
- HIV
- Pancreatitis
- Diabetes mellitus
- Gout
- Collagen vascular disorders (e.g. SLE)
- Vasculitis and hypertension
- Organ transplantation
- Burns
- Haemodialysis
- Damage from radiation, bisphosphonates or denosumab
- Idiopathic, familiar

Alcoholism accounts for about 10 % of cases with osteonecrosis. Chronic alcohol intake predisposes to bone infarction by interference with lipid metabolism, hypofibrinolysis, fat embolism and fatty liver. In alcoholics, the femoral head is the most common site of bone infarction.

Patients receiving *steroids* are also at risk of developing osteonecrosis, and many of these patients are also predisposed to fat embolism. The risk of osteonecrosis correlates with the amount of steroids; however, the critical dose and duration are difficult to define, because the susceptibility of steroid-induced bone necrosis varies from patient to patient. The smallest reported dose was 16 mg of prednisone for 30 days. High doses of steroids are used for systemic erythematosus, asthma, multiple sclerosis, rheumatoid arthritis, polymyalgia rheumatic, inflammatory bowel disease and immunosuppression following renal transplantation, and as many as 40 % of these patients develop bone infarcts. Many locations of the skeleton are involved: the femoral head, distal femur, proximal humerus and tibia. Often the medullary shafts of femur and tibia are involved, and as many as 90 % of patients with osteonecrosis have multiple sites of involvement.

Individuals who work in environments of compressed air such as divers and caisson workers also have a high risk developing bone infarction: *dysbaric osteonecrosis*. Rapid decompression allows nitrogen in the tissues to come out of solution and form bubbles, which disrupt fat cells in the marrow and lead to fat embolism.

Subarticular and medullary bone necroses have also been reported in patients with *sickle cell disorders*, occurring in about 50 % of patients. The sickled red cells cause capillary sludging and vascular thrombosis. The acute bone infarcts may be difficult to distinguish from acute osteomyelitis. However, bone infarction is at least 50 times more common in these patients than bacterial osteomyelitis, a further complication of this disorder. A variety of *other disorders* predispose to osteonecrosis. These include:

- Gaucher's disease
- Pancreatitis
- Diabetes mellitus
- Collagen vascular diseases
- Leukaemias
- Gout

Radiation osteonecrosis, a rare disorder, is now almost exclusively seen after external beam radiation therapy for malignant neoplasias. Bone damage occurs in about 5 % of patients treated with this modality. The affected bone may have been the target of radiation, or normal bone was included in the radiation field for treatment of a visceral tumour. The degree of bone damage is dependent from the type of irradiation, the dose and the method of administration. Bone damage does not occur below 3000 rads, but doses above 5000 rads cause permanent bone damage. Osteonecrosis does not usually manifest until 5–10 years after radiotherapy. Pathologic fractures and collapse of joint surfaces are frequent complications. Although any bone can be affected in the irradiation field, certain areas are common: mandibular involvement followed by irradiation of oral cancer; the ribs, clavicle and humerus after treatment of breast or lung tumours; and the pelvis and proximal femurs after irradiation of rectal, prostate or gynaecologic cancers. Long bones adjacent to irradiated soft tissue or osseous sarcomas may be severely affected. In children, the growth plates are also damaged and result in skeletal deformities. The early hallmark of osseous necrosis is marked bone marrow oedema and the loss of osteocytes

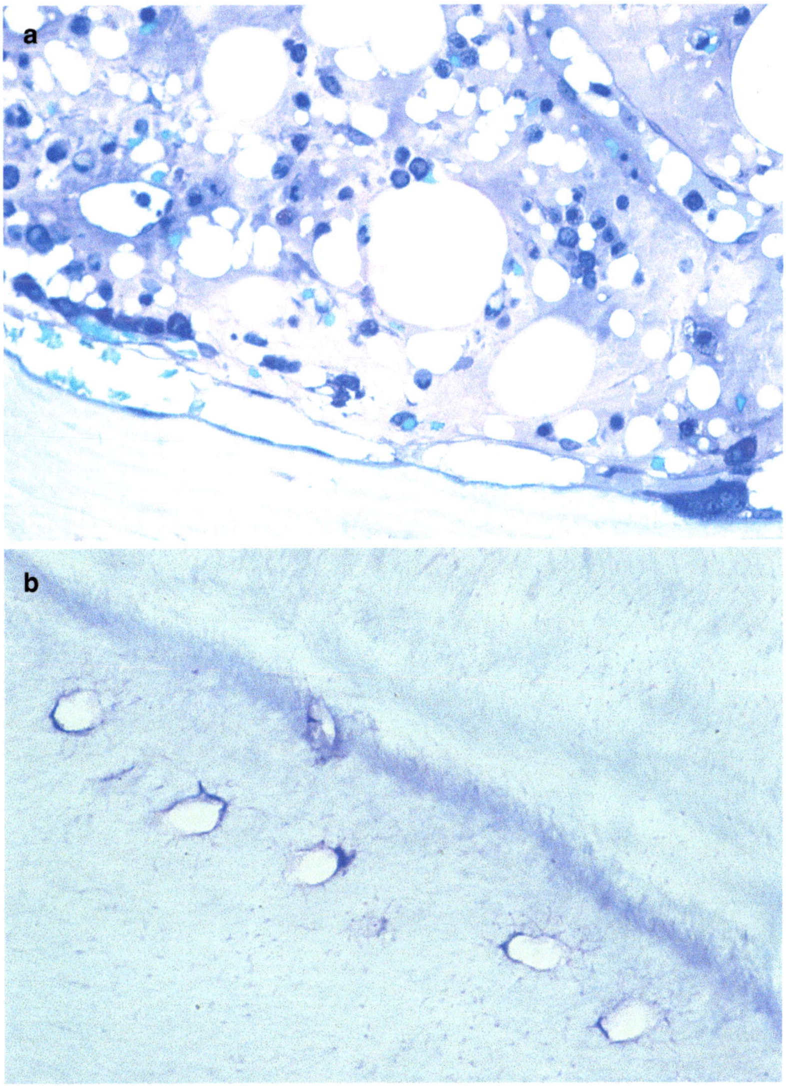

Fig. 71.6 (**a**, **b**) Early radiation damage of bone and marrow tissue: (**a**) marked bone marrow oedema with loss of haematopietic cells, (**b**) death of osteocytes after irradiation of the bone

("osteocyte death") (Fig. 71.6a, b). Loss of nuclear staining of bone cells may be detected within a few days, but empty osteocytic lacunae in the affected trabeculae are rarely seen until a week after the ischaemic or toxic event. The mineral density and trabecular structure may remain unaltered for weeks, so that radiologic alterations do not occur this time. The first radiographic feature is osteopenia, which develops 5 months to 1 year after therapy. Also the bone scan in radiation osteodysplasia shows no increased uptake of radioisotope. The repair reaction begins with the removal by phagocytosis of necrotic tissue from the marrow spaces. Proliferating capillaries and fibroblasts reconstitute the marrow stroma. Some woven bone is formed in the intertrabecular spaces near the necrotic areas. The pathologic fractures resulting from irradiation heal slowly and often require internal fixation. Collapsed necrotic femoral heads are best treated by total joint arthroplasty. The development of postradiation sarcomas is rare (0.2 % in patients who have received up to 7000 rads).

71.4 Osteochondroses

The *osteochondroses* are a heterogeneous group of epiphyseal and apophyseal disorders affecting children and adolescents. Radiologically, they are defined by bone fragmentation and surrounding sclerosis and are believed to be manifestations of osteonecrosis. Trauma to the vulnerable growing bone may be the main cause of these syndromes. Of at least 30 syndromes at particular sites of the skeleton, four disorders are characterised by osteonecrosis (Table 71.3):

Table 71.3 Types, locations and age distribution of frequent epiphyseal osteonecroses

Type of necrosis	Skeletal site	Age of manifestation (years)
Calvé	Vertebra	1–12
Scheuermann	Vertebra	14–17
Perthes	Femoral head	6–16
Kienböck	Carpal lunate	14–18
Osgood-Schlatter	Tibial apophysis	12–17
Köhler I	Os naviculare pedis	3–8
Köhler II	Os metatarsale II	12–18

- Legg-Calvé-Perthes disease (capital femoral epiphysis)
- Freiberg's disease (metatarsal II head)
- Köhler's disease (tarsal navicular)
- Kienböck's disease (carpal lunate)

Two other osteochondrotic syndromes, Osgood-Schlatter disease (apophysitis of the tibial tuberosity) and Scheuermann's disease (vertebral endplates), are not characterised by necrotic bone (Fig. 71.7). Scheuermann's disease is now recognised to be caused by herniation of intervertebral disc material into the vertebral body. Isolated herniations of vertebral disc material are known as Schmorl's nodes, common in elderly patients with osteoporosis. In contrast, Scheuermann's disease affects adolescents between the ages of 13 and 17, and the process is multifocal. A family history of this disorder is present in 25 % of cases, suggesting a heritable weakness of the vertebral endplates in these patients. Radiographically this disorder is characterised by irregular or disrupted endplates with adjacent lytic lesions.

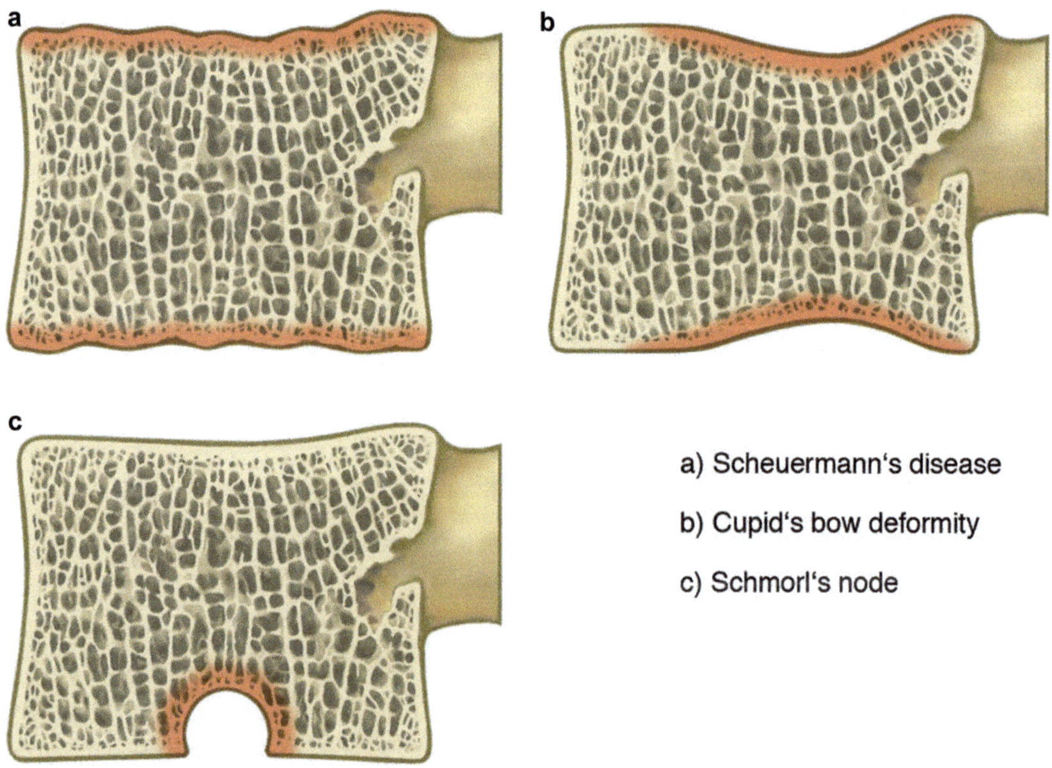

Fig. 71.7 Types of vertebral deformities

The vertebral bodies become wedged; the disc spaces are narrowed especially in the anterior zone and resulting in varying degrees of kyphosis. Involvement of at least three contiguous vertebrae is required to establish the diagnosis.

71.5 Diagnosis

In the early stages, MRI and bone scans are diagnostic and most sensitive, but X-rays of avascular necrosis in the early stages can be normal for months or even years after the onset of symptoms. Early X-ray signs include subtle osteoclerosis and local bone loss. The femoral head may show subchondral lucency (the "crescentic sign"), followed by bone collapse and arthrotic changes. A CT scan may be useful to quantify the degree of bone collapse, which may predict the response to treatments. Bone scan discloses skeletal reconstitution with or without fracture.

71.6 Treatment

The degree of disability that results from osteonecrosis depends on the following questions:

- Which bone is affected?
- What part of the bone is affected?
- How large is the area involved?
- How effectively the bone rebuilds itself?
- How effectively will be the treatment with drugs or core decompression?

If left untreated, the healing processes will be ineffective, and the osseous tissue breaks down faster than the repair mechanisms can build up new bone. The disease will progress, the bone tissue collapses, and the joint surface will be damaged leading to arthritis and massive pain. Medical treatment of ischaemic bone disease includes non-weight-bearing for osteonecrosis affecting load-bearing bones, vasoactive drugs such as prostacyclin and especially intravenous N-containing bisphosphonates (ibandronate or zoledronate) to reduce the surrounding oedema and to prevent the collapse in early stage of osteonecrosis. Surgical treatment includes core decompression to reduce the intramedullary pressure within the ischaemic bone and so improving circulation. Endoprosthetic replacement is the procedure of choice in patients with advanced joint destruction.

Infections of Bone

72

72.1 Definition

Infections of bone are known as *osteomyelitis* and are usually caused by bacteria, although they may result from many other microorganisms such as mycobacteria or fungi. Locations in children and adults are illustrated in Fig. 72.1.

The clinical syndrome associated with the initial invasion of microorganisms is called *acute osteomyelitis*.

> About 80 % of osteomyelitis cases result from contiguous spread or from open wounds and is often polymicrobial.

If the acute osteomyelitis remains subclinical and the defence mechanisms of the patients confine the infection to a local area of the bone, the situation is called *subacute osteomyelitis*. Microorganisms find their way into bone by two mechanisms:

- "Haematogenous osteomyelitis" via the bloodstream from an origin elsewhere in the body
- "Secondary osteomyelitis" via direct invasion from an open fracture or an adjacent tissue infection (dermatitis, tonsillitis, otitis media)

Osteomyelitis without immediate diagnosis and therapy has two main consequences for the patients:

- The infection destroys the bone, with the consequence of instability and fractures of the bone involved.
- Reactive bone alterations insulate the microorganisms and make the eradication of the infection extremely difficult.

If the infection cannot be completely cured, the continuous interaction of microbial growth and bone reaction results in *chronic osteomyelitis*.

> Common symptoms of osteomyelitis are localised bone pain and tenderness with or without constitutional symptoms. Diagnosis is made by radiography and cultures. Treatment is with antibiotics and surgery.

72.2 Haematogenous Bacterial Osteomyelitis

This type of blood-borne bone infection is usually caused by *Staphylococcus aureus* (about 90 %) and almost always begins in the metaphyseal region of long bones. Patients are usually children younger than 15 years. Five steps are distinguished in the development of this type of osteomyelitis:

- Fenestrated capillaries in the metaphysis permit organisms to pass from the blood to the

R. Bartl, C. Bartl, *Bone Disorders*, DOI 10.1007/978-3-319-29182-6_72

Fig. 72.1 Locations of osteomyelitis in (**a**) children and (**b**) adults

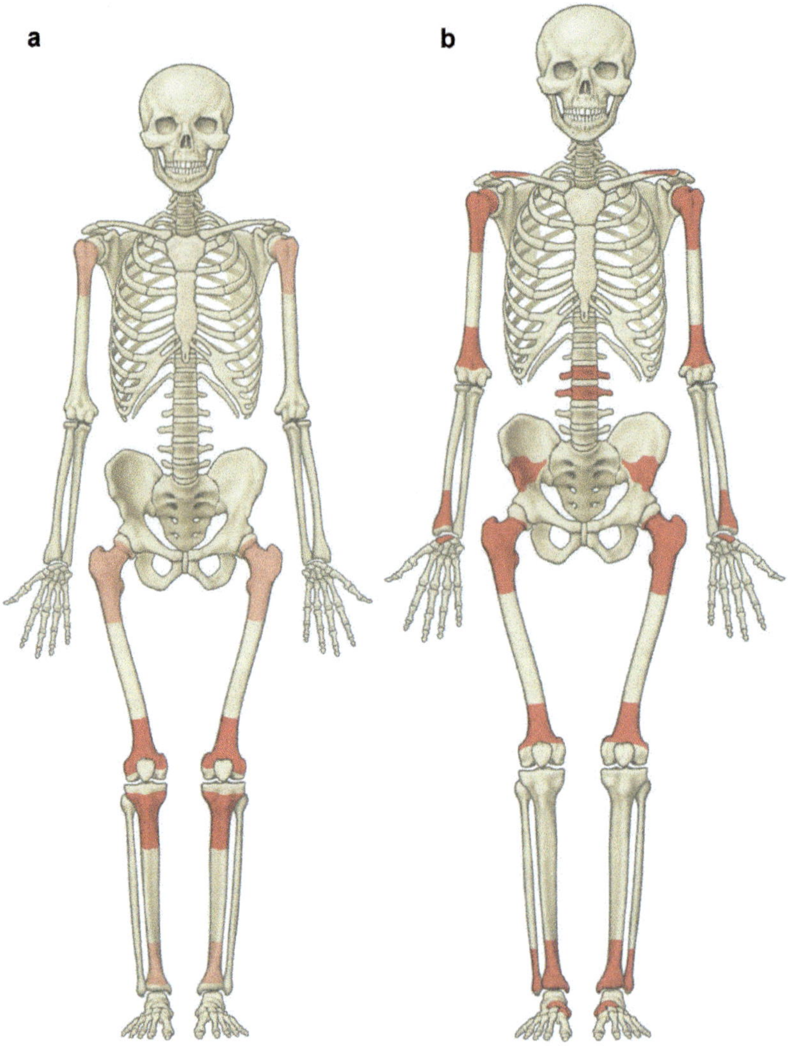

marrow and to the bone surface. Especially *Staphylococcus aureus* has receptors to bone surface such as sialoprotein and collagens.
- After initial binding, bacteria secrete a coat of mucopolysaccharides, which causes a tight adhesion to bone and favours bacterial survival by inhibiting phagocytosis by immune cells and penetration of antibiotics.
- Cytokines released from immune cells activate osteoclasts to resorb bone.
- In addition to osteoclastic bone destruction subperiosteal abscesses disrupt blood vessels and cause segmental cortical necrosis ("sequestra").
- The periosteum, which has an external blood supply, remains viable and produces reactive new bone and encases the abscess and the sequestra.

In the usual presentation of *acute osteomyelitis*, children and young adults present with fever, bone pain and loss of function of the joint involved. Severe local bone tenderness together with a septic or sterile effusion in the joint is a characteristic sign of osteomyelitis. Laboratory evaluation shows a marked leucocytosis and an elevated erythrocyte sedimentation rate (or an increased CRP).

The bone scan is a very sensitive indicator of acute osteomyelitis and is positive already within 2–4 days after the onset of symptoms. However, the bone scan is nonspecific, and similar changes can be caused also by neoplasms. The plain radiograph is more specific, but the changes are not apparent until 10–14 days after the onset of symptoms. The first change is usually a poorly defined lytic region in the metaphysis. Later, a sequestrum appears as a sclerotic area within the region of bone destruction. The amount of periosteal new bone parallels to the amount of bone destruction. Adults develop osteomyelitis in long bones, and the abscess is often intracortical with intracortical lucency on X-rays. The treatment of acute osteomyelitis requires extensive antibiotic therapy and in most cases surgical drainage of pus. A needle aspiration and biopsy at the site of maximum bone tenderness should be made to isolate the organisms for microbiological studies. Parenteral administration of tested antibiotics for at least 4–6 weeks is usually necessary to obtain an acceptable rate of cure, followed by an oral antibiotic therapy.

Occasionally, patients may be asymptomatic with vague pain and low-grade fever for months. This syndrome is known as *subacute osteomyelitis* or *Brodie's abscess*. Radiographs show a well-delineated metaphyseal lytic area surrounded by a sclerotic rim of new bone. It is most commonly seen in the tibia. MRI and CT scans are also useful for diagnosis.

Chronic osteomyelitis is the long-term infection of bone due to failure to eradicate osteomyelitis (Fig. 72.2). Most cases of chronic osteomyelitis result from open fracture-related secondary osteomyelitis. In fact, about 5 % of open fractures result in this syndrome. The progression usually becomes clinically evident within 1 year of the primary infection. The characteristic feature is a smouldering bone destruction and sequestration. The dead bone fragments harbour the microorganisms and protect them against both host defence mechanisms and antibiotics. Clinically, patients have episodes of pain accompanied by the extrusion of sequestra and pus from bone to the skin. In less than 1 % of the cases, sinus tracts may develop squamous cell carcinoma. Radiographs show signs of bone destruction and repair that alter the shape of the bone contour. A CT may be helpful to localise the sequestra. Chronic osteomyelitis always requires aggressive surgical treatment. Removal of all infected bone and soft tissue and reconstruction of resulting tissue defects are necessary.

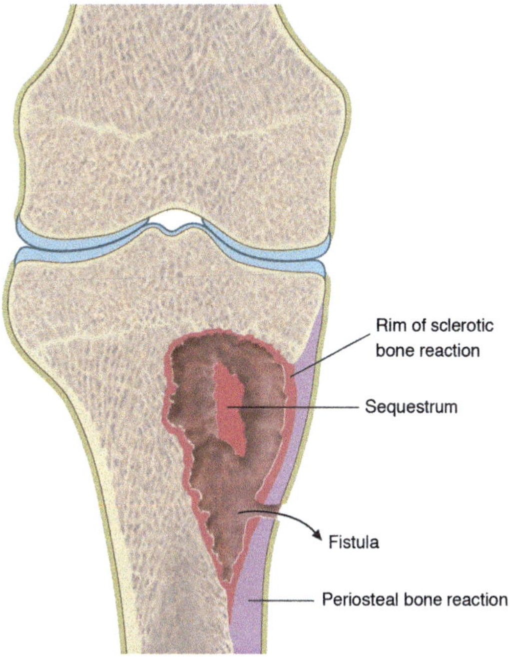

Fig. 72.2 Chronic osteomyelitis with central lytic zone, sequestrum with fistula and extensive periosteal bone reaction

72.3 Secondary Osteomyelitis

Secondary osteomyelitis may be caused by an adjacent soft tissue infection, a contaminated open fracture, decubitus of a diabetic patient or a complication of puncture or bone surgery. Any bone may be invaded by microorganisms. This type of osteomyelitis often presents diagnostic problems, and a bone biopsy with a microbiologic culture is the only way to establish the diagnosis.

72.4 Vertebral Osteomyelitis

Unlike haematogenous osteomyelitis of childhood and young adults, which typically affects the metaphyseal region of long bones, in adults usually the spine is involved, also called *spondylitis*. Microorganisms invade the vertebrae via arterial blood or via backflow through the venous plexus of Batson. Infection begins in the endplates and then erodes the disc spaces and the vertebral bodies. As in children, *Staphylococcus aureus* is the most common agent, but also gram-negative organisms are often the causative agent. Common risk factors are genitourinary tract surgery and infection, diabetes mellitus or intravenous drug abuse. The main clinical feature is back pain and tenderness. An increased level of CRP is often a critical laboratory test. The most diagnostic radiographic feature of vertebral osteomyelitis is narrowing of the disc space and destruction of the adjacent vertebral endplates, helping to distinguish from neoplasm or osteoporotic compression fracture. CT and MRI are very sensitive in early detection of vertebral infection.

72.5 Osteomyelitis in Patients at Risk

Five groups of patients are at higher risk of developing symptomatic osteomyelitis:

- Patients with *acquired immunodeficiency syndrome* (AIDS), which develop bone infections with a wide range of organisms including fungal and mycobacterial species. Infections occur in the end stage of disease, often with a fulminant course.
- Patients on long-term *haemodialysis* also have an increased frequency of osteomyelitis, often due to a bacteraemia originating in infected catheters. Bone pain may also be attributed to renal osteopathy in end-stage renal disease.
- Patients with *sickle cell anaemia* are also at risk of developing osteomyelitis due to repeated episodes of sepsis caused by micro-infarction of the gut. Osteomyelitis may be extremely difficult to distinguish from bone infarction, a frequent complication of this haematologic disease. Positive blood cultures and a subperiosteal abscess on ultrasound favour the diagnosis of osteomyelitis.
- *I.V. drug abusers* often show unusual locations of infection, for example, the symphysis pubis ("osteitis pubis") and the sternocostal and sternoclavicular joints.
- Patients with *diabetes mellitus* and deep decubitus ulcers are predisposed to osteomyelitis.

72.6 Specific Infections of Bone

Tuberculosis with involvement of bone and joints results from dissemination from the primary lesion, which in half of these patients is the lung. About 5 % of patients with tuberculosis have bone or joint involvement. Three main presentations are observed:

- Involvement of the spine, also known as "tuberculous spondylitis". Two thirds of patients with vertebral collapse develop kyphosis, which may result in paraplegia ("Pott's disease").
- Involvement of the hip and knee, also known as "tuberculous arthritis".
- Involvement of the bones of hands and feet.

There are five features that favour a diagnosis of skeletal tuberculosis:

- It is not uncommon in children,
- Its clinical manifestations usually develop slowly and insidiously.
- It is particularly likely to appear in the spine, hip and knee.
- The involvement in large joints is usually monoarticular.
- If more than one joint is affected, the contralateral joint is almost never affected.

The main complaints and findings are:

- Mild to severe pain, especially in the hip and cervical spine
- Swelling due to joint effusion and to thickening of the periarticular tissues

- Local heat without redness of the skin
- Muscle spasm or local muscle atrophy
- Limitations of movement of the joint, especially if the cartilage is eroded
- Local tenderness, especially in diaphyseal tuberculosis
- Local cold abscesses
- A limp in association with coxitis
- Contractures and subluxations of large joints
- Gibbus deformity of the vertebral column

Fungal organisms (*Candida*, *Cryptococcus* and *Aspergillus*) can also cause bone and joint infections, especially in immunocompromised patients or those receiving long-term corticosteroid therapy. Radiologically fungal infections produce nonspecific osteolytic defects, and the spine is the most commonly involved site.

Syphilitic infection of bone is rare, and three manifestations can occur:

- Synovitis
- Periostitis
- Osteomyelitis

In biopsy, lesions show the typical *gumma*, a central necrosis surrounded by chronic inflammation (plasma cells and vasculitis).

Chronic recurrent multifocal osteomyelitis, a syndrome characterised by malaise, bone pain and multiple bone lesions, appears spontaneously over a period of years and is often associated with autoimmune disorders. One definite syndrome is called *SAPHO* and is described in detail in another chapter. The active disease is painful and self-limiting, but may be present for many years.

73 Oral Bone Loss due to Periodontitis and Systemic Osteoporosis

Bone loss in the oral cavity occurs due to many conditions which may be grouped into diseases of bacterial aetiology and oral bone loss associated with systemic disease (e.g. osteoporosis). *Periodontitis* (parodontitis, paradontosis) is an inflammation of the tissues (the gums) surrounding the teeth, which leads to resorption of the alveolar bone and can progress to abscess formation with loosening and shedding of teeth. Inflammation of the gums with loosening of the teeth is a clear indication of an immediate DXA, dental investigation and appropriate treatment.

73.1 Oral Bone Loss and Systemic Osteoporosis

It has been long postulated that oral bone loss may be related to systemic conditions predisposing the patient to osteoporosis. Indeed, some of the same risk factors are present. In postmenopausal women, an association between systemic measures of osteoporosis (DXA of hip and spine) and oral bone mineral density was demonstrated in several studies. There is also evidence that loss of teeth may be related to systemic bone mass. Some studies also reported a relationship between systemic bone loss and residual ridge resorption.

73.2 Pathogenesis of Periodontitis

Periodontal inflammation is due to bacteria in the plaques on the teeth causing inflammatory reactions and resorption of the alveolar bone of the jaws (Fig. 73.1). Matrix metalloproteinases participate in the destruction of the periodontal tissues by splitting extracellular molecules. Mediators of inflammatory reactions such as prostaglandin (PGE_2), interleukin-1 (IL-1) and TNF are also involved in the resorption of the alveolar bone. Other participants in the process are collagenases, macrophages and osteoclasts. The diagnosis usually is not in doubt. Rarely, however a specific cause may be found as, for example, Gorham's disease presenting as an osteolytic lesion confined to the mandible. The patient was successfully treated with the BP zoledronate.

73.3 Clinical Findings

Examination of the inside of the mouth reveals inflammations, possibly even purulent, of the gums leading to resorption of the alveolar bone surrounding the teeth, which are loosened and may fall out on pressure.

R. Bartl, C. Bartl, *Bone Disorders*, DOI 10.1007/978-3-319-29182-6_73

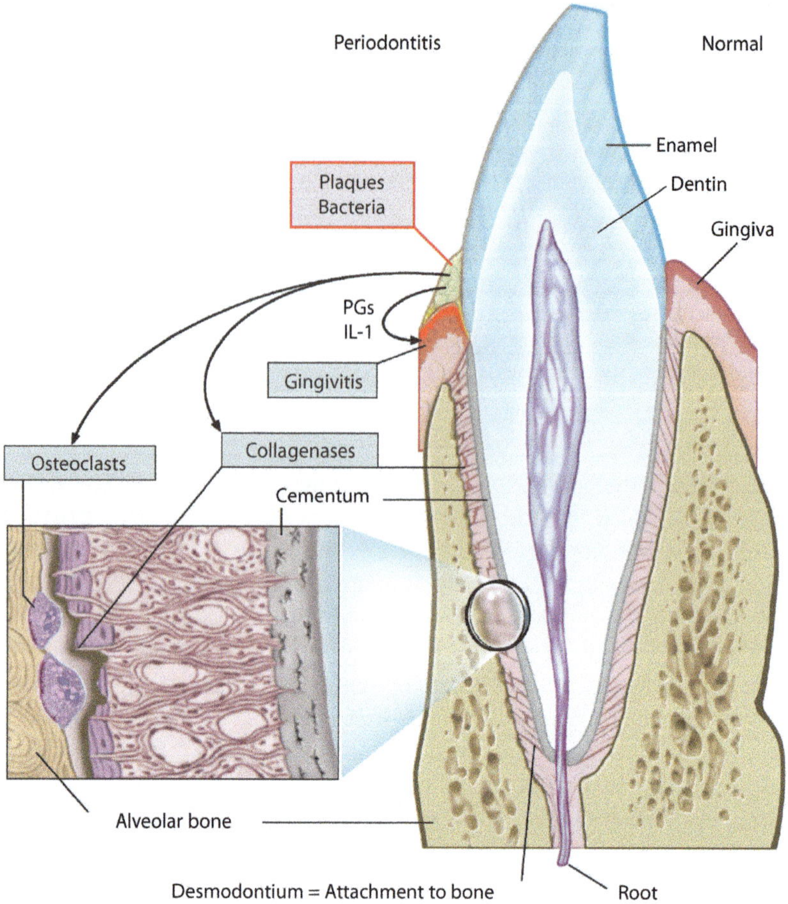

Fig. 73.1 Pathogenesis of alveolar bone loss induced by periodontitis

73.4 Treatment Strategies

Elimination of the dental plaque harbouring the bacteria is an essential prerequisite for successful treatment. This is accomplished by mechanical removal, cleansing and topical application of antibiotics such as tetracycline or metronidazole. Non-steroidal anti-inflammatory drugs decrease the level of prostaglandin in the area of the inflamed gums and thereby reduce the loss of alveolar bone.

BP minimise resorption and loss of alveolar bone in the inflamed areas. They inhibit both osteoclastic activity and collagenases (metalloproteinases). This has been demonstrated in many studies using oral alendronate preparations. Local application of BP in toothpaste has also been tested. Topical application of etidronate decreases plaque formation and thereby also bacterial infections. Many clinical studies have examined a possible connection between systemic osteoporosis and buccal bone loss leading to loosening and loss of teeth. Presumptive mechanisms include the following: all the bones of the skeleton are affected in generalised osteoporosis, including those of the jaws; therefore, a systemic low bone mass in the skeleton includes the jaw bones so that there is a propensity for the teeth to fall out.

Systemic factors which influence systemic bone loss also modify the local tissue reactions to a periodontal infection.

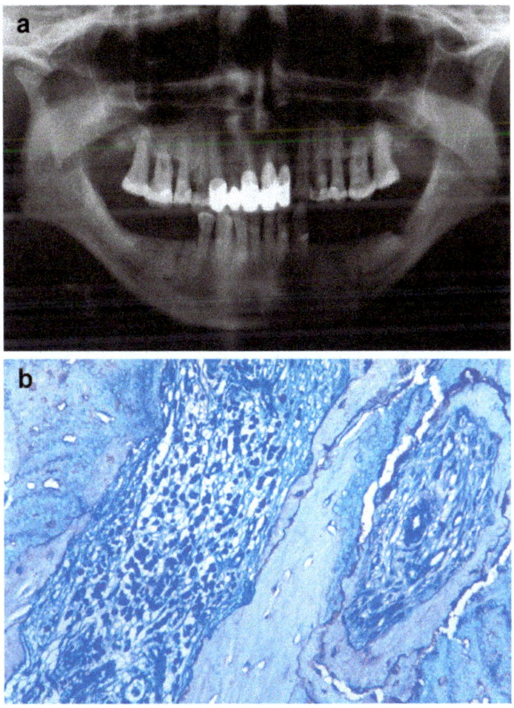

Fig. 73.2 (**a**, **b**) Osteonecrosis of the jaw (ONJ) in a patient with metastatic breast cancer under long-term treatment with IV bisphosphonate: (**a**) X-ray showing necrotic area in the left side of the mandible, (**b**) histology from this area demonstrating necrotic bone tissue with empty osteocytic lacunae and inflammatory reaction in the surrounding marrow, Giemsa staining

Cases of *osteonecrosis of the jaw* have been reported following treatment with high-dose bisphosphonates, almost exclusively in cancer patients treated intravenously, and in the presence of additional risk factors, such as immunosuppression, chemotherapy, corticosteroids and poor oral hygiene (Fig. 73.2a, b). Whereas the majority of BP-associated osteonecrosis of the jaws have been observed in patients receiving high-dose, long-term intravenous BP therapy, only some patients on oral therapy have been reported as case reports. In a study of 335 patients, treatment with alendronate was not associated with a higher incidence of complications secondary to dental procedures, and no cases of osteonecrosis of the jaw were observed. The incidence of tooth loss was decreased more than 40 % in the patients treated with oral alendronate. Therefore, the large number of women routinely taking oral BP and the very small risk of developing osteonecrosis should be considered with due regard for the benefit in retarding alveolar bone loss and treating systemic osteoporosis.

74 Local Osteodysplasias

74.1 Osteopoikilosis

Osteopoikilosis is a hereditary bone disease that causes increased bone density. However, unlike the diffuse bone density of most other sclerosing bone dysplasias, osteopoikilosis is characterised by multiple discrete round or oval radiodensities (*spotted bone disease* or "osteopathia condensans disseminata") (Fig. 74.1a, b). Each lesion is an enostosis, a "bone island". Hundreds of these spots, about 2–5 mm in size, are clustered in epiphyseal and metaphyseal areas of the skeleton and seem to be the result of focal abnormal bone remodelling. The radiodense lesions are scattered symmetrically throughout the skeleton, a feature that helps distinguish this disorder from metastatic carcinoma. The bone tissue in these spots is lamellar and shows evidence of remodelling. These bone lesions are asymptomatic. Some patients with osteopoikilosis have multiple small dermal or subcutaneous fibromas, and the association with these skin lesions suggests an underlying connective tissue disorder.

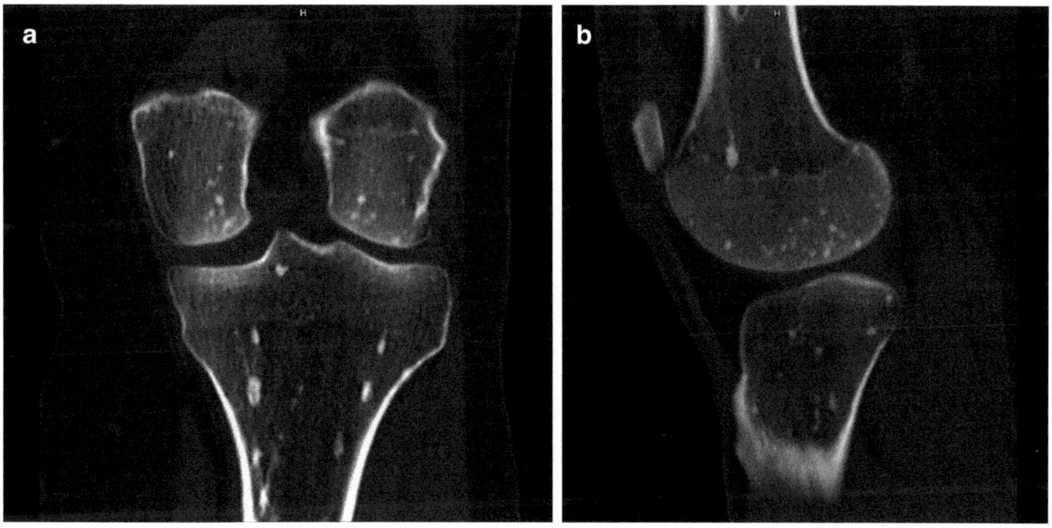

Fig. 74.1 (**a**, **b**) Osteopoikilosis ("spotted bone disease") with multiple discrete round or oval radiodensities

R. Bartl, C. Bartl, *Bone Disorders*, DOI 10.1007/978-3-319-29182-6_74

74.2 Melorheostosis

This form of periostosis (also called "flowing hyperostosis") is derived from the Greek words "melos" (limb) and "rheos" (flow) and describes the characteristic results of bone formations which on the outer side of the affected bones "flow down" *like wax flowing down a candle* (Fig. 74.2). There are at least two adjacent, frequently several bones infected, and, as a general rule, of only one limb. Irregular, dense and eccentric endosteal and periosteal hyperostoses with infestation of one or more bones are found in the X-ray image. The lower limbs are especially affected. These changes are painful, often with neighbouring skin changes, and they increase rapidly in childhood. Surgical correction of contractures is difficult and gives only a temporary pain relief. Figure 8.7 shows an unusually severe bone lesion (maceration preparation) of the femur with bizarre periosteal deposits and calcifications of soft tissues. More rare local dystrophies of the bone are found in specific reference books, cited in the appendix of this book.

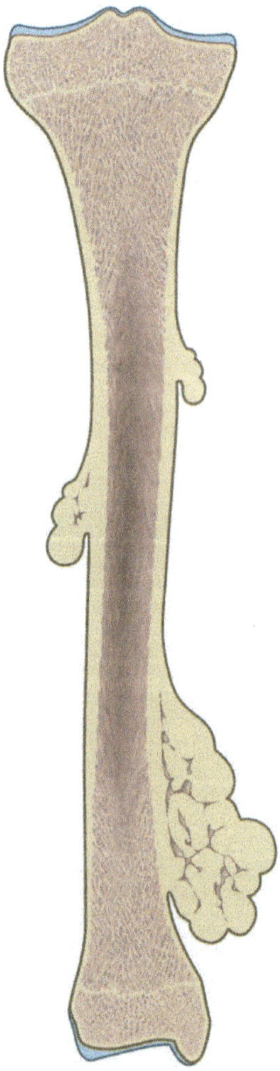

Fig. 74.2 Melorheostosis characterised by painless irregular cortical hyperostoses following the long axis of bone (result of the deposition of periosteal and/or endosteal new bone)

74.3 Dysostoses

Dysostoses are *developmental disorders of individual bones* without evidence of an underlying connective tissue system disease. They are divided into 3 groups according to their *main location*:

- Predominantly cranial and craniofacial involvement (e.g. Apert syndrome)
- Predominantly axial participation (e.g. Klippel-Feil syndrome)
- Predominantly peripheral participation (e.g. Poland syndrome)

Part XIII

Extraskeletal Mineralisation

75 The Patient with "Extraskeletal Mineralisation"

Calcification in soft tissues is caused by deposition of calcium compounds in radiologically detectable quantities. Joints close to soft tissue, fasciae or muscles are affected according to the underlying disease or trauma. This degenerative process is also called *calcification* and *calcinosis*. With migration of fibroblasts and other connective tissue cells into the mineral deposits, an increasing conversion of inorganic calcium compounds to organic bone tissue may occur, together with connective tissue proliferation and mineralisation of the newly produced bone matrix. It is then called an *ossification*.

> The amorphous deposits of calcium-phosphate crystals are termed "calcification". "Ossification" is characterised by formation of true bone in non-osseous soft tissue, partly developing from amorphous mineral deposits. Typical examples are calcifications and ossifications in the shoulder.

Calcinoses or ossifications can be divided into six groups, according to their origin:

- Dystrophic calcifications
- Calcifications in connective tissue diseases (SLE, scleroderma)
- Calcifications in disorders of the mineral homeostasis
- Metastatic calcifications due to increased calcium-phosphate concentrations in the extracellular fluid
- Ectopic calcifications (after burns and muscle injuries)
- Myositis ossificans progressiva

Heterotopic calcifications are observed in the walls of arteries of the bone marrow in patients with arteriosclerosis, primary HPT and renal osteodystrophy (Fig. 75.1). Calcifications may also occur on the heart valves of patients with Marfan syndrome.

Heterotopic ossification occurs mainly in muscles and primarily after trauma, for example, after hip surgery with or without implantation of a prosthesis. It can also occur after shoulder surgery, after brain injury or in paraplegia. Historically, heterotopic ossification was the first of this group for which treatment with a bisphosphonate (etidronate) was successfully tried. *Myositis fibrodysplasia ossificans* is a congenital disorder, and *fibrodysplasia ossificans progressiva* is the severe variant of this genetic disorder. Severe ossification has also been observed in joints and adjacent soft tissues in disseminated idiopathic skeletal hyperostosis (DISH). In *myositis ossificans circumscripta* heterotopic bone

R. Bartl, C. Bartl, *Bone Disorders*, DOI 10.1007/978-3-319-29182-6_75

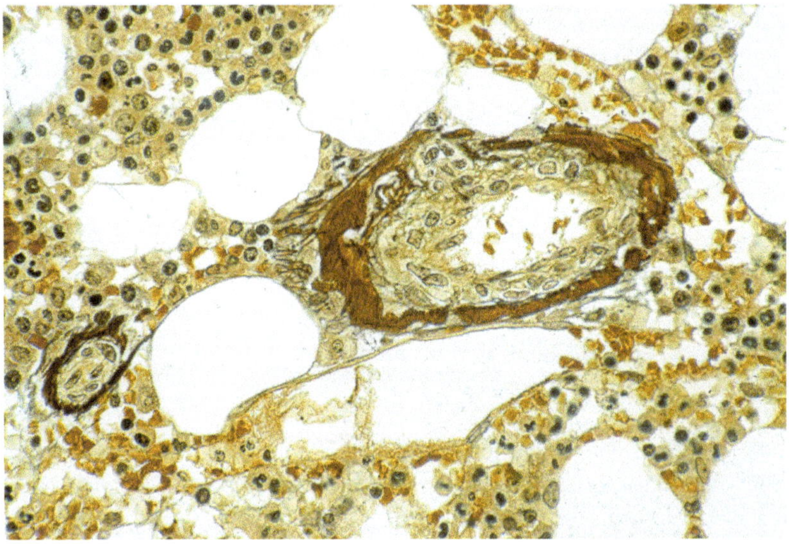

Fig. 75.1 Iliac crest biopsy of a patient with pHPT showing calcification of the walls of a small (*left*) and a large (*right*) arterial blood vessel. Gomori staining

tissue – similar to fracture callus – is found in skeletal muscle following trauma and is characterised by the intramuscular proliferation of fibroblasts, bone tissue and occasionally cartilage. *Neurogenic heterotopic ossification* forms in 25 % of patients paralysed from a spinal cord injury or in patients with closed head trauma.

Heterotopic calcification may be found in vessel walls in arteriosclerosis as well as in primary hyperparathyroidism. It may also occur in the cardiac valves. In the urinary tract, it may result in stone formation and nephrocalcinosis (Table 75.1). Calcification is also observed in calcinosis universalis and dermatomyositis. Some disorders manifest ectopic calcification around or in joints, with normal concentration of calcium and phosphorus. In these cases local tissue factors are important in initiating this *dystrophic calcification*. The main basic disorders are:

- *Ochronosis*, with homogentisic acid depositions in the cartilage.
- Gout, both primary metabolic and secondary (e.g. leukaemia, drugs, renal disease).
- *Pseudogout*, with normal serum uric acid.
- *Scleroderma*, with soft tissue calcification especially at pressure areas (e.g. ischial tuberosities).
- *Tumoral calcinosis*, showing painful, large lobulated calcified swellings about the larger joints. There may be bone atrophy due to pressure on the nearby bone, especially at the elbow.

Table 75.1 Conditions causing nephrocalcinosis

Renal tubular acidosis
Hyperparathyroidism
Idiopathic hypercalciuria
Sarcoidosis
Multiple myeloma
Carcinomatosis
Cushing's syndrome
Hypervitaminosis D

76 Heterotopic Calcifications

76.1 Dystrophic Calcifications

They develop in local tissue lesions. Degenerative, partly necrotic connective tissues with reduced blood flow and acid pH values are a "calcium captor" and store calcium salts at a different rate. The main causes of dystrophic calcification are:

- *Tissue trauma*: Haematoma calcifications seen in roentgenographs as cloudy, amorphous shading may lead to ossifications. Often calcifications arise in inflammatory and degenerative disorders in the area of muscle attachments and bursae. Painful calcifications are found near the joints of shoulder, hip, knee and elbow ("tennis elbow", epicondylitis).
- *Infectious and parasitic disorders*: Abscess calcifications are often found in patients with tuberculosis. Parasites behave like a foreign body causing a calcification in the adjacent soft tissue. Echinococcus cysts and calcifications around these lesions are examples.
- *Tumour calcifications*: *They* may occur in patients with both benign and malignant neoplasias and are not a proof for or against malignancy. Causes of local calcification in tumour tissue are rather reactions like tumour necrosis, inflammation, haemorrhage, circulatory disorders or fatty tissue degeneration. Bone metastases of mucus-forming neoplasias also show a tendency to calcifications.

76.2 Calcifications in Collagen Disorders

Calcifications, an expression of the underlying systemic disease, occur generalised ("calcinosis generalisata") or in localised areas ("calcinosis circumscripta") of the skin or deeper subcutaneous tissue. For differential diagnosis, the spectrum of "connective tissue diseases" must always be taken in consideration.

- *Scleroderma*: 40 % of patients (mainly female patients) with scleroderma develops a calcinosis circumscripta and 32 % of patients a calcinosis generalisata. The crumbly calcifications are mainly localised in periarticular sites; they start in the subcutaneous fatty tissue and later spread into deeper connective tissues and muscles.
- *Dermatomyositis*: Increased intramuscular calcifications are present in adults. "Juvenile dermatomyositis" is an idiopathic inflammatory disease of the skin and muscles together with vasculitis of the small vessels. Muscle weakness and calcifications in necrotic soft tissues are noticeable.
- *Lupus erythematosus*: Occasionally calcifications are found near the joints of the fingers.
- *Raynaud's syndrome*: Calcifications are located in the cutis and subcutis of the acra.
- *Rheumatoid arthritis*: Calcifications are nodular, less dense and periarticular (fingers and toes).

R. Bartl, C. Bartl, *Bone Disorders*, DOI 10.1007/978-3-319-29182-6_76

Ectopic calcification in the fingers is often associated with scleroderma, Raynaud's disease, SLE, dermatomyositis and epidermolysis bullosa. As these cases are accompanied by spasm and narrowing of the small arteries, an insufficient blood supply may lead to bone resorption of the terminal phalanges. Tissue calcification can also occur in hypercalcaemic variants of sarcoidosis.

76.3 Calcifications in Disorders of Mineral Homeostasis

The basis of this group of disorders is an abnormal calcium and/or phosphate level in the serum. Calcifications are very different with respect to size, shape and spreading and allow no conclusions to be drawn concerning the basic disorder.

Soft tissue calcification appears in patients with hyperparathyroidism and while on dialysis. This often occurs in the hand (Fig. 76.1) or shoulder.

Tumour calcinosis is a rare autosomal recessive metabolic disorder, characterised by a progressive deposition of amorphous calcium phosphate crystals in periarticular soft tissues. Biochemically a hyperphosphataemia and elevated levels of 1,25 $(OH)_2$ vitamin D are found with a raised reabsorption of phosphate in the tubules of the kidney. The age of onset is different, usually between 5 and 20 years of age. Round nodes of chalk deposits are found in the periarticular regions (Table 76.1). Basic disorders causing calcifications of the ligaments along the spine are summarised in Table 76.2. Painful deposits may need a surgical removal. For therapy, aluminium hydroxide, calcitonin and bisphosphonates have been used with varying degrees of success. At least, the symptoms can be reduced.

Vitamin D intoxication and milk-alkali syndrome cause generalised calcinosis of the periarticular tissue in various internal organs. Also in patients with primary, secondary and tertiary

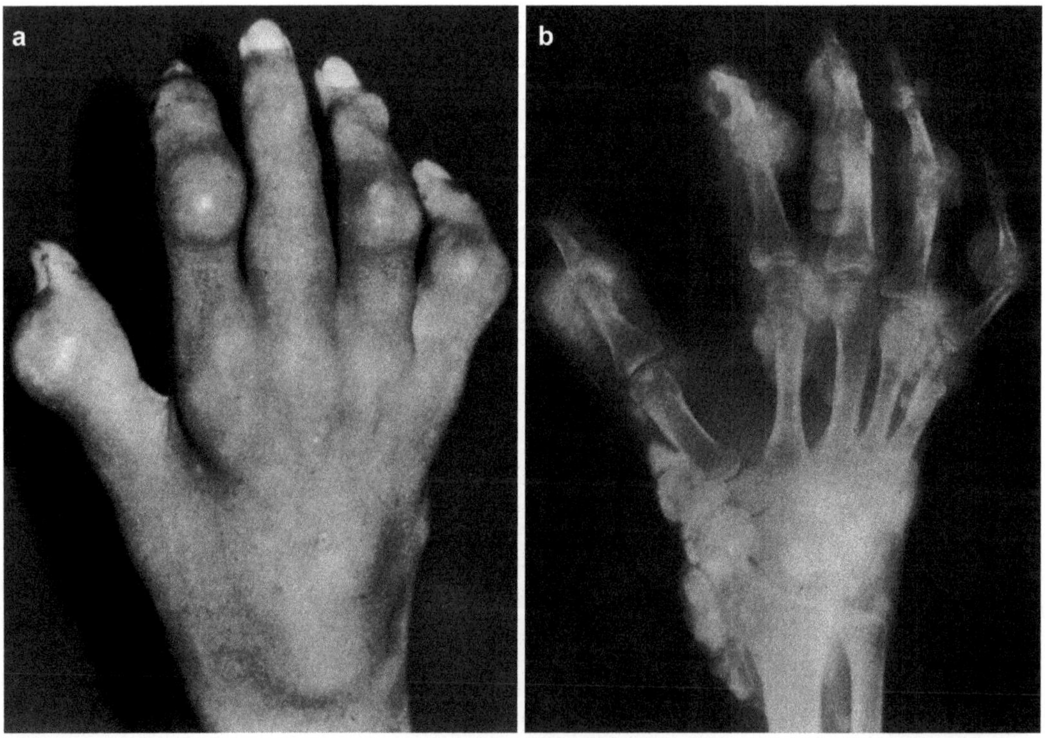

Fig. 76.1 (**a, b**) Severe and multiple soft tissue calcifications in the hands while on dialysis (With kind permission of Springer, from [38])

Table 76.1 Basic disorders with periarticular and intraarticular calcifications

Metastatic calcification
Chronic renal failure
Hyperparathyroidism
Hypervitaminosis D
Dystrophic calcification
Infections (e.g. tuberculosis)
Degenerative
Diabetes mellitus
Ochronosis
Gout
Calcinosis
Pseudogout
Scleroderma
Tumoural calcinosis

Table 76.2 Ligamentous calcification along the spine

Ankylosing spondylitis
Diffuse idiopathic skeletal hyperostosis (DISH)
Spondylarthrosis
Fluorosis
Acromegaly

hyperparathyroidism, soft tissue calcifications may occur as well as calcifications in the walls of small and large arteries.

Lipocalcinogranulomatosis is a system disease of the bursa apparatus on the basis of a calcium metabolism disorder. Storage of cholesterol in the bursa is followed by storage of calcium carbonate and calcium phosphate.

Paraneoplastic hypercalcaemia (bone metastases, multiple myeloma) and *extensive destructive bone disease* (osteomyelitis, osteonecrosis) may also show massive soft tissue calcifications.

76.4 Alkaptonuria (Ochronosis)

Ochronosis is a congenital disorder that indirectly affects the skeleton. This disorder is characterised by black urine and severe arthropathy due to pigment deposition. Large amounts of homogentisic acid are stored in the bone marrow, cartilage, discs, menisci and sclerae. Orthopaedic complications usually begin in early adulthood, and the spine is usually the first region to be affected by pigment depositions. The disc spaces are narrowed and calcified. Involvement of large joints begins later with black ochronotic pigment in the articular cartilage. Ultimately, patients develop severe secondary osteoarthritis with extensive intraarticular calcified loose bodies.

77 Heterotopic Ossifications

77.1 Pathogenesis

"Heterotopic ossification" is also referred to as "heterotopic bone", "ectopic ossification", "myositis ossificans circumscripta" or "fibrodysplasia ossificans progressiva". According to the WHO definition, it is a "non-neoplastic change" following surgery, trauma, burns or neurologic injury. The bone lesion is located on the outer surface of the bone or in soft tissues (muscles) but always at a distance to the periosteum. The abnormal tissue is characterised by a connective tissue proliferation and formation of new bone ("osseous metaplasia"). Three zones are typical:

- In the central zone, fibroblastic tissue with polynuclear cells
- In the middle zone, osteoid
- In the outer zone, increasing maturation with mineralised lamellar bone

Two clinical categories of ectopic ossification ("myositis ossificans") can be distinguished:

- C*ongenital generalised progressive heterotopic ossification* with autosomal dominant inheritance and abnormalities of the skeleton
- A*cquired localised heterotopic ossification* as a result of traumatic brain injury, spinal cord injury, trauma of the musculoskeletal system, after burns or frostbites, after infectious diseases or induced by carcinoma

Further heterotopic ossifications are found *after surgery at the hip joint*, especially after hip replacement. Ossifications are observed in 15–50 % of cases, but in only a few cases, pain and restriction of movement are present. However, massive forms may lead to severe functional limitations.

> Heterotopic bone is observed in four main clinical entities:
>
> - Myositis ossificans circumscripta
> - Head trauma or spinal cord injury
> - Total hip arthroplasty
> - Fibrodysplasia ossificans progressiva

Heterotopic ossifications, joint destructions ("haemophilic arthropathy") and erosive pseudotumours may affect patients with severe haemophilia. In patients with *para- and tetraplegia*, calcifications of the muscles, tendons and joint capsules are observed.

77.2 Treatment Strategies

Unfortunately, no satisfactory treatment is available as yet. Surgical removal of large deposits, non-steroidal anti-inflammatory drugs, radiotherapy, dissolution and local glucocorticoid injections have all been tried. In practice, radiation

R. Bartl, C. Bartl, *Bone Disorders*, DOI 10.1007/978-3-319-29182-6_77

and indomethacin are most commonly used today for therapy of heterotopic calcification. In high-risk patients, the incidence of heterotopic bone can be reduced by prophylactic *low-dose irradiation*. Experimental trials have shown that *bisphosphonates* (BP) inhibit mineralisation and calcification of many soft tissues as well as heterotopic ossification. Unfortunately, they have not been successful in clinical situations, but so far only etidronate has been tested. Prevention of calcification of synthetic heart valves is a possible future application for etidronate. BP could also be considered for prevention of heterotopic ossification using the following protocols:

- Ibandronate: Monthly infusion of 3–6 mg
- Pamidronate: Monthly infusion of 60 mg
- Etidronate: 2 mg daily for a maximum period of 4 months

Higher doses of etidronate should not be given for extended periods because of the risk of osteomalacia. Currently, radiation therapy and indomethacin are the treatments used for heterotopic ossification.

Non-steroidal anti-inflammatory drugs (NSAIDs) and local irradiation (1000 rads in five divided doses) are the classic treatment and prophylaxis options in painful ectopic calcification and ossification.

Part XIV

Drug-Induced Bone Disorders

78 Corticosteroid-Induced Osteoporosis

A detailed drug history is of vital importance, because many drugs and substances can adversely affect the skeleton. A comprehensive list of drugs associated with increased risk for osteoporosis in adults has been outlined by the National Osteoporosis Foundation (Table 78.1).

Table 78.1 Drugs associated with an increased risk of generalised osteoporosis (alphabetical list)

Aluminium antacids
Antibiotics
Anticonvulsants
Antihypertensives
Aromatase inhibitors
Chemotherapeutics
Diuretics
Glucocorticosteroids
GnRH agonists
Heparin
Immunosuppressants
Isoniazid
Lithium
Loop diuretics (e.g. Lasix)
Proton pump inhibitors
Tamoxifen
Thyroid hormone
Warfarin

78.1 Pathogenesis

Steroid-induced osteoporosis is nearly always due to long-term therapy with one of the steroid hormones, only rarely to an endogenous Cushing's syndrome. It should also be stressed that the underlying disorder itself often causes osteoporosis, which is then aggravated by the steroid therapy. Examples are Crohn's disease, rheumatic disorders, collagenoses, organ transplants, bronchial asthma, malignant lymphomas, multiple myeloma and others.

The use of corticosteroids over a period of days or weeks, even in very high doses, will not result in clinically significant bone loss. But bone loss is evident within months of the start of steroid therapy. When treated over long periods of time – possibly years – about 50 % of these patients will suffer from manifest osteoporosis (Fig. 78.1). Continuing bone loss is particularly likely in patients requiring more than 10 mg/day of prednisone. Children, young men and postmenopausal women are particularly vulnerable. A few patients may have an individual sensitivity to corticosteroids. Initial bone density measurement is recommended in all patients so that a baseline is established for later comparison.

Corticosteroid-induced osteoporosis has the following characteristics:

- It occurs in 30–50 % of patients on long-term steroid therapy.
- Osteoporosis affects the trabecular bone; therefore fractures occur preferentially in vertebral bodies, ribs, femoral neck and pelvis (Fig. 78.2).

R. Bartl, C. Bartl, *Bone Disorders*, DOI 10.1007/978-3-319-29182-6_78

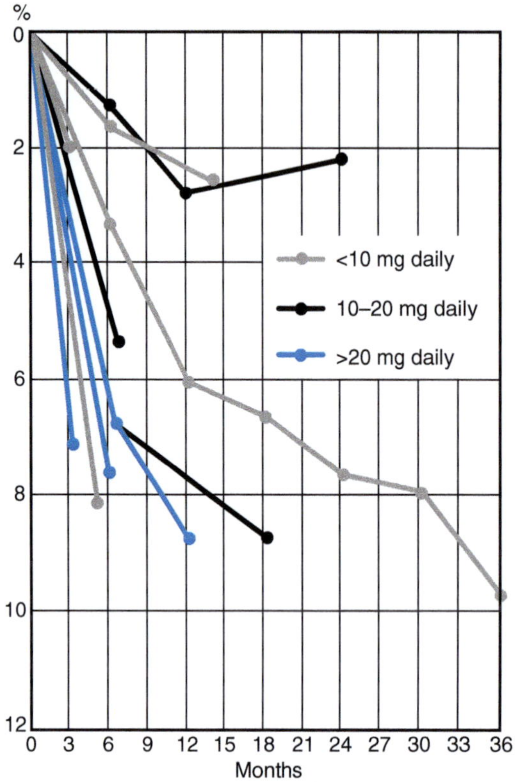

Fig. 78.1 Loss of spinal BMD from start of corticosteroid therapy. Results of ten studies (Modified from van Staa et al. 2002)

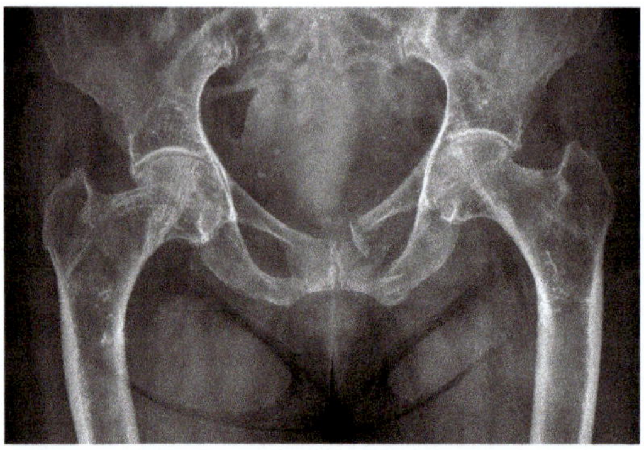

Fig. 78.2 Marked osteoporosis and fractures of the pelvis under long-term glucocorticoid therapy

- The rate bone loss is rapid – "fast losers", "very high turnover osteoporosis". A loss of up to 20 % of the bone mass may occur in the first year of steroid therapy.
- Dramatic bone loss may result from even low doses of prednisone (7.5 mg or its equivalent).

Glucocorticoids have a multifaceted *effect on the bone* (Fig. 78.3):

- Inhibition of osteoblast proliferation, differentiation and function
- Increased apoptosis of osteoblasts
- Stimulation of osteoclastic activity
- Decreased intestinal absorption of calcium
- Increased renal excretion of calcium
- Increased parathormone secretion
- Decreased secretion of calcitonin
- Decrease in number of bone remodelling units
- Occurrence of aseptic bone necroses
- Increased production of collagenases
- Decreased production of corticotropin and gonadotropin

In addition, interactions of glucocorticosteroids with other factors also contribute to the pathogenesis of steroid-induced osteoporosis:

- Increased sensitivity of osteoblasts to PTH and to active vitamin D
- Decreased production of prostaglandin E
- Decreased local production of IGF1
- Effect on IGF-binding proteins

Various guidelines have been recommended for the therapy and prevention of corticosteroid-induced osteoporosis.

> The results of many reviews suggest that the risk of fracture appears shortly after the start of therapy and at relatively low daily doses above 5 mg/day.

It is also likely that the BMD threshold for fractures in corticosteroid-induced osteoporosis differs from that in postmenopausal osteoporosis. Bone loss may be substantially reversible after stopping therapy, and it is independent of underlying disease, age and sex. Patients with

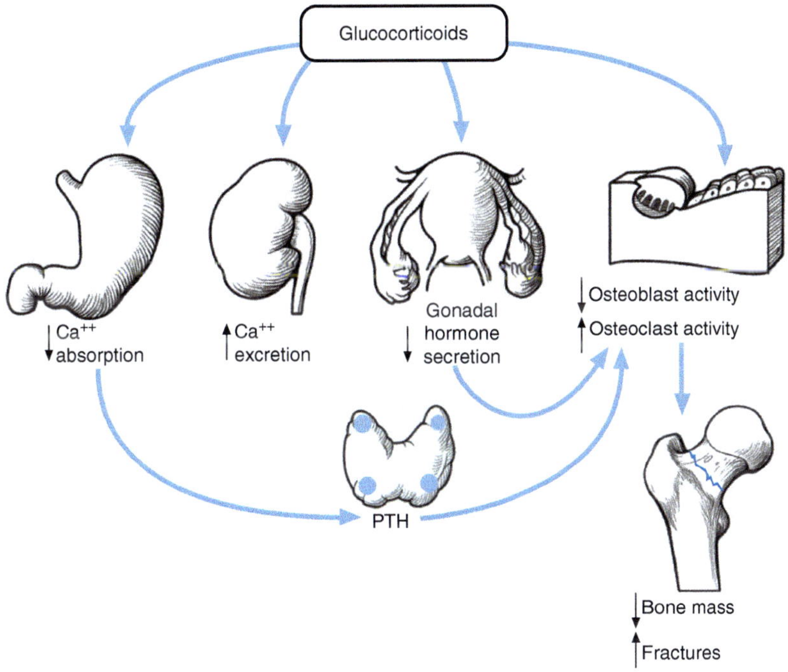

Fig. 78.3 Negative effects of glucocorticoids on calcium homeostasis, on the activity of bone cells and on bone mass

obstructive pulmonary disease showed increases in fracture risk comparable to those of the patients with arthropathies.

Users of *inhalation corticosteroid therapy* (*ICS*) also had higher risks of fracture, but this may be related to the underlying respiratory disease rather than to inhaled corticosteroid therapy. However, a quantitative systematic review has found deleterious effects of ICS on BMD. Budesonide appeared to be the ICS which had the least damaging effects on the bone, followed by beclomethasone dipropionate and triamcinolone.

As a general rule, one can assume that with oral therapy of more than 6 months duration, and at a dose of more than the equivalent of 7.5 mg prednisone/day, a significant loss of bone will occur so that bisphosphonates are indicated for prevention. At higher doses the loss of bone may rise to 15 % or more per annum so that when prescribing glucocorticoids the following *recommendations* should be followed:

- Check for the shortest possible duration of treatment to avoid adrenal cortical atrophy.
- Use glucocorticoids with the shortest half-life.
- Utilise local application whenever possible (creams, sprays, etc.).
- Emphasise physical activity and muscle training.
- Prescribe vitamin D at 1,000 IU daily.
- Make sure the patient ingests 1,000 to 1,500 mg calcium daily with food or supplements.

78.2 Treatment

Therapy of corticosteroid-induced osteoporosis is the same as that of postmenopausal, but early use of preventive measures against corticosteroid-induced osteoporosis is highly recommended. In a recent trial, no difference was found between treatment with vitamin D or calcitriol; but alendronate was superior to either for treatment of glucocorticoid-induced bone loss. Therefore the following recommendations for prevention and treatment are given:

- Physical activity and muscle training.
- Calcium and vitamin D supplements.
- Check and treat steroid-induced diabetes mellitus.
- Check for hypogonadism and treat as needed. Administration of testosterone to men whose testosterone levels are decreased by steroid therapy may increase BMD in the lumbar spine by 5 % in 12 months.
- Start early with a modern nitrogen-containing bisphosphonate (e.g. alendronate once weekly 70 mg or risedronate once weekly 35 mg).

Patients with problems of intestinal absorption, e.g. Crohn's disease, or after a transplant are preferably treated with infusions of a nitrogen-containing bisphosphonate (zoledronate 5 mg annually). Before therapy is started, bone density should be measured at the lumbar spine and at the femoral neck. One of the following *treatment strategies* can then be applied according to the results:

- Normal bone density (*T*-score 2.0 to −1.0) and no additional risk factors: Calcium-rich diet, vitamin D and muscle training. DXA control measurement at half-yearly intervals
- Osteopenia and osteoporosis (T-score < −1.0): Strategy as above plus a modern BP orally or by infusion

Avascular osteonecrosis is a characteristic complication of hypercortisolism, most frequent in the femoral head, the humeral head and the femoral condyles.

Transplantation Osteoporosis 79

The number of transplants of solid organs such as the kidney, liver, heart, lung and pancreas is rising steadily together with an increase in the length of the patients' survival times. For example, 98 % of kidney, 87 % of hepatic and 69 % of heart transplant patients live longer than a year. Half of all transplant patients eventually develop osteoporosis with fractures and this substantially reduces their quality of life. Even now, as shown by a recent study, the fracture rates remain intolerably high with 20–40 % of the patients. The major cause of the fractures is the bone disease which could have preceded the transplant and the subsequent conditions which follow it. In the absence of preventive measures, increased bone loss begins in the immediate postoperative period due to immobilisation and immunosuppression and continues thereafter due to many additional factors, such as possible neuropathy, reduced mobility, and lack of exercise, nutritional factors and above all the immunosuppressive therapy which the patients have to take. Patients who had diabetes before the transplant had significantly increased post-transplant fractures in the absence of prophylactic measures.

Pathogenesis of transplant osteoporosis is complex and only partly understood. General risk factors (inactivity, vitamin D deficiency, menopause, andropause, alcohol and nicotine) and some medications (diuretics, anticoagulants, corticosteroids and other immunosuppressive agents) are frequently involved. In addition, in many cases the diseased organ probably damaged the bone for long periods prior to transplantation. Biochemical markers of bone resorption are always elevated in the pre-transplantation phase. But the post-transplantation occurrence of fractures is due to immunosuppression with glucocorticoids, cyclosporin A and tacrolimus (FK506). Azathioprine increases the number of osteoclasts but not their resorptive activity. Loss of bone is especially prominent during the first year post-transplant. Put briefly, these recognised *pathogenic factors* are:

- Prior osteopenia/osteoporosis
- Immunosuppressive drugs
- Calcium and vitamin D deficiency
- Hypogonadism
- Poor mobility
- Poor nutrition

During the first month after *cardiac transplantation*, the levels of testosterone decreased but normalised during the second month. The levels of gonadotropins also decreased, suggesting an adverse effect of prednisone on the hypopituitary-gonadal axis. Subsequently, low testosterone levels are common. Therefore these patients must be checked and treated also for BMD to avoid effects of hypogonadism and osteoporosis. Today, the situation is changing, especially if the patients underwent assessment of bone density before the transplant and a programme for preservation of the bones was initiated. This includes proper nutrition, calcium and

R. Bartl, C. Bartl, *Bone Disorders*, DOI 10.1007/978-3-319-29182-6_79

vitamin supplements, early mobilisation, targeted exercise therapy and antiresorptive treatment with one of the N-containing BP. Studies on anabolic therapy, for example, with PTH, have not been published to date.

It should be noted that *kidney transplant patients* require special attention: the presence of renal osteodystrophy, possibly with low bone turnover or even adynamic bone disease, is a contraindication for bisphosphonates. Vitamin D supplements are particularly important in kidney transplant patients as they may reduce post-transplant hyperparathyroidism. Results of a prospective trial of alfacalcidol alone, of alendronate alone and of the two together in renal transplant recipients showed that the combination was more effective in improvement of bone mass than the separate use of either one alone. Pre-transplantation administration of vitamin D could also have a beneficial effect on the immune system and reduce the possibility of rejection. In addition these patients are even at risk for cancer if the pre-transplant levels of vitamin D were low.

The presence of *pre-transplant diabetes* is also a significant risk factor for post-transplant fractures. Since the survival time of transplanted patients has now increased, it is important to stress that long-term preventive therapy must also be given!

Lifestyle, nutrition and risk factors: Previous experience has shown that long before a transplant, bone density should be measured, and if required, appropriate therapy should be instituted well before transplantation: bisphosphonates, calcium, vitamin D or its active metabolites and muscle training. This should prevent bone loss before transplantation. In the post-transplantation period, up to 20 % of the bone mass may be lost, particularly from the vertebral bodies and the femoral neck. Patients with liver, heart and lung transplants have a particularly high rate of loss. N-containing bisphosphonates and calcitriol are the first choice for preventive therapy. Vitamin D-induced hypercalciuria must be avoided in patients with kidney transplants. In patients with hypogonadism, oestrogen or testosterone should be given. Calcium-rich diet and special exercises are also recommended for healthy bones. Calcitonin and fluoride, tested in clinical trials, were not found to be effective. Other factors such as sex and age may also impinge on osteoporosis. For example, the early rapid loss of bone in men following renal transplantation can be prevented by BP given i.v. at the time of transplantation and a month later.

80 Tumour-Therapy-Induced Osteoporosis

Many treatment protocols in oncology lead to manifest osteoporosis. Irradiation causes local atrophy of the bone and bone marrow due to the toxic effects on bone and bone marrow cells, while chemotherapy and hormone therapy induce systemic rarefaction of both trabecular and cortical bones. Moreover, these iatrogenic effects may even be increased by a direct effect on the bone of the tumour itself, which could well have preceded the deleterious effects of the therapy.

The *causes* of osteoporosis during treatment of neoplasias are:

- Therapy-induced hypogonadism
- Glucocorticoids in chemotherapy protocols
- Toxic effects of chemotherapy
- Radiotherapy – also of the CNS in children because of brain tumours or acute leukaemias
- Immobilisation
- Nutritional disturbances

Tumour therapy with induction of secondary hypogonadism

Any chemotherapy with this effect will eventually also cause severe osteoporosis. Two groups of tumours are distinguished:

- Sex hormone-dependent neoplasias such as breast or prostatic cancer. Here the hypogonadism is part of the treatment strategy and substitution therapy cannot be given.
- Sex hormone-independent tumours such as Hodgkin's disease and other malignant lymphomas. In these cases hypogonadism is an unwanted side effect.

80.1 Hypogonadism and Breast Cancer

Premenopausal patients with breast cancer develop irreversible ovarian insufficiency within the first year of chemotherapy. BMD of the lumbar spine decreases by 8–10 % and of the hips by 4–6 % within 2 years of chemotherapy. However, if bisphosphonates are given at the same time as chemotherapy, this bone loss can largely be avoided. Moreover, therapy of ovarian insufficiency is integrated into the treatment schedule especially of patients with oestrogen receptor-positive tumours. This is achieved by means of gonadotropin-releasing hormone (GnRH) analogues, inhibitors of aromatase (especially those of the third generation) and oestrogen antagonists. Such antihormone therapy entails a considerable long-term risk of osteoporosis. *Tamoxifen*, a synthetic anti-oestrogen, has an antiresorptive effect on the bone but cannot make up for the lack of oestrogen stimulation of bone formation. In contrast, *aromatase inhibitors* markedly suppress plasma oestrogen levels by inhibiting aromatase, the enzyme responsible for the synthesis of oestrogens from androgenic substrate. Unlike tamoxifen, aromatase inhibitors have no stimulatory effect on the bone. Consequently, non-steroidal aromatase inhibitors of the third

R. Bartl, C. Bartl, *Bone Disorders*, DOI 10.1007/978-3-319-29182-6_80

generation have been shown to increase the risk of osteoporosis by a profound lowering of circulating oestrogen levels. Short-term use of letrozole (an aromatase inhibitor) has been shown to be associated with an increase in bone-resorption markers; and adjuvant therapy with anastrozole (also an aromatase inhibitor) is associated with a higher incidence of fractures than therapy with tamoxifen (ATAC study). The steroidal aromatase inhibitor exemestane, however, significantly prevents bone loss and enhances bone mechanical strength. The steroidal action of exemestane's principal metabolite 17-hydroexemestane may account for the observed bone-preserving effects.

Development of osteoporosis under non-steroidal aromatase inhibitors or chemotherapy can be prevented or modified with concurrent use of bisphosphonates. Therefore, all patients with breast cancer should have a BMD (DXA of lumbar spine and hips) before commencing therapy. If osteopenic, *preventive therapy* with bisphosphonates should be instituted:

- Clodronate 1,600 mg daily per os will increase bone mass and most probably also decrease both skeletal and visceral metastases.
- Alendronate (10 mg) or risedronate (5 mg) daily orally can also be used as a single therapy for the prevention and treatment of osteoporosis.
- Alendronate (70 mg) or risedronate (35 mg) once weekly if authorised instead of the daily dose.
- Ibandronate (150 mg) once monthly.
- Alternatively ibandronate 3 mg i.v. at three-monthly intervals according to the severity and type of osteoporosis.
- And last, but certainly not least, zoledronate 5 mg i.v. annually is recommended and has already been tested in clinical studies.

It is worth emphasising that patients with osteoporosis and a history of breast cancer should not receive hormone substitution therapy, but only an aminobisphosphonate orally or intravenously. Raloxifene can also be given.

80.2 Hypogonadism and Prostate Cancer

Attainment of hypogonadism is one of the aims of therapy, particularly in all forms of metastatic cancer and a high postoperative PSA level. Possible modes of treatment are orchidectomy, GnRH analogues and anti-androgens. Patients who have received such treatments are at great risk of developing osteoporosis, and the appropriate diagnostic and therapeutic measures are indicated as for patients with mammary cancer.

80.3 Hypogonadism in Hodgkin's Disease and Other Malignant Lymphomas

Hypogonadism resulting from therapy of malignant lymphomas is the most frequent in the group of non-hormone-dependent neoplasias. Irreversible ovarian insufficiency and early menopause are induced in 30–60% of women after radiotherapy and intensive chemotherapy. Because of the low proliferative index of Leydig cells, men are less likely to develop severe osteoporosis, though some degree of bone loss will be manifest later in life. BMD measurements at diagnosis should also be made in patients with lymphomas so that bisphosphonate therapy, if needed, can be given to prevent development of osteoporosis.

80.4 Antitumour Therapy with Direct Effect on the Bone

Many protocols applied in oncology contain substances which, when given systematically, effect bones adversely and cause osteoporosis. However, the degree of damage and extent of bone loss depend on the frequency and/or duration of the cycles of chemotherapy. Measurement of BMD indicates when osteoporosis should be forestalled and/or treated.

80.5 Protocols Including Corticosteroids and Other Drugs

Patients with malignant lymphomas and multiple myeloma receive chemotherapy protocols which include high doses of corticosteroids, but these are given intermittently, not continuously. In contrast to women with ovarian insufficiency, patients without hypogonadism did not suffer bone loss although high cumulative doses of prednisone were given. One possible explanation may be the relatively short exposure time, in addition to which the negative impact on the bone of bone marrow infiltration is reduced by the therapy, in lymphomas and especially in multiple myeloma. It should also be remembered that modern BP have antitumour effects, for example, on myeloma cells, which contribute to their positive influence on remodelling of the bone, on osteoporosis and other osseous lesions.

80.6 Therapy Protocols Including Methotrexate and Doxorubicin

Many chemotherapeutic agents have not yet been investigated for their possibly harmful effects on the bone. An exception is methotrexate given for rheumatoid arthritis: increased resorption of the bone together with decreased formation has been reported with an ensuing high renal excretion of calcium and reduction in BMD. One of the direct consequences of methotrexate appears to be a drop in the recruitment of osteoblast precursors. Children treated with methotrexate (e.g. in acute lymphatic leukaemia) are especially liable to considerable resorption of the bone, though with cessation of methotrexate therapy, the resultant osteopenia is reversible. Clinical studies of the bone in patients with breast cancer treated with protocols containing methotrexate (CMF protocol) have not yet been reported.

80.7 Therapy with Ifosfamide

This alkylating agent combined with cisplatin is used mainly for solid tumours. Depending on the amount given, it causes reversible or permanent damage of the proximal renal tubuli, resulting in metabolic acidosis, loss of phosphate and hypercalciuria, which in turn lead to the clinical picture of osteoporomalacia. However, there is no information as yet as to whether or not ifosfamide itself has a direct toxic effect on bone cells.

80.8 Treatment Strategy

The problem of osteoporosis in patients with malignancies is underestimated. Usually, an osteologist is only consulted when the patient has already sustained one or more fractures. This unsatisfactory situation could be avoided by timely "osteoprotection" which starts with a BMD measurement when the diagnosis is established and appropriate steps are taken depending on the results. These steps include the basic and specific measures outlined above.

The choice, dose, duration and intervals of bisphosphonate therapy are determined by the severity of bone loss and the patient's risk factors. When carefully chosen and correctly administered, the bone deficit can be eradicated and a positive bone balance with increases up to 10% in bone density obtained. A broad spectrum of bisphosphonates is available.

Oral administration:

- Alendronate: 10 mg daily
- Alendronate: 70 mg once weekly
- Risedronate: 5 mg daily
- Risedronate: 35 mg once weekly

Intravenous administration:

- Ibandronate: 3 mg infusion/injection every 3 months
- Pamidronate: 30 mg infusion every 3 months
- Zoledronate: 5 mg infusion annually
- Clodronate: 600 mg infusion every 3 months

In summary, intravenous administration has some important advantages.

For supportive treatment when i.v. chemotherapy is given at 4–6 week intervals:

- Avoids gastrointestinal side effects
- Avoids problems of gastrointestinal absorption
- Avoids problems of compliance

81 Drug-Induced Osteoporomalacia

Bone formation and mineralisation require calcium and phosphate together with active metabolites of vitamin D. Drugs affecting the vitamin D system may cause both osteoporosis and osteomalacia by several mechanisms:

Blockers of Vitamin D Production The elderly and institutionalised individuals with limited nutrition and sunlight exposure are at particular risk.

Inhibitors of Vitamin D Absorption Vitamin D, a fat-soluble vitamin, is absorbed in the jejunum and ileum, in combination with bile acids. Therefore, bile acid-binding resins such as cholestyramine and colestipol interfere with this process and inhibit vitamin D absorption.

Interference with Vitamin D Metabolism To be active, vitamin D must first be metabolised in the liver and then in the kidney. Drugs such as anticonvulsants or rifampicin induce drug-metabolising enzymes in the liver which then accelerate the catabolism of vitamin D and its metabolites. Some reports have shown that 20–65 % of patients with epilepsy receiving anticonvulsants such as phenytoin or phenobarbital developed osteoporosis and/or osteomalacia, especially if they were institutionalised. These patients were at an increased risk of fractures during their epileptic seizures. Patients taking these anticonvulsants require higher doses of vitamin D to achieve a positive calcium balance, with doses up to 4000 IU per day. Anticonvulsants such as sodium valproate do not induce the hepatic drug-metabolising enzymes and therefore have no impact on vitamin D metabolism.

Antagonists of Vitamin D Action Glucocorticoids interfere with intestinal calcium absorption, but they are not direct antagonists of vitamin D at the receptor level. There are no known drugs that directly interfere with the actions of active vitamin D at the target-tissue level.

Inhibitors of Phosphate Absorption Hypophosphataemia is a major cause of osteomalacia, and the most important drug-induced form is caused by excessive ingestion of aluminium-containing antacids, which inhibit intestinal phosphate absorption.

Inhibitors of Bone Mineralisation Aluminium-induced osteomalacia is mainly found in patients on haemodialysis and on total parenteral nutrition. Etidronate, the first bisphosphonate, also induced disturbances in mineralisation when given in higher doses. However, no reports have been published of osteomalacia caused by nitrogen-containing BP. Bone biopsies of patients treated with alendronate for more than 7 years have shown no evidence of demineralisation. Fluoride in high doses often showed evidence of abnormal mineralisation, and this defect is aggravated by concomitant low calcium and vitamin D intake.

R. Bartl, C. Bartl, *Bone Disorders*, DOI 10.1007/978-3-319-29182-6_81

82 Antiepileptic Drug-Related Osteopathy

It is well known that antiepileptic drugs (AEDs) have long-term effects on the state (health) of the bones, specifically with respect to bone density, vitamin D metabolism as well as other risk factors for fractures. However, these aspects of AED therapy have not been adequately investigated in the studies published to date.

> It is therefore important to stress that patients with epilepsy on AEDs have an increased risk for bone loss, defects in mineralisation and fractures.

A patient on long-term therapy with an AED has two to three times greater risk of fracture than the control, and as demonstrated in the studies, 4–70 % of the patients, i.e. 50 % on average, have demonstrable osteopathies. The type, the dosage and the duration of the antiepileptic therapy determine the type of osteopathy, and this is valid for the enzyme-inducing as well as for the non-enzyme-inducing medications.

The *pathogenesis* of AED-related bone disease remains controversial and multifactorial:

- Accelerated hepatic vitamin D metabolism by enzyme-inducing AEDs
- Altered vitamin K metabolism
- Lowered calcitonin levels in AED users
- Reduction of insulin-like growth factor (IGF)-I and IGF-binding protein 3 (IGFBP-3)
- Direct inhibition of intestinal calcium absorption
- Reduced exercise levels, poor dietary calcium intake and reduced sunlight exposure
- Increased falls during seizure and at other times
- Lower levels of endogenous oestrogens
- Increased levels of sex-hormone-binding globulin
- Inhibition of osteoblast-like cells

The *enzyme inducers* such as phenytoin, primidone, phenobarbital and carbamazepine have been particularly well investigated with regard to their effects on the metabolism of vitamin D. However, loss of bone may occur in the absence of vitamin D deficiency. Moreover, combinations of osteoporosis and osteomalacia are frequently seen and must be taken into consideration when specific therapy is recommended. The question of what, if any, effect on the bone is exerted by modern AEDs, such as lamotrigine, gabapentin and levetiracetam, is still under consideration.

Before administration of therapy, every patient should be thoroughly investigated, including bone density by DXA and lever of 25(OH) D in the serum to establish baseline values – similar to the approach to patients when long-term therapy with systemic corticosteroids is contemplated. Moreover, in addition to the clearly defined treatment of any osteopathy already present, patients with epilepsy should be advised on how to minimise epileptic attacks and falls.

R. Bartl, C. Bartl, *Bone Disorders*, DOI 10.1007/978-3-319-29182-6_82

In light of all the above, the following therapeutic measures are recommended:

- Careful choice and dosage of the AED to reduce the frequency of epileptic attacks.
- Physical activity in particular for muscular development, maintenance and improvement in coordination.
- Appropriate lifestyle to benefit the bones – no smoking!
- Nutrition – including a minimum of 1000 mg calcium daily.
- Vitamin D_3 2000 IU daily, but more than 4000 or 5000 or even up to 15,000 IU daily if osteomalacia is already present at diagnosis. The patient's serum should be monitored. Patients on phenytoin need higher doses of vitamin D. Alternatively vitamin D may also be taken as weekly or monthly capsules of 20,000 IU or given as intramuscular injections of 100,000 IU every 3 months.
- Active vitamin D metabolites, e.g. alfacalcidol or calcitriol, should only be given in cases of marked osteomalacia or if patients cannot accept high doses of vitamin D_3.
- Nutrition rich in vitamin K (such as dark green vegetables) or vitamin K supplements are given in rare cases for the prevention of phenytoin-induced bone loss.
- When impending or manifest osteoporosis is diagnosed initially, nitrogen-containing BP or other medications can be given, as recommended by the FDA or other responsible authorities in individual countries.

83 Other Drugs Associated with Osteoporosis

Systemic osteoporosis has also been observed in patients receiving various medications:

- High-dose and long-term *heparin* and *warfarin* therapy is associated with an increased risk of osteoporosis, and there may be a prolonged effect on the bone after cessation of therapy. The use of low-molecular-weight heparin and of newer antithrombotic agents such as fondaparinux is probably associated with fewer skeletal effects.
- *Thiazolidinediones (TZDs)* are widely used in the treatment of type 2 diabetes. Administration of rosiglitazone resulted in significant bone loss and suppression of biochemical markers of bone formation. In women, there was a significant increase in the incidence of fractures. This drug class effect is positively associated with duration of treatment; men and women are equally affected.
- *Selective serotonin receptor uptake inhibitors* (SSRIs) are widely described antidepressants and are associated with reduced bone mass and increased fracture risk. However depression itself may be associated with increased risk of osteoporosis.
- *Long-term and high-dose acid-suppressive medications* (proton pump inhibitors, PPI, e.g. omeprazole) increase fracture risk, though the mechanism remains unknown. Reduced intestinal calcium absorption seems unlikely to be solely responsible for the development of increased fracture risk within 1 year of starting therapy. Inhibition of the osteoclastic proton pump would be expected to have beneficial effects on bone resorption.

Drugs protecting against osteoporosis:

- In several studies, a significant protective effect of *beta-blocker* therapy on fracture risk has been reported, although this finding has not been universal.
- In *thiazide* users, reduced fracture risk and increases in bone density have been reported. Increased renal calcium reabsorption may play a role in these effects.
- *Statins* inhibit an important enzyme in the mevalonate pathway, thus inhibiting osteoclastic activity. However, benefits on fracture risk and BMD were only small in some studies.

R. Bartl, C. Bartl, *Bone Disorders*, DOI 10.1007/978-3-319-29182-6_83

Part XV

Bone and Bone Marrow

The "Bone and Marrow" System

84

Owing to the calcification and ossification of its extracellular compartment, the bone is converted into an extremely hard structure enabling optimal implementation of its four major functions:

- It constitutes the means for direct locomotion and movement.
- It provides support and protection for softer, vulnerable tissues.
- It participates in the homeostasis of minerals.
- It houses the bone marrow which provides the formed elements of the blood.

The bone and the marrow are closely interrelated organs. They share the same vascular system, and there are many interrelations between stromal elements and cellular lineages (e.g. monocytes and osteoclasts). Therefore, it is not astonishing that disorders of one invariably affect the other to a lesser or greater degree. The haematological conditions in which alterations in the trabecular bone have been observed are:

- Haemolytic and aplastic anaemias
- Myelodysplastic syndromes
- Chronic myeloproliferative disorders
- Acute leukaemias
- Chronic lymphoproliferative disorders
- Multiple myeloma
- Systemic mastocytosis

> In the development of animals, cancellous bone was first found in primitive vertebrates. At the stage of frogs and amphibians, there was the first shift of blood formation to the medullary cavities, which were before filled with loose connective tissue.

During childhood, when replacement of the embryonic cellular marrow by adipose tissue is completed in the skeleton, the marrow cavities of the axial skeleton are adapted for homing the different cell lines of haematopoiesis (Fig. 84.1). The spongiosa and cortex, the specialised blood vessels, the stroma of the marrow and the haematopoietic tissue form a complex anatomical and functional unit (Fig. 84.2). For example, the haematopoietic lineages need the cancellous bone framework and the specialised sinus system with its thin walls in order to release mature blood cells into the circulation (Fig. 84.3). Conversely, the bone and cartilage need haematopoiesis for recruitment of bone cells and the vascular system for supply of proteins, minerals, oxygen and energy.

The skeleton is not only responsible for mechanical tasks and mineral homeostasis, but also for the protection and design of the soft and vulnerable blood-forming tissue and the undifferentiated stem

R. Bartl, C. Bartl, *Bone Disorders*, DOI 10.1007/978-3-319-29182-6_84

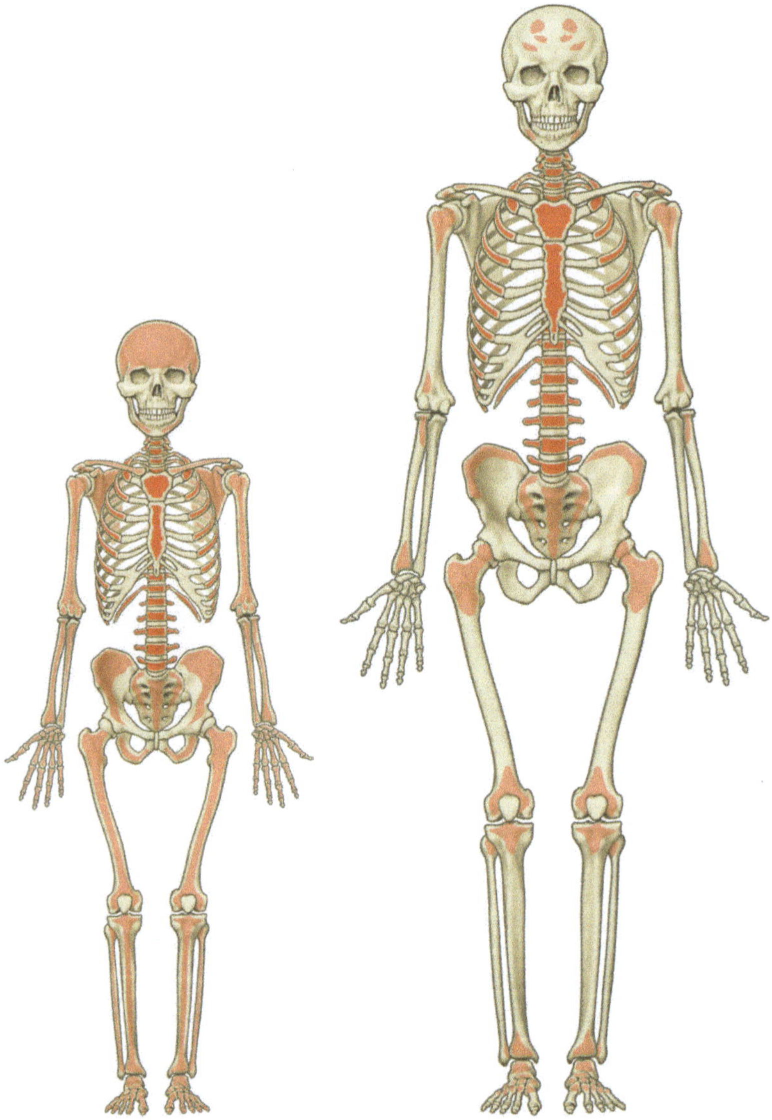

Fig. 84.1 Distribution of haematopoiesis (*red marrow*) in the skeleton in a child and an adult

cells. In return, haematopoiesis provides precursors of bone cells which differentiate on the surface of the bone to osteoclasts and osteoblasts, controlled by hormonal and neural influences. The following *cell systems in the bone marrow* have an influence on normal bone remodelling and regeneration:

- Haematopoietic stem cells (HSCs), starting point for osteoclasts
- Mesenchymal stem cells (MSCs), starting point for osteoblasts and osteocytes
- Endothelium and perivascular cells, in collaboration with the endosteal osteoblast
- Sympathetic and sensory nervous systems, which affect bone remodelling
- Arteries, capillaries and endosteal sinus system, responsible for blood supply
- Adipocytes, with inhibition effects on HSCs
- Macrophages and monocytes, including osteoclasts entrusted with bone-resorbing functions
- B and T lymphopoiesis for immune-competent functions
- Stroma and connective tissue cells including fibrocytes, entrusted with organisational and structuring functions in the marrow cavities

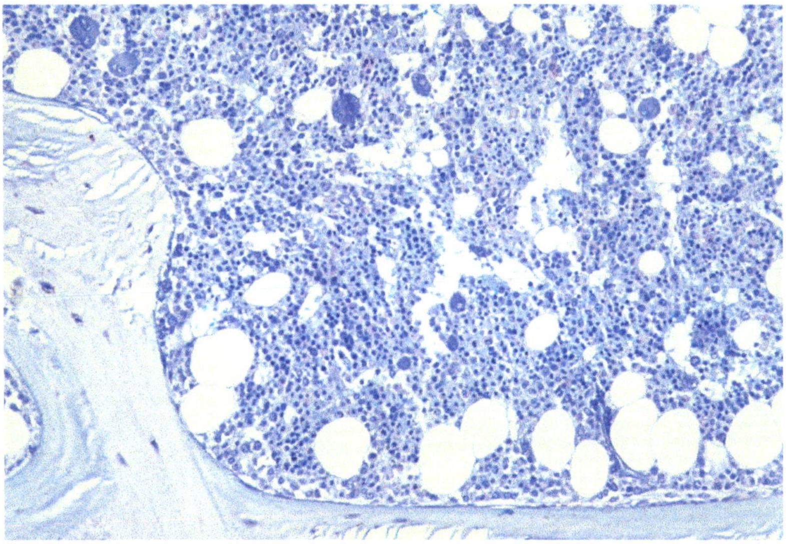

Fig. 84.2 Normal architecture of the bone marrow with granulopoietic precursors at endosteal surface, erythrons and megakaryocytes around the central sinusoids. Giemsa staining

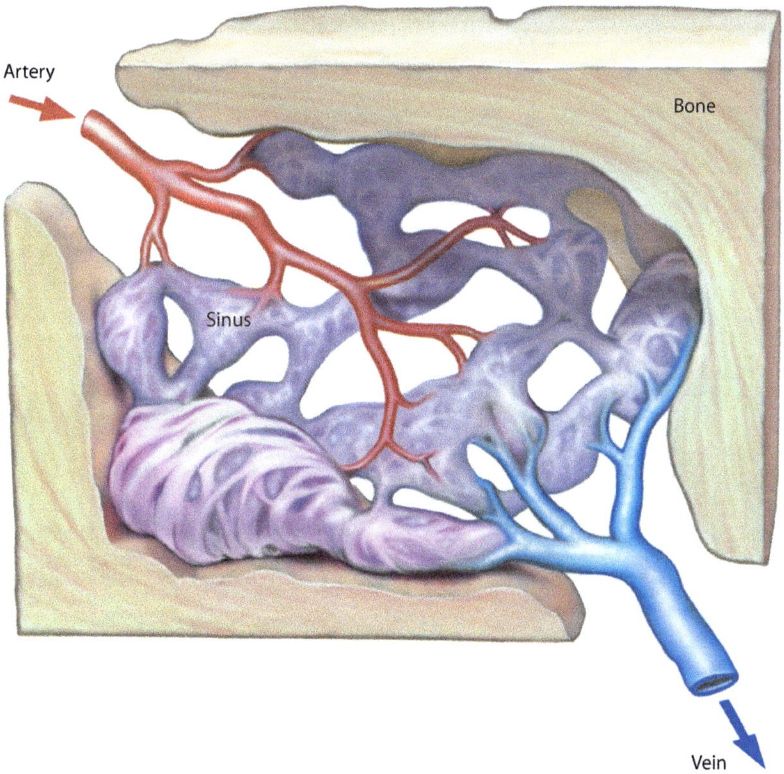

Fig. 84.3 Vascular system in the bone marrow

85 The Patient with "Myelogenous Osteopathy"

Neumann and Bizzozero published almost simultaneously in 1868 that the bone marrow and the bone are closely interrelated organs. The term "haematic osteodysplasia" was first introduced by Gaensslen in 1938 to describe the effects on the skull caused by congenital haemolytic anaemias, i.e. the typical "hair-on-end" appearance of the cranial bones. Subsequently, Rohr in 1940 and Markoff in 1942 used the term *myelogenous osteopathy* and *osteogenous myelopathy* for osteoporosis, osteolysis and osteosclerosis occurring in myelogenous disorders and the suppression of haematopoiesis due to diseases of the bones, respectively. Based on thousands of evaluated iliac crest biopsies, Burkhardt has distinguished eight different *pathogenetic mechanisms of myelogenous osteopathy*, which may occur alone or in combination:

- *Osteoporosis due to marrow atrophy*, with simultaneous depletion of bone trabeculae, haematopoiesis and small vessels
- *Suppression osteoporosis*, with loss of bone trabeculae caused by reactive or neoplastic expansion of cells in the marrow cavities
- *Haematic osteodysplasia* with hyperplasia of erythropoiesis, the sinusoidal system and the endosteal osteogenesis in the growing skeleton as a result of maximum stimulation of blood formation
- *Ischaemic osteopathy*, with cystic and sclerotic lesions after marrow necrosis caused by circulatory disorders
- *Destructive osteolysis*, caused by extensively growing tumours and accompanied by osteoclastic bone remodelling
- *Compression osteopathy*, due to the pressure of a cyst, haemangioma or haematoma
- *Osteomyelosclerosis syndrome*, due to fibrosis and osteoblastic reactions and triggered by myeloproliferative syndromes with an atypical megakaryopoiesis
- *Myelogenous pseudohyperparathyroidism,* increased bone remodelling, triggered by humoural products (parathyroid hormone-like activity) of haemoblastoses and reticuloses

There are also different histologic patterns in osseous abnormalities depending on the underlying conditions of the bone marrow:

- *"Low-turnover" versus "high-turnover" osteopathy.* When the marrow is hypoplastic or aplastic, there is a marked decrease in the number of sinusoids and of stromal elements including the bone-lining cells; this may be the main cause of osteopenia and osteoporosis in aplastic anaemias. Thin trabeculae surrounded by fat cells, with virtual absence of endosteal sinusoids, osteoblasts and osteoclasts are characteristic for this type of cancellous bone atrophy. When the marrow is hypercellular, as in haemolytic anaemias and myeloproliferations, the endosteal sinusoids, the bone-lining cells and the adjacent mesenchyme are also hypoplastic, corresponding to inactive osteoporosis.

R. Bartl, C. Bartl, *Bone Disorders*, DOI 10.1007/978-3-319-29182-6_85

Activation of osteoclasts has been ascribed to the production of osteoclast-activating factors (OAFs) by myeloma, lymphomas or leukaemic cells. Production of osteoblast-inactivating factors has also been postulated.

- *"Thin trabeculae" versus "coarse trabeculae" osteoporosis.* Not only the degree of marrow cellularity but also the different proliferating haematopoietic cell lines influence osseous reactions. While in polycythaemia vera the trabeculae are attenuated but with normal microarchitecture and connections, a coarsening of the trabecular network with fewer connections and correspondingly large marrow spaces is characteristic of chronic myeloid leukaemia.
- *"Generalised" versus "focal" osteopathy.* The mode of spread of marrow infiltrations is a major parameter determining the pattern of osseous lesions. Processes with diffuse marrow infiltration (leukaemias) are characterised by a systemic osteopathy in bones which otherwise contain a trabecular network and red marrow, while in patients with focal, nodular or patchy infiltrations (granulomatous disorders, Hodgkin's disease, hairy cell leukaemia, nodular types of myeloma or lymphomas), local osseous lesions or even circumscribed osteolytic lesions are found.

There are, of course, still a large number of other factors, e.g. renal, gastrointestinal, neurological and endocrine disorders, which influence different bone reactions and complications and which are described elsewhere in this book. Table 85.1 shows the frequencies of bone changes (X-rays and iliac crest biopsies) in important haematologic neoplasias (own results).

Table 85.1 Bone reactions in skeletal radiology and iliac crest biopsy in haematologic neoplasias (own results)

Parameter	PV	CML	AL	NHL	HD	MM
Patients, number	210	190	200	510	85	300
Skeletal X-ray						
Normal (%)	72	69	89	72	84	32
Osteoporosis (%)	22	27	3	23	10	24
Osteolyses (%)	2	4	6	4	4	22
Osteosclerosis (%)	4	0	2	1	2	2
Bone biopsy						
Normal (%)	69	60	63	65	72	52
Osteoporosis (%)	27	27	23	28	19	44
Osteosclerosis (%)	4	3	4	7	9	4
Bone turnover, increased (%)	15	8	3	4	53	80

PV polycythaemia vera, *CML* chronic myeloid leukaemia, *AL* acute leukaemia, *NHL* non-Hodgkin's lymphomas, *HD* Hodgkin's disease, *MM* multiple myeloma

Anaemias and Bone Reactions 86

With the description of facial abnormalities in haemolytic anaemia, Cooley in 1927 first described the relationship of hyperplastic erythropoiesis and increased bone remodelling with malformation of the skeleton. Especially in severe *congenital haemolytic anaemias,* such as sickle cell anaemia, thalassaemia major and hereditary spherocytosis, there are classic but quite similar osseous abnormalities due to marrow expansion ("haematic dysplasias"). The whole bone may be affected, but the most prominent changes occur in the axial skeleton homing the red marrow (Fig. 86.1). Abnormalities are striking in the skull with widening of the diploic space and thinning of the outer table. Radial spicules of the bone lead to a "hair-on-end appearance" or "brush head" (Fig. 86.2). Osseous expansion also occurs in the face and causes striking facial abnormalities. Also vertebral body deformities are common, with wide marrow cavities and thin cortices. There is, however, no close correlation between the severity of the anaemia and osseous abnormalities on skeletal X-ray. Local lesions are also caused by microvascular occlusions (aseptic necrosis, infarcts and osteomyelitis).

In adults with hyperplastic erythropoiesis (haemolytic anaemia, pernicious anaemia), only signs of low-turnover osteoporosis are observed (Fig. 86.3), but no malformation of the skeleton. A relationship between bone marrow aplasia and

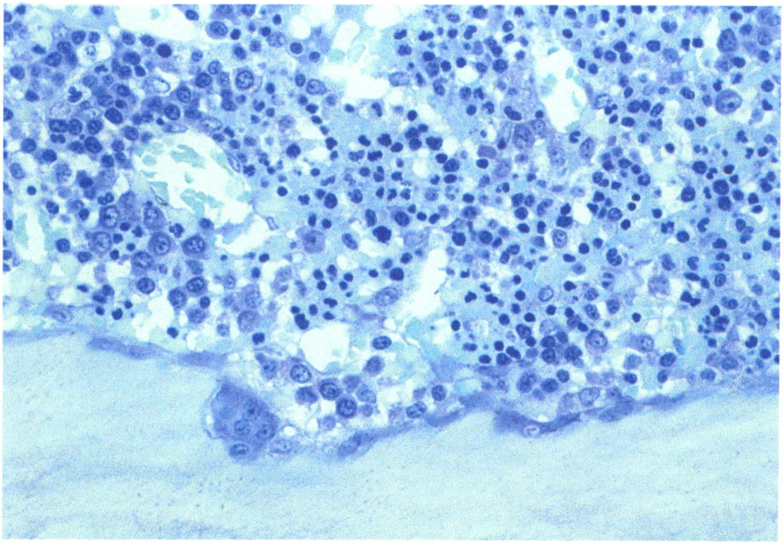

Fig. 86.1 Congenital haemolytic anaemia with hyperplastic erythropoiesis and increased osteoclastic bone resorption. Giemsa staining

R. Bartl, C. Bartl, *Bone Disorders*, DOI 10.1007/978-3-319-29182-6_86

bone loss had already been assumed by Pommer in 1923. In 1967 Burkhardt pointed out the relationship between inflammatory capillary damage and atrophy of the marrow and bone and coined the term *marrow atrophy-associated osteoporosis* in rheumatic disorders and aplastic anaemias (Fig. 86.4).

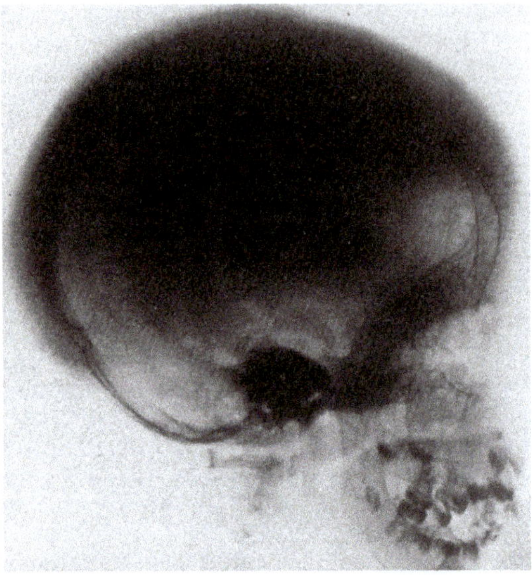

Fig. 86.2 X-ray of the skull of a young patient with sickle cell anaemia, showing a widening of the diploic space with the characteristic "hair-on-end appearance"

Haemochromatosis is characterised by an excessive accumulation of iron in the tissues. Symptoms are caused by damage of internal organs and include hepatomegaly, liver cirrhosis, skin pigmentation, diabetes mellitus, arthralgias and cardiomyopathy. The following subtypes are distinguished:

- Primary haemochromatosis, a hereditary form with a mutation in the HFE gene
- Secondary haemochromatosis (haemosiderosis, e.g. in thalassaemia, sideroblastic anaemia or in patients with frequent transfusions and massive iron deposits in the RES)

However, iron deposits in the bone marrow are strikingly low and rarely cause osseous abnormalities. The iron deposits in the skeleton are too low to be visible in roentgenograms.

As a result of massive bone marrow hyperplasia, hereditary haemolytic anaemias are always accompanied by osseous abnormalities. Bone infarcts and osteomyelitis may also occur.

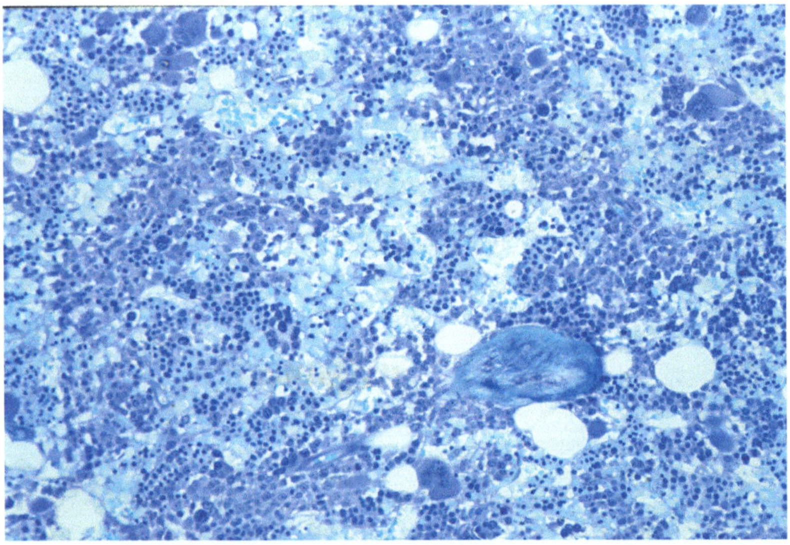

Fig. 86.3 Haemolytic anaemia with hyperplastic anaemia and marked osteoporosis, low turnover. Note "button phenomenon". Giemsa staining

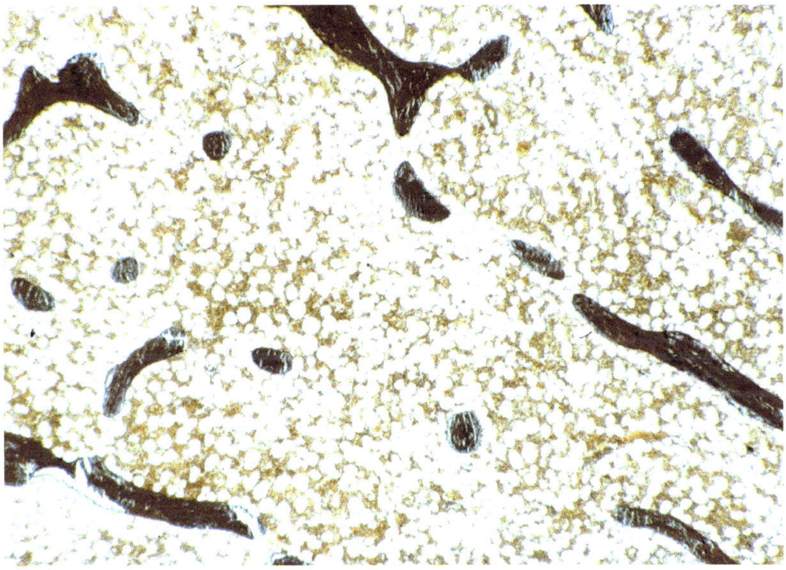

Fig. 86.4 Hypocellular marrow showing extensive replacement by fat cells and osteoporosis, low turnover. Gomori staining

Leukaemias and Lymphomas of the Bone

87

Acute leukaemia (AL) is the most common malignant disease of childhood, and the lymphoblastic subtype (ALL) accounts for about 80 % of the cases. Radiologically the skeleton is affected in approximately half the cases, with the following forms of lesions:

- Osteolytic lesions 30 %
- Diffuse osteopenia 16 %
- Periosteal reaction 20 %
- Metaphyseal bands 17 %
- Mixed lesions 18 %

The first roentgenological abnormalities may be horizontal radiolucent bands in the metaphyses of long bones. Periosteal reactions of long bones often reflect the infiltration of the cortex by leukaemic cells. With increasing tumour load and expansion in the rigid marrow cavities, generalised thinning of the cortex and the trabeculae causes systemic osteoporosis. In the terminal phase, massively destructive confluent lesions may be observed, and pathology fractures are then common.

Adults with acute leukaemia rarely show bone abnormalities (less than 10 % of cases). The median trabecular bone volume was within normal range. The osteoid volume and the bone remodelling, however, were decreased, indicating an inactive bone surface. During the course of treatment, osteoporosis, lytic lesions and osteosclerotic reactions due to extensive marrow necrosis have been observed.

In *chronic myeloid leukaemia (CML)*, skeletal abnormalities are considered uncommon. Osteolytic lesions have been reported in chronic myelomonocytic leukaemia. Generalised demineralisation is by far the commonest abnormality in the bone. Osteolytic lesions and/or hypercalcaemia is most frequently observed in the accelerated and blastic phase. Osteosclerotic lesions in CML and polycythaemia vera (PV) are usually signs of transformation to MF/OMS.

Although the individual *malignant lymphomas (MLs)* are histologically distinct and present with different clinical manifestations and radiologic features, they have enough in common to be considered together. Destruction of the bone and hypercalcaemia are relatively infrequent in lymphomas of the bone, except for Hodgkin's disease (HD), chronic lymphocytic leukaemia (CLL) and some T-cell lymphomas. The lymphokine lymphotoxin has been shown to be a potent bone-resorbing agent in vitro. Interleukin-1 may play an important role in stromal and osseous reactions, for example, in HD. Hypercalcaemia associated with certain lymphomas may be caused by the increased synthesis of calcitriol by lymphoma cells. In patients with chronic lymphocytic leukaemia (CLL) (Fig. 87.1a, b) and Waldenstrom's disease, osteoporosis occurred in about 15 %, and osteosclerosis was found in 7 % of patients. Active remodelling, as indicated by the presence of osteoblasts and osteoclasts, was minimal and rare. In ML of high-grade malignancy, osteolytic lesions have been found in about one third of patients.

R. Bartl, C. Bartl, *Bone Disorders*, DOI 10.1007/978-3-319-29182-6_87

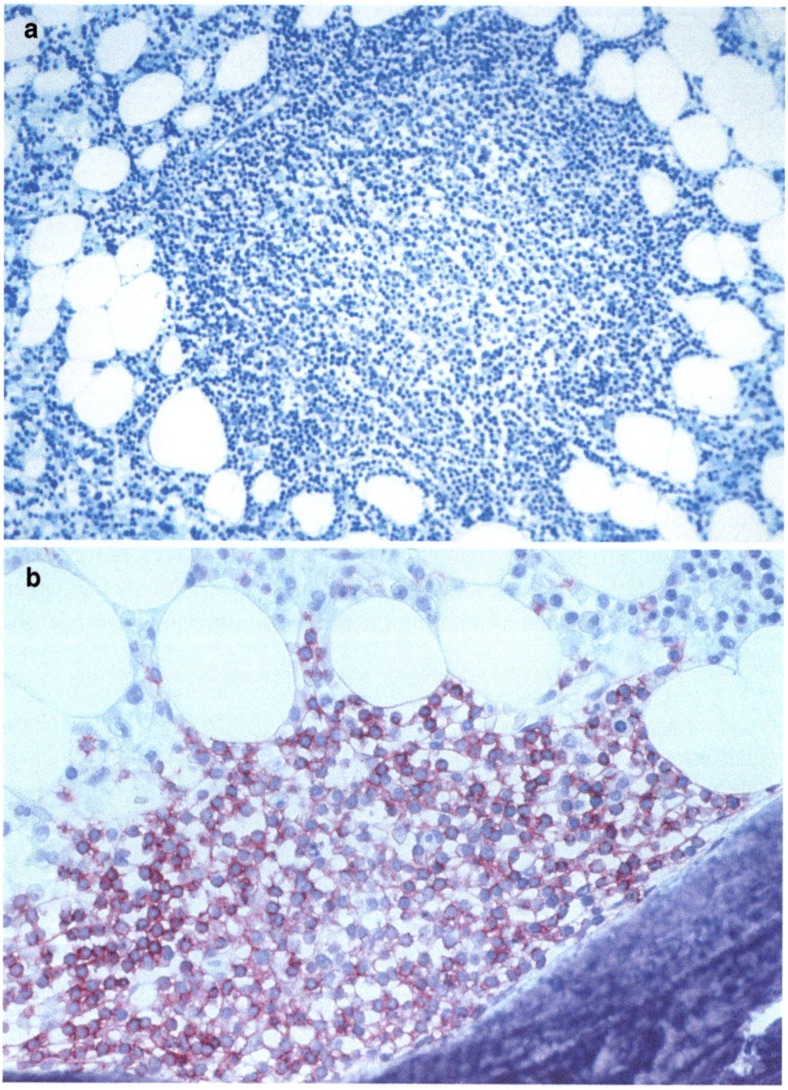

Fig. 87.1 (**a**) Reactive lymphoid follicle in the central part of a marrow cavity, with germinal centre, Giemsa staining. (**b**) Immunohistology of ML lymphocytic in the paratrabecular region and proof of monoclonality. No osseous reaction

Today the overall incidence of *Hodgkin's disease (HD)* at initial presentation is very rare. HD arising primarily in the bone is also a very rare occurrence. Bone involvement signifies stage IV lymphoma. The axial skeleton is more frequently involved (77 %) than the appendicular skeleton (23 %). Bone lesions were predominantly lytic in about 50 % of cases, with marked osteoclastic activity and surrounded by a lymphogranulomatous tissue with low content of lymphocytes but with a large number of Reed-Sternberg and Hodgkin's cells. Osteosclerotic reactions were observed in 20 % of the biopsies involved, especially in areas with a high content of lymphocytes and with inflammatory reactions, culminating in the appearance of an "ivory" vertebra. In 12 % of the positive biopsies, areas of osteoclastic resorption and osteoblastic formation were found, mimicking metastatic carcinoma on skeletal X-rays.

Hodgkin's disease in the bone shows a broad spectrum of osteolytic and osteosclerotic reactions, in some cases indistinguishable from the histologic pattern of Garré sclerosing osteomyelitis, fibrotic tissue without evidence of Reed-Sternberg and Hodgkin's cells.

88 Myelofibrosis/Osteomyelosclerosis Syndrome (MF/OMS)

The normal bone marrow has few fibres, and these are found mainly in association with trabecular bone surfaces and blood vessels. Fibrosis of the bone marrow takes place in response to many different toxic, inflammatory, osteolytic and malignant processes and is always of collagen type III. The basic disorders associated with bone marrow fibrosis are:

- Chronic myeloproliferative disorders (CMDs)
- Myelodysplastic syndromes (MDSs)
- Lymphoproliferative disorders (LPDs)
- Hodgkin's disease (HD)
- Bone metastases
- Inflammatory reactions
- Hyperparathyroidism
- Paget's disease

Reactive fibrosis on the basis of a myeloproliferative disorder (MPD) is called *myelofibrosis (MF)* or, when primitive bone is present, *osteomyelosclerosis (OMS)*. Variable amounts of this poorly mineralised bone (collagen type I) are randomly interwoven with the fibrous tissue (collagen type III) which occupies the intertrabecular cavities (Figs. 49.4 and 88.1). The extent of overall osseous increase is variable even in the same biopsy, and three grades of bone sclerosis in

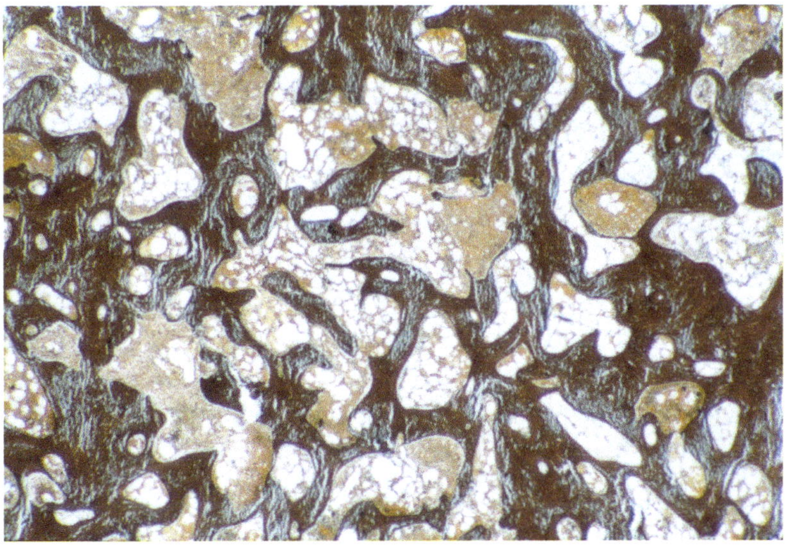

Fig. 88.1 Osteomyelosclerosis with a network of fibres in the empty, small marrow spaces

R. Bartl, C. Bartl, *Bone Disorders*, DOI 10.1007/978-3-319-29182-6_88

OMS are distinguishable, from small foci of primitive bone via increased appositional and woven bone in equal proportions to almost complete replacement of normal trabecular architecture by a network of poorly mineralised primitive bone. Transformation to MF and OMS was observed in about half of the patients with MPD.

Cases in the MPD with proliferation of megakaryocytes have a particular tendency to develop MF/OMS. Agnogenic myeloid metaplasia is the term applied to MF/OMS when the cause or the preceding disease is unknown and there is extramedullary haematopoiesis in the liver and spleen. It is now thought that most (if not all) cases are a consequence of preceding MPD with particularly numerous and atypical megakaryocytes.

The frequencies of the main underlying MPD in OMS patients were:

- Chronic myeloid leukaemia (CML) 39 %
- Polycythaemia vera (PV) 28 %
- Idiopathic thrombocythaemia (IT) 8 %

In MPD, the fibrosis and sclerosis is thought to be due to a combination of mechanisms including:

- A chronic inflammatory reaction mediated by immune complexes
- Production of megakaryocyte and platelet-derived growth factors (PDGF) and collagenase-inhibiting factor (platelet factor 4)
- Production, release and activation of transforming growth factor-β (TGF-β)

Other growth factors are also involved, as well as matrix proteins.

Myelofibrosis/osteomyelosclerosis affects usually adults and most present with anaemia, hepatosplenomegaly and bone pain.

The radiological findings reflect the pathological changes, and the pelvis, ribs, spine and proximal ends of femora and humeri are the most frequently affected skeletal sites. Diffuse osteoporosis may be the initial finding in the early stages. As new bone is deposited in the marrow cavities, the radiographs show islands of increased density. In the later stages, extremely dense bone may occupy the entire spongiosa.

In about 30 % of the patients with OMS, we observed marked discrepancies between the considerable increase of poorly mineralised woven bone in the biopsy and the osseous changes on X-rays.

Pain induced by osteomyelosclerosis also responds rapidly and for long periods to intravenous bisphosphonate (BP) therapy. This indicates that relief of pain by BP is not due exclusively to inhibition of osteoclasts, but that the BP also act on other cells such as T lymphocytes and stromal cells and thereby exert an effect on the RANKL/OPG system.

89 Disorders of the Mononuclear Phagocyte System

Storage diseases are the consequence of inherited enzyme deficiencies that lead to accumulation of the substances that are incompletely catabolised in the cells of the mononuclear phagocyte system in organs such as the liver, spleen and bone marrow. Many of these products are derived from lipids of the cell membrane.

89.1 Gaucher's Disease

This is due to a defective lysosomal glucosidase (glucocerebrosidase) which splits beta-glucose-cerebrosides. There are different levels of enzymatic activity in the mononuclear phagocyte system, and these in turn influence the time of appearance of the disease so that three types are recognised: infantile, juvenile and adult. All patients have hepatosplenomegaly, myelophthisic bone marrow involvement and severe bone complications. Episodes of "bone crisis", also called "aseptic osteomyelitis", are one of the most painful manifestations of Gaucher's disease. Bone marrow transplantation has been tried in patients with bone marrow failure due to replacement (Fig. 89.1a). Enzyme replacement is now available.

Skeletal X-ray shows two different types of abnormalities:

- Generalised osteoporosis and cortical thinning due to expansion of the infiltrated marrow spaces.
- Focal osteonecrosis due to loss of local blood supply. Infarcts can be massive in size and multiple, with patchy osteosclerosis. Flaring of the distal femur (Erlenmeyer flask deformity) is the most typical finding, together with marrow infarctions and subchondral bony collapse resulting from osteonecrosis.

The "Gaucher cell" is large and has the appearance of crumpled silk or tissue paper (Fig. 89.1b). "Pseudo-Gaucher cells" are similar in appearance to Gaucher cells and have been observed in the bone marrow in CML (Fig. 89.1c).

89.2 Niemann-Pick Disease

This lipid storage disease is due to sphingomyelinase deficiency, with accumulation of lipids in the spleen, liver, lymph nodes and bone marrow. The "Niemann-Pick cell" is large with a clear

R. Bartl, C. Bartl, *Bone Disorders*, DOI 10.1007/978-3-319-29182-6_89

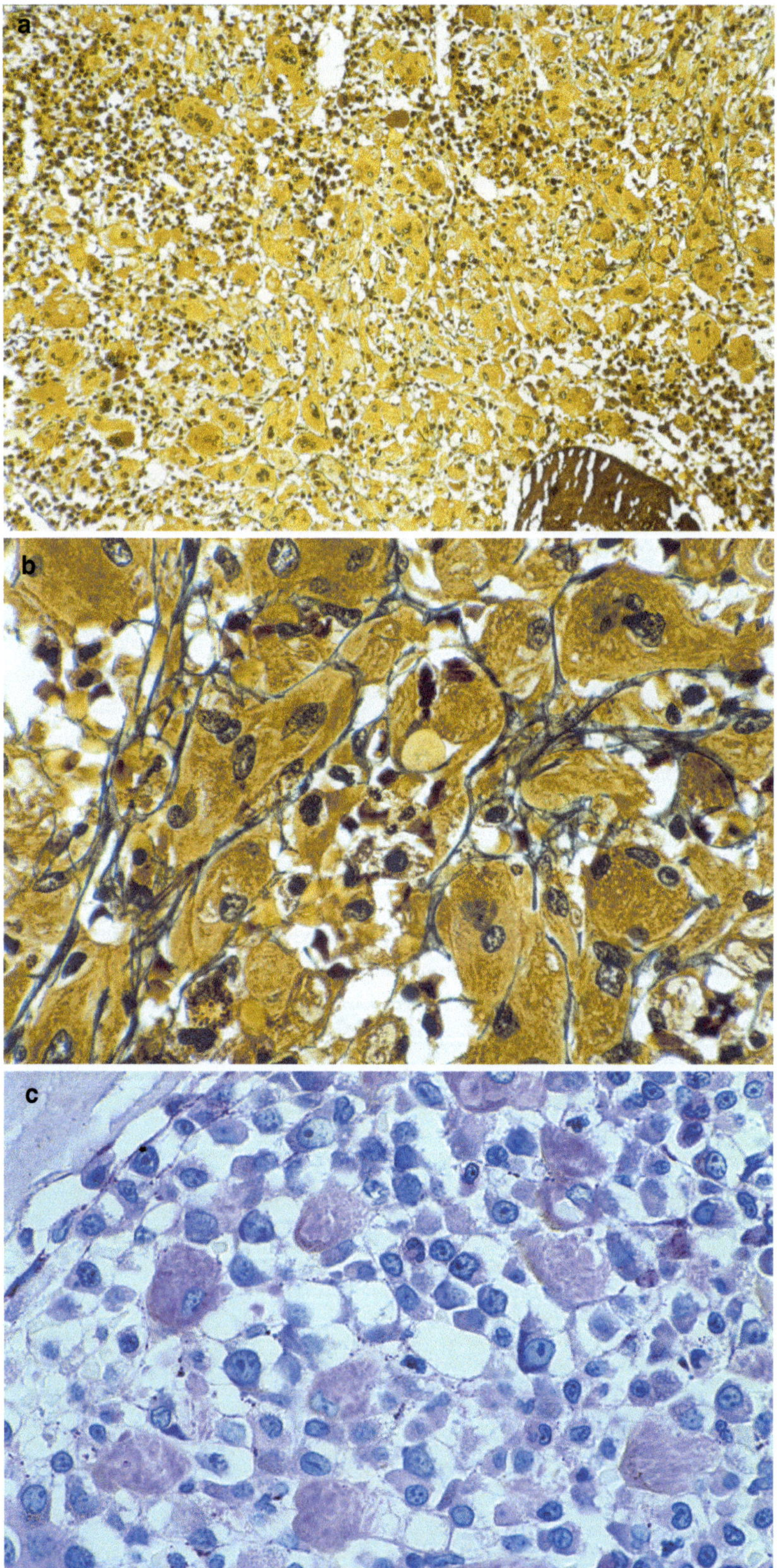

Fig. 89.1 (**a**–**c**) Iliac crest biopsy of a patient with Morbus Gaucher: (**a**) aggregate of typical Gaucher cells alternating with areas of normal haematopoietic tissue (upper left), (**b**) at higher magnification typical wrinkled silk or tissue-paper appearance of Gaucher cells. All Gomori staining. (**c**) Iliac crest biopsy in a patient with CML showing large "pseudo-Gaucher" cells. PAS staining

cytoplasm in histologic sections. Most cases run a rapidly fatal course, and only rare patients survive as long as a year after diagnosis has been made. Because of the rapid course, few osseous abnormalities such as cortical expansion of long bones have been reported.

89.3 Fabry's Disease

This is also called "angiokeratoma corporis diffusum" and is inherited in an X-linked recessive manner. The storage cells have a foamy appearance, and in the bone marrow, they may induce a marked perivascular and paratrabecular fibrosis with osteoclastic bone resorption. Diffuse angiokeratomatous skin lesions are frequently associated.

89.4 Mucopolysaccharidoses and Mucolipidoses

These are a group of inborn errors of metabolism in which the activity of one of the exoglycosidases is deficient. The clinical entities are characterised by variable degrees of skeletal dysplasia, and the most common variants are Hurler's syndrome, Hunter's syndrome, Morquio disease and Scheie disease.

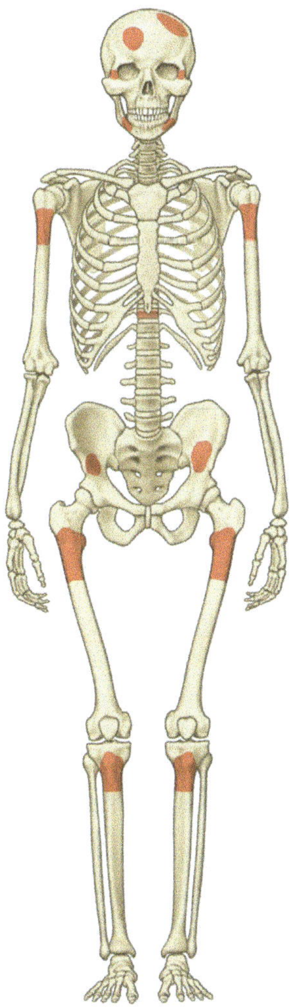

Fig. 89.2 Topography of eosinophilic granulomas

89.5 Histiocytosis X (Langerhans Cell Histiocytosis)

Today the cause of this syndrome is assumed to be an immature clonal Langerhans cell. Three related diseases are under this heading:

- *Eosinophilic granulomas of the bone* occur in the skeleton as circumscribed lytic lesions varying in size from 1 to 5 mm^2. The most common locations are the skull, femur, pelvis, ribs and spine (Fig. 89.2). The inner and outer tables of flat bones are eroded, often with a central sequestra, thus simulating pyogenic osteomyelitis. Occasionally, lesions show a "hole in a hole" pattern because of the different rates of bone destruction of the inner and outer cortical surfaces. A bone biopsy from an involved site shows eosinophils, plasma cells, lymphocytes, fibroblasts and storage cells. The foci may heal with a margin of sclerosis.
- *Hand-Schüller-Christian disease*, a more extensive and serious variant, comprises about 10 % of all cases of histiocytosis X. It is classically known as a syndrome consisting of osteolytic lesions in the skull, exophthalmos and diabetes insipidus. The osteolytic lesions are scattered throughout the skeleton with an affinity to the skull ("the geographical skull") and to other flat bones.
- *Abt-Letterer-Siwe disease* is a disseminated variant with a very poor prognosis, occurring in less than 2 % of the entire group. Multiple

destructive lesions in the haematopoietic areas of the skeleton are prominent.

- *Erdheim-Chester disease*, also known as lipid granulomatosis, is another disorder characterised by a proliferation of histiocytes in the bone and other organs. Foamy lipid-laden histiocytes accumulate in the bone marrow and induce fibro-inflammatory reactions. Most patients have bone pain and tenderness. A patchy or diffuse osteosclerosis is most prominent in the diaphysis and metaphysis. The cortices are also thickened because of periosteal new bone formation. The cause of Erdheim-Chester disease is unknown, although this disorder resembles to Langerhans granulomatosis.

Systemic diseases that most commonly affect the skeleton fall into two major groups:

- Proliferative disorders of the haematopoietic system with diffuse and symmetric osseous abnormalities
- Proliferative disorders of the reticuloendothelial system (also called mononuclear phagocyte system) with multifocal and asymmetric bone lesions.

90 Systemic Mastocytosis (SM)

An *increase of marrow mast cells* together with plasma cells and lymphocytes has been observed in a variety of conditions: inflammations, wound and fracture healing, oedema and fibrosis (Fig. 90.1). Immunocytic and lymphocytic marrow infiltrations often have a high content of mast cells. Certain tumours may contain numerous mast cells. Mast cell proliferation near osseous surfaces is also a consequence of primary and secondary HPT. There is also a relation between mast cells and postmenopausal osteoporosis, suggesting that mast cells accelerate trabecular bone loss.

Systemic mastocytosis (SM, mast cell disease) is characterised by a proliferation of mast cells in various organs and tissues. Bone loss results from the excessive degranulation of mast cell products, including IL-1, IL-3 and IL-6, which all promote osteoclast differentiation. Histamine and other mediators released by mast cells may increase bone formation and cause the typical picture of patchy osteosclerosis. A mutation of the tyrosine kinase c-kit, present in over 90% of patients with mastocytosis, contributes to bone resorption. The hyperplasia of mast cells that defines systemic mastocytosis in most cases is not neoplastic. The indolent course and the granulomatous features in SM suggest an immunological, non-neoplastic pathogenesis favouring the designation of "mast cell granulomatosis".

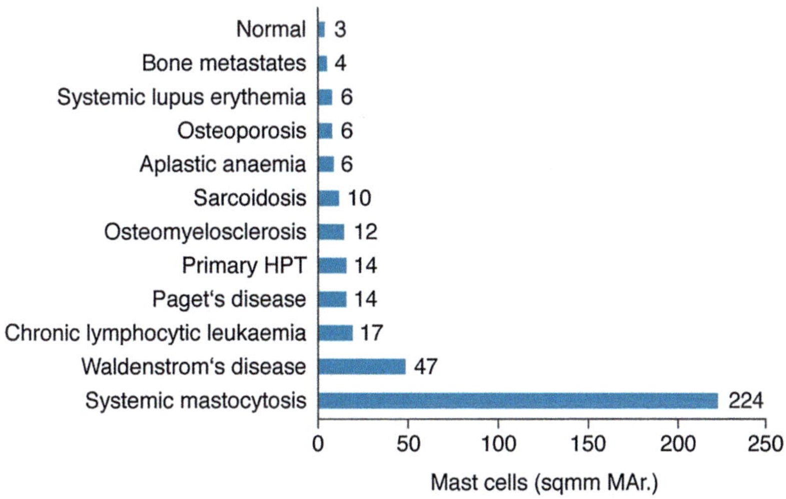

Fig. 90.1 Conditions with increase in mast cells in the bone marrow

R. Bartl, C. Bartl, *Bone Disorders*, DOI 10.1007/978-3-319-29182-6_90

In our observation period of 10 years, only 4 out of 100 patients with SM died. Malignant forms, usually leukaemic or sarcomatous, developed in only 4 cases.

It is localised to the skin (urticaria pigmentosa), systemic in distribution (systemic mastocytosis), sarcomatous (mast cell sarcoma) or even leukaemic (mast cell leukaemia).

Several *classifications* of mastocytosis have been published and a consensus classification describes four variants:

- An indolent type, which constitutes the majority of patients and without major influence on life expectancy
- A haematological type, which is associated with basic myeloproliferative and myelodysplastic disorders
- An aggressive type, in which the extent of mast cell proliferation in parenchymal organs determines the prognosis
- Mast cell leukaemia or sarcoma, rare and fatal diseases

The characteristic *histologic lesion* is the presence of mast cell granulomas. These are located predominantly in the endosteal and perivascular regions (Fig. 90.2). The granulomas consist of spindle-shaped mast cells variably granulated, lymphocytes, plasma cells, eosinophils and sea-blue histiocytes, all within a network of fibres and capillaries (Fig. 90.3a–d).

Skeletal changes are noted in approximately 70% of patients with SM, and they may be osteolytic, osteoporotic, osteosclerotic, circumscribed and/or diffuse. They are more frequent in the skull, vertebrae and pelvis than in long bones. Often, the osseous lesions may resemble metastatic malignant bone disease. Bone marrow mastocytosis is also an important "occult" cause of secondary osteoporosis.

The *clinical picture* is dominated by liberation of mast cell products: itching, flush, diarrhoea, intestinal bleeding, abdominal cramps, pancreatitis, muscle and bone pain and tachycardia.

Serum tryptase may be normal and the measurement of the 24-h urine excretion of *N*-methyl histamine represents a valuable non-invasive parameter to bone marrow biopsy in establishing diagnosis and evaluating the degree of mast cell load. The diagnosis however can only be confidently established by histologic evaluation of bone marrow biopsies that demonstrate the pathognomonic features of atypical mast cells in granulomatous lesions.

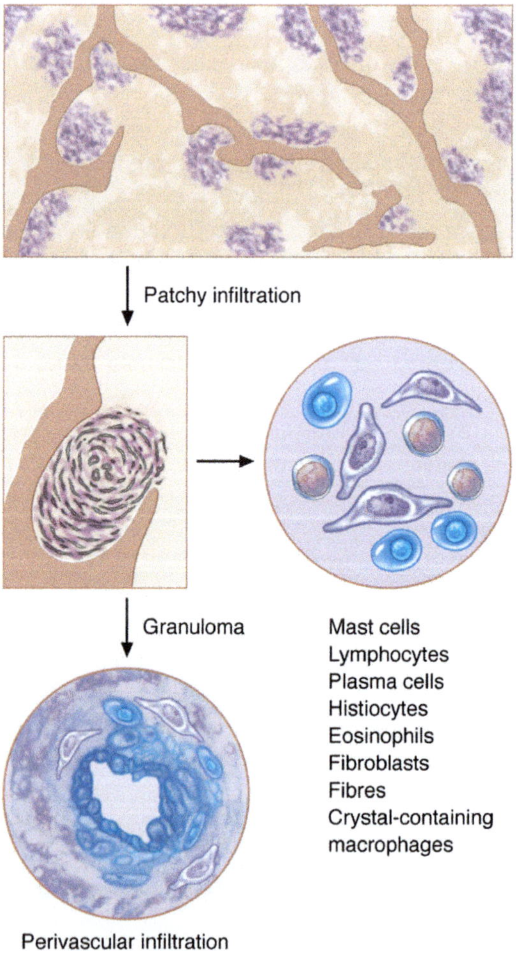

Fig. 90.2 Systemic mastocytosis in the bone marrow. There is a patchy involvement: paratrabecular, intertrabecular and perivascular granulomas consisting of a heterogeneous cell population, though the majority are mast and lymphoid cells

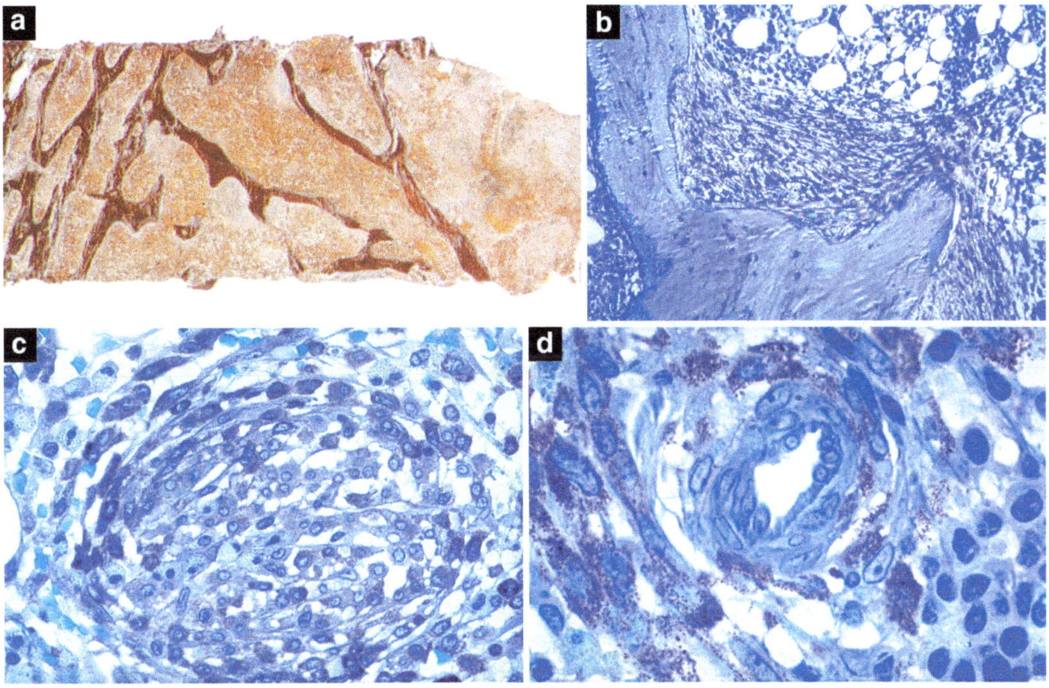

Fig. 90.3 (**a**) Iliac crest biopsy of a patient with systemic mastocytosis, Gomori staining. (**b**) Higher magnification of round- and spindle-shaped mast cells with variable granulation in a mast cell granuloma, endosteal orientation within a deep resorption bay, Giemsa staining. (**c**) Larger mast cell nodule (granuloma) with lymphoid cells in the centre, Giemsa staining. (**d**) Arteriole with mast cell infiltration, Giemsa staining

Treatment is supportive. Antiproliferative drugs, radiotherapy and prednisone have been used, but without major success. Severe bone pain and bone loss from advanced bone involvement has been reported to respond to intravenous bisphosphonates.

91 Multiple Myeloma

91.1 Definition

Multiple myeloma (MM) is a malignant haematologic disorder caused by a monoclonal proliferation of plasma cells and their precursors: B lymphocyte neoplasia with terminal differentiation. The plasma cells produce a monoclonal protein either a complete immunoglobulin (G, A, D or E) or fragments thereof (e.g. light chains, Bence-Jones protein).

91.2 Pathogenesis

Multiple myeloma constitutes about 1 % of all malignancies and about 10 % of all haematologic neoplasms. Its incidence is about three cases per 100,000 people annually. The peak frequency lies between 55 and 75 years with a median age of 65 years, though in recent years the number of younger people has shown a tendency to increase.

The initial malignant transformation takes place in immature B lymphocytes, which originate in the bone marrow or in the lymphatic system and enter the circulation before settling down in the skeleton, occasionally in other organs. Multiple myeloma is a typical disease of the bone/bone marrow system. Once established, the myeloma cells activate monocytes, T lymphocytes and stromal cells by a battery of cytokines which also influence the growth and manifestations of the myeloma itself. These cytokines and other factors mediate complex interactions between the multiple myeloma, the bone marrow stroma and the bone cells; finally, these interactions result in osteoclastic destruction of bone (Fig. 91.1).

Interleukin-6 (IL-6) plays a key role in these processes. It is produced by bone marrow stromal and endothelial cells, osteoblasts and osteoclasts. IL-6 stimulates the growth and inhibits apoptosis of myeloma cells.

> Overall, the mechanisms responsible for the growth and development of multiple myeloma involve the activities and interactions of the tumour cells with stromal and bone cells.

When soluble IL-6 receptors (sIL-6R) as well as IL-1 are also present, inhibition of bone formation and stimulation of bone resorption are particularly pronounced. The latest studies have shown that myeloma cells increase IL-6 production by osteoblasts either through indirect cell contact or by means of soluble factors. All these interactions are presumed to be responsible for the osteoclastic bone lesions. Soluble VCAM-1 ligands produced by stromal cells also stimulate myeloma cells to produce substances which trigger osteoclastic bone resorption. Angiogenesis plays an additional important role in the pathogenesis of MM. Myeloma cells themselves produce vascular endothelial growth factor (VEGF),

R. Bartl, C. Bartl, *Bone Disorders*, DOI 10.1007/978-3-319-29182-6_91

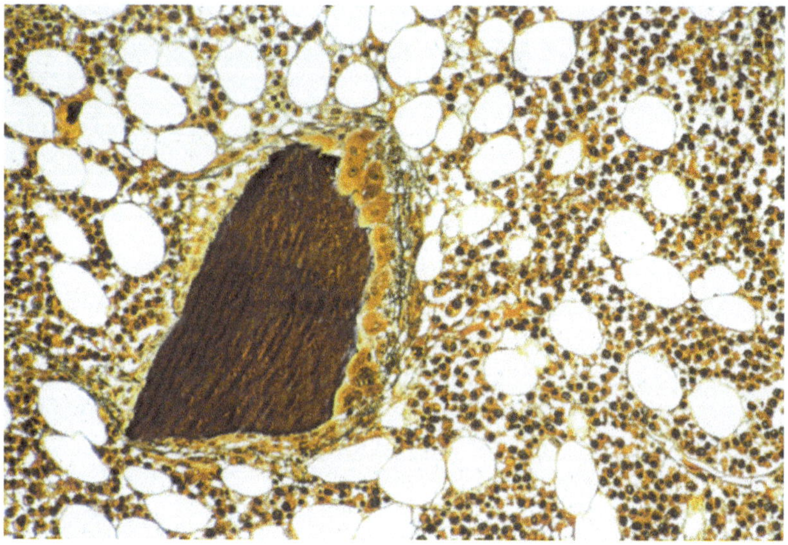

Fig. 91.1 Massive osteoclastic bone resorption of an ossicle with myeloma cells in the vicinity. Gomori staining

receptors for which are located on the surface of bone marrow stromal cells. Moreover, it has been demonstrated that VEGF increases IL-6 production by stromal cells in MM.

Adhesion molecules (integrins) are also important for proliferation of myeloma cells. These molecules are demonstrable on the surface of osteoclasts, myeloma cells and endothelial cells. Tumour cells with high levels of integrins are particularly invasive. It is of interest that lack or inhibition of integrins on the osteoclasts leads to their inactivation and thereby possibly to osteopetrosis in special circumstances. On the other hand, intercellular contact between osteoclasts and myeloma cells generates resistance to the antitumour effects of some chemotherapeutic agents, e.g. doxorubicin, while osteoclastic resorption and the life span of the myeloma cells are both increased. TRANCE, a new member of the TNF family, released by the interaction of myeloma and stromal cells, also activates osteoclastic resorption as well as stimulating the myeloma cells. Numerous experimental studies have now demonstrated the crucial role of the "microenvironment" and the RANKL/osteoprotegerin system not only for the growth of the myeloma itself but also for development of its resistance to radio- and chemotherapy.

In summary, four main pathogenic mechanisms are now held responsible for the osteolytic and osteoporotic effects of MM (Fig. 91.2):

- The surface expression of RANK ligand on myeloma cells stimulates osteoclasts.
- Other pro-osteoclastogenic factors (IL-6, IL-11, TGF-β) secreted by myeloma cells activate osteoclasts and bone resorption.
- Myeloma cells protect themselves against osteoprotegerin by means of phagocytosis and intracellular lysis.
- Myeloma cells produce DKK-1 which inhibits stromal cell differentiation into osteoblasts and thereby prevents new bone formation.

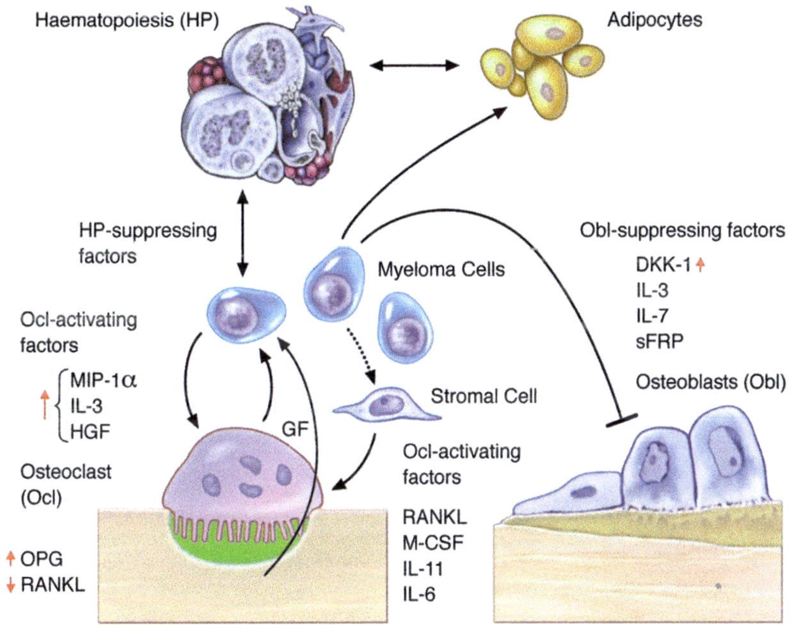

Fig. 91.2 Pathogenetic mechanisms of myeloma bone disease

91.3 Clinical Findings

Kahler's classical triad of bone pain, cachexia and proteinuria are all symptoms of an advanced stage of MM which today is observed far less frequently at diagnosis because now the disease is far more frequently exposed at an early or incipient stage. This is mainly due to the regular health checks many people undergo, because at this early stage the myeloma is mainly asymptomatic. The subsequent course is insidious and variable. The first objective manifestations are weakness, fatigue, decreased capability, lack of appetite and weight loss – all nonspecific indications of a malignant condition.

Frequently an elevated ESR, a pathologic M-peak on protein electrophoresis or a cytopaenia discovered incidentally by a routine check-up during a symptomless stage provides the impetus for further investigations. As the condition develops, it evokes symptoms by the interactions of tumour products leading to organ damage.

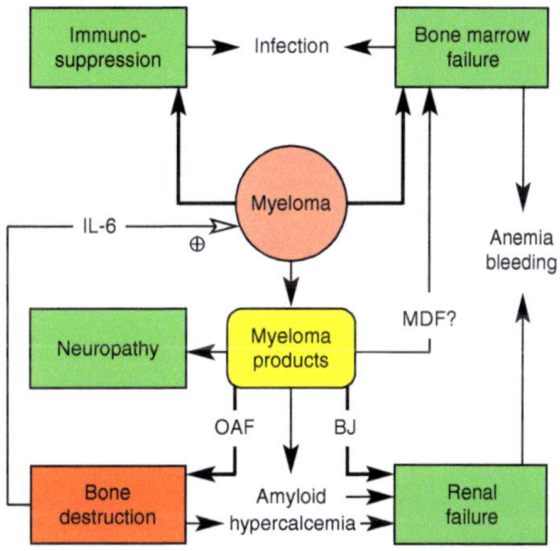

Fig. 91.3 Pathophysiology of multiple myeloma (MM). *OAF* osteoclast-activating factor, *BJ* Bence-Jones protein, *MDF* myelopoiesis depressing factor, *IL-6* interleukin-6 secreted by osteoclasts

The first relatively specific signs are bone pain, spontaneous fractures and increased liability to infections. The significant physiologic mechanisms and the complications of MM are summarised in Fig. 91.3.

91.4 Diagnosis of Skeletal Manifestations

Multiple myeloma is not only a malignant disease of the bone marrow, it is also a generalised disorder of bone characterised by skeletal destruction. The skeleton must therefore be carefully examined together with investigation of haematopoiesis and of the myeloma itself.

A retrospective study showed that in the year before myeloma was diagnosed, 16 times more fractures were observed than expected, particularly spinal, pelvis or rib fractures, all regions harbouring the red bone marrow.

These investigations should ideally be completed before organ complications have developed so that early preventive and supportive measures can be undertaken.

Bone-specific findings and symptoms at the time of diagnosis:

- Bone pain 55 %
- Osteolyses 45 %
- Osteoporosis 40 %
- Spontaneous fractures 18 %
- Hypercalcaemia 16 %.

Systematic X-ray examination of the axial skeleton is essential for initial diagnosis and for monitoring. Bones most frequently affected are those of the skull (Fig. 91.4), thoracic and lumbar vertebrae, followed by other bones which enclose haematopoietic bone marrow. The structure of the osseous lesions is determined by the basic growth pattern of the MM within the bone marrow: osteolyses with the nodular type and osteoporosis with the interstitial type. Osteosclerosis has been found in less than 3 % of myeloma patients.

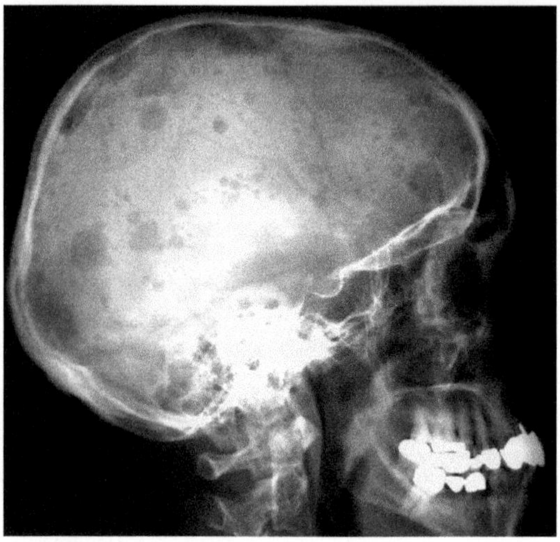

Fig. 91.4 X-ray of skull illustrating typical punched-out lesions in a patient with multiple myeloma (MM)

MRI is becoming increasingly important for early detection and prognostic evaluation of multiple myeloma, particularly in the axial skeleton.

Today early diagnosis and accurate staging of myeloma depend on MRI of the vertebral column. Bone scans are not suitable for diagnosis of MM since there is no activation of osteoblasts, in contrast to the situation in many metastasising tumours.

Even in the presence of completely normal X-ray findings, MRI will reveal small focal or nodular infiltrations of plasma cells in the vertebral bodies, thereby complementing the findings in bone biopsies taken from the iliac crest. MRI is equally indispensable in the investigation of a suspected solitary plasmacytoma.

Bone density measurements should be made by DEXA or QCT at diagnosis to provide a baseline so that potential bone loss, for example, during glucocorticoid therapy, can be monitored and the success of therapy with bisphosphonates can be assessed.

Parameters of bone metabolism (calcium, phosphate, alkaline phosphatase, creatinine and

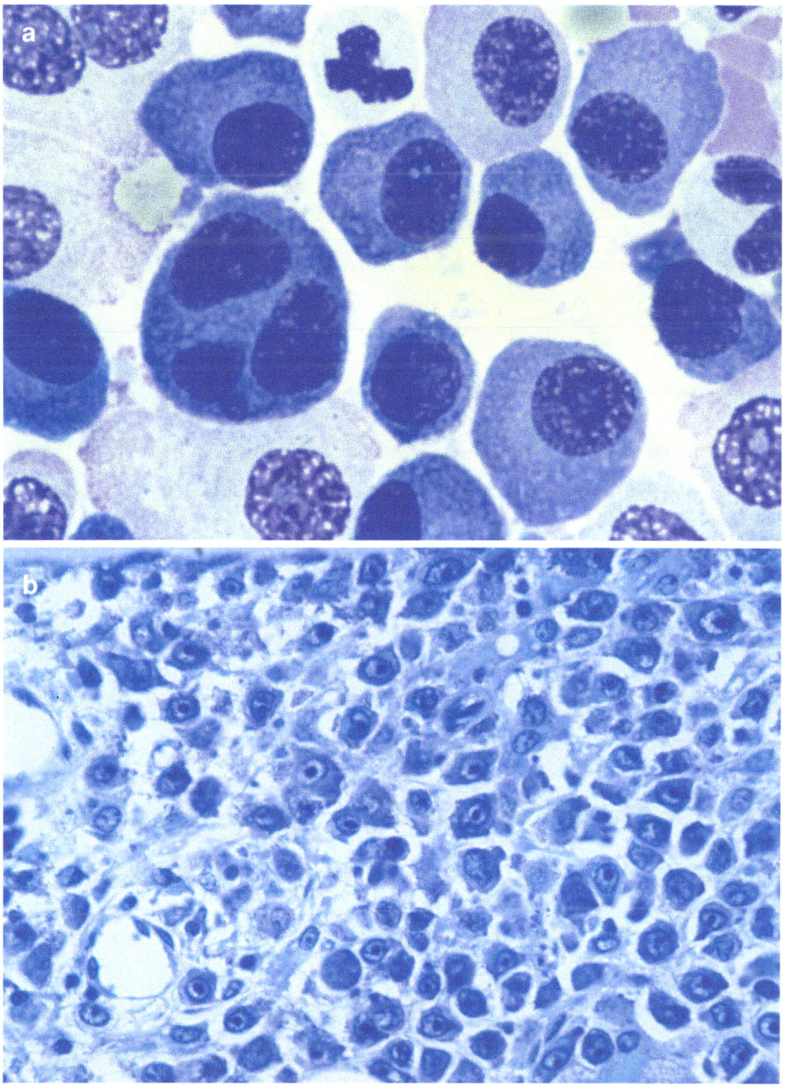

Fig. 91.5 Myeloma cells (**a**) bone marrow aspiration with atypical, heterogeneous and partly nucleolated plasma cells. (**b**) Bone marrow biopsy with large nucleolated plasma cells occupying the marrow space. Giemsa staining

markers of bone resorption such as deoxypyridinoline and telopeptides) should be checked in addition to performing a complete blood count and routine biochemical investigations, including indicators of hepatic and kidney function.

Bone and bone marrow biopsy and aspiration enable estimation of the type of plasma cells, the labelling index, quantity of infiltration, residual haematopoiesis, stromal elements, structure and microarchitecture of bone and of bone remodelling, all of which are important for a detailed diagnosis and for estimation of prognostic factors (Figs. 91.5a, b and 91.6a, b). Moreover, evaluation of blood vessels and connections between myeloma cells and bone marrow stroma have acquired increasing significance in light of the latest therapeutic possibilities, for example, thalidomide. In addition detailed information on the tumour cells, reactions of the bone marrow and stromal cells and bone and its cells is obtained from a bone marrow biopsy. Furthermore, quantitation of the number and activity of osteoclasts also provides criteria for early preventive therapy with bisphosphonates.

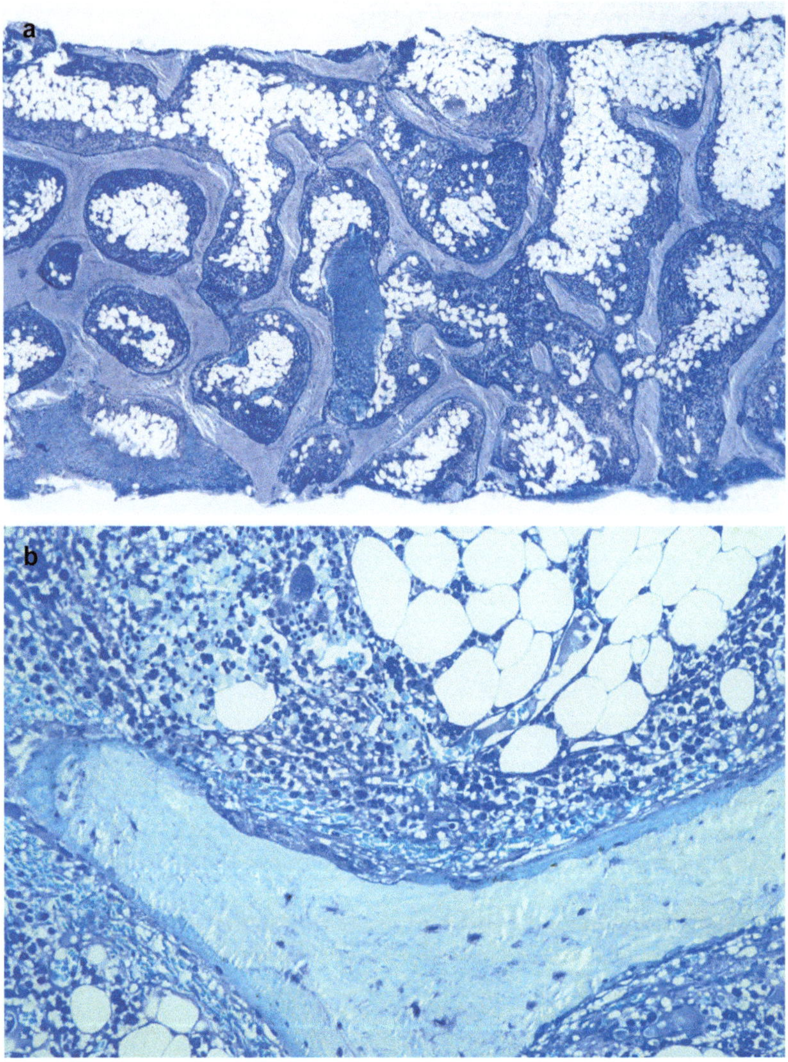

Fig. 91.6 (**a**) Example of paratrabecular infiltration in MM and the effect on bone. Giemsa staining. (**b**) Higher magnification showing that the paratrabecular layer of cells consists almost entirely of myeloma cells activating the osteoclastic resorption. Giemsa staining

The following histologic data are clinically relevant:

- Type of plasma cells (morphologic classification and grading)
- Quantity of plasma cells (morphologic staging)
- Growth pattern (diffuse, nodular)
- Haematopoiesis (quantity and maturation/dysplasia)
- Angiogenesis (normal vessels, neoangiogenesis, amyloidosis)
- Stromal components (fibrosis)
- Resorption of bone (osteolysis, osteoporosis)
- Mineralisation defect (increased osteoid, osteomalacia)
- Number and activity of bone cells (osteoclasts and resorption bays, osteoblastic seams)
- Deposition of iron

When the histologic growth pattern of the myeloma is correlated with osteoclastic bone remodelling, two groups can be distinguished:

- *Paratrabecular* and/or nodular growth patterns with high-grade osteoclastic resorption (Fig. 91.6a, b)
- *Interstitial* loose infiltration without apparent increased osteoclastic resorption

The first is associated with a distinctly less favourable prognosis, and therapy with bisphosphonates is clearly indicated. Change to an interstitial type under bisphosphonate therapy carries a more favourable prognosis with it.

91.5 Myeloma Variants

Variant forms of multiple myeloma (MM) are occasionally encountered. These can readily be distinguished if the methods described above are applied. The variants include:

- Smouldering and indolent MM
- Plasma cell leukaemia
- Nonsecretory MM
- Osteosclerotic MM
- Light chain amyloidosis (Fig. 91.7a, b)
- POEMS syndrome (polyneuropathy, organomegaly, endocrinopathy, M protein, skin manifestations)

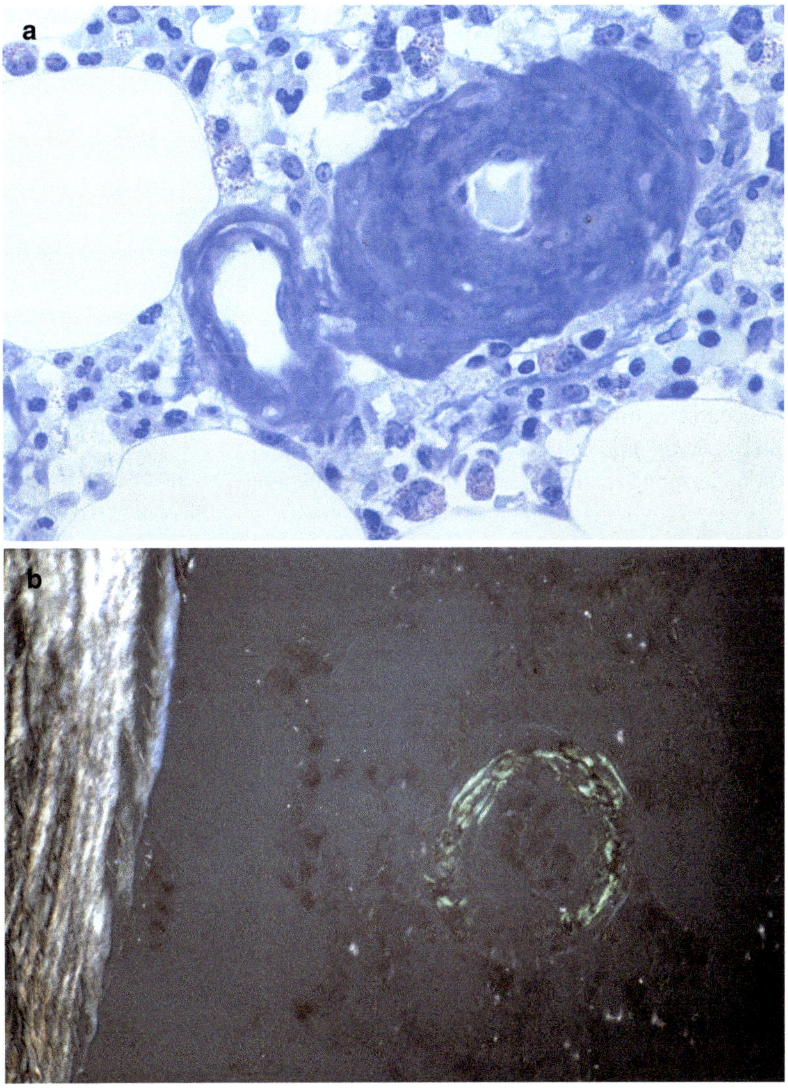

Fig. 91.7 Light chain amyloidosis: (**a**) Small artery and arteriole showing amyloid deposition in their wall. Giemsa staining. (**b**) Biopsy section stained with Congo red and viewed in polarised light: amyloid in arterial wall shows characteristic green fluorescence

- Light chain deposition disease
- MGUS (monoclonal gammopathy of undetermined significance)
- Waldenstrom's macroglobulinaemia

Patients with MGUS, a monoclonal abnormality of an immunoglobulin that may progress to multiple myeloma, also have a 2.7-fold increased risk of axial fracture.

91.6 Treatment Strategies

Cures have only been achieved in rare cases of solitary plasmacytoma or in younger patients treated by bone marrow transplantation. Therefore, in the vast majority of patients, the aim of therapy is to attain the longest survival with the best possible quality of life. To achieve this goal, skeletal destruction must be prevented, and this constitutes the most cogent argument for prompt administration of bisphosphonates as soon as the diagnosis is made.

The median *survival time* of a newly diagnosed patient with multiple myeloma is 30 months from the time of therapy. Nevertheless, the course of disease is very variable. For example, patients with rapidly progressive MM who do not respond to therapy may survive for only a few months. On the other hand, there are patients with asymptomatic MM who have a smouldering course lasting for many years without any chemotherapy or who survive for up to 20 years with only short periods of therapy. Therefore, it is now necessary to provide detailed information for a variety of therapeutic options which include the following questions:

- When to treat?
- Bone marrow or stem cell transplantation?
- Which therapy protocol?
- Duration of primary chemotherapy?
- Quality of remission?
- Duration of remission?
- Early recognition of impending relapse – MRD (minimal residual disease)
- Definition and methods for recognition of MRD
- Which second-line chemotherapy on relapse?
- Administration of thalidomide?
- Which supportive measures?
- How to investigate and to treat complications?
- Vertebroplasty and kyphoplasty in cases with advanced spinal disease.

The possibility of high-dose chemotherapy followed by bone marrow or stem cell transplantation should be considered early on.

91.7 Bisphosphonates

Though chemotherapy reduces the tumour mass considerably, it does little to repair osteolytic bone lesions or to prevent further loss of bone. First-generation BP also showed little effect. On the other hand, modern BP such as ibandronate or zoledronate given intravenously in placebo-controlled trials were effective in the treatment of *skeletal-related events* (SREs). The broad range of indications for therapy with BP in myeloma should be taken into account when planning the management of each patient.

Results of previous clinical experience as well as of clinical trials have highlighted the following indications for bisphosphonate therapy in multiple myeloma:

- Hypercalcaemia
- Bone pain
- Osteoporosis
- Osteolytic lesions
- After radiotherapy for osteolyses

The protocols used for therapy of skeletal-related events (SRE) are given below:

Pamidronate 60–120 mg infusion every 3–4 months
Clodronate 600–900 mg infusion every 3–4 months
Ibandronate 6 mg infusion every 3–4 months or 50 mg orally daily
Zoledronate 4 mg infusion every 3–4 months

These are practical guidelines only and must be regarded as such. A comparative study has been carried out with pamidronate and zoledronate: a 5 min infusion of 4 mg zoledronate was as effective as 90 mg pamidronate in prevention of SRE. In case of dehydration and/or hypercalcaemia, infusion of a BP should be carried out after rehydration and slowly to avoid renal damage, which is almost the rule in myeloma. Therefore, it is best always to choose BP with the longest half-life in the serum to minimise the possible renal damage.

The significance of BP therapy in multiple myeloma lies in *prevention* of skeletal complications. Institution of BP therapy at the time of diagnosis will lead to significant abrogation or at least to a clearly delayed appearance of skeletal complications, such as osteolysis, osteoporosis, fractures, hypercalcaemia and bone pain.

Furthermore, it has been demonstrated conclusively that the aminobisphosphonates exert an antiproliferative effect on tumour cells: that is, they inhibit growth of myeloma cells both directly and indirectly as described below. Therapy with zoledronate or ibandronate triggered a number of activities which were even enhanced when dexamethasone or chemotherapy with paclitaxel was added:

- Increased apoptosis of myeloma cells
- Reduction of osteoclastic and stromal cell production of IL-6
- Anti-angiogenic effect on blood vessels and stromal cells (changes similar to those seen after therapy with thalidomide)
- Cytotoxic effect on myeloma cells through activation of T lymphocytes
- Interference with cellular interactions such as:
- Inhibition of matrix metalloproteinase-1 secretion (stimulated by IL-1)

91.8 Denosumab and Bortezomib

Denosumab, a human monoclonal antibody against RANKL, is already used successfully for the prevention of SREs in patients with bone metastases and is now being tested in studies with MM. A recently published study shows benefits of denosumab with solid tumours and with MM, including cases with resistance towards bisphosphonates.

Denosumab 120 mg s.c. every 4 weeks

A red hand letter pointed out that denosumab therapy can cause severe symptomatic hypocalcaemia. In addition, all patients must receive vitamin D and calcium, except for existing hypercalcaemia. Special care must be taken with patients with renal insufficiency. In reverse, severe symptomatic hypercalcaemia is observed after discontinuation of denosumab, known as a "rebound"-effect.

Bortezomib a proteasome inhibitor, directly influences the activity of osteoblasts and osteoclasts through suppression of RANKL and DKK-1 in blood of myeloma patients. Clinical studies have shown activation of the osteoblasts and the suppression of the osteoclasts. Another interpretation is a direct suppression of the myeloma cells by bortezomib with secondary normalisation of the osteoblast and osteoclast function. Bortezomib is administered intravenously in cycles, alone or in combination with other substances.

Bortezomib 1.3 mg/body surface 4 times i.v. in 3-weekly cycles

MM in particular is a typical example demonstrating the close collaboration of tumour cells and osteoclasts with its high rate of skeletal complications (SREs). By early use of nitrogen-containing BP or denosumab, skeletal complications and tumour proliferation can be reduced (Fig. 91.8a, b).

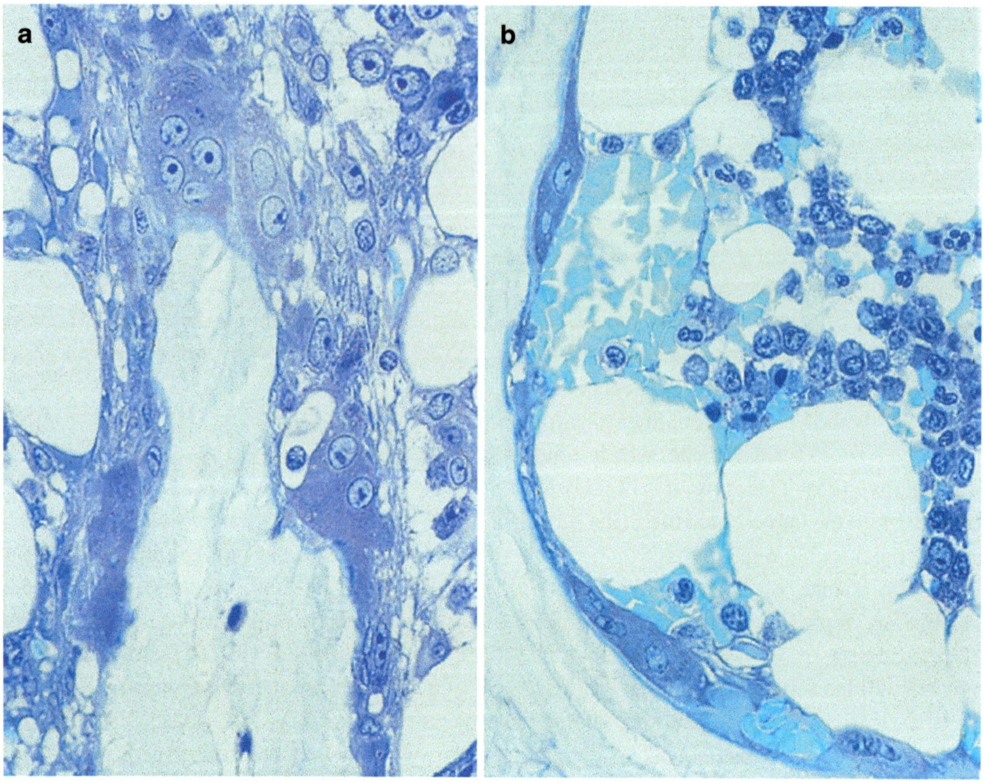

Fig. 91.8 Effect of intravenous BP on destruction of bone and on proliferation of myeloma cells. (**a**) Massive osteoclastic bone resorption with polymorphic, nucleolated myeloma cells in the vicinity. (**b**) The same patient after several infusions of ibandronate. Demonstration of unequivocal decrease in bone resorption with flat, inactive osteoclasts, absence of resorption lacunae, and mainly unremarkable plasma cells in the surrounding areas. All Giemsa staining

Part XVI

Bone and Cancer

Recent studies have raised the question of a possible connection between osteoporosis and cancer, as demonstrated by a report of a cohort of 23,935 men and women with osteoporosis who were investigated for risk of cancer. The patients were divided into two groups: up to 70 years of age who appeared were at increased risk of cancer, and the second group: older than 70 years who appeared to be at decreased risk of cancer. The results suggested that the risk factors associated with earlier or later onset of osteoporosis were also related to an increased or decreased risk of cancer, respectively.

92 Tumour-Induced Hypercalcaemia (TIH)

92.1 Definition and Pathogenesis

Hypercalcaemia is found in about 1 % of all hospitalised patients and caused by malignancy in 46 % of all cases and by pHPT in 35 %. In the remaining 19 %, other conditions are responsible. These include sarcoidosis, immobilisation and medications such as thiazides or active metabolites of vitamin D. Patients with mild hypercalcaemia have no symptoms. The term "hypercalcaemic syndrome" refers to a constellation of symptoms independent of the aetiology including renal, gastrointestinal and neuropsychiatric changes.

> The "hypercalcaemic syndrome" has a wide clinical spectrum, from asymptomatic to lethal.

It is characterised by severe dehydration which is caused by the following sequence of events: hypercalcaemia – hypercalciuria – polyuria – polydipsia – polyuria. Nausea and vomiting further increase the fluid and electrolyte loss. The result is hypopotassaemia together with disturbances of cardiac rhythm. Moreover, fatigue, depression and a general deceleration of cognitive function indicate additional neuropsychiatric involvement. In severe cases the condition may progress to a hypercalcaemic crisis with somnolence and coma.

All patients with cancer are subject to hypercalcaemia in the advanced stages of a malignancy, in particular patients with breast cancer or with multiple myeloma, less frequently with neoplasms of the lung or prostate.

> Hypercalcaemic episodes occur in 30 % of patients with metastatic tumours and in 50 % of patients with multiple myeloma.

Hypercalcaemia of malignancy is characterised by elevation of serum calcium with suppression of normal parathyroid secretion. The increase in serum calcium is due to aggressive local osteolyses, increased renal excretion and increased tubular re-absorption of calcium. Two types of TIH are recognised:

- *Osteolytic hypercalcaemia*: Tumour cells in the bone marrow secrete osteoclast-stimulating factors (IL-6, TGF), which stimulate massive osteoclastic resorption with release of calcium from the bone.
- *Humoral hypercalcaemia*: Many tumours produce parathyroid hormone-like substances (PTHrP) which bind to PTH receptors in bone and kidney and trigger the normal physiological effects of PTH (paraneoplastic syndromes). In addition, granulomas, e.g. in tuberculosis, sarcoidosis and sarcomas, and tumour-induced production of

R. Bartl, C. Bartl, *Bone Disorders*, DOI 10.1007/978-3-319-29182-6_92

active vitamin D metabolites (e.g. in lymphomas) can lead to hypercalcaemia.

92.2 Treatment Strategies in TIH

BP have greatly simplified the treatment of hypercalcaemia. A single 2 h infusion of one of the following is generally effective, especially those with high potency, e.g. ibandronate and zoledronate (Fig. 92.1):

Clodronate 1500 mg
Pamidronate 90–120 mg
Ibandronate 6 mg
Zoledronate 4 mg

After rehydration, the BP is infused slowly (1–4 h) in plenty of fluid (e.g. 500 ml of physiological saline), in order to avoid renal damage. The therapeutic activity comes into effect after a delay of 2–4 days (longer with pamidronate), and normal levels of calcium are obtained within 4–7 days and maintained for a period of several weeks, depending on the aggressivity of the tumour and which of the BP was used (zoledronate 88 %, ibandronate 78 %, pamidronate 70 %). Generally, the period of normalisation ranges from 2 to 4 weeks, with a success rate of 70–95 %. If a satisfactory result is obtained with zoledronate, then the second infusion should be given 7 days later. Treatment is repeated if and when elevation of serum calcium recurs. Four milligrams of zoledronate via 15 min infusion is the dose recommended for initial treatment of hypercalcaemia of malignancy (HCM) and 8 mg for relapsed or refractory hypercalcaemia. The median durations of complete responses were 32 (4 mg) and 43 (8 mg) days, respectively.

Patients with renal failure should receive 30–50 % lower doses, and longer infusion times are recommended (e.g. pamidronate 0.5 mg/min). Disturbances of renal function and/or local side effects at the site of infusion have not been reported for ibandronate. Moreover, as the hypercalcaemia is normalised, an improvement in renal function is also achieved. BP therapy is less effective and of shorter duration when there is a high level of PTHrP. The extraskeletal effects of PTHrP are not influenced by BP therapy. In life-threatening situations, when the level of calcium must be lowered rapidly, the combination of a BP with calcitonin is recommended, because this reduces the serum calcium level within a matter of hours by increasing the renal excretion of calcium. The calcitonin acts rapidly and bridges the gap till the BP begins to exert its effect.

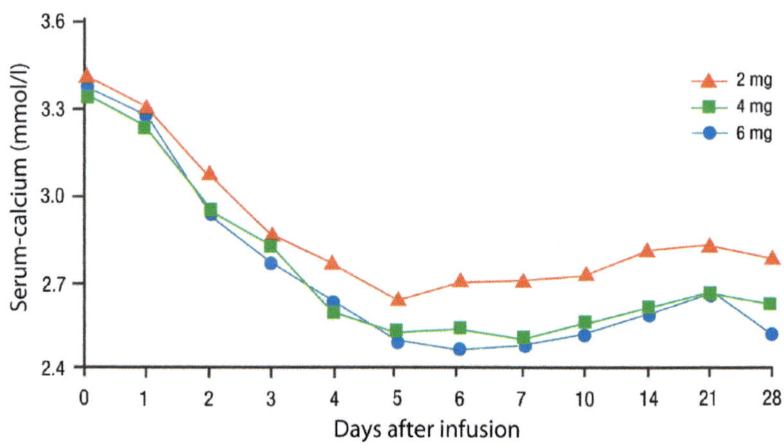

Fig. 92.1 Effect of different doses of ibandronate on hypercalcaemia

93 Tumour-Induced Bone Pain (TIBP)

93.1 Definition and Pathogenesis

Bone pain is the most frequent symptom in patients with osseous metastases. More than 50 % of these patients experience bone pain before or at the time of diagnosis of skeletal metastases. The pain is constantly present and may increase in intensity. Multiple myeloma and osteomyelosclerosis are also often accompanied by severe bone pain. Bone pain has a complex aetiology, incompletely understood. Mechanical factors include:

- Increased pressure in the bone marrow
- Bending or distortion of bone
- Stretching of the periosteum and/or endosteum
- Destruction of bone

Inflammatory, humoral and neural factors also play a role. Prostaglandins, histamine, serotonin, bradykinin and other cytokines can all act as triggers or as modulators. Bone pain is mediated primarily by stimulation of nociceptors (pain receptors) in the periosteal and endosteal sheaths of the bones. It can also be caused by irritation and lesions of the afferent nerve fibres within the bone marrow. These fibres regulate blood flow through bone, bone marrow and sinusoids. Sensory nerve fibres are also present, as demonstrated, for example, by the pain induced when bone marrow is aspirated. Results of recent studies have implicated the RANKL/OPG system as a major factor in triggering bone pain. Moreover, tumour cells themselves secrete cytokines which stimulate T lymphocytes and osteoclasts which leads to further release of inflammatory mediators as bone is resorbed. Generalised bone pain is also caused by the increased pressure resulting from bone marrow infiltration (metastatic, leukaemic) or by oedema of the bone marrow. Paraneoplastic bone pain is mediated indirectly by the tumour by way of the hormone-like substances it secretes.

93.2 Treatment

The treatment of bone pain in patients with malignancies should be an integral part of the overall management. Bone pain in cancer patients may have various causes:

- Due to the tumour itself (85 %)
- Due to therapy (17 %)
- Associated with the tumour (9 %)
- Independent of the above (9 %)

The first aim is elimination of the cause of the bone pain by specific therapy of the condition diagnosed if possible, for example:

- Vitamin D for osteomalacia
- Antibiotics for osteomyelitis
- Radiotherapy for focal neoplastic lesions

R. Bartl, C. Bartl, *Bone Disorders*, DOI 10.1007/978-3-319-29182-6_93

Treatment of tumour-induced bone pain also includes:

- Physical therapy (exercises, physiotherapy)
- Central and peripheral analgesics
- Additional medications (antidepressants, tranquilisers, muscle relaxants)
- Invasive therapy (peridural or intrathecal opioids)
- Antineoplastic therapy (chemo- and radiotherapy)
- Antiresorptive therapy (BP, calcitonin)

The alleviation of tumour-induced bone pain by BP has been demonstrated in several placebo-controlled clinical trials. The effect is often felt within a day and may last for weeks or months, depending on the dose administered. However, not all physicians, even experts in the field, are aware of the alleviation of bone pain by BP. Markers of bone resorption correlate closely with the analgesic effect. Success of BP therapy is indicated by:

- Reduction of pain intensity
- Reduction in use of analgesics
- Reduction in need for radiotherapy
- Reduction in surgical interventions

The following *protocols* are recommended for tumour-induced bone pain:

- Clodronate: 600 mg infusion every 3–4 weeks
- Clodronate: 1600 mg orally daily
- Pamidronate: 60–120 mg infusion every 3–4 weeks
- Zoledronate: 4 mg i.v. infusion every 3–4 weeks
- Ibandronate: 2–6 mg infusion every 3–4 weeks
- Ibandronate: 50 mg orally daily

Until recently, BP were given when bone pain was presumably caused by osteolytic lesions (Fig. 93.1). Pain induced by osteoblastic metastases, osteomyelosclerosis or systemic mastocytosis also responds rapidly and for long periods to BP therapy. In practice, all large studies of metastatic carcinoma and multiple myeloma have confirmed the analgesic effects of BP on pain due to osteolytic as well as osteoblastic and mixed metastases. This indicates that relief of bone pain by BP is not due exclusively to inhibition of osteoclasts, but that the BP also act on other cells such as T lymphocytes and stromal cells and thereby exert an effect on the RANKL/OPG system.

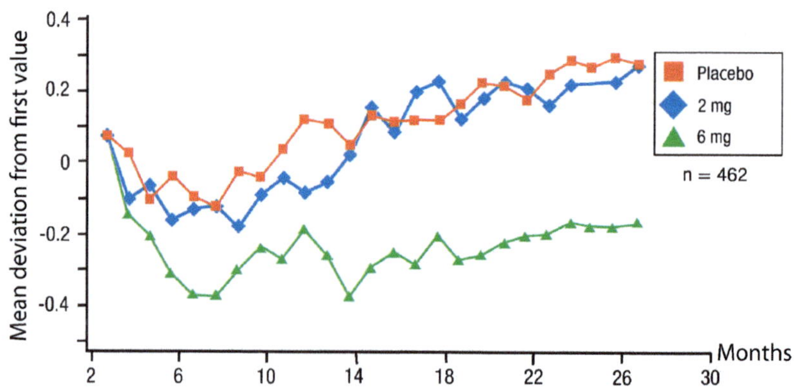

Fig. 93.1 Decrease of pain under therapy with ibandronate in patients with breast cancer

94 Bone Metastases: Incidence and Development

Metastasis is a fundamental problem in clinical oncology. Once established in the skeleton or elsewhere, the malignancy is systemic and can no longer be cured by surgery alone. This is the reason that tumours are regarded as systemic from the moment osseous or other metastases are detected. Some even consider all malignant tumours as systemic from the moment they are established and certainly as soon as they have attained a clinically detectable size.

Skeletal metastases can remain dormant and symptomless for many years. But when they begin to spread, metastases cause a drastic reduction of the patient's quality of life due to complications such as pain, immobility, fractures, spinal cord compression, hypercalcaemia and haematopoietic insufficiency. The situation is made even worse by the fear, depression and hopelessness which inevitably accompany the physical condition.

> Prevention of metastatic spread is as yet unattainable simply because it has already occurred in many patients before the tumour itself was diagnosed. Studies have shown that over 10 % of patients with breast cancer have metastases which have been dormant for over 10 years.

Cases of recurrence of metastatic spread after more than 20 years (or even longer) have also been reported. What intrinsic and/or extrinsic factors enable malignant cells to survive in a state of "hibernation" or "dormancy" and what events/circumstances trigger their subsequent awakening and renewed growth have not yet been completely elucidated. The lungs, liver and bone marrow act as filters for disseminated circulating malignant cells and are the most frequent sites for haematogenic spread. And of these, the bone/bone marrow environment offers ideal conditions for establishment of metastases.

However, the frequency of metastatic involvement of the skeleton at autopsy varies from 25 to 85 % probably due to differences in the method and thoroughness of search.

> Skeletal metastases are found at autopsy in 70–85 % of patients with tumours of the breast, prostate and lung, but fewer than half of these had been recognised clinically during the patients' lifetime.

The overall impression from previous studies is that up to 90 % of all patients who die of malignant tumours had skeletal metastases.

R. Bartl, C. Bartl, *Bone Disorders*, DOI 10.1007/978-3-319-29182-6_94

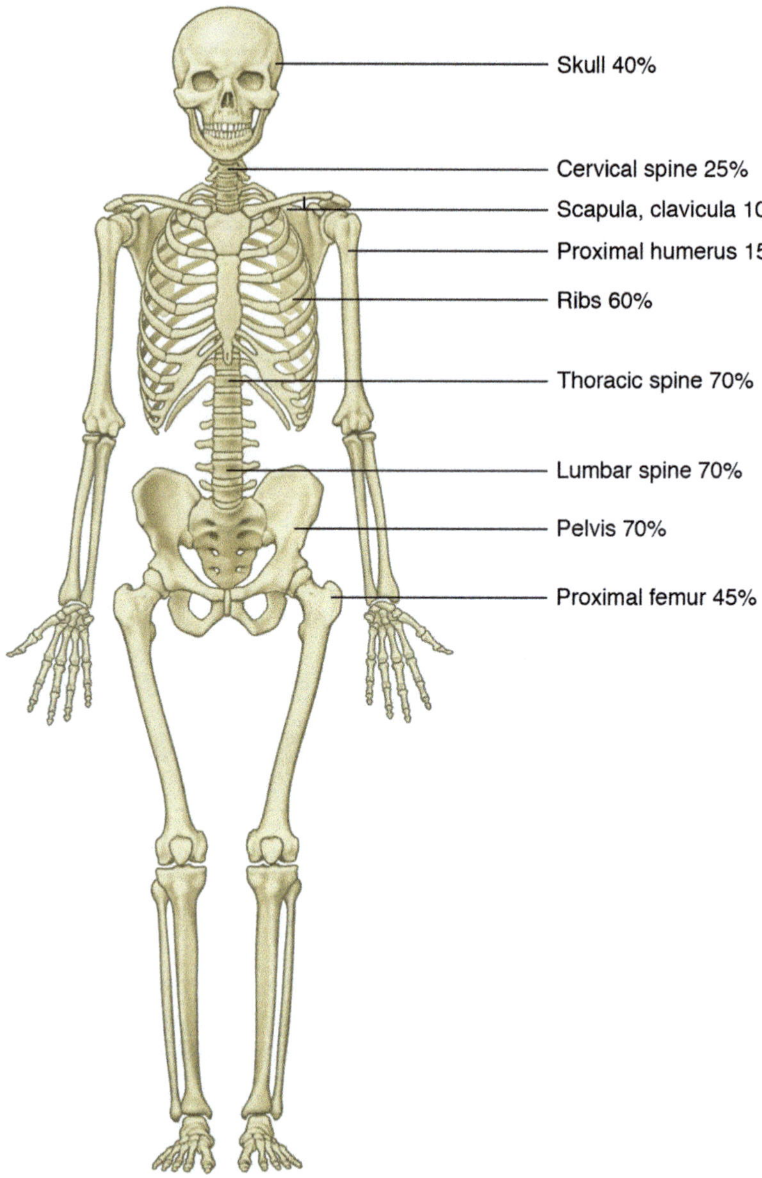

Fig. 94.1 Regional distribution of bone metastases within the skeleton

Certain tumours exhibit *osteotropism*, that is, a particular affinity to metastasise to the bones. These include tumours of the breast, prostate, lung, kidney and thyroid, and they are responsible for over 80% of all metastases in bone. Figure 94.1 shows the regional distribution in the skeleton.

Metastases "home" to bones which house red haematopoietic marrow (Fig. 94.2a–c). Several factors are responsible for this proclivity:

- The extensive vascular system
- Thin vascular walls, often without a basal membrane
- The slow blood flow through the sinusoids in the bone marrow
- Collagen fragments and minerals derived from normal bone resorption which are chemotactic for tumour cells
- Shedding of platelets into the marrow sinusoids and subsequent release of growth factors

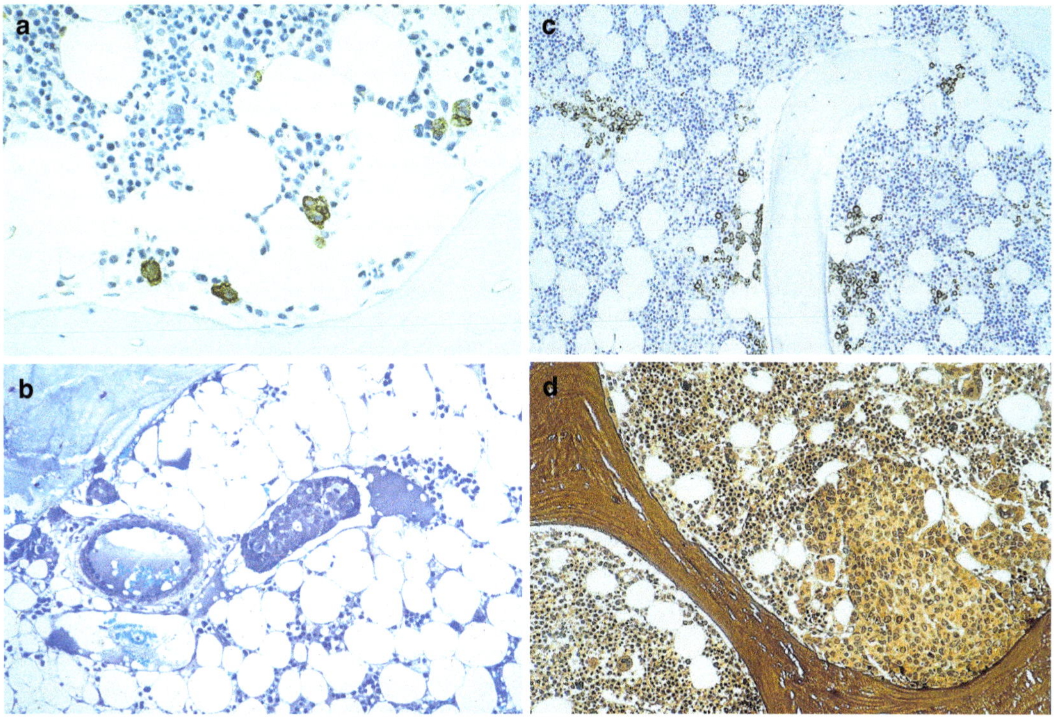

Fig. 94.2 Initial stages in the process of establishment of metastases in the bone marrow: (**a**) dissemination of tumour cells in the bone marrow and incipient adhesion to the surface of the bone (immunohistology), (**b**) large intravascular tumour embolus and small interstitial clusters of tumour cells in hypocellular bone marrow, Giemsa staining. (**c**) Cluster of tumour cells in the centre of a bone marrow cavity (*left*) as well as attached to the surface of a trabecula (immunohistology), (**d**) development of a micrometastasis with induction of stroma, attached to the surface of a trabecula, Gomori staining

These are ideal conditions for intravascular tumour cells to migrate into the surrounding tissues and to implant, i.e. establish themselves (*seed and soil hypothesis*) (Fig. 94.3). A greater understanding of the molecular mechanisms of skeletal metastases is expected to lead to development of more targeted therapy. Some progress has already been made with respect to factors released by the tumour cells, the bone cells and the environmental mesenchymal cells. Tumour cells produce predominantly growth factors and cytokines that stimulate either osteoclasts or osteoblasts. Growth factors released from the bone matrix support and maintain the tumour cells themselves – a kind of vicious cycle is established whereby the environment and the metastases support each other (Fig. 94.4). The elucidation of this process has suggested new therapeutic avenues of approach – to inhibit tumour growth by targeting the bone marrow microenvironment.

As outlined above, an *osseous reaction* with markedly increased remodelling, particularly resorption, occurs in 93 % of patients with skeletal metastases, and bone turnover markers are used for diagnosis, prognosis and as predictors of skeletal complications in many solid tumours. Two types of bone resorption in metastatic bone disease are known: osteoclastic and expansive by the tumour cells themselves (Figs. 94.5 and 94.6a, b). The type of osseous reactions to the metastases depends on the primary tumour. Usually osteoclastic resorption is accompanied by osteoblastic formation. Metastases of breast cancer exhibit this mixed osteoclastic/osteoblastic reaction, while the metastases of prostatic carcinomas evoke an almost exclusively osteoblastic reaction with production of woven bone (Table 94.1).

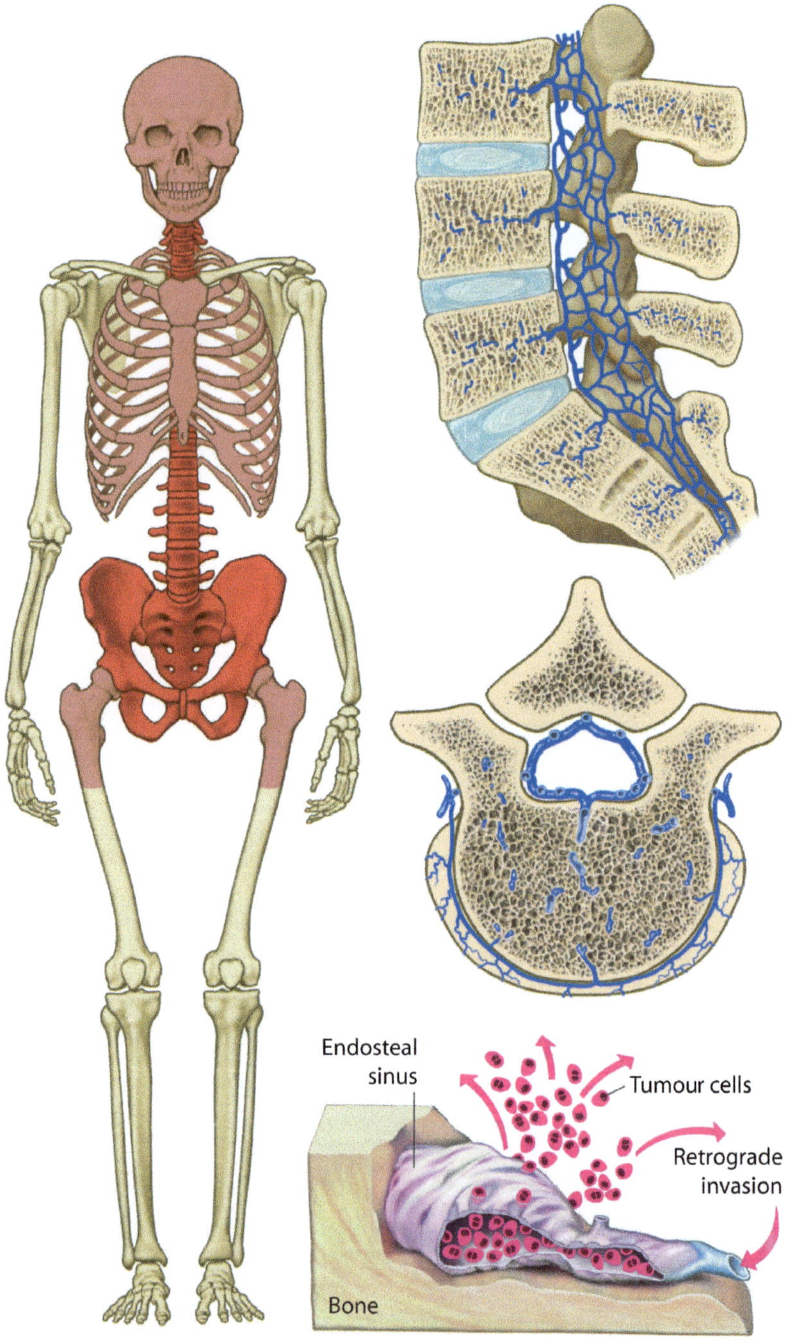

Fig. 94.3 Retrograde spread of tumour cells via the venous complex (Batson's) in the vertebral column. This is a common route for metastases to the axial skeleton. The tumour cells invade the bone marrow by way of the endosteal sinuses, which are the terminal vessels of the venous system in the bone marrow

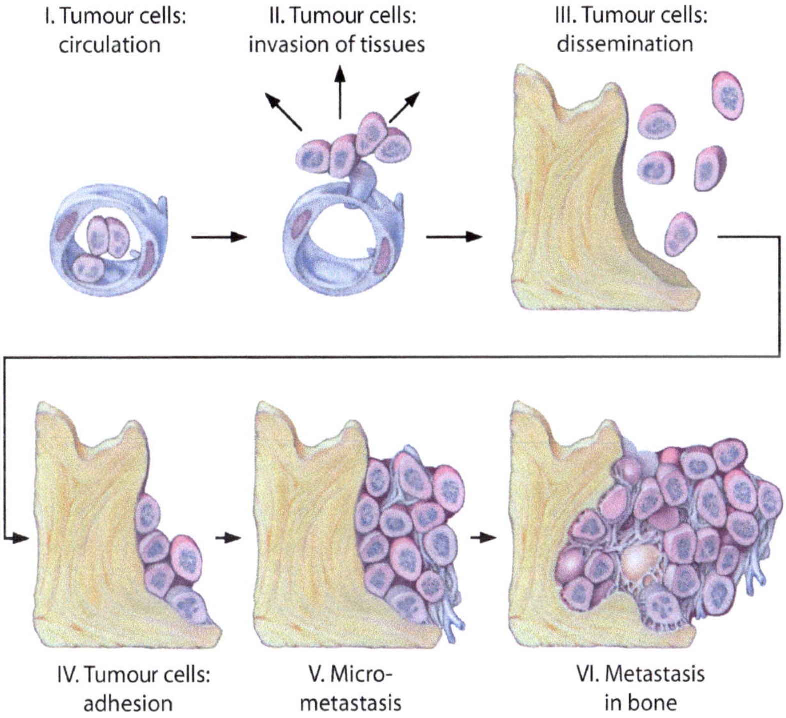

Fig. 94.4 Six stages in establishment of bone metastases

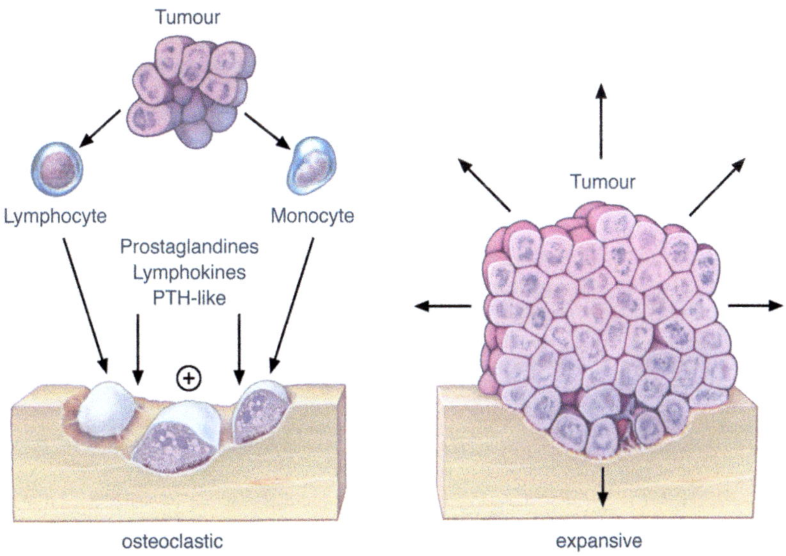

Fig. 94.5 Mechanisms of tumour osteolysis: cells and factors involved in metastatic osteolysis

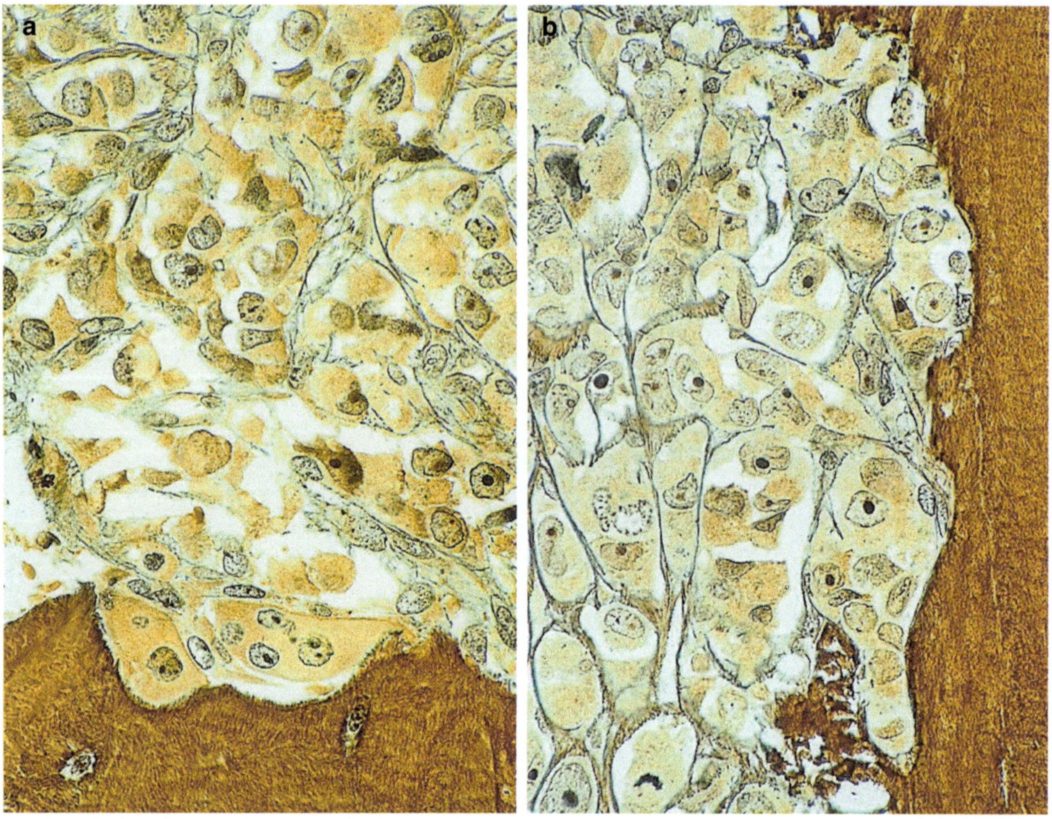

Fig. 94.6 Iliac crest biopsies illustrating (**a**) osteoclastic and (**b**) direct tumour cell osteolyses in metastatic bone disease. All Gomori staining

Table 94.1 Histologic bone reactions in various primary tumours (% of cases with metastatic bone disease)

	Breast	Prostate	Bronchus
Normal	5	0	28
Osteoporosis/lysis	20	7	18
Mixed form	41	38	27
Trabecular sclerosis	22	0	26
Woven bone	12	55	0

95 Skeletal Metastases of Breast and Prostate Cancer

95.1 Bone Reactions in Breast Cancer

Mammary carcinoma is the most frequent malignant tumour in women. It affects one out of ten women and is fatal in 30 % of cases, and over 75 % of patients will have osseous metastases with progression of the disease. The average survival after the appearance of osseous metastases is approximately 2–3 years. The prognosis is much worse (only a few months) when visceral metastases have occurred.

Destruction of bone and replacement of haematopoietic tissue by the tumour or by the cytotoxic effects of chemotherapy or both lead to the following complications:

- Bone pain: 60–80 %
- Osteoporosis: 40–50 %
- Pathologic fractures: 10–30 %
- Hypercalcaemia: 10–30 %
- Bone marrow failure: 20 %
- Spinal cord compression: 10 %.

95.2 Treatment Strategies in Metastatic Breast Cancer

Before beginning therapy for breast cancer, certain goals are set:

- *Prevention of development of metastasis by tumour cells* already dispersed in the body. Treatment of micrometastases and prevention of skeletal destruction once bone marrow involvement has been detected, for example, by MRI, bone scan or bone biopsy. The efficacy of BP in this setting has already established.
- *Prevention and treatment of osteoporosis.* It should be noted that bone loss may be due to the patient's age, to the disease itself and to therapy, any or all of which can cause osteoporosis resulting in pathologic fractures. Recent studies have indicated that this bone loss can be prevented by bisphosphonates and skeletal integrity maintained.
- *Treatment of pre-existing skeletal complications*, as in patients with advanced breast cancer or complications associated with radiotherapy or other procedures (palliative treatment). Administration of bisphosphonates after radiotherapy can accelerate the recalcification of osteolytic lesions after radiation.

Prophylaxis with BP is becoming ever more significant, also in view of the minimal side effects of these drugs. On completion of radio- and chemotherapy, after surgery, treatment with aromatase inhibitors, anastrozole or letrozole, is initiated. BP therapy is continued as long as this treatment is continued, up to 5 years. Results of a study with zoledronic acid 4 mg given biannually by i.v. infusion for 5 years have documented the prevention of

R. Bartl, C. Bartl, *Bone Disorders*, DOI 10.1007/978-3-319-29182-6_95

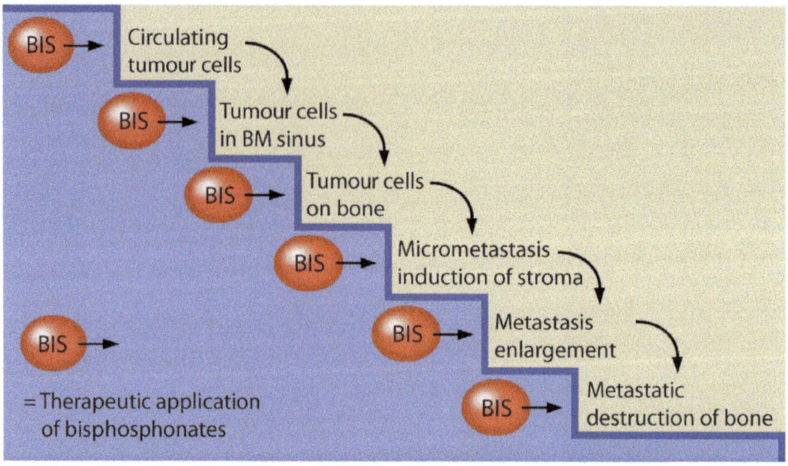

Fig. 95.1 Cascade of reactions in the development of skeletal metastases and the inhibitory effect of bisphosphonates (BIS)

bone loss in these postmenopausal patients on therapy with letrozole after the first year of therapy.

95.3 Bisphosphonates for Prevention of Metastasis

BP form an integral part of the management of breast cancer (Fig. 95.1). Clinical studies of patients treated with clodronate over a 3-year period have shown a 50 % reduction in skeletal metastases. The survival time of patients on long-term therapy with clodronate or ibandronate was significantly increased. However, these studies did not produce uniform results with respect to visceral metastases and survival. It is clear that patients who had circulating tumour cells or high levels of bone sialoprotein (BSP) benefit most from this type of adjuvant therapy. BSPs are produced by osteoclasts and tumour cells and play an important part in cell-matrix interactions in bone, e.g. adhesion of osteoclasts to collagen type I.

95.4 Bisphosphonates for Prevention of Skeletal Complications

Micrometastases – as well as larger established metastases – are demonstrable by MRI, by tumour markers in blood and by bone biopsy. At this point, these metastases have not evoked any osseous reactions demonstrable by bone scan or X-ray, and administration of BP can prevent their establishment and development on and in the bones (Fig. 95.2).

95.5 Bisphosphonates for Treatment of Skeletal Complications

BP have strong antiresorptive effects and also some degree of osteoreparative (recalcification) effect (Fig. 95.3). They can prevent unwanted bone loss following radiotherapy. Administration of BP leads to increased formation of callus which accelerates healing of bone defects. 1000 IU vitamin D daily (after exclusion of hypercalcaemia!) promotes mineralisation of the newly formed bone. However, since complete restoration of normal bone structure in large osteolytic lesions can take years, it is all the more important to prevent them. Previous studies have shown that BP can prevent skeletal-related events (SREs) (new osteolytic lesions, pathologic fractures, hypercalcaemia, spinal cord compression and bone pain) and thereby reduce the need for surgery and radiotherapy. Clinical studies on the renal safety and on the efficacy of BP in patients treated for over 10 years have now been published.

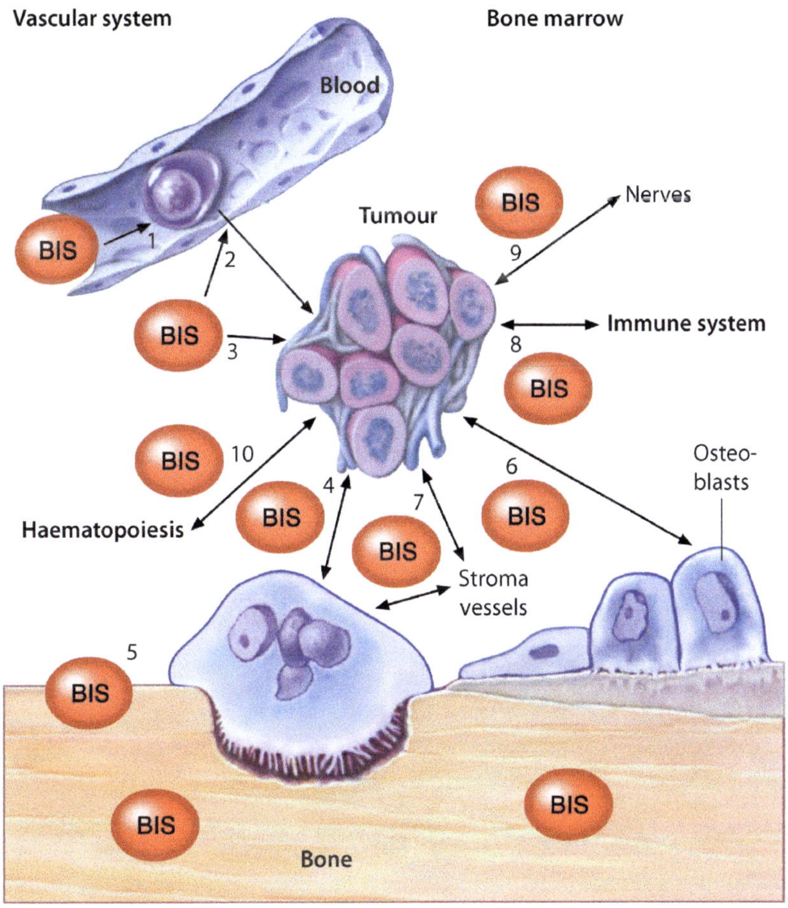

Fig. 95.2 Ten actions of bisphosphonates (BIS) on metastases in bone

A modest increase in survival of premenopausal patients was also observed. Administration of a BP such as clodronate together with irradiation of an osteolytic lesion is thought to have an additive effect. The presence of visceral metastases, though probably predictive of a shorter survival, is no justification for not giving BP. In addition, numerous articles from many countries have now confirmed the efficacy of BP for skeletal protection in patients with breast cancer. Many have emphasised the efficacy of early administration of BP, for example, immediately following neoadjuvant chemotherapy, to evaluate effects on cellular apoptosis, on proliferation and on angiogenesis, in addition to the effects on the actions of the bone cells for prevention of the osteoblastic and or osteolytic effects stimulated by the tumour cells.

Treatment of skeletal complications is best achieved by monthly intravenous N-containing BP or subcutaneous denosumab:

Pamidronate: 90 mg infusion monthly
Ibandronate: 6 mg infusion monthly
Zoledronate: 4 mg infusion monthly
Denosumab (XGEVA®): 120 mg subcutaneous injection monthly

The optimal duration of BP therapy has not yet been established. A diet rich in calcium and a vitamin D supplement should also be prescribed after exclusion of hypercalcaemia. Hypocalcaemia was more frequent with denosumab versus zoledronate. Therefore, low serum calcium levels and vitamin D deficiency should

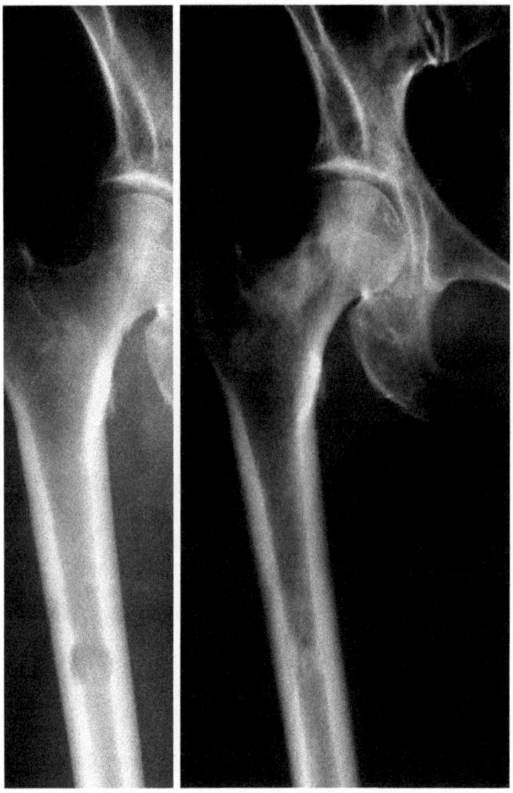

Fig. 95.3 Recalcification of osteolytic lesions of the femur under bisphosphonate and chemotherapy in a patient with metastatic breast cancer

be corrected before initiating treatment with denosumab, and corrected serum calcium levels should be monitored during treatment.

95.6 Bone Reactions in Prostatic Cancer

Ten to twenty percent of the patients with prostatic cancer have bone metastases at time of diagnosis, and some may be small. Consequently whole-body MRI has been advocated for complete as possible detection of skeletal metastases of prostate cancer. Moreover, the simultaneous demonstration of associated skeletal complications is an advantage. Whereas osteolytic lesions predominate in multiple myeloma and breast cancer, metastases of prostatic cancer are characterised by their osteoblastic reactions evoked by a number of mediators (Figs. 95.4a, b, 95.5, and 95.6).

In spite of the preponderance of bone formation, BP are also indicated both as a preventive and a palliative measure due to the significant role played by the osteoclasts because of the "coupling" of processes involved in bone remodelling even in these metastases. Moreover, experimental studies have shown that tumour cells can produce the receptor activator of RANKL, which activates osteoclasts. Matrix metalloproteinases, which degrade bone matrix, are also secreted by prostatic tumour cells. Moreover, after therapy with BP, a rapid and prolonged alleviation of pain, together with a reduction in requirements of analgesics, has been reported by patients with prostatic skeletal metastases. The improvement in the pain score also coincides with a decrease in resorption products in blood and urine. The considerable risk of osteoporosis due to therapeutic hypogonadism constitutes another justification for the early initiation of BP therapy. The effects of androgen deprivation therapy are far reaching including changes in body composition: lean mass, fat mass and muscle mass, as well as reduction in BMD. Encouraging results have already been obtained with high doses of parenteral clodronate, alendronate, pamidronate and ibandronate.

> BP treatment of painful osseous metastases due to hormone refractory prostate cancer resulted in a significant decrease of pain and a corresponding significant reduction in the daily consumption of analgesics in 75 % of patients.

Each parameter correlated with an increase in the Karnofsky index, mainly due to better mobility. Therefore, BP have a definite role in the palliative management of symptomatic hormone refractory prostate cancer. It has already been established that therapy with BP decreases the risk of skeletal complications in men with androgen-independent prostate cancer and bone metastases. Moreover, preliminary trials of chemotherapy (taxane) together with a BP (zoledro-

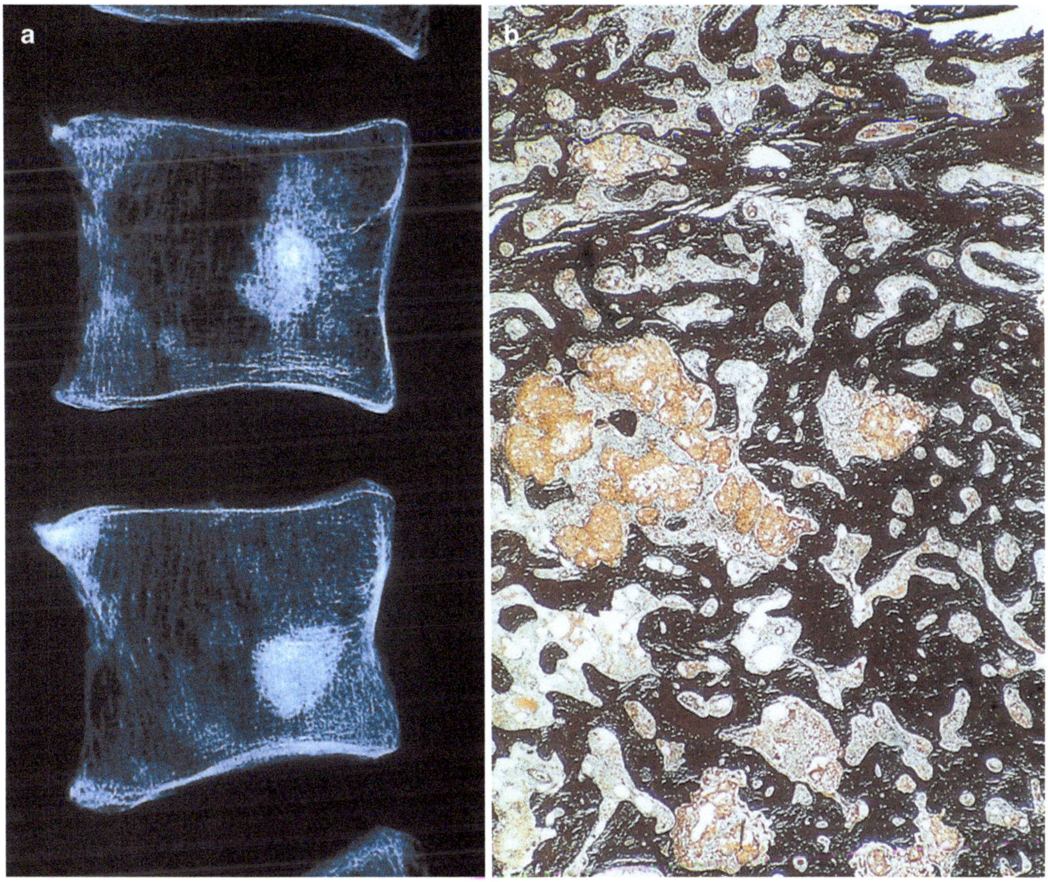

Fig. 95.4 (**a**, **b**) Osteosclerotic metastases in a patient with prostatic carcinoma. (**a**) Within vertebral bodies in the lumbar spine. (**b**) Small metastatic foci are walled in by an osteosclerotic reaction in a patient with prostatic carcinoma (section of iliac crest bone biopsy)

nate) have shown good results, as have preliminary results of therapy with denosumab, a human monoclonal antibody to RANKL.

Consensus Guidelines have been published for introduction of BP into the management of metastasising cancers (Berensen 2005). Studies on the benefits of zoledronate in prevention of skeletal complications have already been published. In addition, studies aimed at prevention of skeletal metastases are currently under way with ibandronate. A retrospective analysis of patients with non-small cell lung cancer treated with zoledronate for 21 months showed a statistically significant correlation between the therapy and increased survival. It should also be mentioned that zoledronate is the only BP that has demonstrated statistically significant long-term benefits in patients with renal cell carcinoma. New Consensus Guidelines on the use of BP in solid tumours have just been published.

Finally, a word of caution: the possibility of bisphosphonate-induced *necrosis of the jaws (ONJ)* must not be forgotten when giving potent BP especially i.v. The patient must be fully informed, consultation with the dentist is strongly recommended and a consent form must be signed before therapy is started, particularly if used for indications not yet completely authorised. Therefore, it is advisable to check whether administration of BP for prevention of metastases in patients with the tumours mentioned above has already been authorised, as for example, zoledronate for treatment of patients with bone metastases in the USA. The efficacy of BP for prevention of skeletal metastases is now being

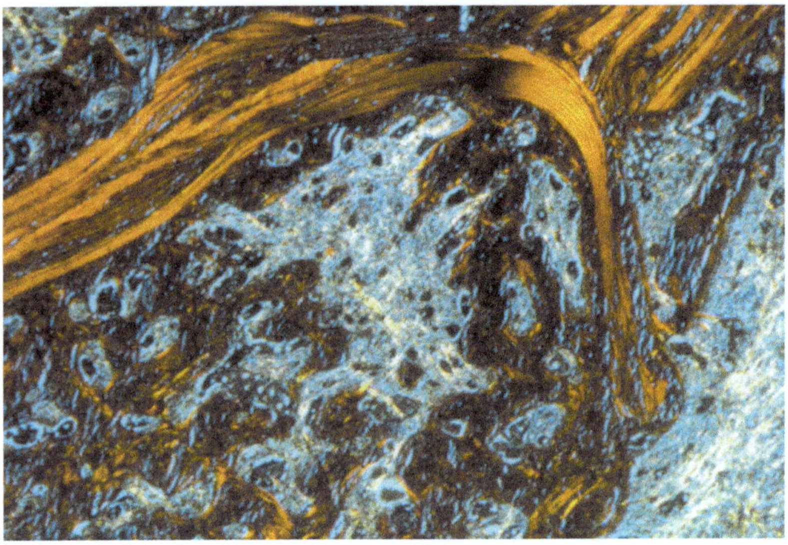

Fig. 95.5 Diminution of marrow space by woven bone deposited on the lamellar trabecula as well as in the marrow space in a patient with skeletal metastases of prostate carcinoma, Gomori staining polarisation

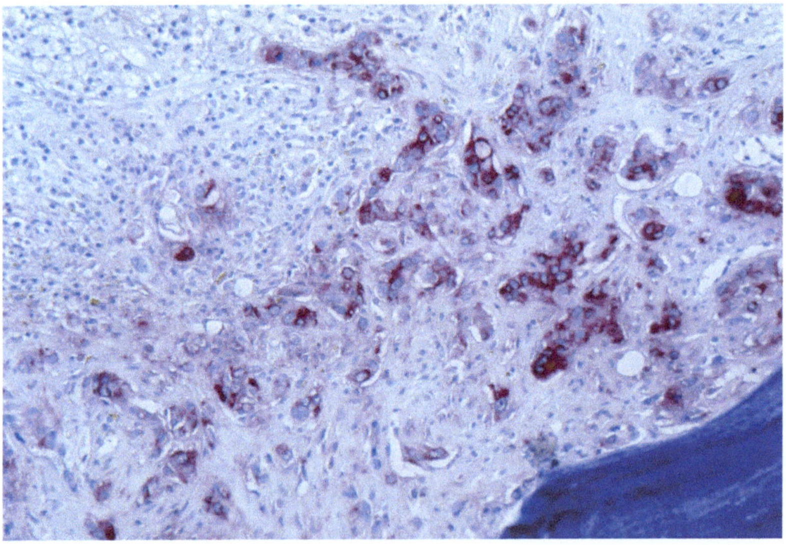

Fig. 95.6 Tumour cell clusters of a prostate carcinoma in the bone marrow in a patient with metastases of unknown primary tumour. Immunohistology (PSA), plastic embedded

investigated in many clinical trials, and results are awaited. Treatment-induced bone loss can also occur in cancers other than those mentioned above, for example, certain sarcomas.

One last important group is the *long-term cancer survivors*, who should be regularly monitored for the state of the skeleton, so that timely preventive therapy can be given if and when required. This applies to children as well as to adults. Finally, in certain specific cases, tumour-induced skeletal destruction may require a completely different approach, for example, in the case of malignant vertebral compression fractures: radionuclide therapy for the malignant cells and injection of polymethylmethacrylate to support the vertebral body. Studies for the optimal treatment of such fractures are underway.

96 Other Tumours with Osteotropic Metastases

96.1 Bronchial Carcinoma

Bone marrow biopsies demonstrated that at least 15 % of patients with adenocarcinoma of the lungs already have bone marrow metastases at the time of diagnosis. Autopsy studies have shown an incidence of 35 %. These metastases evoke variable osseous reactions. Relatively few studies on the effects of bisphosphonates have been carried out, possibly because of the short survival times – a matter of months – of patients with bronchial cancer once metastases are established. However, the studies that have been published have shown a positive effect of bisphosphonates on reduction of SREs as well as delay in time to occurrence of the first SREs (Fig. 96.1). Moreover, in these patients, a prolongation of even a few months to occurrence of the first SRE is significant, and BP reduce skeletal morbidity regardless of SRE history. The rapid analgesic effect of BP (within 2 days) was also observed in these patients. Recent studies have emphasised the need for early identification of patients at risk and the beneficial role of the latest BP in the management of patients with advanced metastatic bone disease. It is also of interest that BP induced apoptosis in cells derived from adenocarcinomas of the lungs in experimental and in "in vitro" investigations. This has promising implications for future therapy.

96.2 Renal Cell Carcinoma

Since the cells of these tumours have retrograde access to the vertebral venous plexus, bone marrow metastases are relatively frequent (25 % of cases). Tumour-induced hypercalcaemia was observed in 3–17 % of the patients with renal cell carcinoma. However, large clinical studies have not yet been carried out, though a positive effect of BP would be expected here also. In the event of bone pain, hypercalcaemia or osteolysis, intravenous administration of N-containing BP is indicated. Experimental data have demonstrated that bisphosphonates also prevent metastasis of renal carcinoma. However, adequate clinical studies are difficult to perform because of the low number of patients with renal carcinoma.

When complications of skeletal metastases occur in patients with carcinomas and sarcomas (bone pain, hypercalcaemia, osteolyses, etc.), the following regimens are recommended:

Clodronate	1600–3200 mg orally daily
Pamidronate	90–120 mg infusion monthly
Ibandronate	6 mg infusion monthly or 50 mg orally daily
Zoledronate	4 mg i.v. monthly

R. Bartl, C. Bartl, *Bone Disorders*, DOI 10.1007/978-3-319-29182-6_96

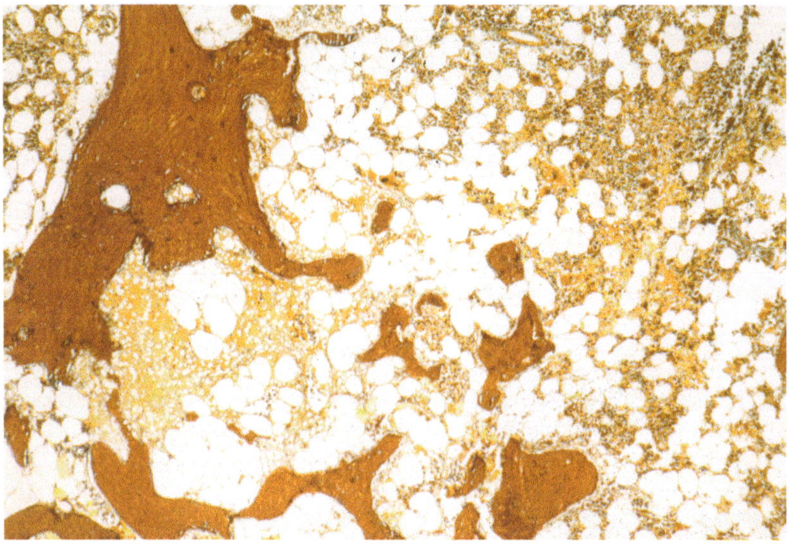

Fig. 96.1 Marginal osteosclerosis around a bone marrow metastasis area (*left*) after BP therapy and chemotherapy. Gomori staining

The biological effect of ibandronate 50 mg orally daily has been shown to correspond to that of ibandronate 6 mg given i.v. monthly.

96.3 Other Tumours with Implications for Skeletal Involvement

96.3.1 Neuroblastoma

The bones are the second most common site of metastases in neuroblastoma. As in breast cancer and in multiple myeloma, the tumour cells themselves activate osteoclasts to resorb bone and thereby cause lytic lesions. Inhibition of osteoclast activation by BP has already been demonstrated in preclinical trials, and results of clinical studies are awaited.

96.3.2 Ewing's Sarcoma

Experimental studies have shown that zoledronate induced apoptosis and inhibited proliferation in human Ewing sarcoma cells. See also Chap. 97.

96.3.3 Giant Cell Tumour of Bone

This is an aggressive primary neoplasm of bone. Osteolytic lesions are produced by osteoclast-like giant cells stimulated by the neoplastic stromal cells which constitute the main neoplastic component of this malignancy. BP inhibit the osteoclastic activity and also induce apoptosis of osteoclasts. See also Chap. 97.

96.3.4 Endometrial Carcinoma

This is an example of a cancer which usually does not metastasise to bone. Skeletal metastases are occasionally seen in patients who had been treated for primary tumours which usually do not metastasise to bone.

97 Primary Bone Tumours and Tumour-Like Lesions

97.1 Introduction

Osteologic practice occasionally includes problems of diagnosis and therapy of bone tumours. Clinical signs common to many bone disorders are also present in patients with primary bone tumours: swelling, tenderness, pain on motion, stiffness and pathologic fractures. The most prominent constitutional symptoms are loss of weight, anorexia and fever. Primary bone tumours are rare (about 1 % of all malignancies) and deceptive in their presentation, clinical and radiologic feature are often nonspecific, and histologic pictures of malignant neoplasms can be easily confused with benign conditions. Therefore, the aim of this chapter is to raise awareness of these diagnostic problems in order that the diagnosis is made early and the effective therapy can be started. It is also important to emphasise that patients with possible malignant bone tumours are referred to *centres familiar with these neoplasms*, including osteologists, oncologists, surgeons, radiologists and histopathologists. Only by the cooperation of these specialists mistakes in diagnosis can be avoided, and early treatment can be started without delay.

97.2 Definition and Epidemiology

A *primary bone tumour* is any neoplasm that arises from the tissues present within bone. Neoplasms arising from osteoblasts, cartilage cells, fibrous tissue, fatty tissue, vessels or neural tissues of bone are referred to as *sarcomas*. The vast majority of primary bone tumours are benign, and many of them are asymptomatic and are detected only incidentally at radiographic investigation for other reasons. The most common benign bone tumour, often asymptomatic, is an osteochondroma. The incidence of malignant bone tumours is, however, well documented in national cancer registries. Excluding the most common haematopoietic neoplasms (multiple myeloma, malignant lymphomas, leukaemias), the yearly incidence in the USA has been estimated to be $8/10^6$, and more than 75 % of malignant bone tumours are osteosarcoma (35 %), chondrosarcoma (26 %) and Ewing's sarcoma (16 %).

The incidence of bone tumours also shows a striking *age-specific distribution*. Benign tumours show a clear association with youth but are often diagnosed at a more advanced age, and most of them do not require any treatment. Malignant bone tumours have an incidence peak between 10 and 20 years (osteosarcoma and Ewing's sarcoma) and a steady increase in incidence from 40 to 80 years (chondrosarcoma).

Anatomic site distributions are also characteristic: benign tumours are often located in region of the knee (31 %), followed by the hip and pelvis (13 %) and the shoulder girdle (13 %). Malignant bone tumours often are located in the distal femur (22 %), pelvis (20 %), spine (18 %), shoulder (12 %) and skull (13 %).

R. Bartl, C. Bartl, *Bone Disorders*, DOI 10.1007/978-3-319-29182-6_97

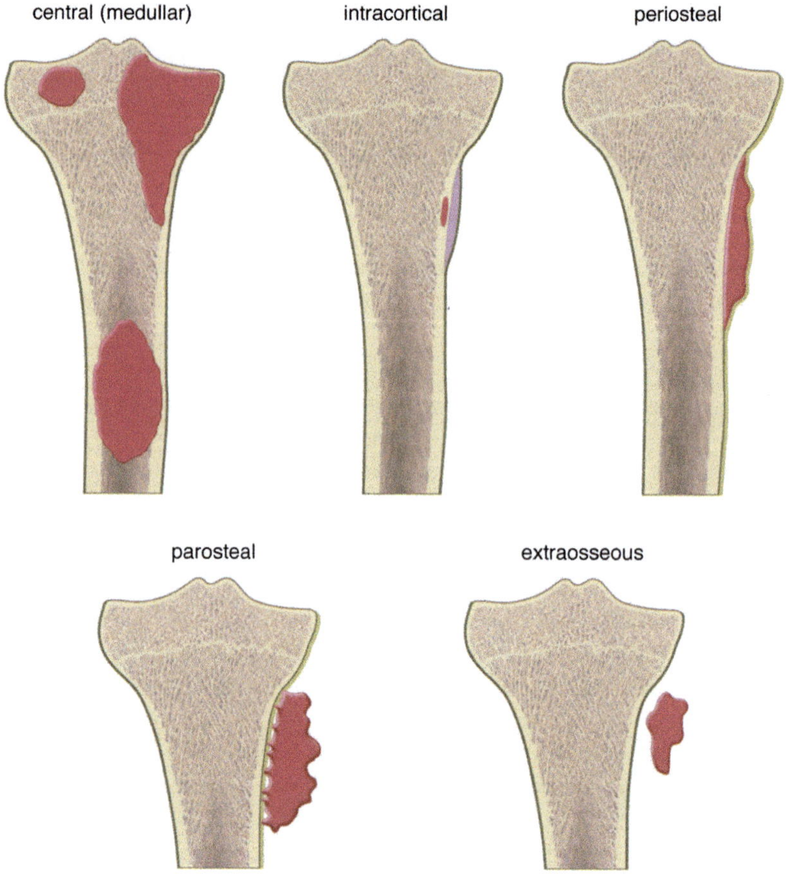

Fig. 97.1 Illustration of locations of primary bone tumours

Awareness of age and site distributions as well as localisations of the tumours (Fig. 97.1) and patterns of bone infiltration is indeed essential for a definite diagnosis, and in the case of an unusual site or age group, the diagnosis should be carefully reevaluated.

Bone tumours typically cause pain and swelling, and especially persistent and progressive pain associated with a mass is suspicious. Plain radiographs are the first investigation, and some signs suggest malignancy:

- Irregular tumour borders
- Lytic lesions
- Multiple bone destructions ("moth-eaten" features)
- Destruction and expansion of the cortex
- Soft tissue extension
- Some periosteal reactions ("onion skin", "hair on end", "Codman triangle")

Certain tumours have characteristic sites in the skeleton:

- Ewing's sarcoma appears first in the diaphysis of a long bone.
- Osteosarcoma appears in the metaphysis of a long bone.
- Giant cell tumour affects the epiphysis.

CT and MRI help in defining the location and extent of a bone tumour and sometimes help to suggest a diagnosis. But usually biopsy is essential for definite diagnosis. In centres with experience in bone biopsies, an accurate diagnosis is possible in >90 % of cases.

97.3 Morphologic Diagnosis of Primary Bone Tumours

Morphologic findings (histology, immunohistology, cytology, electron microscopy, cytogenetic and molecular investigations) form the basis for the definite diagnosis of bone tumours, and the final diagnosis integrates clinical, laboratory and imaging findings.

Correct morphologic diagnosis of bone tumours includes special problems:

- Their rarity needs sufficient diagnostic experience of the pathologist.
- There is a wide spectrum of bone lesions with overlapping features.
- There are problems of definite distinction between reactive, inflammatory, metabolic and developmental changes.

Planning for the biopsy is best done jointly by the orthopaedic oncologist, the musculoskeletal radiologist and the bone pathologist. Needle biopsies can achieve a diagnostic accuracy of 90 % at experienced centres, and therefore to avoid the risk of sampling error, some centres prefer incisional biopsies. Moreover, bone tumours frequently involve children or young adults, and the diagnosis often has dramatic consequences in terms of surgical and adjuvant therapy.

The correct diagnosis of the pathologist needs complete clinical, imaging and biopsy informations:

- Clinical and familial history
- Signs and symptoms of the tumour
- Abnormal serologic tests
- Exact anatomic site of the tumour (solitary or multicentric)
- Clinical evidence of metastases
- Type of surgical procedure (fine-needle aspiration, core needle biopsy, open surgical biopsy, curettage, resection, amputation)

The analysis of radiographs is based on five questions:

- Which bone is affected (long bones, flat bones)?
- Where in that bone is the lesion located (medullary, periosteal, metaphysis, diaphysis, epiphysis)?
- What type of bone destruction is present (trabecular and/or cortical, marginated, zone of transition between tumour and normal bone, osteolytic, moth eaten or permeative)?
- What type of matrix mineralisation is present (stippled, rings and arcs, solid, cloud-like, ivory-like) (Fig. 97.2)?
- What type of periosteal reaction is present (expanded, solid, buttress, lamellated, parallel speculated, Codman angle) (Fig. 97.3)?

97.4 Classification of Bone Tumours

It must be remembered that secondary malignant infiltration in the system bone marrow (bone metastases of carcinomas) and haematologic neoplasias (multiple myeloma and lymphomas/leukaemias) are much more common than primary malignant bone tumours. This chapter is concerned with primary tumours of bone, based on the revised World Health Organization (WHO) classification and definition of bone tumours. The 4th edition of the WHO was published in 2013 and has incorporated more cytogenetic and molecular data. A revised WHO classification is shown in Table 97.1.

97.5 Cartilage-Forming Tumours

A *chondroma* is a benign tumour characterised by formation of mature cartilage. Most chondromas are solitary lesions located centrally within the medullary cavity (enchondroma) and are asymptomatic. Sometimes they provoke expansion of the bone, destroy the cortex (periosteal subtype) and produce swelling, pain and pathologic fractures. In multiple chondromas (enchondromatosis) (Fig. 97.4), the risk of malignant transformation is greater than in any other benign cartilage lesion (up to 30 %).

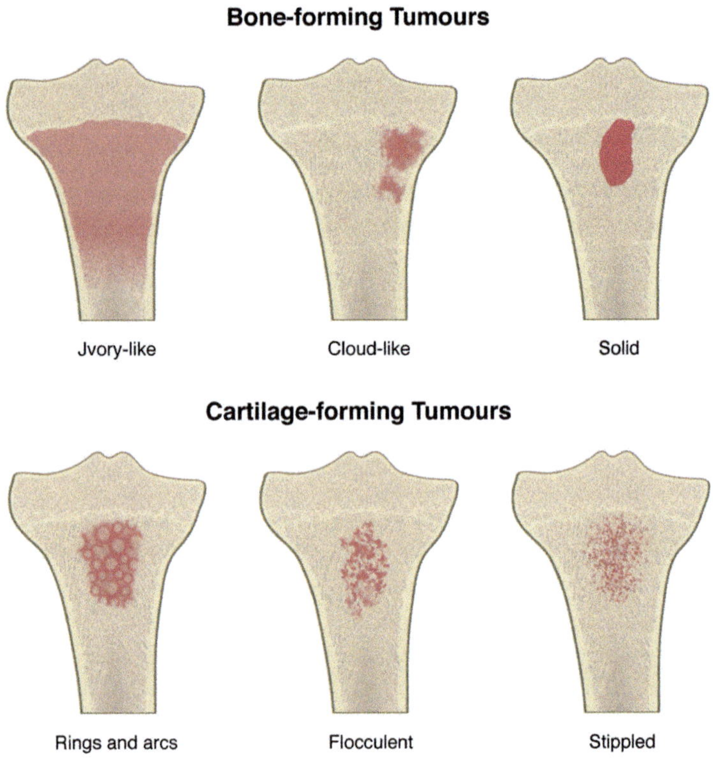

Fig. 97.2 Mineralised matrix patterns of primary bone tumours (Modified from M. Davies, Imaging of Bone Tumors and Tumor-Like Lesions. Springer 2009)

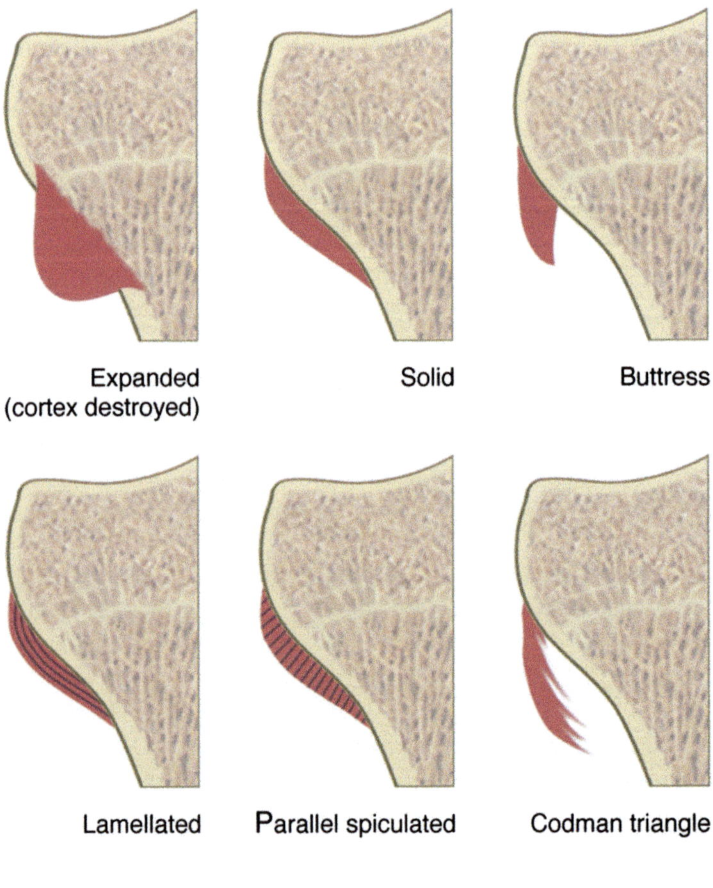

Fig. 97.3 Types of periosteal reactions in patients with primary bone tumours (Modified from M. Davies, Imaging of Bone Tumors and Tumor-Like Lesions. Springer 2009)

Table 97.1 WHO classification of bone tumours

Bone tumours	Benign	Intermediate	Malignant
Chondrogenic tumours	Chondromas	Chondroblastoma	Chondrosarcomas
	Osteochondroma	Chondromyxoid fibroma	Osteochondromyxoma
	Chondroblastoma		
Osteogenic tumours	Osteoma	Osteoblastoma	Osteosarcomas
	Osteoid osteoma		
	Osteoblastoma		
Osteoclastic giant cell-rich tumours	Giant cell lesion	Giant cell tumour of bone	
Ewing's sarcoma of bone			Ewing's sarcoma
Vascular tumours	Haemangioma	Haemangioendothelioma	
	Lymphangioma	Haemangiopericytoma	Angiosarcoma
	Glomus tumour		Malignant haemangiopericytoma
Other connective tissue tumours	Benign fibrous histiocytoma	Desmoplastic fibroma	Malignant fibrous histiocytoma
	Lipoma		Liposarcoma
			Fibrosarcoma
			Leiomyosarcoma
			Undifferentiated Sarcoma

The following figures of primary bone tumours and tumour-like lesions include sketches based on radiographs showing and emphasising the most characteristic morphologic and diagnostic features. These informative illustrations have been published in the year 1980 in the book Kuhlencordt F, Bartelheimer H. eds. Klinische Osteologie B. (Remagen W, Morscher E, Rösli A. *Primäre und sekundäre Tumoren der Knochen und Gelenke*, pp.1317–1438). Heidelberg: Springer 1980 (figures reprinted with kind permission of the publisher Springer).

Radiologically chondromas appear as small osteolytic areas with well-defined boundaries thinning the cortex. The lesion is usually located in the metaphysis of the upper humerus (Fig. 97.5) and distal femur. Mottled calcifications are characteristic but may be absent in some cases.

An *osteochondroma* is a cartilage-capped bony projection on the external surface of a bone. It is the most frequently occurring bone tumour (about 40 % of all benign bone tumours and 20 % of all bone tumours). The most commonly involved locations are the long bone in the metaphyseal region near the active growth plate

Chondroblastoma is a relatively rare benign tumour characterised by chondroblast-like cells but may grow to an enormous size. Local pain, swelling, tenderness and limitation of movement are the most frequent complaints. On X-ray, the characteristic feature is an oval, sharply limited area located in the epiphysis (Fig. 97.6). Most chondroblastomas are cured with curettage and packed with cancellous bone.

Chondrosarcoma is malignant tumour characterised by the formation of pleomorphic cartilage tissue. Chondrosarcomas comprise 20–25 % of all bone sarcomas, with a peak incidence in the fourth and sixth decade of life. They may be subclassified into primary and secondary central, secondary peripheral and periosteal variants. They have a predilection

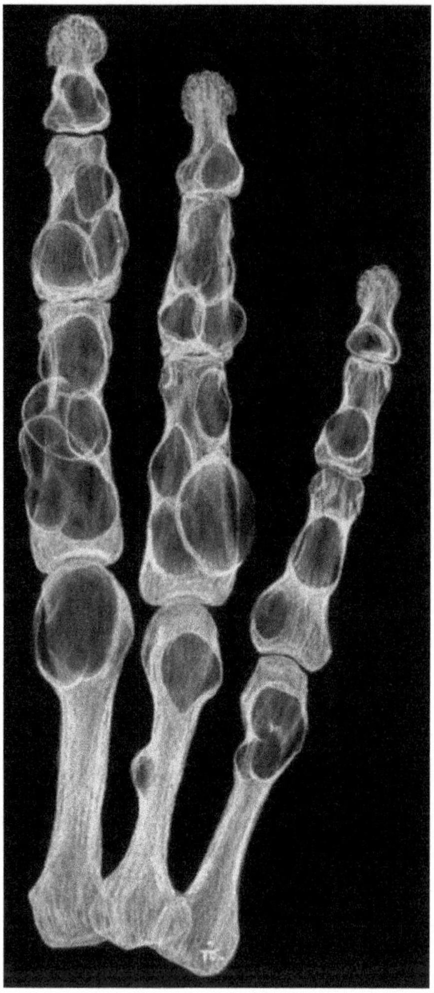

Fig. 97.4 Multiple enchondromas (enchondromatosis) with osteolytic round or ovoid lesions with well-defined boundaries, expanding and thinning the cortex (With kind permission of Springer, from [55])

for the diaphyseal portions of long bones (femur) (Figs. 97.7 and 97.8a–e) and the flat bones (scapula) (Fig. 97.9). Chondrosarcomas have an indolent history and present as pain and swelling. Radiographically, the lesion has a lobular appearance with calcifications of the cartilaginous matrix. Most chondrosarcomas are resistant to chemotherapy, and surgical resection is the mainstay of therapy.

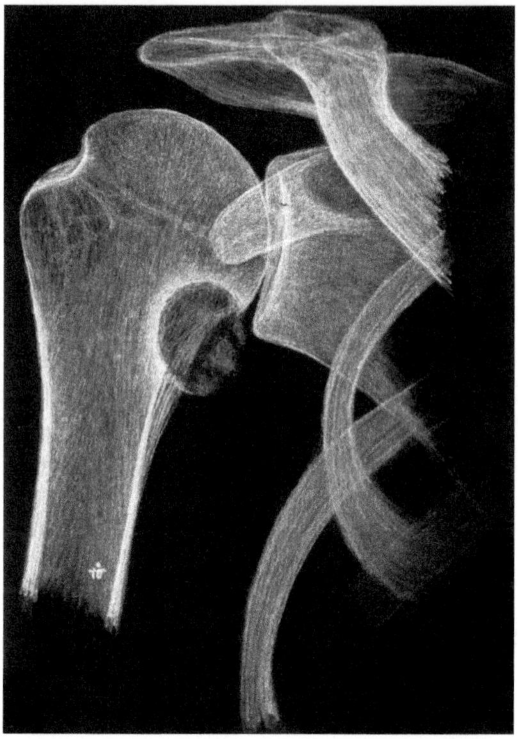

Fig. 97.5 Periosteal chondroma of the proximal humerus with erosion of the cortex, endosteal reactive sclerosis and mottled calcifications in the cartilaginous tumour mass (With kind permission of Springer, from [55])

97.6 Bone-Forming Tumours

Osteoma is a benign lesion consisting of mature bone tissue with lamellar structure and showing very slow growth. It is found in all age groups, and three subtypes are distinguished:

- Conventional, classic osteomas ("ivory exostosis")
- Parosteal osteomas (juxtacortical)
- Medullary osteomas (enostosis, "bone islands")

The classic osteomas involve almost exclusively bone of intramembranous formation, particularly the external table of the skull (Fig. 97.10). Osteomas are often asymptom-

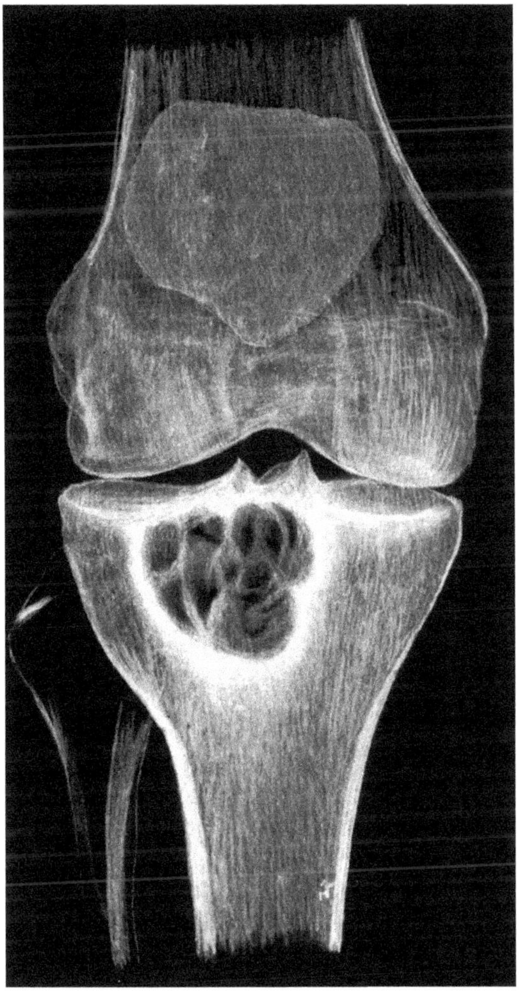

Fig. 97.6 Chondroblastoma with oval and round, sharply limited area of osteolyses located eccentrically in the epiphysis of the proximal tibia. Note marked reactive sclerosis (With kind permission of Springer, from [55])

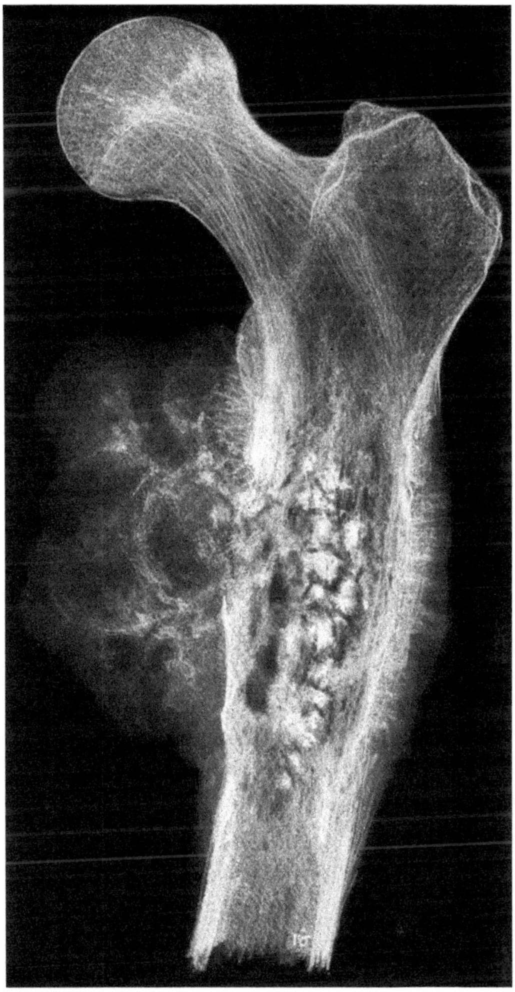

Fig. 97.7 Chondrosarcoma of the femur situated in the metaphysis and extending in the medullary cavity of the diaphysis. It shows a thickening and expansion of the cortex and stippled calcifications in the huge radiolucent areas. Destroyed periosteal osseous lamellae with spiculae and Codman angles proximal and distal (With kind permission of Springer, from [55])

atic, with a slowly increasing swelling. Multiple osteomas are part of the Gardner's syndrome, a familial disease consisting of the triad of colonic polyposis, osteomas and soft tissue tumours. Multiple enostosis is a hereditary disease, also referred to as *osteopoikilosis*. Radiologically osteomas are characterised by a dense, well-defined image, usually less than 3 cm in diameter.

Osteoid osteoma is a benign, osteoblastic lesion (less than 1 cm of size), with a demarcated outline and a surrounding zone of reactive bone formation (Figs. 97.11 and 97.12). According to the location of the nidus three variants may be distinguished:

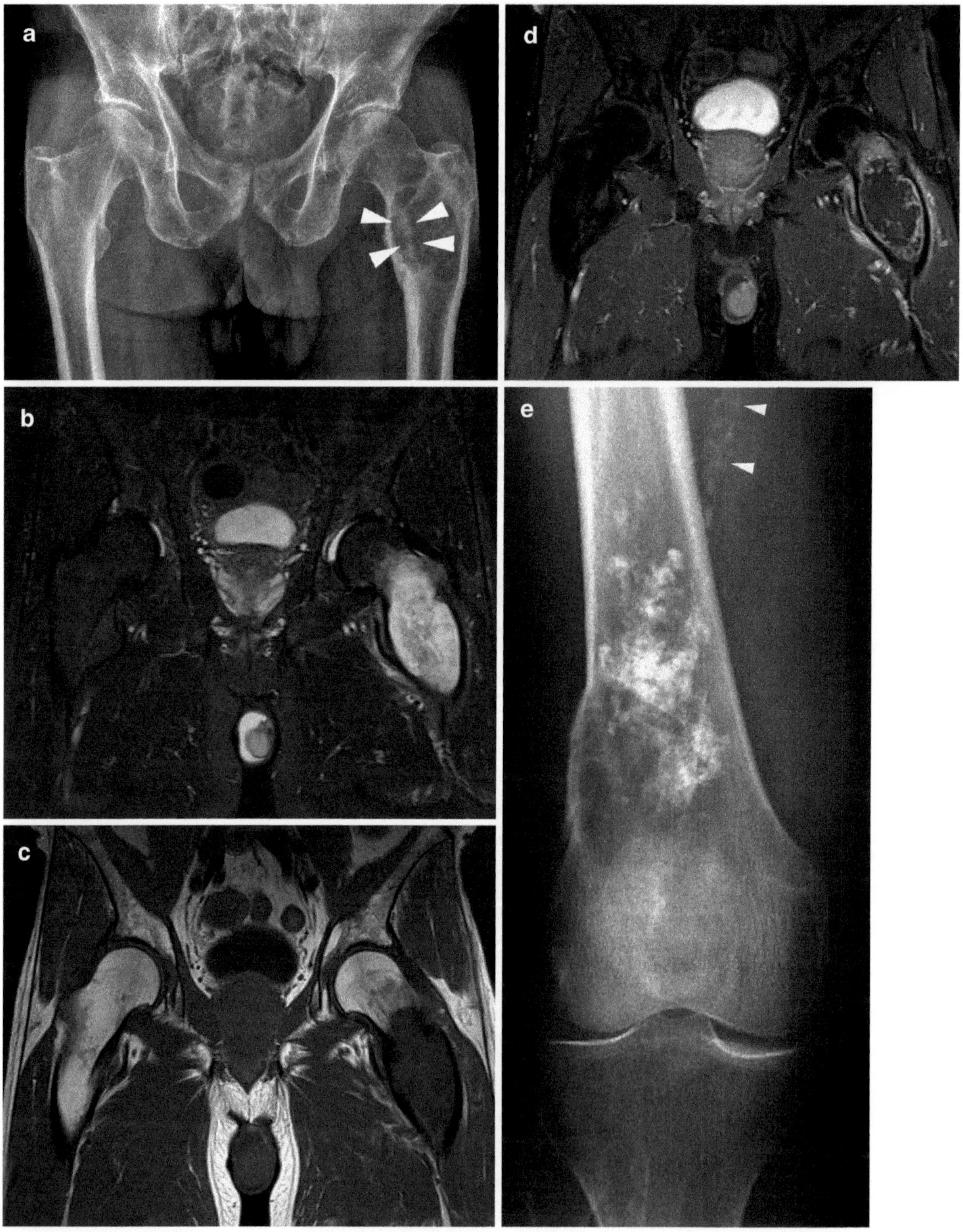

Fig. 97.8 (**a**–**e**) A 75-year-old male patient (**a**–**d**) with chondrosarcoma in the left proximal femur (**a**–**d**): the plain film radiograph (**a**) shows the typical, in this case rather less pronounced intralesional calcifications (*arrowheads*) which are present in up to 94 % of the cases and can be delineated in about two thirds of the radiographs. In the non-calcified parts of the tumour, MRI shows a high signal intensity in STIR sequence (**b**), while in T1w images (**c**), the tumour has an iso- or slightly hyperintense signal intensity compared to muscle. After administration of contrast agent, fat-saturated T1w images (**d**) show a heterogeneous contrast enhancement with a septal and peripheral rim-like enhancement (Courtesy: Tobias Geith). An 83-year-old female patient with chondrosarcoma (**e**): plain film radiograph shows typical calcifications within the chondrosarcoma in the distal right femur and cortical bulging. Also note calcifications due to atherosclerosis (*arrowheads*) (Courtesy: Tobias Geith)

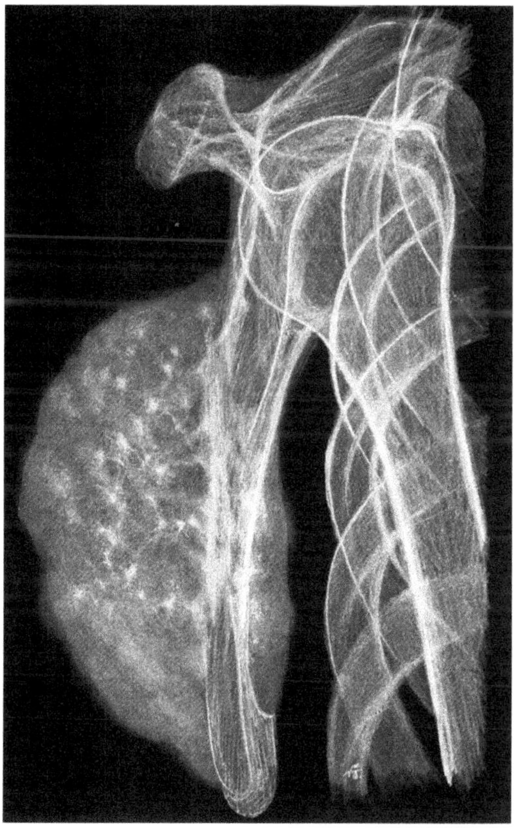

Fig. 97.9 Chondrosarcoma of the scapula with involvement of the flat bone and extraosseous growth. Note the fine, stippled and ring-shaped calcifications in the radiolucent tumour mass (With kind permission of Springer, from [55])

- Cortical
- Medullar (cancellous)
- Subperiosteal

Histologically, it consists of a highly vascularised tissue of immature bone and osteoid. This common, benign tumour is typical of adolescence and young adult age. Common locations are the femur and tibia. Pain is a constant and permanent symptom, not relieved by rest and often more intense at night. Pain is exacerbated under alcoholic beverages and is dramatically relieved with *aspirin*. Treatment consists of complete surgical removal of the nidus. Radiologically guided core resection and photocoagulation are alternatives in order to avoid pathologic fractures.

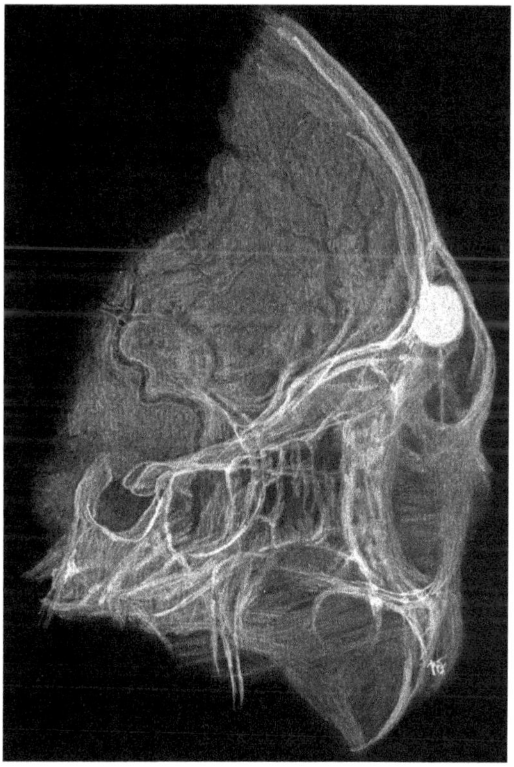

Fig. 97.10 Osteoma in the dorsal wall of the sinus frontalis characterised by a dense, radiopaque, structureless and well-delineated image, usually less than 1 cm in diameter (With kind permission of Springer, from [55])

Osteoblastoma is similar to the osteoid osteoma but with a nidus greater than 2 cm (Fig. 97.13). Three subtypes can be distinguished:

- Medullary and cortical osteoblastoma
- Periosteal osteoblastoma
- Multifocal sclerosing osteoblastoma

The tumour frequently occurs in the vertebral column and the sacrum. Pain is frequently present for more than 2 years. Treatment depends on the stage and location of the tumour. In aggressive variants, wide excision is indicated, sometimes together with radiotherapy.

Osteoclastoma (giant cell-rich tumour) affects young adults and occurs in the epiphysis of long bones and extends into the soft tissues. Histologically, giant cell-rich tumours consist of multinucleated giant cells resembling osteoclasts

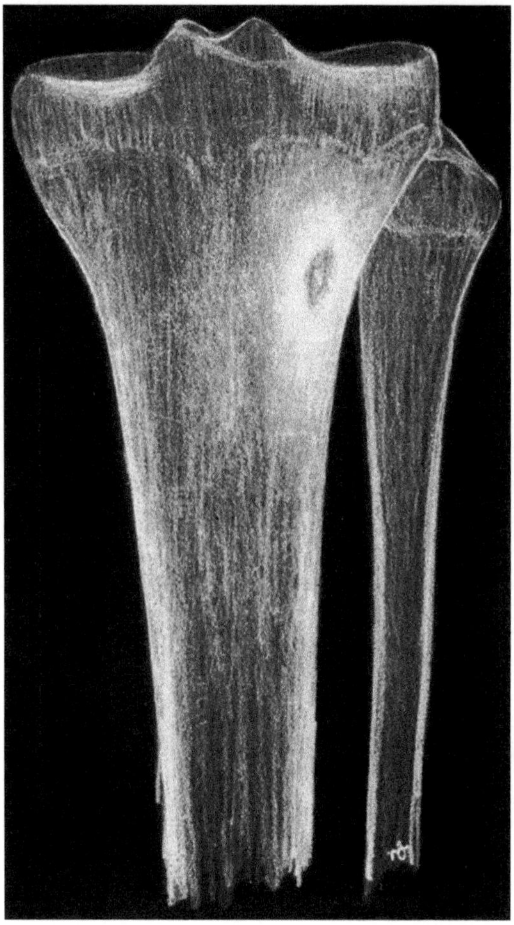

Fig. 97.11 Osteoid osteoma with the characteristic small rounded area of osteolysis ("nidus") surrounded by a marked hyperostosis (With kind permission of Springer, from [55])

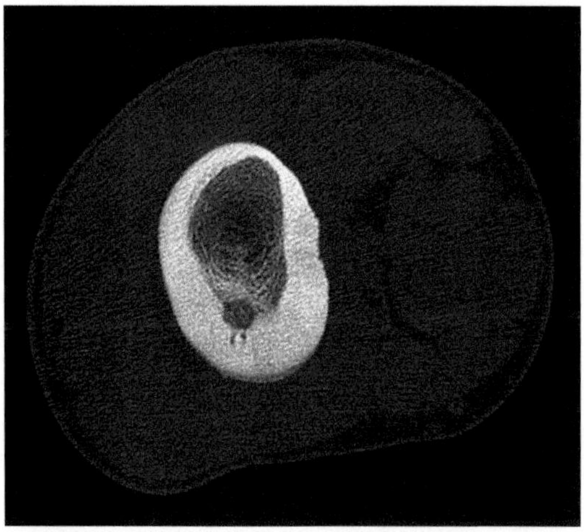

Fig. 97.12 A 14-year-old boy with osteoid osteoma in the left femoral diaphysis. Note the cortical thickening around the nidus. CT, bone window (Courtesy of Tobias Geith)

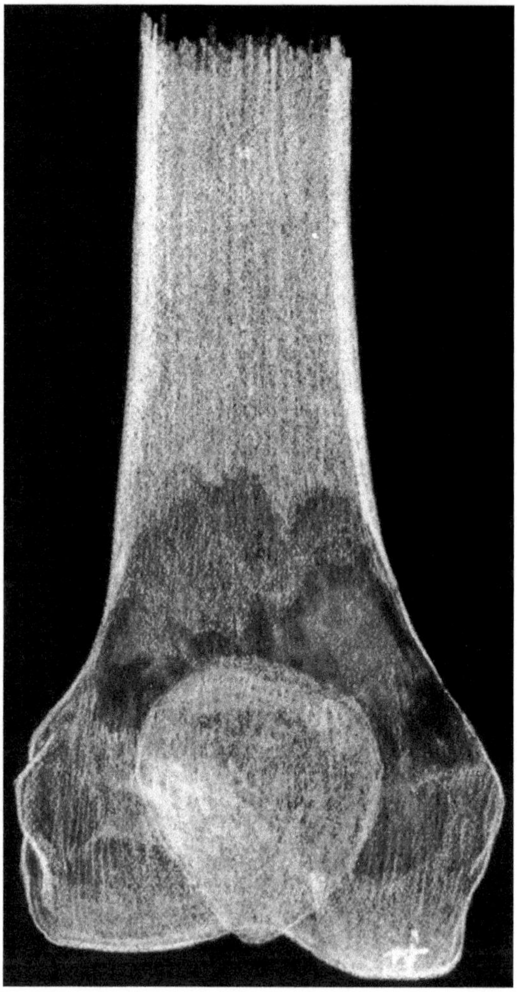

Fig. 97.13 Osteoblastoma of the distal femur, a single large osteolysis, attenuating the cortex and resembling an aneurysmal bone cyst. Fine calcifications in the osteoid tissue (With kind permission of Springer, from [55])

and admixed with mononuclear stromal cells. Rarely giant cell tumours metastasise, but they are notorious for their tendency to recur. They appear lytic on X-ray. Usually they are treated with curettage and bone grafting or packing with methyl methacrylate.

Osteosarcoma accounts for almost 45 % of all bone sarcomas and is a spindle cell neoplasm that produces osteoid or bone. Conventional and juxtacortical parosteal variants are distinguished. About 60 % of all osteosarcomas occur in children and adolescents, mostly located in the metaphysis of long bones (Figs. 97.14 and

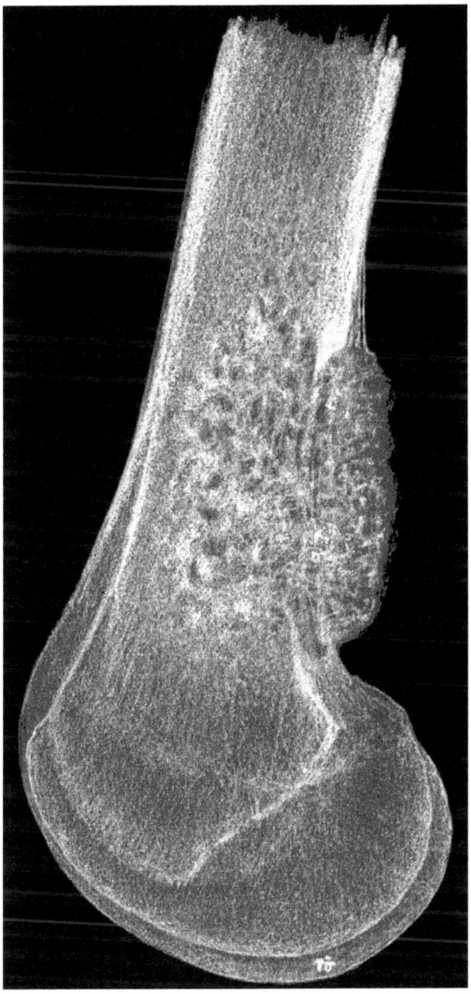

Fig. 97.14 Osteosarcoma of the distal femur revealing a large destructive lesion with a moth-eaten appearance, a speculated periosteal reaction with filiform spicules ("sunburst appearance") and a cuff of periosteal new bone formation at the margin of the extraosseous soft tissue mass ("Codman triangle"). Codman triangle may also be seen in osteomyelitis, chondrosarcoma and Ewing's sarcoma (With kind permission of Springer, from [55])

97.15a–i). Pain and a palpable mass are characteristic, with a rapid course. The skin above the tumour tends to be warm due to the intensive vascularity. Treatment consists of chemotherapy and surgery, with survivals after 5 years of about 60–70 % of patients. Osteosarcoma is radioresistant, and therefore radiation therapy has no place in the treatment strategy. Periosteal and parosteal variants (Fig. 97.16) have a rather favourable course, under wide en bloc resection.

97.7 Ewing's Sarcoma

Ewing's sarcoma constitutes 10–15 % of all bone sarcomas and has a peak incidence in the second decade of life (Figs. 97.17 and 97.18a–e). Almost all Ewing's sarcoma cases are associated with a translocation between chromosomes 11 and 22, which results in a fusion protein between the EWS and FLI1 genes and which promotes tumorigenesis. The neoplasm is characterised by a tissue with a rather uniform appearance composed of densely packed small cells with round nuclei, but without distinct cytoplasmic outlines or prominent nucleoli (Fig. 97.19). They typically involve the diaphyseal region of long bones and flat bones, but no part of the skeleton is immune from Ewing's sarcoma. Pain is usually the first symptom, together with a firm swelling or a pathologic fracture. X-ray may show a characteristic "onion peel" periosteal reaction with a generous soft tissue mass. The disease is very aggressive, and it is therefore considered a systemic disease. Common sites of metastases are the lung and bone marrow. Systemic chemotherapy is the preferred primary treatment, often being used before surgery.

97.8 Other Rare Bone Tumours

A *haemangioma* is a benign lesion of newly formed blood vessels, with a frequency as high as 60 % of all bone tumours. The common sites are the spine, the cranium (Fig. 97.20) and more rarely in other bones. Most haemangiomas are asymptomatic and do not require treatment. Surgery or radiotherapy may be required in cases with neurologic symptoms or pain.

Haemangioendothelioma and *haemangiopericytoma* are more aggressive but non-metastasising, and most patients complain of pain or swelling.

Haemangiosarcoma is a malignant tumour characterised by irregular vascular structures (Fig. 97.21). Radical surgery is the therapy of choice.

Benign fibrous histiocytoma, desmoplastic fibroma, fibrosarcoma (Fig. 97.22*) and malignant fibrous histiocytoma* are all characterised by

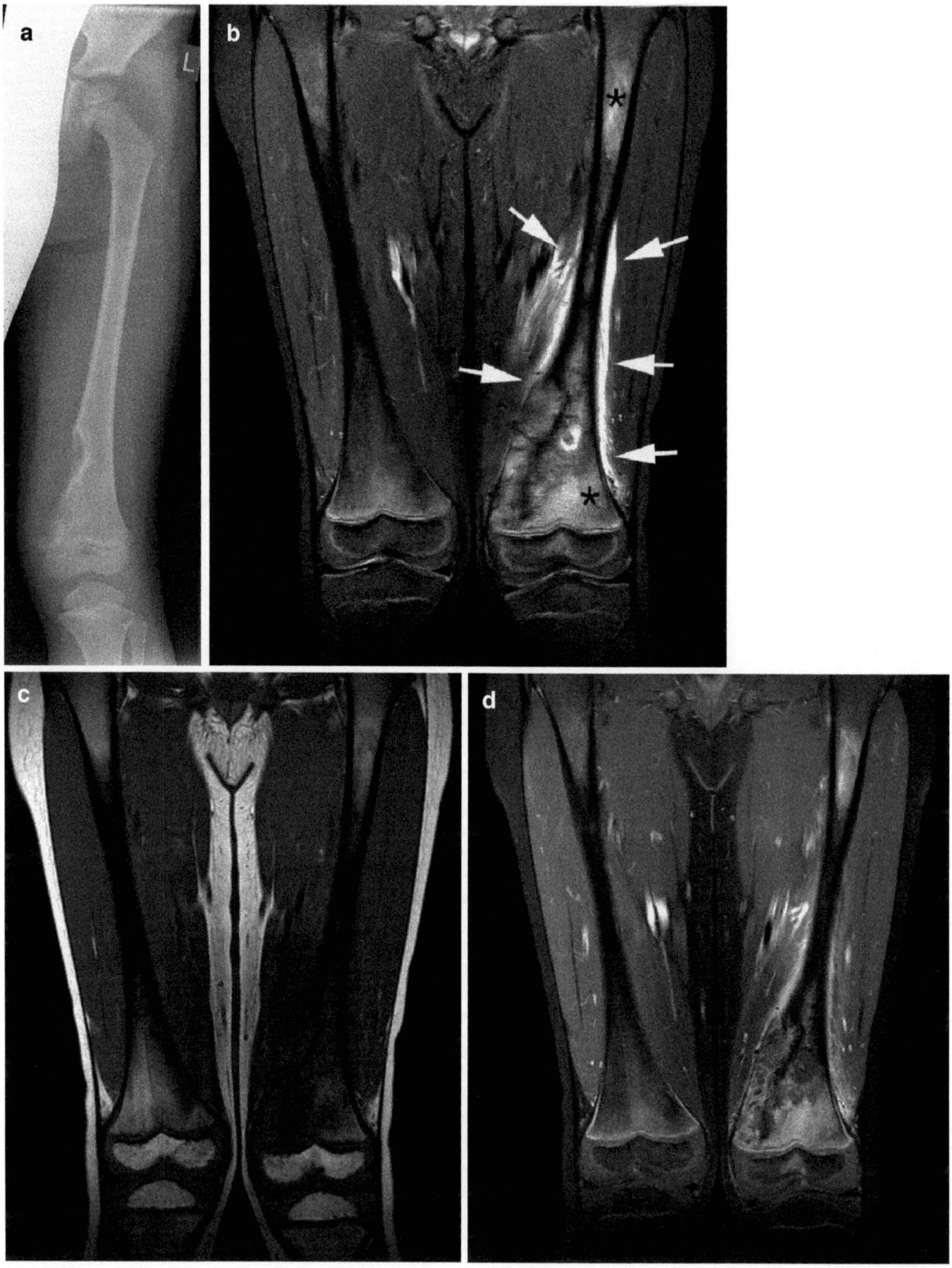

Fig. 97.15 (**a**–**i**) A 4-year-old boy with osteosarcoma of the left distal femur (**a**–**e**) The plain film radiograph (**a**) shows medullary and cortical bone destruction. MRI shows a high signal intensity of the tumour in STIR sequence (**b**) and an extensive peritumoural oedema in the surrounding soft tissues (*arrows*) and bone (*asterisks*). T1w images (**c**) show an intermediate signal intensity, while after contrast administration T1w fs images (**d**) show enhancement in the solid parts of the tumour. PET-CT (**e**) reveals a high glucose utilisation in the solid parts of the tumour (Courtesy: Tobias Geith). A 36-year-old male patient with periosteal osteosarcoma in the right distal femur (**f**–**i**): The plain film radiograph (**f**) shows extensive calcifications in the tumour. On MRI, there is cortical destruction and an inhomogeneous mass with inhomogeneous high signal intensity on PDw (**g**), inhomogeneous signal intensity on T1w (**h**) and inhomogeneous contrast uptake in fat-saturated T1w (**i**) (Courtesy: Tobias Geith)

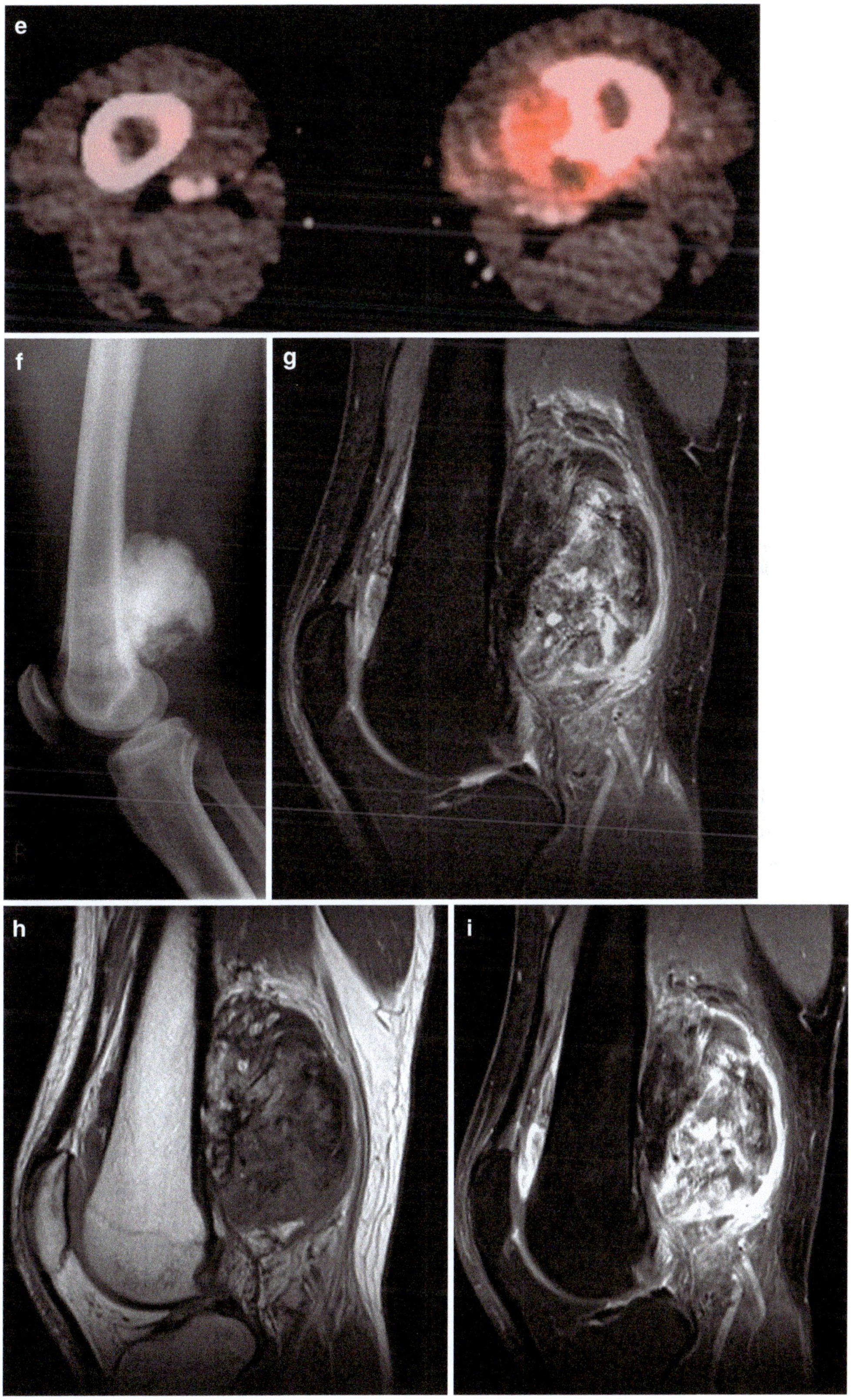

Fig. 97.15 (continued)

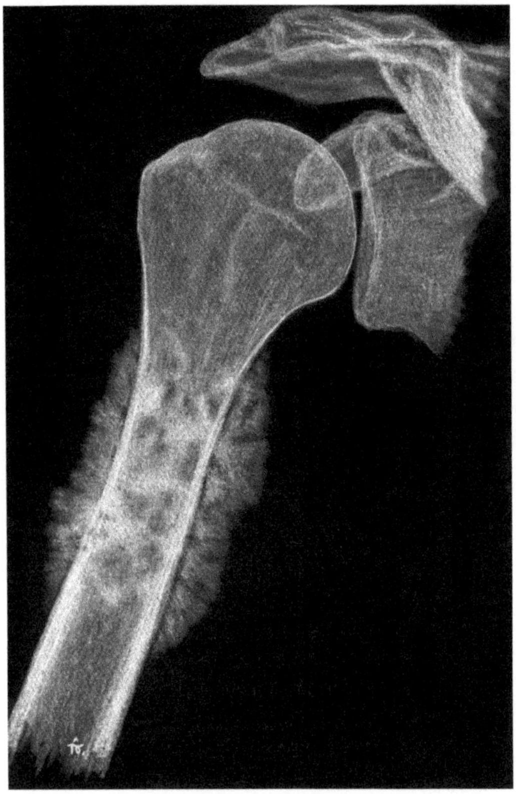

Fig. 97.16 Parosteal osteosarcoma in the upper end of the humerus, infiltrating the periosteum in the lateral and distal region of the tumour (With kind permission of Springer, from [55])

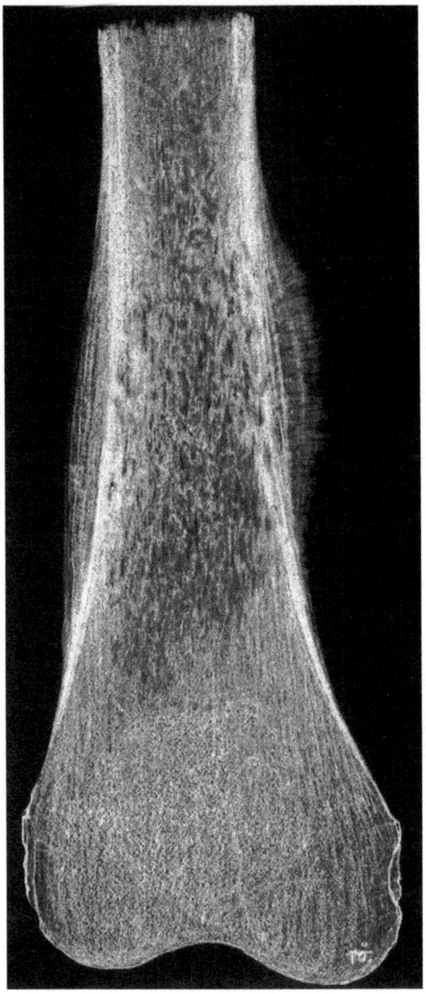

Fig. 97.17 Ewing's sarcoma of the distal femur with irregular central areas of bone destruction and an enlarged cortex. The cortex is covered by the formation of periosteal lamellated "onion peel" reactive bone and radial spicules (medial areal) (With kind permission of Springer, from [55])

the presence of fibrous tissue or collagen fibres. These tumours are usually not radiosensitive, and radical surgery is the treatment of choice.

Malignant lymphomas of bone comprise about 3 % of malignant bone tumours and affect adults of advanced age. They can develop as isolated solid tumours with a predilection of the axial skeleton or as bone marrow infiltrations ("stage IV") of a systemic lymphoproliferative disorder. Radiation therapy in combination with chemotherapy is the treatment of choice.

97.9 Conditions Simulating Primary Bone Tumours

Solitary bone metastases of carcinomas (in particular carcinomas of the breast, prostate, lung, thyroid and kidney) are the most common conditions simulating primary bone tumours. In addition, *other benign lesions* may cause diagnostic problems, and these include various bone cysts (aneurysmal bone cyst (Fig. 97.23), unicameral bone cyst), exostoses, heterotopic ossifications, myositis ossificans, fracture callus, osteoporotic vertebral collapse, systemic mastocytosis, osteomyelitis, osteonecrosis, histiocytosis X (Fig. 97.24), eosinophilic granuloma (Fig. 97.25), amyloidomas, reactive periostitis, SAPHO syn-

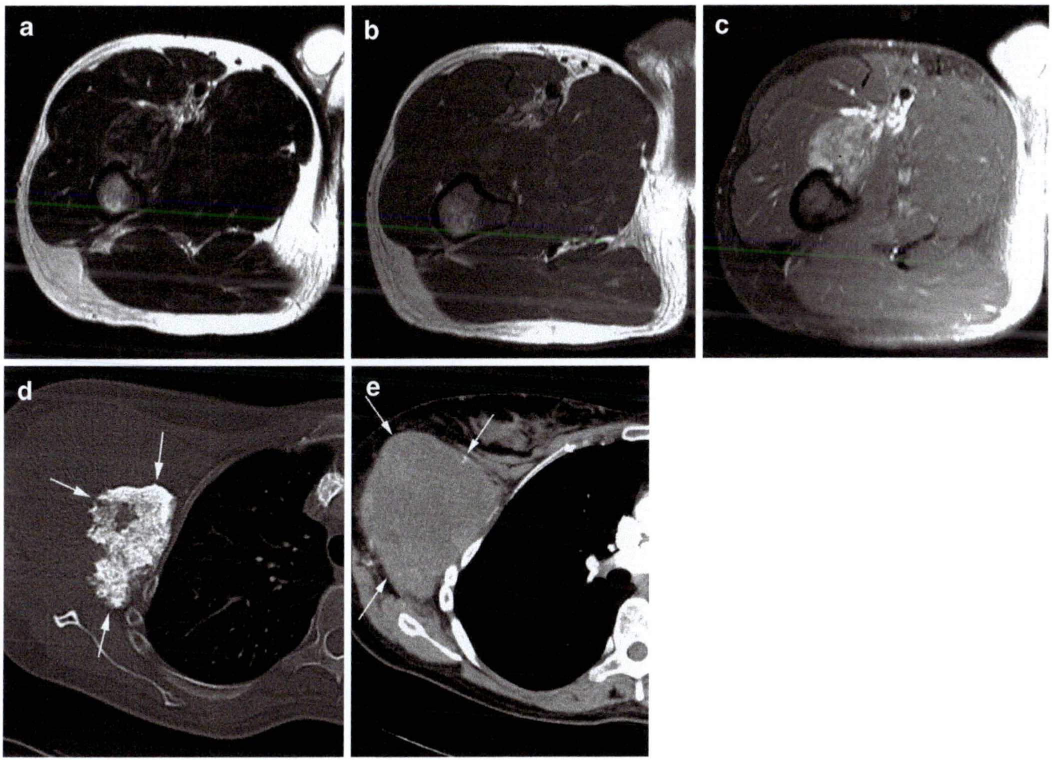

Fig. 97.18 (**a**–**e**) A 21-year-old male patient with Ewing's sarcoma (**a**–**c**): T2w MRI (**a**) shows a heterogeneous signal intensity. T1w images show a hypointense to intermediate signal (**b**). After contrast administration, fat-saturated T1w images (**c**) show a heterogeneous but distinct enhancement (Courtesy: Tobias Geith). A 44-year-old female patient with Ewing's sarcoma of the right upper thoracic wall (**d**–**e**): CT in bone window (**d**) shows central dense calcifications in the tumour. CT in soft tissue window (**e**) shows a large mass with slight contrast uptake (Courtesy: Tobias Geith)

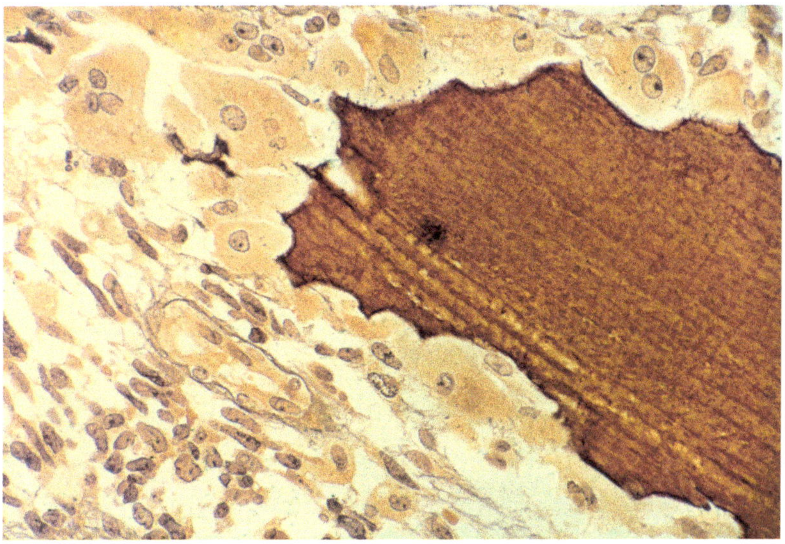

Fig. 97.19 Iliac crest biopsy showing active osteoclasts activated by adjacent tumour cells in a patient with metastatic Ewing's sarcoma. Gomori staining

Ewing's sarcoma is now a curable tumour, even in the presence of metastases or local recurrence, especially in children.

drome, Paget's disease, haemorrhage and "brown tumours" in patients with pHPT. *Fibrous dysplasia* is a fibro-osseous aberration of the skeleton, probably a developmental disorder of the mesenchyme of bone tissue. The fundamental abnormality is an osteoclastic bone resorption and replacement of bone and marrow by masses of fibrous tissue, within which bone may develop later (Fig. 97.26a, b).

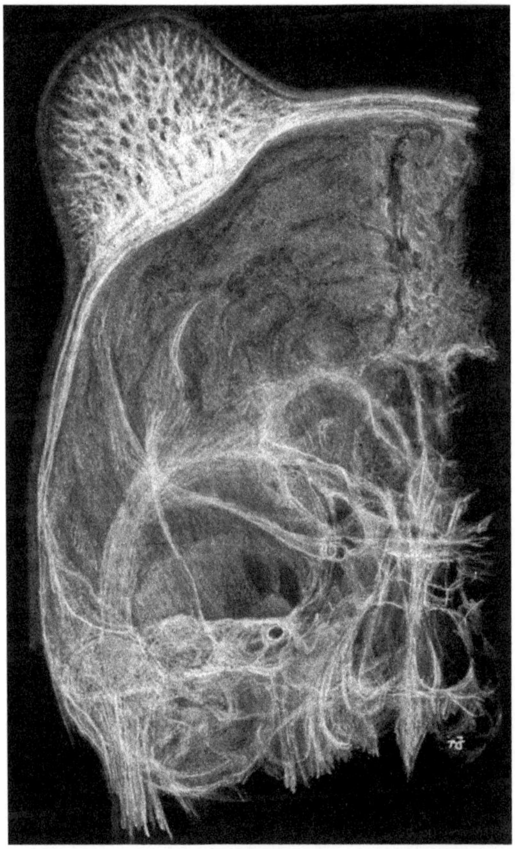

Fig. 97.20 Haemangioma of the cranium, a radiolucent defect with periosteal reaction. "Sunburst" or "sunray" patterns are often noted in cranial bones (With kind permission of Springer, from [55])

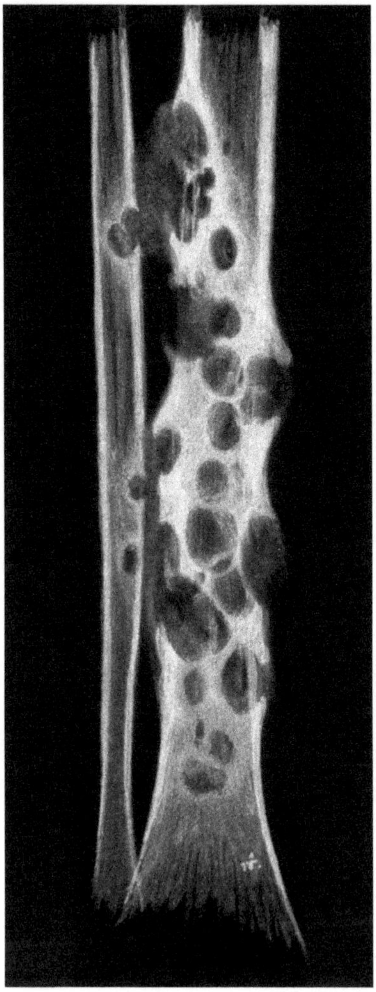

Fig. 97.21 Haemangiosarcoma of the tibia, multifocal lesions already infiltrating the fibula (With kind permission of Springer, from [55])

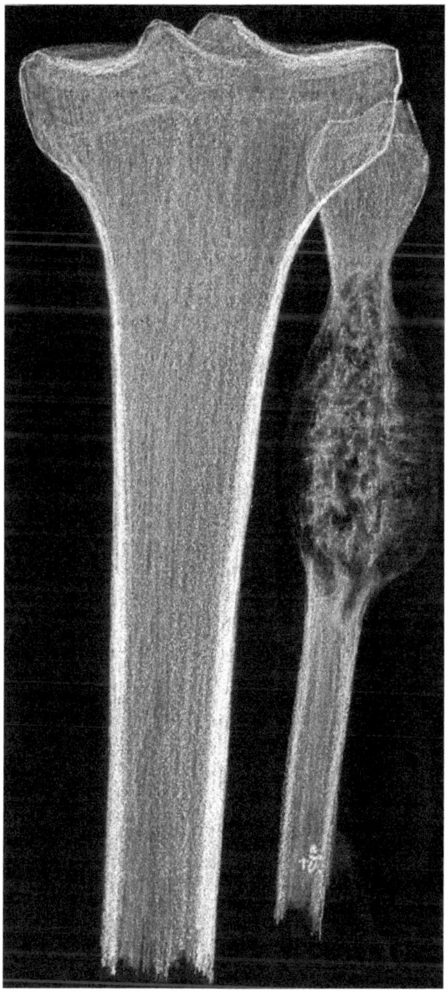

Fig. 97.22 Fibrosarcoma of the fibula, a radiolucent, destructive and expanding lesion ("moth-eaten" structure) with ill-defined borders, located in the metaphyseal region with extension into the diaphysis (With kind permission of Springer, from [55])

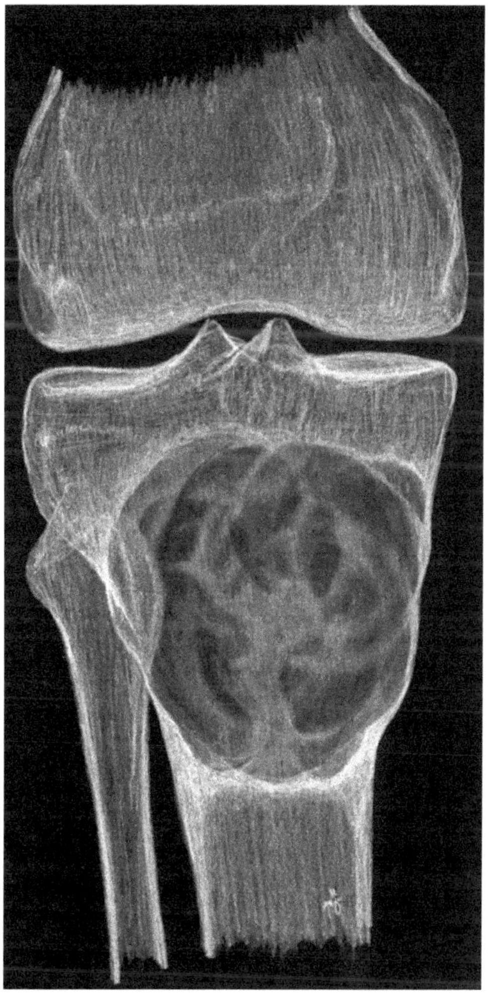

Fig. 97.23 Large aneurysmal bone cyst in the metaphyseal region of the proximal tibia with expansion of the thin cortex (With kind permission of Springer, from [55])

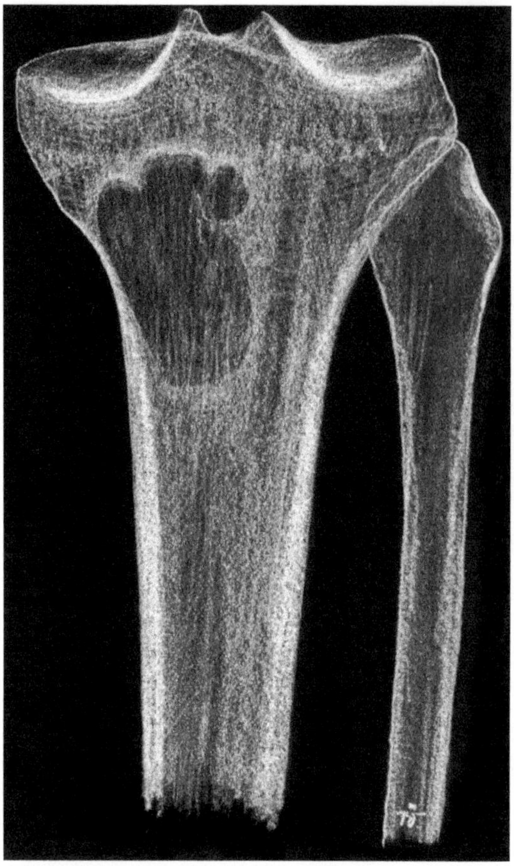

Fig. 97.24 Histiocytosis X of the proximal tibia (metaphysis). Lytic lesion with moderate sclerotic reaction of the surrounding bone (With kind permission of Springer, from [55])

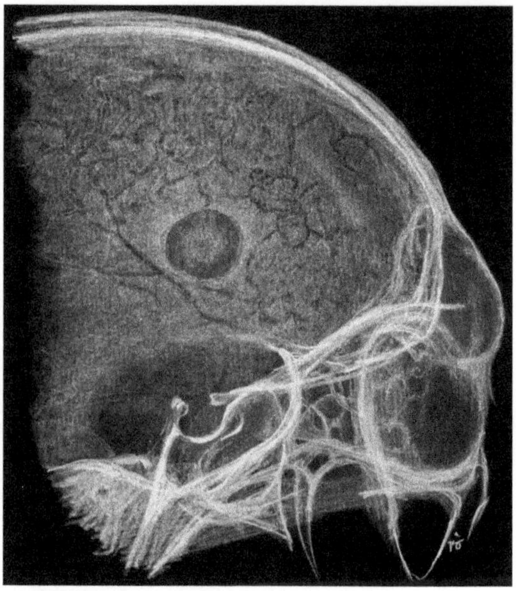

Fig. 97.25 Eosinophilic granuloma of the skull. Round osteolytic lesion with moderate sclerotic bone reaction and a central sequestrum (With kind permission of Springer, from [55S])

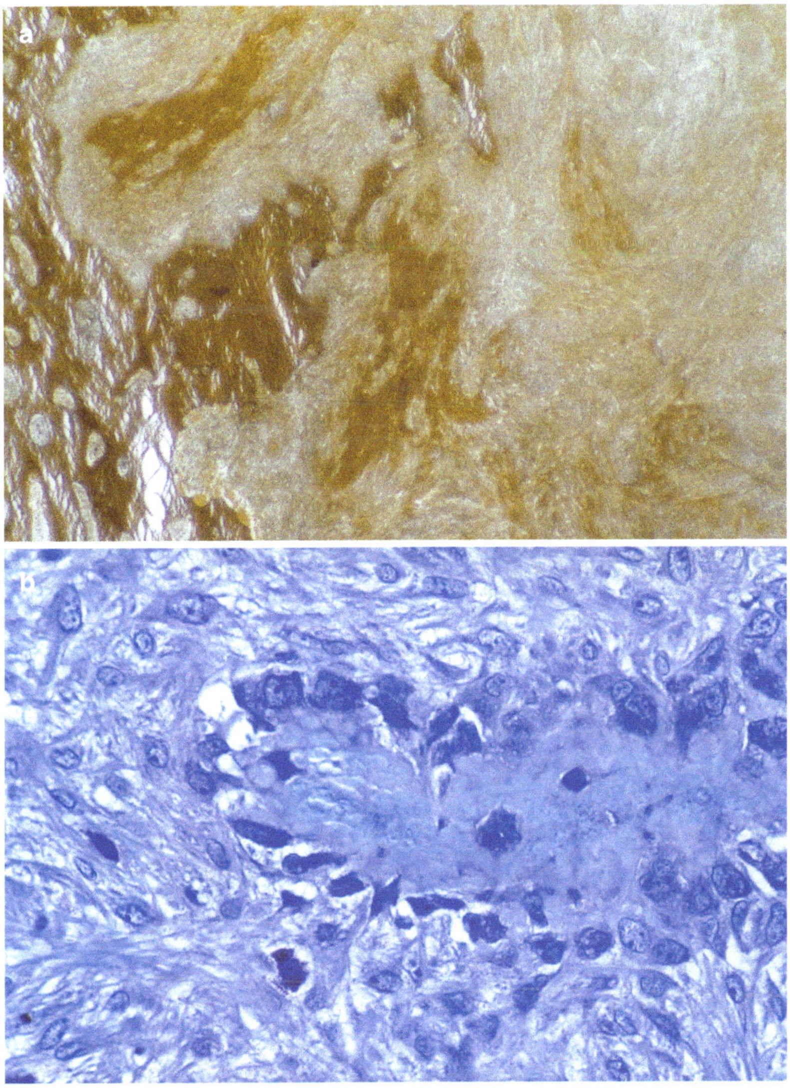

Fig. 97.26 Fibrous dysplasia: (**a**) cortical and subcortical area illustrating marked porosity of cortex and subcortical residue of trabecular bone. Note substitution of ossicles by primitive, poorly mineralised woven bone. Gomori staining. (**b**) Higher magnification of focus of osteoblastic bone formation. Giemsa staining

Part XVII

Bone and Joints

98 The Normal Joint

The human body has about 327 joints which vary greatly in size and function. Diarthrodial joints have a joint capsule that encloses the bone ends of a joint space (Fig. 98.1a–c). The bone ends are covered by articular cartilage, and the joint space is partially lined by a synovial membrane. The fluid is secreted by the synovial membrane and is mainly a transudate of water and solutes from bone marrow vessels. Hyaluronic acid and glycoproteins are added by the lining cells of the synovial membrane. The cartilage of articular surfaces is known as hyaline cartilage and consists of chondrocytes scattered throughout an abundant extracellular matrix (Fig. 98.2a, b). Collagen type II is the most abundant organic component of hyaline cartilage. The deepest zone of cartilage directly adjacent to subcortical bone is calcified. Supporting tissues of the joint allow frictionless motion of one bone end against the other. Joint motion and loading are necessary to maintain healthy articular cartilage. Immobilisation and casting lead to atrophy and degeneration of the cartilage.

R. Bartl, C. Bartl, *Bone Disorders*, DOI 10.1007/978-3-319-29182-6_98

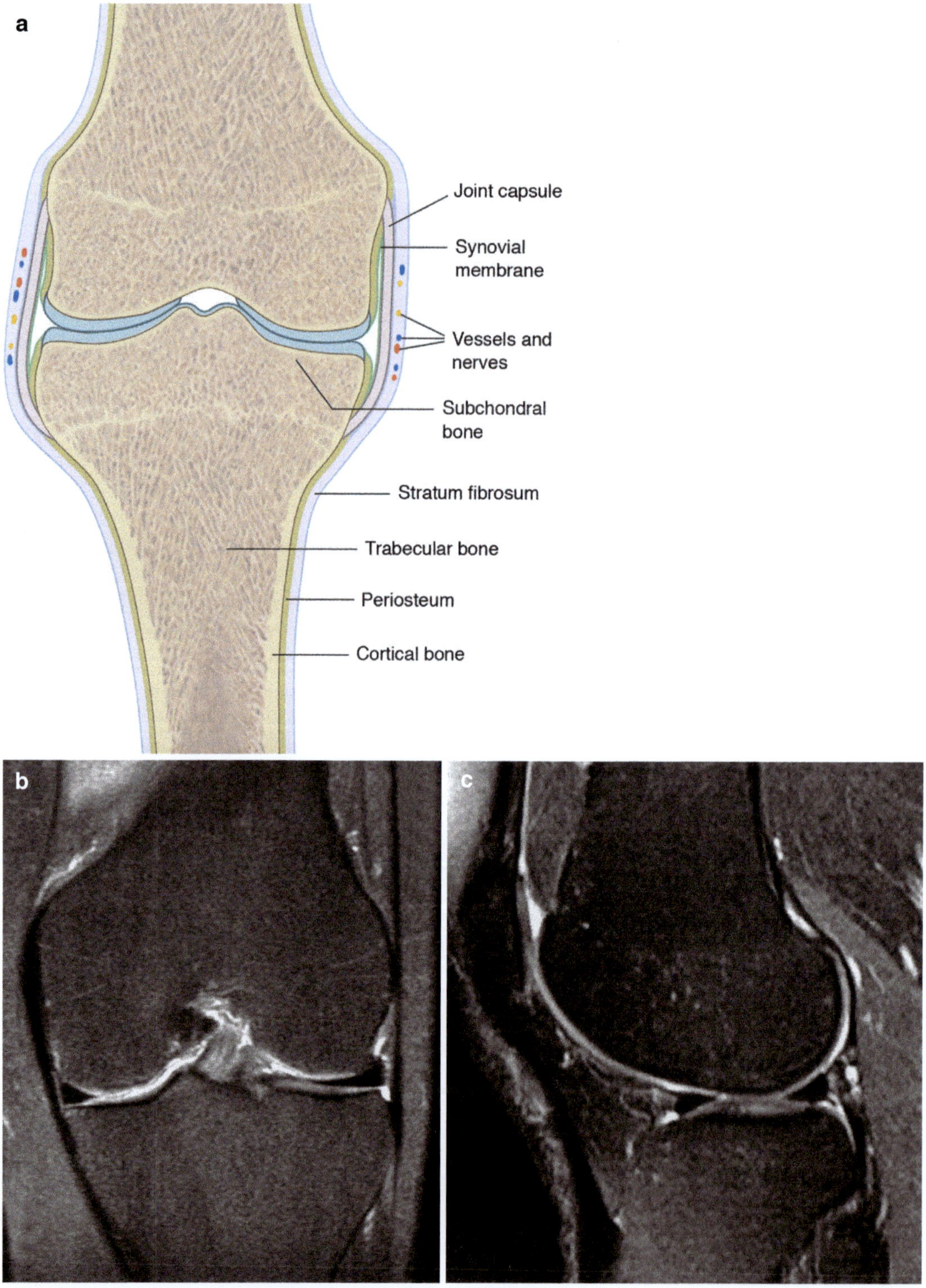

Fig. 98.1 (**a–c**) Illustration (**a**) and MRI, T2 weighted (**b**, **c**) of a knee joint demonstrating the diversity of connective tissue structures. The subchondral bone is dark because of a high-mineral and low-water content and can be seen below the very thin grey layer of cartilage

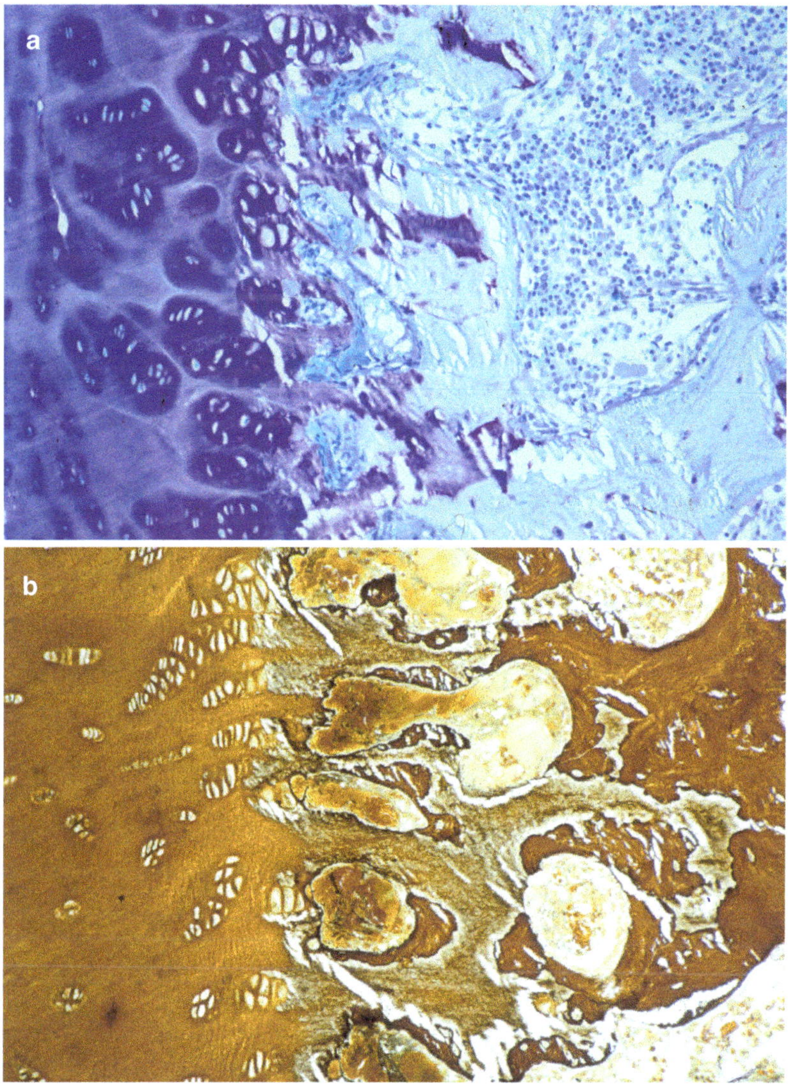

Fig. 98.2 (**a**, **b**) Histology of the epiphyseal growth plate with cartilage and chondrocytes (*left*), subchondral bone with osteoblastic seam (*middle*) and bone marrow with haematopoiesis and small vessels (*right*). Giemsa (**a**) and Gomori (**b**) staining

Motion and loading have two positive effects on cartilage:

- Cartilage tissue has no blood supply, and therefore pressure is necessary to force nutrients and oxygen from the synovial fluid into the cartilage.
- Chondrocyte deformation is required to maintain homeostasis of the extracellular matrix. Cartilage contains no nerves and therefore receives no direct regulatory messages from the body.
- Cartilage is also impermeable to cellular or humoral immune responses.
- Mechanical stresses on chondrocytes are an important factor that regulates the balance between synthesis and breakdown of the matrix.

Pathogenesis of Bone Disorders in Joint Diseases

99

The functioning of the joint depends on the "frictionless" interaction of the components involved (cartilage layers, synovium, synovial fluid, subcortical bone, adjacent bone marrow, ligaments, muscles and menisci) (Fig. 99.1). This functional unit, joint-bones-synovia-muscles, can be affected by different factors (traumatic, degenerative, infection, autoimmunological, neurogenic and metabolic).

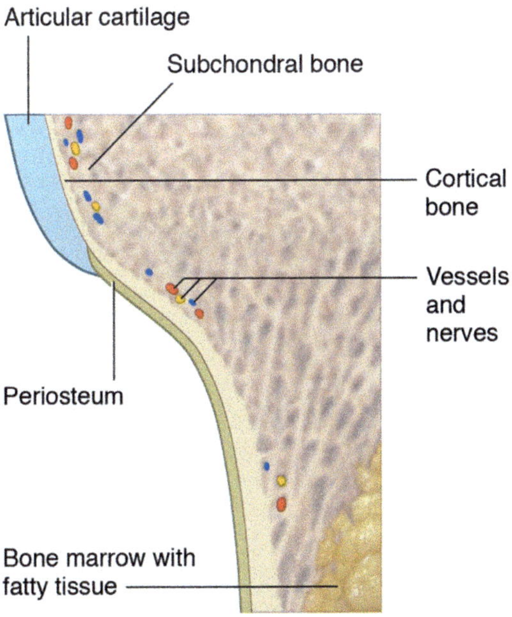

Fig. 99.1 Illustration of the functional unit "cartilage-bone-periosteum"

Cartilage destruction is at the centre of all joint destruction.

The mechanisms, however, that lead to joint damage show comparable results. Excessive use of joints however does not inevitably lead to osteoarthritis. In fact, distance runners and ballet dancers actually have a lower incidence of osteoarthritis of the "overused" joints. However, they may develop secondary osteoarthritis due to joint trauma and disrupted joint mechanics. In persons predisposed to develop osteoarthritis, overuse may accelerate, but not cause its development.

There are two main theories which cause the development of osteoarthritis:

- A defect in the articular cartilage matrix leads to premature failure.
- Primary abnormalities in the subchondral bone lead to secondary failure of the cartilage.

Age-dependent but also disease-related changes make the supply of nutrition to the cartilage cell worse through changes in the molecular structure. Inflammatory cytokines and enzymes

R. Bartl, C. Bartl, *Bone Disorders*, DOI 10.1007/978-3-319-29182-6_99

contribute to a destruction of cartilage with inflammatory reaction on neighbouring tissue. These changes can be traced in the X-ray image, above all in MRI. It leads to reparative processes as in subchondral sclerosis of the articular surface osteophytes at the edges of the joint.

Radiological signs of osteoarthritis are:

- Joint space narrowing
- Subchondral bone sclerosis
- Subchondral cystic bone defects and erosions
- Bone marrow oedema in the subchondral region (MRI)
- Joint deformities and limb axis deviation

As there are no nerve endings, even severe morphological changes of the cartilage tissue might not be accompanied by pain. The accompanying inflammation of the adjacent tissues (synovitis and bone marrow oedema) triggers the typical pain.

Within the *rheumatological spectrum*, the following four groups are distinguishable:

- Inflammatory/articular: Rheumatoid arthritis
- Inflammatory/extra-articular: Polymyositis, polymyalgia rheumatic
- Non-inflammatory/articular: Osteoarthritis
- Non-inflammatory/extra-articular: Fibromyalgia syndrome

100 Subchondral Cysts

Acquired subchondral cysts are caused by trauma to the cartilage or subchondral bone. These lesions include:

- Osteoarthritis cysts
- Intraosseous ganglia
- Posttraumatic cysts

Injury to the articular cartilage stimulates granulation tissue proliferation in the marrow of the subchondral zone. Small foci of myxomatous material develop and finally form cysts with local bone resorption. The result of this degenerative/inflammatory process is a subchondral radiolytic defect:

- *Osteoarthritic cysts* often complicate late rheumatoid arthritis. The subchondral cysts occur near the areas of maximal joint space narrowing and are usually present on both sides of a joint. The hip and the knee are the most common joints to develop these cysts. They vary in size from a few millimetres to several centimetres.
- *Intraosseous ganglia* are regarded as a distinct entity because patients lack osteoarthritic signs. They occur in middle-aged patients and most frequently involve the medial malleolus of the distal tibia, the proximal tibia and the acetabulum. Radiographically these lesions are distinct lytic defects in the epiphysis beneath the subchondral zone. Intraosseous ganglia are treated successfully by removal and curettage of the myxomatous tissue. A rare lesion, "periosteal ganglion", develops beneath the periosteum in the tibia.
- *Posttraumatic cysts* develop in subchondral bone following severe articular injury with concomitant bone marrow oedema. Sometimes the cysts may cause an osteochondral fracture, best visualised by CT and MRI. The distal femur, the proximal tibia and the talus are the most common locations of this process. Posttraumatic subchondral cysts may be treated with evacuation of the myxomatous contents and curettage of the lining.

R. Bartl, C. Bartl, *Bone Disorders*, DOI 10.1007/978-3-319-29182-6_100

101 Bone Reactions in Rheumatic Disorders

101.1 Inflammatory-Induced Bone Loss in Rheumatic Disorders

Inflammatory joint disorders comprise of a broad group of disorders, which are characterised by inflammatory-destructive processes. They cause damage to the structure and function of articular and periarticular tissues. The entire skeleton and extraarticular organs/tissue could also be involved. Typical examples are rheumatoid arthritis (RA), systemic lupus erythematosus (SLE), ankylosing spondylitis, Crohn's disease and psoriatic arthritis.

With RA and SLE, the *synovium* is the target of the autoimmune process with the result of a proliferation of the synovium and production of potent inflammatory cytokines and mediators. As a result of the inflammation, there is a destruction of joint tissue. In contrast to RA, spondyloarthropathies lead to additional calcifications and ossifications.

> "Rheumatism" is an umbrella term for many inflammatory and degenerative diseases of connective tissue, which together have a "flowing" pain character (Greek: "Rhine" = flow). Over 1000 disorders with different pathogenesis and localisations are grouped together with the term "rheumatism".

101.2 Rheumatoid Arthritis (RA)

Rheumatoid arthritis (RA, synonym: primary chronic polyarthritis, PcP) is a systemic inflammatory disorder characterised by symmetrical polyarthritis. RA is the most common inflammatory arthritis, affects about 1 % of whites and often results in severe disability. Women are affected two to three times more frequent than men. Most joint destruction occurs within the first 4–5 years. About 10 % of patients have an acute onset, with the development of polyarticular disease within a few days. The most helpful, though not diagnostic laboratory test in the diagnosis is the *serum rheumatoid factor*.

> Four forms of pathological bone remodelling can be distinguished:
>
> - Focal marginal articular erosion (typical sign of RA)
> - Subchondral bone loss
> - Periarticular osteopenia/osteoporosis
> - Systemic osteoporosis

Inflammatory changes also occur in the subchondral bone causing a diffuse osteopenia (Fig. 101.1). The layer between the "pannus" and the bone surface is characterised by resorption lacunae, filled with polynuclear

R. Bartl, C. Bartl, *Bone Disorders*, DOI 10.1007/978-3-319-29182-6_101

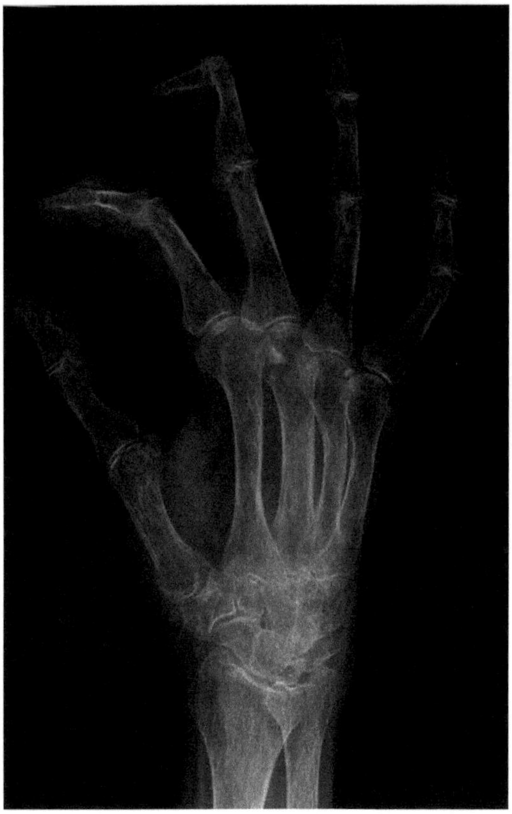

Fig. 101.1 Severe systemic and localised bone loss in a patient with rheumatoid arthritis

cells and typical osteoclasts. It is very likely that these osteoclasts are also responsible for triggering the adjacent bone marrow oedema. Histologically, inflammatory cells are found especially in the periarticular bone marrow with signs of oedema and vasculitis. These inflammatory cells secrete a broad spectrum of cytokines and hormones (RANKL; IL-1, IL-6, IL-11, IL-15 and IL-16; monocytes of CSF; TNF-α; prostaglandins and PTHrP). RANKL, produced in synovial fibroblasts and T-cells, is of particular importance. The role of RANKL is shown by the fact that treatment with *denosumab* successfully suppressed the formation of articular bone erosions in patients with RA. A positive "side effect" of denosumab is the simultaneous effective treatment of accompanying local and systemic osteoporosis.

Periarticular bone loss in RA has three causes:

- Painful joints often lead to disuse atrophy of the adjacent bone.
- Cytokines released from the inflamed synovial membrane directly activates osteoclasts.
- Many patients with RA are on long-term steroid therapy that leads to systemic osteoporosis.

Another feature of subchondral bone loss in patients with RA is the inability to repair bone. The inflamed synovium cells produce TNF-α and *dickkopf*-1 (DKK-1), which block the formation of bone. The development of the periarticular bone erosion is triggered by immobilisation and glucocorticoid treatment as well as by cytokines of inflammatory cells in the adjacent bone marrow.

Bone destruction in RA is caused by a complex network of inflammatory cytokines and lymphocyte activation, resulting in chronic inflammation of the synovium.

The damage of the systemic bone remodelling is caused by many proinflammatory cytokines from the inflamed synovium/bone marrow, which get into the blood circulation and act like hormones. Thus, circulating OPG/RANKL in RA patients causes continuously increased bone erosion. An anti-TNF therapy with infliximab coincided with a decline of the serum RANKL levels and a reduced bone loss.

Drug therapy is the mainstay of the management of RA, and steroidal and non-steroidal anti-inflammatory drugs are used in almost all patients. Some patients respond to DMARDs (e.g. methotrexate or cyclophosphamide) or biologic agents that bind and neutralise TNF. *Surgery* is indicated in cases of severe joint destruction and functional limitation.

101.3 Ankylosing Spondylitis (AS)

The ankylosing spondylitis (AS, Morbus Bechterew-Marie-Strümpell) is a systemic condition with inflammation of the axial skeleton (especially the sacroiliac joint) and is closely associated with the HLA-B27-allele. This association of the seronegative spondyloarthropathies with HLA-B27, an antigen present in only 8 % of the general population, suggests that these disorders share a common pathogenesis.

Most patients with ankylosing spondylitis are men, and about 90 % of affected individuals are HLA-B27 positive. One proposed pathogenesis of AS is that a triggering microbial infection, with *Yersinia* or *Klebsiella* organisms, elicits an antibacterial immune reaction that cross-reacts with the HLA-B27 molecule itself.

As with RA, synovial hyperplasia, lymphocytic infiltrates and pannus formation can be seen. In contrast to RA, patients with AS show an increased bone formation and enchondral ossification in the joint area. The reason for which seems to be increased levels of BMP-2 and BMP-6 in these region. Part of the *radiological evidence* of sacroiliitis with SA is therefore erosion, budlike osteoproliferations and subchondral sclerosis. MRI shows a massive bone marrow oedema in this area. In advanced stages sacroiliitis results in a bony ankylosis of the joint gap and finally into a bamboo-like stiffening of the spinal column ("bamboo back bone") (Fig. 101.2). The development of syndesmophytes is particularly observed in the area of inflamed modified vertebrae. However, an effective anti-TNF therapy does not lead to a standstill.

This finding is explained as the effect of the inflammatory processes on the systemic bone remodelling. A *Reiter syndrome* is established, if

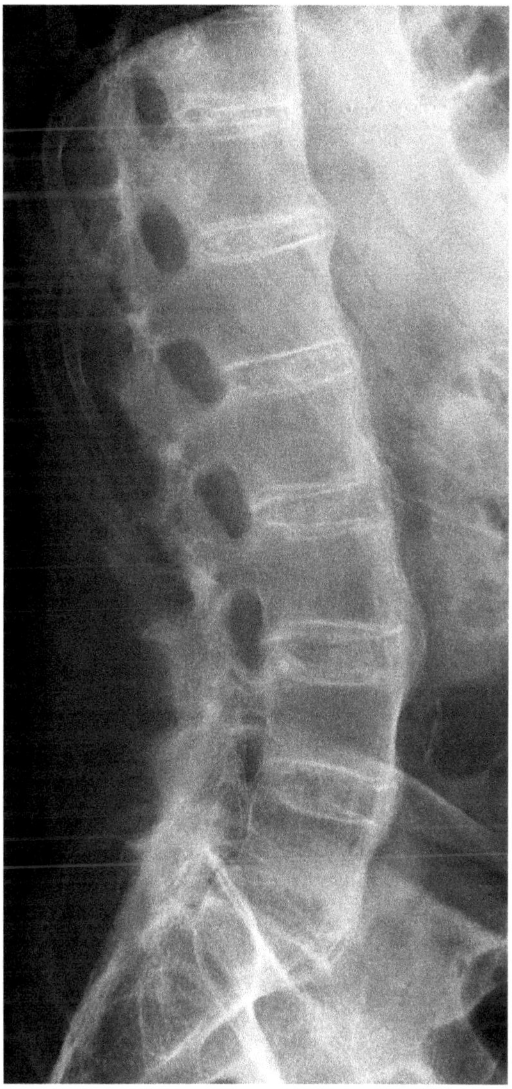

Fig. 101.2 Bamboo-like stiffening of the spinal column

Despite the tendency to excessive joint bone formation, many patients with AS show signs of spinal osteopenia. This excessive loss of trabecular bone is due primarily to the immobilisation in the spinal ankylosis, although a low bone density has also been shown with AS patients without any ankylosis.

in addition to the arthritis, a conjunctivitis, urethritis, uveitis or psoriatic skin changes can also be found.

In most patients, AS can be managed conservatively, and often *non-steroidal anti-inflammatory drugs* together with muscle strengthening and posture exercises are sufficient. Long-term steroid therapy has no role in AS. Administration of *intravenous BP* is indicated in patients with bone marrow oedema and vertebral pain.

101.4 Systemic Lupus Erythematosus (SLE)

Like RA this autoimmune disorder is a systemic inflammatory condition, which also affects and damages many other organs besides the joints. In contrast to RA, in SLE there are no erosive joint changes and no cartilage destruction. The inflammatory reactions of the soft tissues are predominant. In the course of soft tissue calcification, decalcification near joints, joint deformities and epiphysis osteonecrosis also occur. Of interest is the realisation that interferon-α and interferon-β inhibit the osteoclastogenesis and that the high regulation of these genes and their products protects against the development of erosions by SLE.

> Bone destruction in SLE patients is the result of increased osteoclastic activity caused by proinflammatory cytokines and an imbalance in RANKL/OPG. Impaired osteoblastic activity may also play a role in the pathogenesis of osteoporosis in SLE patients.

As with RA and AS, patients with SLE have a higher risk of systemic osteoporosis and "low-trauma" fractures. In addition to the systemic inflammation process, immobilisation, glucocorticoid therapy, renal insufficiency and vitamin D deficiency contribute to the bone loss.

101.5 Systemic Sclerosis (Scleroderma)

With this systemic connective tissue disorder, there is a defective regulation of collagen biosynthesis with accumulation of collagen in the skin and in the connective tissue of many internal organs

> The *CREST syndrome* includes the "calcinosis", the "Raynaud's phenomenon", the "oesophageal dysfunction", the "sclerodactyly" and the "telangiectasia".

The skin and soft tissues are too tight and cause deformities of joints, osteolyses at the fingertips ("rat-bite phenomenon") and signs of arthritis. In addition, hand skeleton *decalcification*, *soft tissue calcification* and *osteolysis* occur in the carpal area. Histological signs of synovialitis but little pannus formation can be found.

Osteoporosis in scleroderma is a highly important, but less observed bone disorder. It concerns not only the hands and feet but the entire skeleton and indicates a systemic disorder. A severe osteoporosis in combination with periarticular soft tissue calcifications should always be considered as evidence of the existence of systemic scleroderma, known as *Thibierge-Weißenbach syndrome*.

101.6 Psoriatic Arthritis

Psoriasis is one of the most common skin disorders, affecting 1–2 % of the population. About 10 % of psoriasis patients suffer from chronic polyarthritis. There is a coexistence of osteodestructive and osteoproliferative joint changes. Describing the attack on the wrist, one can differentiate between a transversal type with attack of a joint series and the axial type with an attack of a finger beam.

There are three clinical forms of psoriatic arthritis:

- Asymmetric polyarthritis involving the interphalangeal joints of the hand
- Severe erosive lesions in the hands, called "arthritis mutilans"
- Sacroiliitis similar to ankylosing spondylitis

Demineralisation in the vicinity of diseased joints is more rarely proven as with RA. Occasionally, a spondylarthritis ankylopoietica evolves with syndesmophytes.

The antiproliferative effect of vitamin D proved to be useful in the treatment of psoriasis.

101.7 Sarcoidosis of the Skeleton (Morbus Jüngling)

Sarcoidosis often shows a diffuse attack of the bone marrow by epithelioid cell granulomas (Fig. 101.3), with differing degrees of damage of the adjacent trabeculae. Osteolysis and local osteosclerosis are observed.

A major complication is *hypercalcaemia*, caused by the formation of active vitamin D metabolites in the granulomas.

Acroosteolyses, areas of sclerosis and signs of arthritis can be found in the hand skeleton, especially in the phalanx.

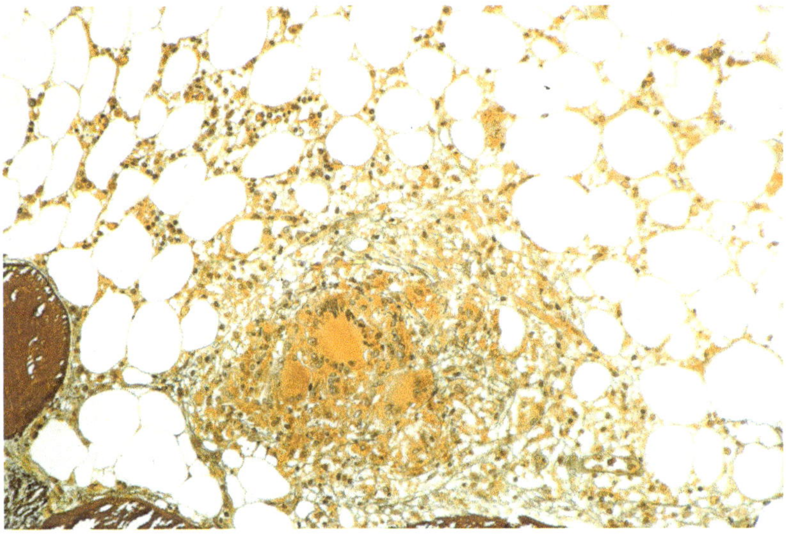

Fig. 101.3 Bone biopsy with an epithelioid cell granuloma in a patient with sarcoidosis. Gomori staining

102 Degenerative, Metabolic and Neurogenic Joint Diseases

102.1 Arthrosis Deformans

Arthrosis deformans (osteoarthritis, degenerative joint disorder) is the most common joint disease and is symptomatic mainly between 40 and 60 years of age. The secondary arthrosis stems from the inferiority of the cartilage tissue, unequal mechanical loading, trauma, inflammation or metabolic disorders. At the beginning, pathogenetically, is the loss of elasticity, changes of the cartilage basic substance (collagen and proteoglycans) and the decrease of chondrocytes. Above all, the spine (cervical and lumbar), knees, hips, hands and feet are above all affected. First radiological changes are loss of cartilage height, cleft in the joint cartilage and subchondral sclerosis. Osteophytes, solitary "scree cysts" and inflammatory reactions ("secondary erosive arthritis") occur with advanced abrasion.

> As there is no causal therapy of the disease process (stopping the cartilage destruction or increasing the collagen synthesis), the treatment is focused on pain relief and functional improvement. Joint replacement is indicated in patients with advanced joint destruction.

102.2 Osteochondrosis Dissecans (OD)

Osteochondrosis appears one sided and prefer weight-bearing epiphyses with convex articular surfaces. The medial femur-condyle and the dome of the talus are most frequently affected. The osteochondral lesion is often accompanied by a painful *bone marrow edema* (Fig. 102.1). A crescent-shaped subchondral sclerosis can be found, radiologically, at an early stage.

102.3 Goutarthropathy and Chondrocalcinosis (Pseudo Gout)

Above all, men over 50 years of age are affected. A hyperuricemia can proceed without symptoms, but may also manifest itself as acute gout arthritis. It produces subchondral osteolysis, also called "Tophus" (Fig. 102.2).

> Each sharply defined, punched-out, round subchondral osteolysis of hand and forefoot should always give rise to the suspicion of gout and be the reason for a determination of uric acid level in the serum.

R. Bartl, C. Bartl, *Bone Disorders*, DOI 10.1007/978-3-319-29182-6_102

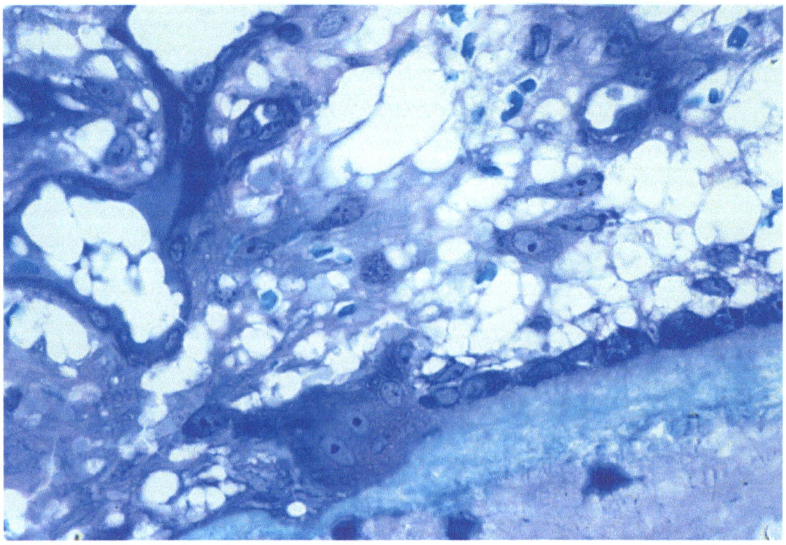

Fig. 102.1 Osteochondrosis dissecans: subcortical area with bone marrow oedema, various vessels and osteoclastic bone resorption. Giemsa staining

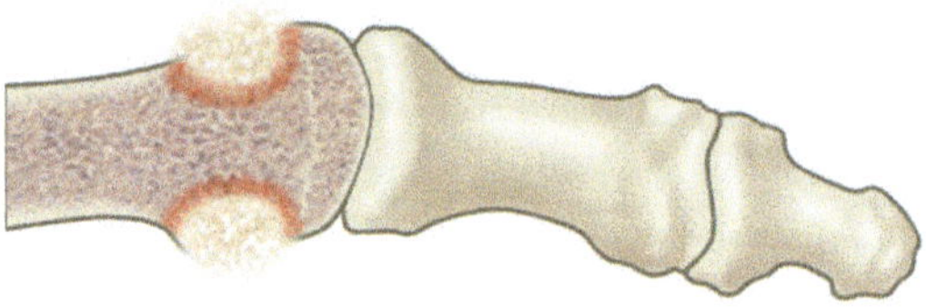

Fig. 102.2 Sharply defined, punched-out and round subchondral osteolyses of a finger in gout

Pronounced tophi are signs of chronic gout and only occur after years. Occasionally they may a bone tumour. Frequently, a lip of subchondral bone overhangs the lytic defect. In contrast to RA there are no osteopenic reactions. Rather, the gout arthropathy goes hand in hand with an osteosclerotic bone response. With *pseudo gout* (chondrocalcinosis), in contrast to the uric acid gout, large joints are attacked. The deposits consist of calciumpyrophosphate crystals and are always suspicious for hyperparathyroidism.

102.4 Neuropathic Joint Disorders

Denervation of a joint results in an unusual form of osteoarthritis characterized either by joint destruction or massive osteophyte formation. The arthropathy in *tabes dorsalis* is the prototype of this group of joint disorders. Similar changes occur in syringomyelia, leprosy, alcoholism, amyloidosis, demyelinating processes and diabetic neuropathy.

Infectious Joint Disorders

103

103.1 Definition and Pathogenesis

Infectious arthritis is caused by various pathogens (bacteria, fungi, viruses), which are mostly blood- borne or by direct pathogenic inoculation (open fractures, after joint punctures, i.v. drug abuse). The large joints are mainly affected. With purulent arthritis, there is, at first, a purulent joint effusion, which leads to panarthritis and finally to the destruction of the joint. From a spondylitis anterior with abscess formation, buckling can develop (Gibbus/hunchback) with neurological symptoms. A typical complication is the *iliopsoas abscess*. The most common pathogen is *Staphylococcus aureus*. Predisposing factors for blood-borne infectious arthritis include diabetes mellitus, chronic renal disease, neoplasia, AIDS, immunosuppressive therapy and cirrhosis of the liver (Table 103.1).

Table 103.1 Risk factors for the development of infectious joint disorders

Pre-existing arthritis (rheumatoid arthritis, gout, pseudogout, osteoarthritis)
Systemic autoimmune diseases (SLE)
Charcot arthropathy
Prosthetic joints
Intraarticular corticosteroid injections
Intravenous drug abuse
Alcoholism
Diabetes mellitus
Liver cirrhosis
Chronic haemodialysis
Cancer
Multiple myeloma
HIV infection
Systemic corticosteroid therapy
Immunosuppressive therapy

103.2 Prosthetic Joint Infection

More than 1 million joint replacements are performed each year in the USA, and the number will increase. Loosening due to infection is more serious and requires extensive revision surgery. Today, the infection rate is only about 1 %. An infected prosthesis requires complete removal of infected prosthetic components, PE inlays, cement and all infected tissues. Joint prostheses may become infected by two mechanisms:

- Wound contamination in the operative phase (*Staphylococcus aureus* >50 %, mixed flora 35 %, gram-negative organisms 10 % and anaerobes 5 %).
- Haematogenous spread of organisms in the postoperative phase (*Staphylococcus*, *Escherichia coli*). Important sources of bacteria are infections of skin, respiratory tract, urinary tract and teeth.

Acute infections occur in the first 3 months after surgery, or they may develop later. Most infections develop within 1 year of surgery.

R. Bartl, C. Bartl, *Bone Disorders*, DOI 10.1007/978-3-319-29182-6_103

Symptoms include prosthesis loosening, pain, swelling and limited motion. An elevated C-reactive protein without another obvious cause is suggestive of infection in a patient with a painful, loose prosthesis. Sepsis may occur and produce increased morbidity and mortality.

Prosthetic joint infections are classified as:

- Early infections (within 3 months after joint replacement, usually related to the implantation surgery)
- Delayed infections (within 3 months to about 1 year after joint replacement)
- Late infections (more than 1–2 years after joint replacement, usually due to haematogenous spread)

Three factors facilitate the growth of the organisms in the periprosthetic region:

- Hardening of the cement may cause necrotic bone, which permits bacteria to grow, safe from circulating host defences.
- Bacteria, especially *Staphylococci*, are able to adhere to foreign biomaterial surface and form a biofilm.
- When bacteria contact an implant, they secret a substance (glycocalyx) which protects them against antibiotics and phagocytosis.
- Some metals in the implant depress macrophages and the immune system.

The main radiologic signs of prosthetic infection are:

- Periosteal reactions
- Scalloping
- Severe radiolucency
- Fistula through the cortical bone
- Severe bone resorption

Peri-implant Bone Loss

104

Total joint arthroplasty of the hip and knee has become one of the most frequent and rewarding operations in orthopaedic surgery. Worldwide more than one million such prostheses are implanted annually. With the steady rise in life expectancy, long-term complications related to implant loosening and peri-implant fractures are on the rise. Efforts to sustain and improve the clinical survival of total joint implants have thus generated great interest. The main challenge of implant integration by the surrounding bone is an adequate load transmission. Following implantation of a femoral stem, the load transmission is more distal in the femur. Due to the changed biomechanics and the stiffness of the implant, the periprosthetic bone reacts with a proximal periprosthetic osteopenia ("stress shielding") (Fig. 104.1). Bone atrophy around the implant components is considered as a potential factor leading to aseptic component loosening limiting the survival of the prosthesis.

104.1 Pathogenesis

Stability of the prosthesis within the surrounding bone is the decisive factor for flawless functioning and longevity of the implants. Periprosthetic osteopenia and peri-implant osteolysis is a multifactorial process stemming from host, implant and surgical factors. Billions of wear particles are generated at material interfaces and are dispersed along the effective joint space, into bone and the adjacent soft tissue, inducing an inflammatory reaction that leads to osteoclast activation and finally causing osteolysis (Fig. 104.2). Over time without proper treatment, osteolysis may progress to aseptic

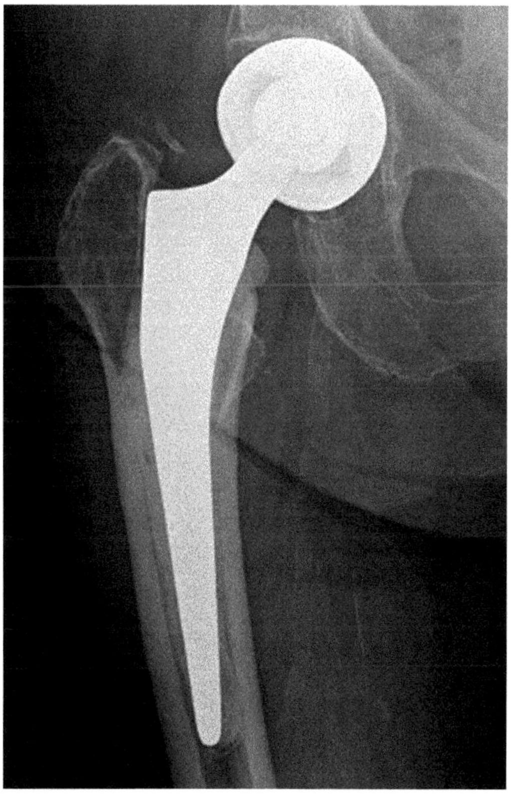

Fig. 104.1 Proximal lateral bone loss in zone 1 following stem implantation due to stress shielding

R. Bartl, C. Bartl, *Bone Disorders*, DOI 10.1007/978-3-319-29182-6_104

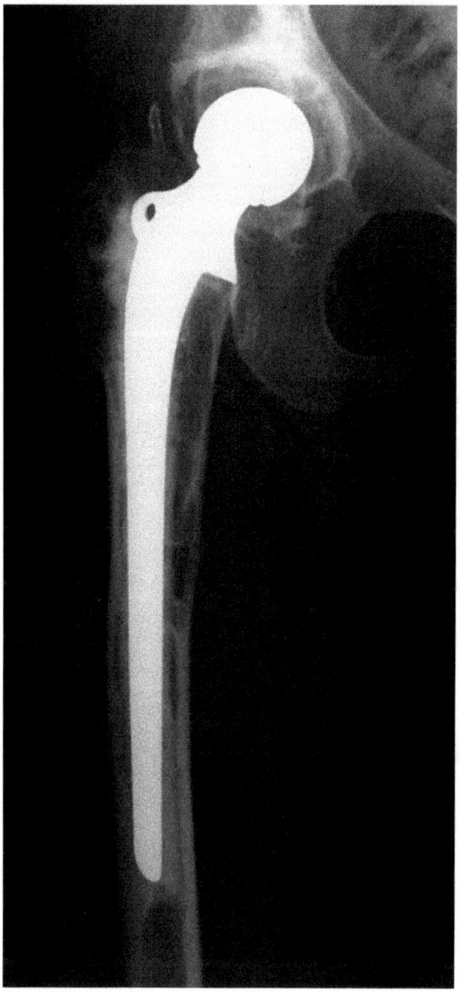

Fig. 104.2 Periprosthetic bone loss with osteolysis around the stem

loosening and failure of the implant. Initially most patients may have no clinical symptoms despite radiographic evidence of osteolysis or bone loss. Usually patients only become symptomatic when implant loosening, implant failure or peri-implant fractures occur.

The main factors involved in peri-implant bone loss leading to aseptic implant loosening following total joint arthroplasty are:

- *Stress shielding:* Insertion of an implant leads to new biomechanical relationships between various regions of the surrounding bone and the implant. Bone regions around the implant receiving high loads of stress result in bone apposition and higher bone density, whereas bone regions receiving lower stress loading react with bone loss (*stress shielding according to Wolffs' law*). Appropriate load transmission is an essential factor in maintaining bone volume. Optimal load transfer is influenced by implant design and stiffness of the implant. Bone loss around the implant due to stress shielding can account for up to 50 % of the former bone stock in underloaded regions mainly in the first 3 months following implantation, which has been demonstrated by DXA measurements (Fig. 104.3)
- *Wear-debris-induced osteolysis:* Integration of the implant into the surrounding bone can be hindered by an inflammatory reaction ("foreign body reaction") induced by macrophages absorbing small particles, mainly polyethylene and metallic wear debris, leading to activation of RANKL and OPG which then trigger osteoclastic activity and stimulate the production of fibrous tissue. The soft tissues that accumulate around the implants are further potent stimulators of osteolysis. Another important factor is the inhibition of osteoblast function mediated by wear particles. Finally, osteolysis and bone loss around the implant occurs.

- *Polyethylene:* Polyethylene particles are mainly generated due to abrasion between the femoral head component and the PE cup inlay, generating a foreign body reaction, if particles are larger than 10 μm.
- *Methyl methacrylate:* Stress at the bone-cement interface causes abrasion, and cement particles become embedded in the soft tissue around the implant.
- *Metal:* Metallic ions enter the soft tissues and even the bloodstream. Titanium and chromium oxide may cause a marked synovitis with an effusion.

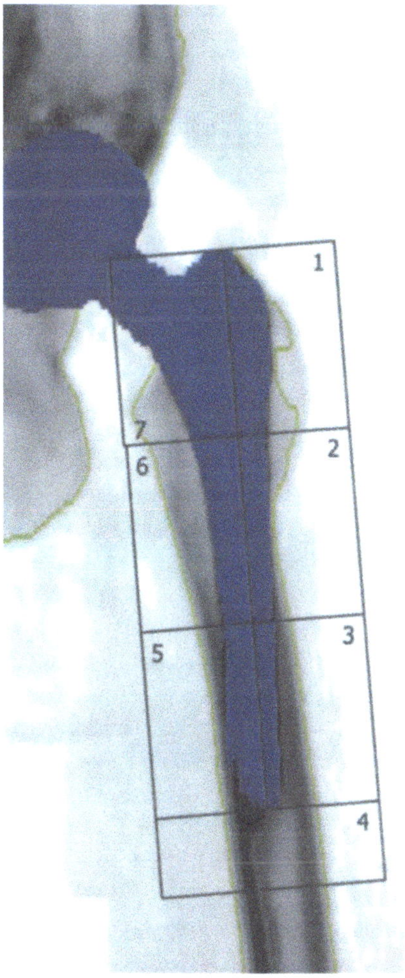

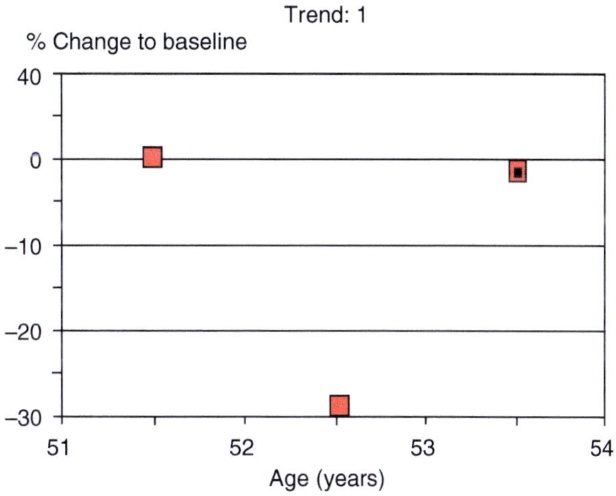

Region	BMD (g/m^2)	BMC (g)	Surface area (cm^2)
1	0.741	1.01	1.37
2	0.946	1.23	1.30
3	1.343	4.10	3.06
4	1.270	5.86	4.61
5	1.414	2.81	1.99
6	1.002	4.21	4.20
7	0.679	1.15	1.70

		Trend: 1	Change to	
Date measure	Age (years)	BMD (g/cm^2)	Baseline (%)	Baseline (%/year)
18.06.2008	53.5	0.741	−1.5	−0.8
20.06.2007	52.5	0.534	−29.0	−28.7
14.06.2006	51.5	0.752	Baseline	Baseline

Fig. 104.3 DXA monitoring of periprosthetic BMD around the stem. Marked bone loss in the first year following implantation. Normalisation of periprosthetic BMD in the second year under intravenous bisphosphonate treatment

- *Micromotion between surfaces:* Implants that do not achieve adequate initial fixation will exhibit micromotion in response to loading. The greater the area of friction, the more osteoclasts are activated causing osteolysis around the implant which leads to *fatigue failure at interfaces*. When the relative micromotion between bone and implant exceeds 150 μm, connective tissue membranes are formed between implant and bone as well as between implant and cement. These membranes hinder the osteointegration of the prosthesis. Many biochemical mediators are involved: cytokines, prostaglandins, metalloproteinases and collagenases.
- *Surgical trauma:* Thermic and mechanical necroses caused by the surgical procedure and cementing techniques alter bone quality. Muscles and tendons that transfer the load on the bone are weakened by the surgical approach.
- *Postoperative immobilisation:* The postoperative decrease in weight-bearing results in a local bone loss. Overall the postoperative bone loss mainly occurs in the first 3–6 months and can reach up to 50 % of the former bone stock.

104.2 Diagnosis

Slight loosening of the implant remains symptomless for long periods. Significant loosening causes considerable pain on weight-bearing and on sudden movements. Pain on rotation of the leg in a patient with a hip implant indicates loosening of the stem, and pain on axial compression may indicate loosening of the cup. Radiolucent lines more than 2 mm wide indicate loosening (Fig. 104.4), but localised and limited osteolysis and incomplete radiolucent lines per se do not constitute evidence of loosening of the implant. Migration of the prosthesis over time is diagnostic: migration of more than 5 mm indicates loosening. Implant migration indicates local bone loss which is a great problem in revision surgery. On standard anteroposterior radiographs, the peri-implant regions of the stem are classified according to Gruen, and the peri-implant zones around the cup in the pelvic bone are classified according to DeLee and Charnley (Fig. 104.5a, b). Bone scans are also useful for detection of regions of high bone turnover around implants, while computed tomography can be used to quantify the amount of bone loss.

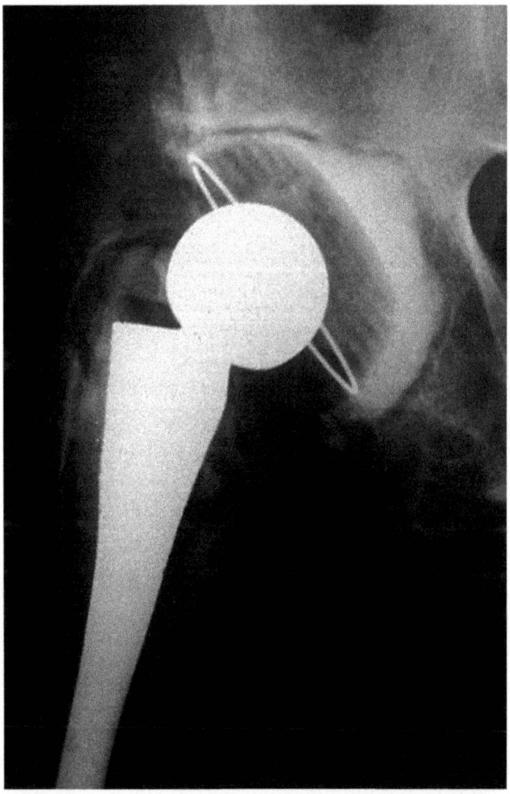

Fig. 104.4 Peri-implant osteolysis showing radiolucent line around the cup indicating aseptic loosening

104.3 Treatment Strategies

Causative therapy consists of replacing the prosthesis. Indications for this are persistent pain, functional limitations and migration of the implant. Accompanying bone loss around the implant can turn this operation into a complicated and more difficult one than the index operation. However, recent advances in technology and in materials for cementing may improve long-term results in the future. Intensive research is underway to improve the survival of the implants including local application of bisphosphonates and implant coating with osteoinductive factors. Implantation of cementless implants is recommended for younger patients with bone of good quality, as less bone is removed, which ensures a more favourable situation if a revision procedure has to be undertaken later.

Various *modifications to improve osteointegration of implants* are under investigation:

- Optimisation of prosthetic design with optimal load transfer to the bone (e.g. short-stem prostheses)
- Improved cementing techniques
- Local application of osteoinductive factors (hydroxylapatite, BMP), as well as PTH to improve osteointegration of the implant

104.4 Bisphosphonates

Early administration of nitrogen-containing bisphosphonates inhibits peri-implant osteoclastic resorption. This has been demonstrated in numerous animal experiments which showed a decrease in bone loss around the implant. Current clinical studies are hampered by short follow-ups. A published meta-analysis of 6 randomised controlled

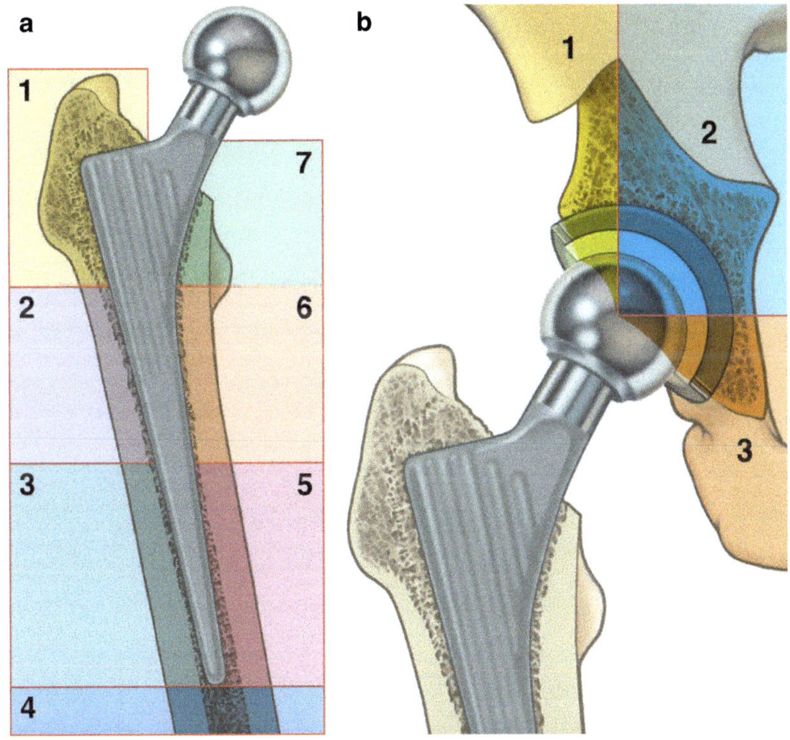

Fig. 104.5 (**a**, **b**) Periprosthetic zones of loosening: (**a**) femoral stem (according to Gruen), (**b**) acetabular cup (according to DeLee and Charnley)

studies showed that bisphosphonates given in the immediate postoperative period prevented peri-implant bone loss and resulted in a higher peri-implant bone mineral density at the end of the study period compared to controls. In a RCT from 2009, a single infusion of 5 mg zoledronate reduced the early migration of the stem and cup following cementless total hip replacement. Currently there is no consensus whether oral or intravenous BP administration leads to superior results. Intravenous application in the early post-operative period leads to a high concentration of the BP in the traumatised bone region around the implant and may lead to more favourable results.

The following treatment protocols can be applied:

- Alendronate 70 mg orally once weekly
- Risedronate 35 mg orally once weekly
- Ibandronate 3 mg intravenously every 3 months
- Zoledronate 5 mg intravenously annually

The following interventions are used to monitor therapy:

- Clinical examination
- Control radiographs
- DXA (bone densitometry)
- Bone markers

A new meta-analysis by Teng et al. in 2015, including four studies, could show that long-term use of bisphosphonates significantly decreased the risk of implant revision following total hip and total knee replacement. To establish the efficacy of bisphosphonates in preventing bone loss after total joint arthroplasty more randomised clinical trials with large numbers of patients, long-term follow-up and clinically relevant endpoints (functional outcomes, revision rates, implant loosening rate) have to be conducted. However, the current results for prevention of peri-implant bone loss with bisphosphonates are very promising. Also new osteoclast inhibitors and osteoanabolic therapies to prevent bone loss around joint and fracture implants are under investigation.

Part XVIII

Bone and Kidney

105 Renal Osteodystrophy (ROD)

105.1 Definition

Because of the importance of the kidney in calcium and phosphorus metabolism, kidney disease adversely affects the bones. Patients with chronic renal insufficiency and patients on long-term dialysis develop complicated bone disorders, also known as *renal osteodystrophy (ROD)* or renal bone disease, often accompanied by severe bone pain, multiple fractures and extraosseous calcifications, all of which considerably reduce the patient's quality of life. The new term *chronic kidney disease-mineral bone disorders (CKD-MBD)* describes a syndrome associated with chronic kidney diseases (CKDs) in which disorders of mineral metabolism and renal osteodystrophy are contributors to the mortality observed in CKD.

> In chronic kidney disease (CKD) fails a multiorgan system involving the kidney, skeleton, parathyroid glands, fatty tissue and cardiovascular system.

The skeletal remodelling abnormalities caused by CKD contribute to the heterotopic mineralisation, especially the vascular calcification, and to the disordered mineral metabolism, especially phosphate and calcium. Abnormalities of bone in the CKD are already seen after a mild reduction in glomerular filtration rate (GFR 40–70 ml/min). Elevated PTH, sclerostin and fibroblast growth factor-23 (FGF23) levels are observed before any changes in the serum phosphorus, calcitriol or calcium. Increased levels of FGF23 indicate that renal injury has already affected bone remodelling and osteocytes. Therefore, to prevent severe bone disease, the nephrologist has to begin early with the management of mineral abnormalities to prevent symptomatic and severe bone disease as long as possible. By end-stage kidney disease, clinically significant skeletal disorders are found in virtually all patients. Prior to the use of renal dialysis, patients died before severe bone changes appeared. Today, however, haemodialysis and renal transplantation support patients with end-stage renal disease long enough for them to develop severe bone disease. Therefore, renal osteodystrophy may be considered an iatrogenic disorder. The most important pathogenetic factors in the CKD-MBD are:

- Increased levels of sclerostin and fibroblast growth factor-23 (FGF23), affecting bone remodelling.
- Klotho deficiency, associated with vascular calcification.
- Hyperphosphataemia, caused by reduction in the fraction of filtered phosphate.
- Calcitriol deficiency, caused by inhibition of vitamin D metabolism in the kidney.
- Hypocalcaemia, caused by decreased intestinal calcium absorption.

R. Bartl, C. Bartl, *Bone Disorders*, DOI 10.1007/978-3-319-29182-6_105

- Hyperparathyroidism, consequence of the factors listed above.
- Hypogonadism, oestrogen and testosterone deficiencies significantly contribute to renal osteodystrophy.
- Other factors such as inflammatory mediators, acidosis, aluminium, leptin and retained catabolites all contribute to the development of CKD-MBD.

Renal osteopathy is an important cause of morbidity, decreased quality of life and an increased risk of fractures. Management focuses on maintaining optimal levels of calcium, phosphorus, vitamin D and PTH.

On a more optimistic note, it has recently been shown that therapy with statins inhibits or prevents decline in creatinine clearance and slows impairment of renal function. Moreover, statins also participate in the regulation of bone turnover. Observational studies have demonstrated that elevated phosphorus, calcium and PTH are associated with an increased risk of death and cardiovascular events (arterial calcifications). These processes are associated with high mortality especially among haemodialysis patients.

Renal osteodystrophy (ROD) consists of a mixture of three histologic features:

- Bone remodelling
- Bone mineralisation
- Bone mass

Typical findings of renal osteodystrophy (ROD) can be recognised on undecalcified bone biopsies:

- High turnover osteopathy with characteristics of secondary hyperparathyroidism
- Osteomalacia with manifestations of severe inhibition of mineralisation
- Low turnover osteopathy with the picture of severe osteoporosis (adynamic bone disease)
- Mixed type with patchy areas of osteitis fibrosa and increased osteoid

Four types of ROD in bone biopsy are reported:

- Osteitis fibrosa
- Osteomalacia
- Adynamic
- Mixed

105.2 Pathophysiology

Many factors influence both the type and extent of osteopathy:

- The renal disorder itself.
- Presence of associated diseases such as diabetes mellitus and amyloidosis.
- Severity of the renal insufficiency.
- Patients' age – young patients are particularly severely affected, especially males up to 40 years. Subsequently there are no differences between the sexes.
- Vitamin D deficiency.
- Dietary restrictions.
- Level of parathyroid hormones.
- Type of dialysis and length of time patient is on dialysis.
- Accumulation of toxic substances (e.g. aluminium, fluoride, iron).
- Glucocorticoid therapy.

The most significant of the above in the mechanism of renal bone disease are:

- Anomalies of vitamin D metabolism
- Degree of secondary hyperparathyroidism
- Deposition of aluminium in bone at the mineralisation front (prevents mineralisation, is now infrequent)
- Immunosuppressive therapy inducing a negative bone balance

105.3 Diagnosis

105.3.1 Symptoms

The most important symptoms are bone pain, low-trauma fractures, skeletal deformities, muscle weakness and anomalies of growth in young patients. Bone pain and fractures can be observed in all patients with ROD independent of the underlying histology. However, low turnover osteomalacia and aluminium-related bone disease are associated with the most severe bone pain and the highest incidence of fractures. In children, growth retardation and bone deformities may be caused by vitamin D deficiency (rickets) or secondary hyperparathyroidism. In adults, skeletal deformities include lumbar scoliosis, thoracic kyphosis and recurrent rib fractures.

105.3.2 Biochemical Investigation

The following parameters of bone metabolism should be measured: calcium and phosphate, alkaline phosphatase and osseous alkaline phosphatase, parathyroid hormone, metabolites of vitamin D 25 and 1,25, aluminium and the Desferal test.

105.3.3 Radiologic Investigation

These may demonstrate characteristic changes seen in osteomalacia (Looser zones) or in secondary hyperparathyroidism (e.g. subperiosteal bone resorption of the phalanges) such as subcutaneous and arterial calcifications, subperiosteal erosions and "rugger jersey" spinal column. Three components of renal osteodystrophy can be identified and classified in histology of bone:

- Alterations of remodelling: osteitis fibrosa cystica or adynamic bone
- Disturbance of mineralisation: osteomalacia, previously associated with aluminium
- Reduction in bone mass: osteopenia, osteoporosis, partly due to glucocorticoids

All the characteristic signs of osteomalacia (Looser zones) (Fig. 105.1) and of secondary hyperparathyroidism may be present (e.g. subcutaneous and arterial calcifications, subperiosteal erosions, osteolytic lesions in the phalanges) (Fig. 105.2). "Brown tumours" are well-defined lytic lesions and usually occur in the metaphysis. The "rugger jersey" sign (three layers) in the cancellous bone of the vertebral bodies is found in 60–80 % of the patients (Fig. 105.3). However, in daily practice the diagnosis may not be straightforward because biochemical and radiological findings do not always match or accurately reflect the extent of damage to the bones.

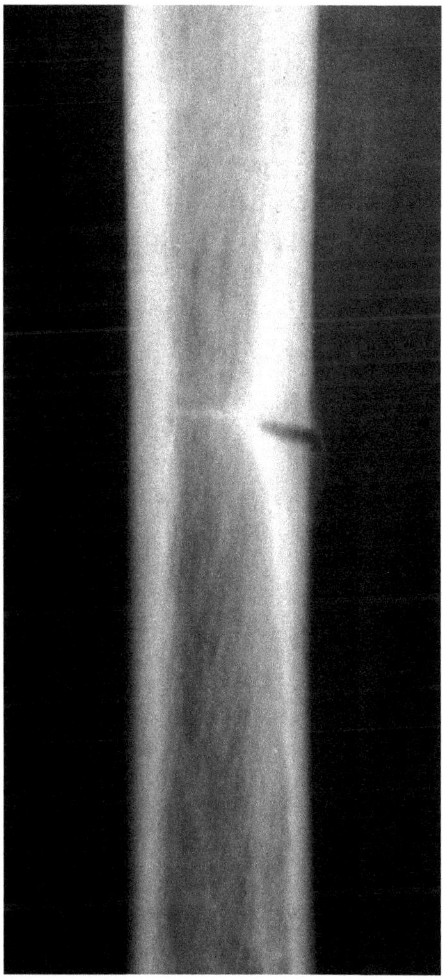

Fig. 105.1 Looser zone of the femur

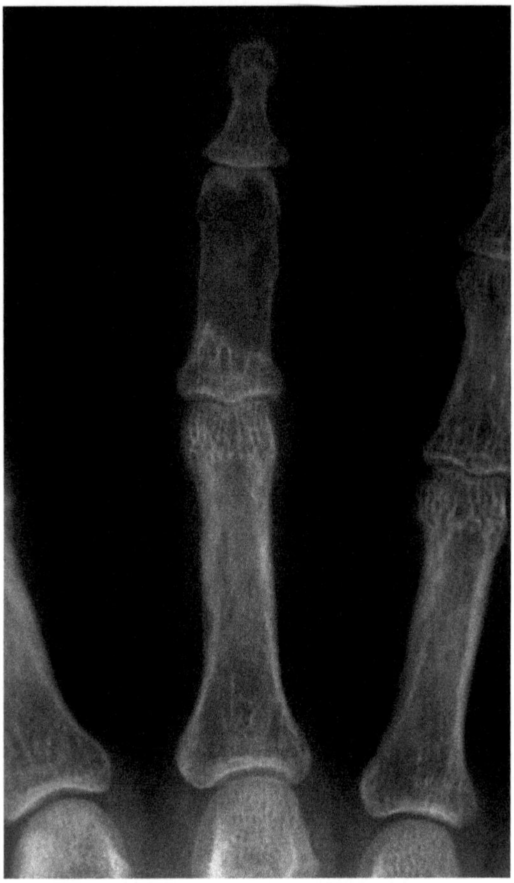

Fig. 105.2 Hyperparathyroid bone disease with marked subperiosteal bone resorption, coarsened trabecular pattern and brown tumours involving the phalanges

105.3.4 Bone Biopsy

A bone biopsy may be essential in situations in which definitive identification of the type of renal osteodystrophy is required for therapeutic decisions, as when parathyroidectomy is considered. Renal bone disease is classified according to three histological features best evaluated in a bone biopsy:

- *Disturbances of mineralisation* (osteomalacia, previously also associated with aluminium) (Fig. 105.4)
- *Anomalies of bone remodelling* (osteitis fibrosa cystica or adynamic bone disease) (Figs. 105.5 and 105.6)
- *Reduction in bone mass* (osteopenia/osteoporosis, possibly partly glucocorticoid-induced) (Figs. 105.7 and 105.8)

Various histomorphometric parameters of bone remodelling such as formation period (FP) and the quiescent period (QP) may permit a clearer identification of osteomalacia and of low turnover conditions. Moreover, detailed studies of bone biopsies have led to the recognition of a variant of adynamic bone disease (ABD) with PTH independent osteoclastic resorption, implicating other factors conducive to osteoclast activation in these cases.

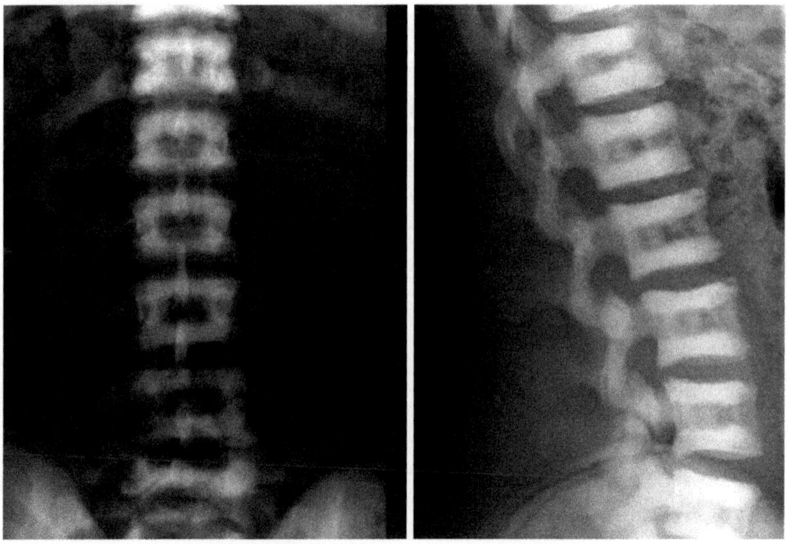

Fig. 105.3 The "rugger jersey" sign (three layers) showing overall loss of bone density with dense bands at the superior and inferior margin of the vertebral bodies

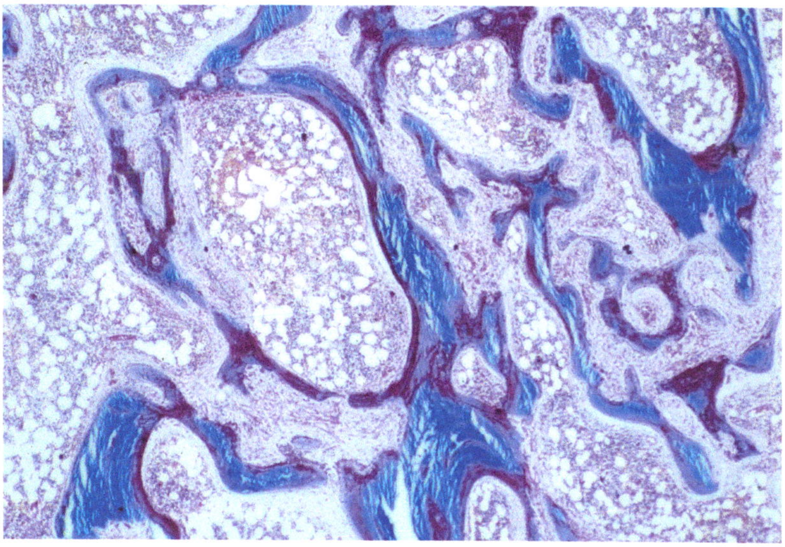

Fig. 105.4 Iliac crest biopsy of a patient with renal osteopathy: characteristics of osteomalacia (osteoid = red) and secondary hyperparathyroidism ("dissection osteoclasia"). Ladewig staining

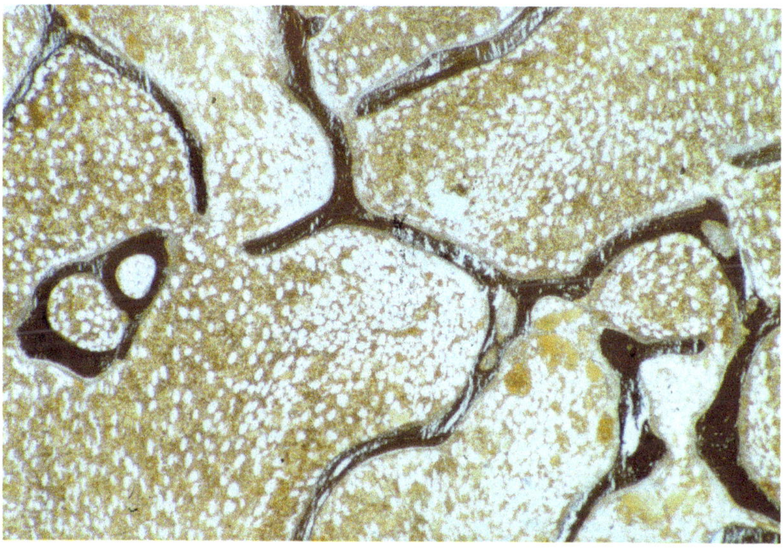

Fig. 105.5 Iliac crest biopsy of a patient with renal osteopathy: small trabeculae showing dissecting bone resorption. Gomori staining

105.4 Treatment Strategies

The goals of treatment of ROD (CKD-MBD) are:

- To attain neutral phosphorus balance
- To control PTH levels in a range that prevents the progression of secondary or tertiary HPT
- To provide adequate vitamin D supplementation
- To reduce the risk of vascular calcification, cardiovascular disease and mortality

Advances in dialysis techniques and the use of active metabolites of vitamin D have radically changed the manifestations and the therapy of renal osteodystrophy over the last 20 years. Previously, osteomalacia and secondary and tertiary HPT were major hurdles, but today severe and therapy-resistant osteoporosis is a major problem. It is characterised by markedly reduced osseous remodelling – adynamic bone disease – previously due to aluminium deposition on bone.

> The effects of the kidney disease on the bone also stimulate cardiovascular disease and mainly cause the high mortality associated with kidney disease.

With early institution of bisphosphonate therapy together with active metabolites of vitamin D, the emphasis is on prevention, since the early management of secondary HPT will decrease the number of patients requiring surgery. Inhibition of bone resorption in high turnover renal osteodystrophy is especially beneficial. In resistant cases with high levels of PTH and enlargement of the parathyroid glands, excision is indicated.

A recent study compared the survival benefit of oral vitamin D in 7203 haemodialysis patients with the survival of 8801 haemodialysis patients who had not received vitamin D, as part of the CORES study carried out in 6 Latin American countries. The study was carried out for a period of 16 months. The results showed that the haemodialysis patients who received the oral active vitamin D daily in low doses, i.e. 1 µg, had the highest survival advantage. The patients who were on active vitamin D showed significant reductions in mortality related to cardiovascular, infectious and neoplastic co-morbidities, compared to the controls. The results of this study confirmed earlier reports on some of the putative actions of vitamin D. However, according to recent studies, the question as to whether all patients with chronic renal disease should receive calcitriol has not yet been definitively answered, and randomised trials are awaited.

> Today the situation has changed due to the increasing application of intravenous nitrogen-containing BP and active vitamin D metabolites.

The aim of therapy is prevention by means of early intervention with BP and active metabolites of vitamin D. Since patients on dialysis require protection of the gastrointestinal tract, intravenous BP therapy is the method of choice. The following protocol is recommended:

- Ibandronate: 3 mg injection every 3 months
- Zoledronate: 5 mg infusion annually

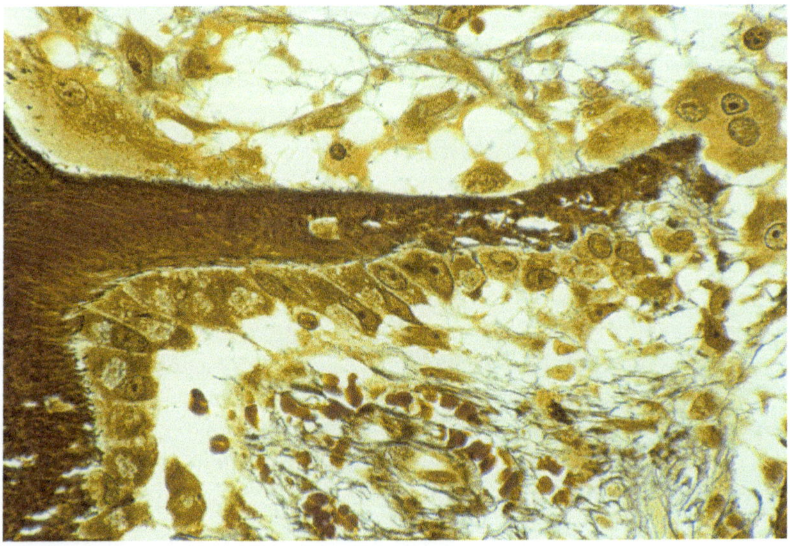

Fig. 105.6 At higher magnification increased osteoclastic activity (*lower half*) and seam of osteoblasts (*upper half*) with endosteal fibrosis. Gomori staining

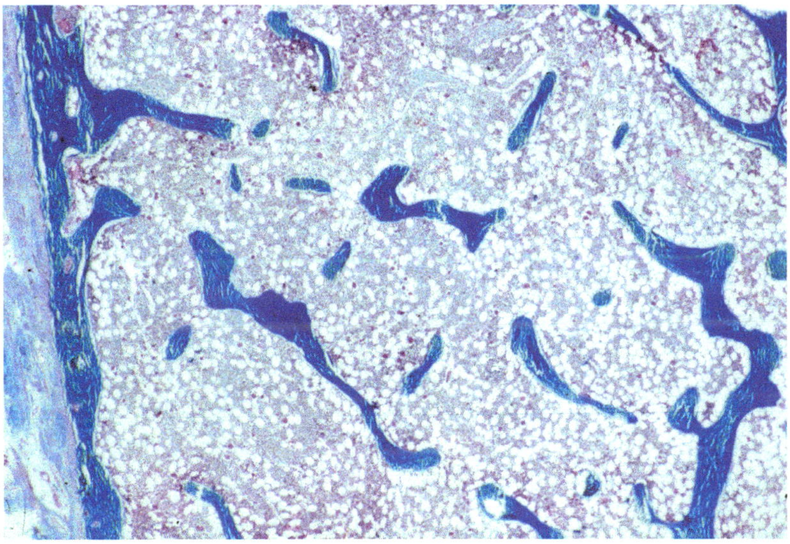

Fig. 105.7 Iliac crest biopsy of a patient with renal osteopathy: marked adynamic osteoporosis, low turnover with button phenomenon and hypoplastic marrow. No increase of osteoid volume or bone resorption. Note very thin cortex (*left*). Ladewig staining

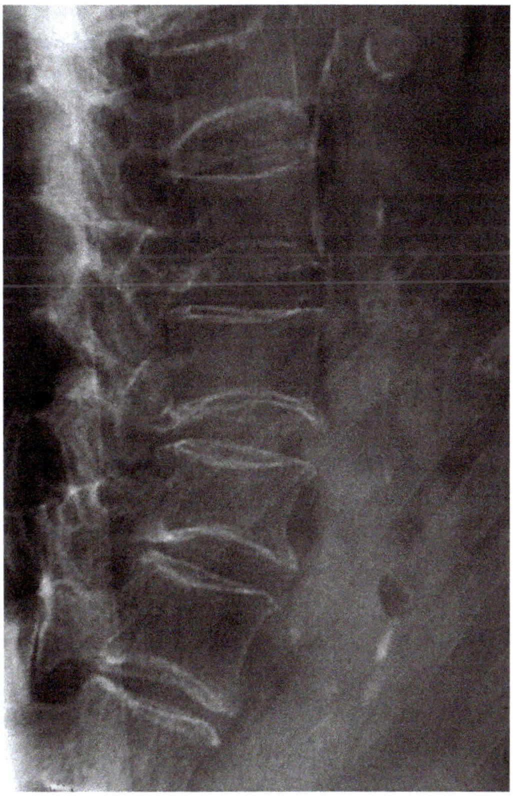

Fig. 105.8 Severe osteoporosis of the lumbar spine with massive calcification of the aorta in a patient with long-term ROD, adynamic bone disorder type

Because of its half-life in the serum of up to 16 h, patients should receive the BP on completion of dialysis. Current recommendations advise against using BP in patients with GFR <35 ml/min. Ibandronate proved to be by far the less toxic BP with respect to renal function. Resistance to BP occurs in patients with high PTH levels and demonstrable enlargement of the parathyroid glands, and parathyroidectomy is indicated in these cases. The monitoring in the immediate post-parathyroidectomy course is necessary to avoid, detect or treat symptomatic hypocalcaemia and hypophosphataemia ("hungry bone syndrome"). These changes of calcium and phosphate reflect increased uptake into bone due to the transition from bone resorption to formation.

Indications for *parathyroidectomy* in ROD patients are:

- Symptomatic or severe hypercalcaemia
- Symptomatic bone disease with spontaneous fractures
- Calciphylaxis
- Persistent HPT after transplantation

Children with renal osteodystrophy require special evaluation and individual therapy for which European Guidelines have been published.

106 Haemodialysis-Associated Amyloidosis

One form of amyloidosis, β_2-microglobulin, is characteristic in renal dialysis patients. Amyloid is deposited in the skeleton and periosteal tissues and is a further manifestation of renal bone disease. About 200 mg of this protein are produced each day on cell surfaces, normally filtered by the glomeruli and catabolised in the tubuli. However, this low-molecular-weight protein does not filter well through dialysis membranes and as a consequence accumulates in tissues. After ten or more years of dialysis, about 70 % of patients are affected. The following manifestations are characteristic:

- Osteoarticular manifestations (carpal tunnel syndrome)
- Soft tissue masses in the shoulder
- Subchondral bone cysts in humeral and femoral heads, in hands and in spine
- Erosive arthropathy

In bone biopsies, amyloid is readily observed in Giemsa-stained sections. It appears as homogeneous dark-blue deposits usually located within the vessel walls (Fig. 106.1a, b) or, more diffusely distributed, in the interstitium (Fig. 106.2a, b). Congo red (Fig. 106.3) and immunohistological stainings are applied for further confirmation and classification. In our series, iliac crest biopsy was positive in 78 % of patients with proven amyloidosis, detected as readily as in biopsies of the rectum or the kidney. Lytic bone lesions appear in combination with dense amyloid deposits in the marrow cavities. Systemic vascular amyloidosis usually leads to haematopoietic hypoplasia and generalised low-turnover osteopenia.

R. Bartl, C. Bartl, *Bone Disorders*, DOI 10.1007/978-3-319-29182-6_106

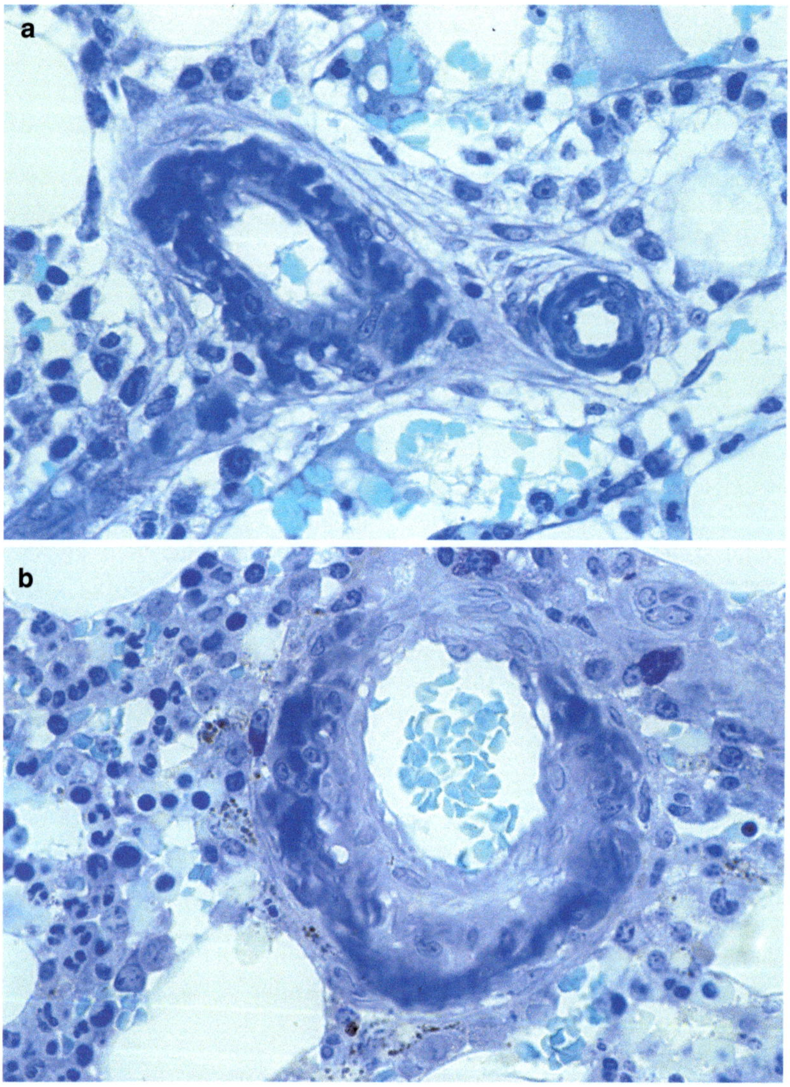

Fig. 106.1 (**a**, **b**) Haemodialysis-associated amyloidosis: (**a**) and (**b**) blood vessels with deposition of amorphous material in their walls. Giemsa staining

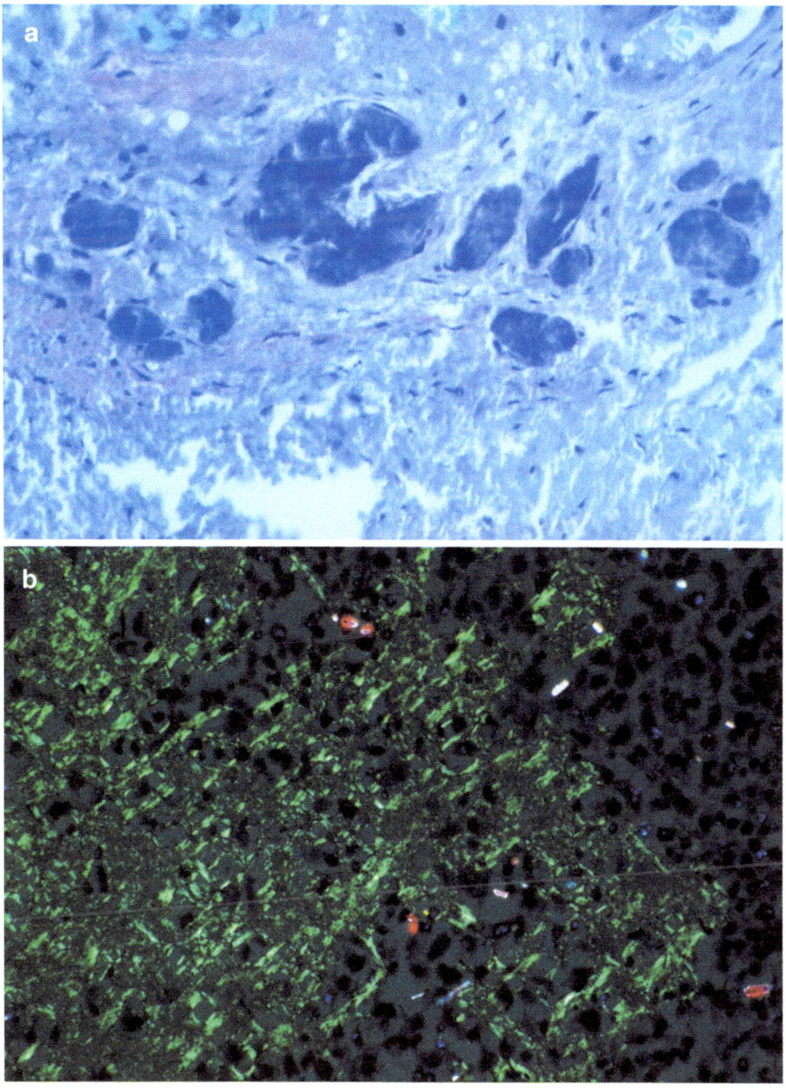

Fig. 106.2 (**a**, **b**) Haemodialysis-associated amyloidosis: deposition of amorphous material in the interstitium. (**a**) Giemsa staining and (**b**) Congo red, polarisation

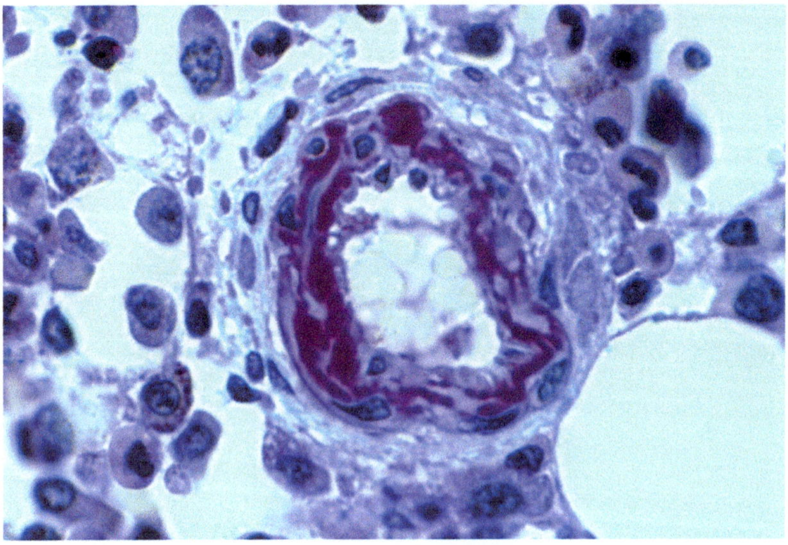

Fig. 106.3 Amorphous amyloid in the vessel wall. Congo red staining

107 Kidney Stones

107.1 Incidence of Kidney Stones

Nephrolithiasis is a common disorder that occurs in about 10 % of the adult population in Western countries. About 1 in a 1000 people must be treated every year and hospitalized due to kidney stone-related colic. Men are, from 5:1 to 2:1, more often affected than women. 80 % of the stones consist of calcium in the form of the crystalline oxalate or phosphate, only 10 % of uric acid and the rest from cystine or magnesium ammonium phosphate ("infection stones"). The main cause for the calcium stones is an unbalanced salt concentration of the urine, caused either through an increased excretion of calcium or a decreased urine volume. In 35 % of cases, the hypercalciuric nephrolithiasis is a family-related disease.

107.2 Risk Factors for Kidney Stones

Increased intake of protein, fat, salt and carbohydrates is a known risk factor for kidney stones. Other risk factors include low fluid intake, especially in warm and hot environments. Hard water (high calcium content) does not correlate with renal stone formation. Reduced calcium absorption has not been linked to a reduction of kidney stones. On the contrary, a calcium-rich diet of 1200 mg daily calcium reduces the risk of calcium oxalate stones by 51 %! However, calcium supplement tablets have no influence on the risk of stones. Other risk factors include an increased consumption of salt, animal protein and oxalate. Obesity, diabetes mellitus and genetics are further important risk factors for kidney stones.

A recently published study showed that a diet with 1200 mg of calcium daily, little animal protein and little salt lowers the oxalate excretion in the urine by 30 % diet. High doses of vitamin C should be avoided, as it also can be metabolised to oxalate. Currently, there is still no drug approved by the FDA against hyperoxaluria.

107.3 Kidney Stones and Bone Reaction

A successful therapy of patients with calcium-containing kidney stones includes four goals:

- Removal and analysis of the urinary stone (diagnosis of kidney stones)
- Avoidance of repeated urinary stone formation (prevention of kidney stones)

R. Bartl, C. Bartl, *Bone Disorders*, DOI 10.1007/978-3-319-29182-6_107

- Exclusion of underlying primary hyperparathyroidism (pHPT) (differential diagnosis)
- Conservation or improvement of reduced bone mass with reduction of the increased fracture risk (prevention of osteoporosis)

This strategy underlies the understanding that stone carriers statistically show a reduced bone density (DXA measurement) and an increased risk of fracture compared to people without kidney stones. A negative correlation between urinary calcium excretion and bone density has been established in both men and women. Additionally, stone carriers showed an increased risk of fracture of the hip, ankle and vertebrae. The majority of the calcium stone carriers is hypercalciuric and extracts the increased calcium in the urine from the skeleton. The existence of an increased bone resorption in stone carriers is verified by raised levels of bone markers and PTH values.

A pHPT must be excluded by differential diagnostics through the determination of calcium and PHT in the serum of all calcium-containing stone carriers. Patients with pHPT and still sufficient vitamin D stores show a greatly increased intestinal calcium absorption with the formation of kidney stones, while patients with pHPT and empty vitamin D stores mobilise calcium from the bones, with the consequence of a distinctive generalised bone reaction in terms of a mixture of hyperparathyroidism, osteoporosis and osteomalacia. Further disorders with higher risk of kidney stone formation are Crohn's disease, gout, diabetes mellitus, obesity and renal tubular acidosis.

107.4 Therapy of Kidney Stones

Thus, it is understandable that early administration of bisphosphonates significantly inhibits the mobilisation of calcium from the bones and thus the calcium excretion by the kidney. Administering thiazide diuretics additionally reduce the calcium excretion by the kidney (increased reabsorption of calcium in the proximal and distal tubules) and thus the risk of recurrences of calcium-containing kidney stones. Patients who "gave birth to the first stone" carry a 40 % probability that a second stone will form in the next 5 years. The exact analysis of the stone is therefore important for effective prevention planning. Hypercalciuric patients should take thiazide diuretics or indapamide to reduce calcium excretion and oversaturation with calcium oxalate. The fluid intake should be >2 l daily; administering potassium citrate reduces the risk of hypocalcaemia. A low-calcium diet is not recommended, in order to avoid a chronic negative calcium balance and thereby a higher risk of osteoporosis. In randomised trials, patients with a low-calcium diet had an even greater risk of recurrence of calcium oxalate stones than patients with a normal calcium diet (1200 mg daily) and a reduced consumption of salt and animal protein. A normal calcium intake is therefore recommended. Control measurements of bone density using the DXA method at intervals of 1–2 years are recommended, and a bisphosphonate therapy should be started early in order to avoid the development of manifest osteoporosis.

Part XIX

Bone and Other Organs/Tissues

108 Bone and Muscles

108.1 Sarcopenia and Bone Mass

A reduction of muscle and bone mass as well as an increase in fat mass are characteristic changes in increasing age. The term "sarcopenia" includes an age-related loss of muscle mass and muscle strength. Muscle loss also significantly contributes to the development of various metabolic and mechanical geriatric syndromes (e.g. diabetes type 2). Sarcopenia develops from the age of 35 years and leads above all to a decline in type II muscle fibres and an increase of intramuscular lipids. The skeletal muscle also produces various growth factors (IGF-1 and MGF), which have an anabolic effect on the skeleton and also support fracture healing. These "myokines" are above all demonstrably increased by muscle building training. In contrast, during physical inactivity and muscular atrophy, myostatin, a negative regulator of muscle mass, leads to muscle loss. Other factors that lead to a decrease in muscle strength and muscle mass include cachexia, AIDS, smoking, protein and vitamin D deficiency, chronic inflammatory processes (e.g. COPD) and glucocorticoids. In addition to sarcopenia, intramuscular lipid, "myosteatosis" increases with age and increasing body fatness.

The skeletal muscle mass correlates closely with bone mass and the corresponding age-related muscle loss goes hand in hand with bone loss and an increased risk of fracture in old age. In addition the fracture risk is increased by the greater tendency to fall in old age. A targeted muscle training with elderly, hospitalised and immobilised people is most important, regardless of age and gender. On the one hand, muscle building leads to increased bone density and on the other hand to a minimised risk of falling and to a reduced fracture risk.

108.2 Muscle Training and Bone Mass

The positive effect of physical activity on bone mineral density and fracture risk is well documented. In older women, a weekly programme of exercise increases bone density and reduces the tendency to fall as well as the risk of fracture. It should be considered that certain training exercises, such as endurance sports, cycling, continuous running or swimming, can lead to a reduction in bone density. All movements that are directed against the force of gravity, e.g. power sports (weight lifting) and sprint training, are worthwhile. The explanation for this seemingly paradoxical behaviour of the muscles is found in the microscopic structure of the muscles.

R. Bartl, C. Bartl, *Bone Disorders*, DOI 10.1007/978-3-319-29182-6_108

There are *two types of muscle fibres*, which are more or less equally distributed in most people:

- Red muscle fibres (type I, ST): slowly working, fatigue-resistant fibres
- White muscle fibres (type II, FT): fast working with short-term high-power and quickly tiring.

Both types of muscle fibre are active at each training session. Depending on the type of activity, different fibre types are dominant. Thus, the muscles of the sprinter Carl Lewis are supposed to have consisted of up to 90 % white muscle fibres. According to the type of sport, the two types of fibre can be specifically trained and strengthened:

- Light jogging, walking, cycling and swimming train above all the slow muscle fibres, which contributes little to the skeletal system.
- Speed and power training as well as weight lifting strengthen mainly the fast muscle fibres with particularly pronounced benefits for the skeletal system.

Vibration training is an interesting development to strengthen muscles and bones. A platform with vibrations of >32 Hz stimulates, above all, the muscle fibres type IIa and thereby the bone structure. The platform is recommended for immobile elderly people as well as people with Parkinsonism, multiple sclerosis, rheumatism and muscle weakness. Higher frequencies have the advantage that disruptive vibrations of the body are avoided.

Muscle and bone mass are correlated and form a functional unit! Strengthening the muscles is the most important preventive measure for the prevention of osteoporosis! At the same time, improving coordination is another important factor for prevention of fractures. Vibration training to strengthen the muscles is useful for people with restricted mobility.

108.3 Immobilisation Osteoporosis

Insufficient physical activity and thereby muscle loss is one of the most important risk factors for osteoporosis. This applies especially to younger bedridden patients, who, within a few months, can lose bone and muscle mass up to 30 % and then need years to restore the original bone density. If, for example, an arm is immobilised after a fracture in plaster for 3 weeks, the affected bones lose up to 6 % of their density. A study on bedridden patients showed that the trabecular bone decreases by an average of 1 % per week. This is true especially for bedridden children. On the commencement of physical activity, the bone mass regenerates at 1 % per month, so that the recovery of bone mass is considerably slower than the bone loss during immobilisation. Examples of *immobilisation with rapid bone loss* are:

- Paralysis after spinal cord injury
- Hemiplegia after cerebrovascular events
- Paraplegia of the lower half of the body
- Myopathies and polyneuropathies with muscle weakness
- Immobilisation after fractures of the lower extremities in children
- Immobilisation from multiple sclerosis

Paraplegia The bone loss after a spinal cord injury can be so pronounced that the smallest force might cause fractures (e.g. during the transfer to a wheelchair or putting on support stockings). After 1 year, you can already find an osteoporosis in the femur neck of 42 % of paraplegics. The spasticity that occurs in most patients with spinal cord injuries has in comparison to patients with flaccid paralysis a significant positive effect on bone density. An early start to training standing upright together with a passive treadmill exercise has a positive influence on bone mass.

Myopathies and Polyneuropathies with Muscle Weakness An example is myasthenia gravis, an autoimmune disease with episodic muscle weakness, which leads to systemic and local osteoporosis, due to reduced bone load wearing and the commonly used glucocorticoid therapy. Regular monitoring of bone density using DXA method is advisable.

Bed Confinement Patients with osteoporosis, who because of a fracture were bedridden for several weeks, suffer from frequent fractures during the subsequent period of mobilisation. The time of postoperative bed rest should be, through use of new surgical techniques, as short as possible, and the bones should be protected against bone loss by application of effective medication (bisphosphonates).

Loss of Gravity Astronauts must perform a special and regular muscle training due to the absence of gravity in outer space. Nevertheless, they lose about 1 % of their bone mass per month. Under space conditions, astronauts experience a ten times higher bone loss than earthbound patients with osteoporosis. The bone loss in astronauts was examined in detail and today serves as a model for immobilisation osteoporosis.

Three mechanisms were detected under zero gravity conditions, which also play an important role in the emergence of osteoporosis on earth:

- Demineralisation of bone substance
- Inhibition of osteoblast activity
- Activation of osteoclasts

Therapeutically, an increased physical activity, targeted gymnastics and an early functional treatment are recommended. Weight and resistance training methods, such as the Theraband, are beneficial for immobilised patients in bed. While bone loss in children and young people can quickly rebuild, with older adults bone recovery can often take many years. As a rule, the bone density levels at the start of the immobilisation phase are not regained. Dependent on the results of the bone density measurement, preventive medication in the form of an early application of oral *BP* comes into use. A BP therapy must be initiated on the basis of osteoporotic results. As a massive bone loss occurs shortly after the onset of paralysis due to the missing load on those bones, a higher i.v. BP therapy should be considered. Options are:

- Alendronate 70 mg weekly
- Risedronate 35 mg weekly
- Ibandronate 3 mg injection per 3 month
- Zoledronate 5 mg infusion per year

109 Bone and Skin

109.1 Drugs and Vitamins

In dermatology, *glucocorticoids* are frequently required, for short- as well as for long-term treatment. The European and US guidelines have been published, in particular for the prevention of corticosteroid-induced osteoporosis in dermatologic patients. The recommendations include calcium and vitamin D supplements and bisphosphonates when therapy for >3 months is contemplated. Supplements of vitamin A have also been recommended.

As protection against the constant challenges of microbial pathogens, the skin has developed antimicrobial peptides (AMPs) such as the *cathelicidins*, which have antimicrobial activity and stimulate host responses, i.e. inflammations, angiogenesis and cytokine release. It has now been demonstrated that vitamin D is directly involved in the regulation of cathelicidin activities, which could be significant in the treatment of various dermatologic conditions.

Vitamin D analogues have been applied as therapy for the hyperproliferative skin disease psoriasis, as well as other infectious and inflammatory skin disorders. However, it should be borne in mind that the skin itself is an organ for vitamin D synthesis, as well as being a target for its application, in autoimmune, infectious and inflammatory diseases of the skin, and to counteract the effects of glucocorticoids as mentioned above. The skin, in addition to being the site of initiation of vitamin D production, is also a target organ of 1,25(OH_2)D. Keratinocytes possess vitamin D receptors (VDR) and are 1,25(OH_2)D responsive. Vitamin D metabolites have also been shown to protect human skin from UV radiation-induced damage and apoptosis of skin cells. The degree of skin pigmentation (melanin content) also affects vitamin D production in the skin. Thus, melanin reduces the efficiency of previtamin D production in response to sunlight. Similar to melanin, topical sunscreens act as a competitor of the photochemical production of vitamin D_3 by absorbing UV radiation. Age is also a variable that influence the production of vitamin D, since the amount of previtamin D decreases as a consequence of advancing age. Sun safety by use of sunscreen and avoidance of excessive sun exposure to prevent serious skin complication are important. However, moderate sun exposure seems to be safe and efficient in preventing vitamin D deficiency. In addition, however, taking vitamin D supplements (1000–2000 IE vitamin D_3 daily) in addition to moderate sun exposure seems to be prudent. Some investigators have regarded the human skin as "the largest peripheral endocrine organ".

> Several dermatologic disorders have a high incidence of skeletal involvement and bone complications, also published under the term "*SKIBO-Diseases*".

R. Bartl, C. Bartl, *Bone Disorders*, DOI 10.1007/978-3-319-29182-6_109

109.2 Psoriasis and Bone

Psoriasis is one of the most common skin diseases, affecting 1–2 % of the population. Joint symptoms develop about 5 % of the patients, and these may precede the skin lesions by months or years. Three clinical types of psoriatic arthritis can be observed:

- Asymmetric polyarthritis involving the joints of the hand
- Severe erosive lesions in the hands
- Sacroiliitis

Psoriasis is a hyperproliferative disorder of the epidermis, characterised by abnormal keratinocyte differentiation and infiltration of immune cells into the dermis. Therefore, psoriasis responds to treatment with vitamin D administered systemically and/or topically. The antipsoriatic effect is due to the antiproliferative and immunosuppressive properties of the hormone 1,25$(OH)_2$D.

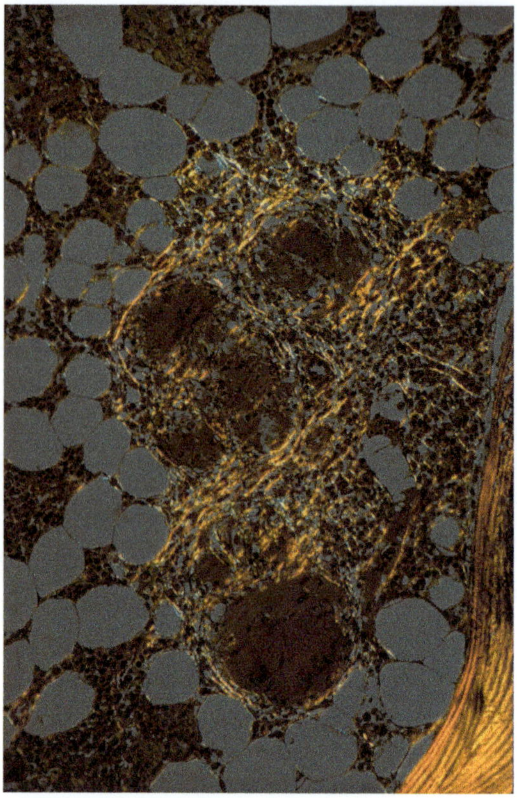

Fig. 109.1 Non-caseating epithelioid cell granulomas in the bone marrow in a patient with sarcoidosis. Gomori staining, polarisation

109.3 Sarcoidosis and Bone

Sarcoidosis is a chronic systemic disorder of unknown aetiology the affects the lymph nodes, lungs, skin and bone. The disease is characterised by the accumulation of non-caseating epithelioid granulomas which distort the normal architecture of the involved organ (Fig. 109.1).

> About 25 % of sarcoidosis patients have joint and bone involvement, and about 30 % of patients with sarcoidosis have characteristic granulomas in their bone marrow biopsies.

Patients with osseous sarcoidosis have skin and pulmonary lesions as well, and therefore the osseous lesions present few diagnostic problems. The hand is the most common location, and the lesions are usually well-defined lytic, sometimes with sclerotic rims. In addition to focal lytic lesions, osseous sarcoidosis may present as systemic osteoporosis or as focal areas of osteosclerosis ("acroosteosclerosis"). Increased osteoclastic bone resorption may cause hypercalcaemia and hypercalciuria in sarcoidosis. It has been shown, that the serum levels of vitamin D metabolites are elevated in hypercalcaemic patients with sarcoidosis, synthesised in the granulomatous tissue.

109.4 Urticaria Pigmentosa and Bone

Urticaria pigmentosa is a term referring to a spectrum of disorders characterised by a proliferation of mast cells in the skin. About 20 % of patients with urticaria pigmentosa have systemic disease in addition to skin lesions. *Systemic mastocytosis* is always accompanied by skeletal lesions, partly osteosclerotic, partly osteolytic, depending on the pattern of spread and topography of the mast cell granulomas (Fig. 109.2). The characteristic histologic lesion in the bone marrow is the mast cell granuloma, which is located in endosteal, perivascular and intertrabecular regions (Fig. 109.3). It consists of variably granulated, mainly spindle-shaped mast cells, together with lymphocytes, plasma cells, eosinophils, sea-blue histiocytes and fibroblasts, all in a framework of fibres and vessels. An immunohistochemical stain for mast cell tryptase can identify the mast cells. Three stages of mast cell infiltration can be distinguished:

- Small solitary granulomas
- Multiple granulomas
- Extensive granulomatous infiltration with fibrosis, replacement of haematopoiesis and increased bone remodelling

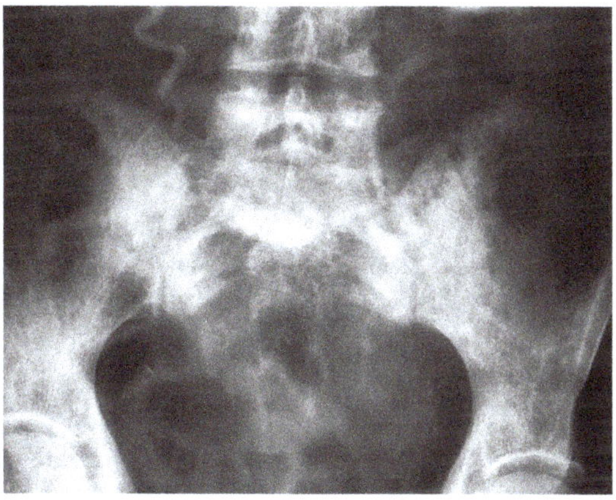

Fig. 109.2 Systemic mastocytosis, with diffuse involvement of the spine and pelvis showing a mixed pattern of osteosclerosis and osteoporosis

Paratrabecular granulomas always induce local osseous reaction: osteolytic, osteosclerotic or mixed.

On X-ray, 70 % of our patients had skeletal lesions: osteopenia in 44 %, multiple osteolysis in 27 % and osteosclerotic lesions in 17 % of the patients.

Moreover, mast cells, because of their ability to produce and secrete heparin and histamines, probably also play a part in the pathogenesis of primary osteoporosis. Local or systemic signs such as urticaria, flushing, nausea and diarrhoea are also caused by the release of these substances.

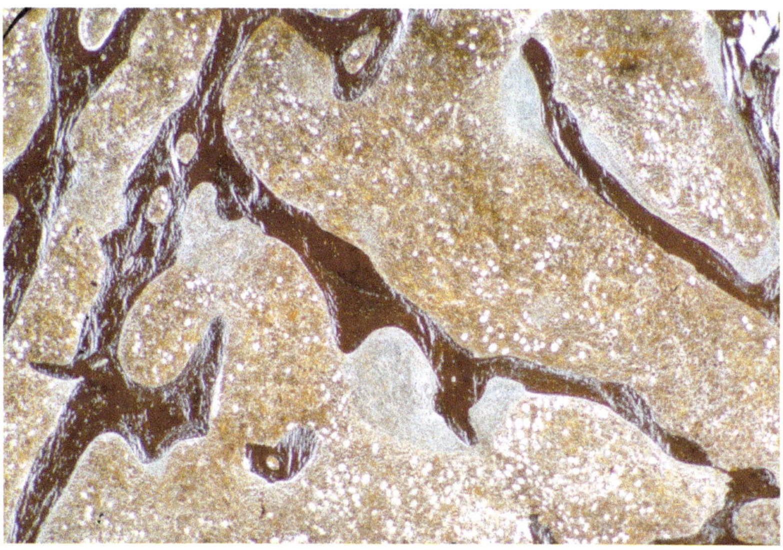

Fig. 109.3 Systemic mastocytosis with multiple paratrabecular mast cell granulomas. Ladewig staining

Systemic mastocytosis, especially during the early or indolent stages, usually requires a bone biopsy for diagnosis.

Biochemical markers have now been tested, and the following three are chosen as probable indicators of systemic mastocytosis: serum tryptase, urinary N(−)methylhistamine and N(−)methylimidazole. However, at this stage, a biopsy is still recommended for confirmation. Vitamin D participates in the regulation of development, differentiation, maturation and function of mast cells. Mast cells play a critical part in various inflammatory disorders, in some neoplasias, and also directly and/or indirectly influence the metabolism of bone cells, as evidenced by the skeletal manifestations which almost invariably accompany mastocytosis. Animal studies have suggested that vitamin D or the more potent analogues could be effective therapeutic agents in disorders of mast cells.

Increases of mast cells in the bone marrow occur in many conditions, characterised by a diffuse or perivascular infiltration of typical mast cell, without evidence of granulomas.

109.5 Systemic Sclerosis and Bone

Systemic sclerosis (SSc) is a chronic systemic disorder of unknown aetiology and is characterised by thickening of the skin (scleroderma) and involvement of multiple internal organs. To investigate the possibility that patients with scleroderma have an increased risk for developing osteoporosis, a survey was carried out with one group of patients suffering from non-inflammatory musculoskeletal disease and another group with rheumatoid arthritis (RA) as controls. The results showed that the patients with SSc and those with RA had the same prevalence of osteoporosis, in addition to which the patients with SSc had a similar or lower BMD, indicating that patients with SSc should be screened for BMD values and treated accordingly. It should be mentioned that many of the clinical manifestations of SSc often go unrecognised indicating that greater awareness is needed. This is also true for the osseous complications, so that the possibility of preventive therapy may be missed. Moreover, the complications themselves, such as cardiovascular, hepatic, thyroid and neurological disorders, may include risk factors for osteoporosis.

110 Bone and Fatty Tissue

110.1 Obesity and Bone Mass

The number of overweight or obese people in the USA (69 %) has reached epidemic proportions. Obesity is a national health problem there and in the meantime also recognised as a problem in Europe. Although obesity correlates with a higher bone mass and bone density, studies have shown that the bone quality in adults and children is inferior and in certain regions of the skeleton higher fracture rates have been observed. Osteoblasts and fat cells (adipocytes) derive from a common mesenchymal stem cells (MSC). Factors that increase adipogenesis typically inhibit the differentiation of osteoblastic cells.

> The characteristic hormone profile, chronically elevated levels of parathyroid hormones, adipokines, low physical activity, changed manner of falling and lifestyles have specific effects on bone quality and fracture risk.

There is also evidence that correlates the decreased bone mass and osteoblastogenesis in old age with an increase of the marrow fat in the bone marrow. In the bone biopsy, it is striking that with increasing age fat cells in the peritrabecular area increase and form a fat cell deposit along the trabecular. Certain antidiabetic drugs such as rosiglitazone increase insulin sensitivity, combined with fat tissue gain, loss of bone mass and increase of the risk of fracture. Glucocorticoids also cause fatty tissue increase (especially visceral fat tissue) at the expense of the osteoblast differentiation. Osteoporosis as well as age-related bone loss go hand in hand with an increase in the proportion of fat in the bone marrow and suggest a modified stromal differentiation from the osteoblast to the adipocyte line. Recent studies have observed that the increase of fat tissue in the bone marrow is accompanied by a lower bone mass.

110.2 Obesity and Risk of Fracture

The "body mass index" (BMI) contributes an important clinical risk factor in the fracture risk estimation model (FRAX®). Obese patients show a higher bone density, but they also show a different distribution of bone mass: the trabecular bone is favoured at the expense of the cortical bone. In this context, the QCT measurement allows a better assessment of the actual situation of the bone than the integral DXA measurement. In addition, obese patients in old age more often show osteoarthritis with calcifications, and thus the actual bone mass can be overestimated in DXA measurement. These changes to the architecture of the bones lead to a higher risk of fracture in certain regions of the skeleton such as the

R. Bartl, C. Bartl, *Bone Disorders*, DOI 10.1007/978-3-319-29182-6_110

humerus and ankle (Fig. 13.1). By contrast, in the area of the hip, vertebrae, forearm and the ankle joint, the fracture risk is lower.

110.3 Weight Loss and Bone Mass

Low body weight and weight loss in old age are associated with a lower bone mass and a higher risk of fracture at the hip. A decrease of body weight by 5 % correlates to an increase in the risk of fracture in the forearm by 33 %. This bone loss can have its cause in a reduced intake of protein, vitamins and calcium, changes of sex hormone levels and less physical exertion.

"Thin women, thin bones". The reason lies in decreased fatty tissue coupled with hormonal disorders and reduced oestrogen production.

111 Bone and Central Nervous System

111.1 Nerval Regulation of Bone and Bone Marrow

Studies in the past decade have demonstrated evidence on the control of bone remodelling and metabolism by the central nervous system (CNS), by neurotransmitters released by bone cells and their stroma and by release of leptin. As shown by semithin sections and immunohistology of bone biopsies, the skeleton is densely innervated by autonomic and sensory nerve fibres (Fig. 111.1). Their main tasks are:

- Regulation of blood flow in the medullary arteries, capillaries and sinusoids
- Regulation of maturation of the haematopoietic cell lineages
- Regulation of the entry of mature blood cells into the circulation
- Regulation of the immune system in the bone marrow
- Regulation of the stromal connective tissue and microenvironment
- Mediators of bone pain and inflammatory processes in the bone marrow
- Regulation of bone remodelling

Bone cells, especially osteoblasts, express receptors for neurotransmitters and neuropeptides such as norepinephrine, acetylcholine and substance. Today, the best characterised brain-to-bone pathway is the sympathetic nervous system (SNS) that mediates and regulates the skeletal effects of leptin and serotonin via a hypothalamic serotonergic relay (Fig. 111.2). Sympathetic nerve terminals form synaptic-like junctions with osteoblasts, which express β2-adrenergic receptors (β2AR). These receptors are activated by norepinephrine released from the sympathetic nerve endings, thus suppressing bone formation and stimulating RANKL expression resulting in increased osteoclastic bone resorption. The sympathetic tone is downregulated by brainstem-derived serotonin.

111.2 The Role of Leptin in Regulation of Bone

The observation that overweight individuals are less susceptible to osteoporosis implies a possible connection between obesity and the skeleton. It was first suggested that the effects of increased weight-bearing might protect bone mass. However, experimental studies have implicated leptin: a hormone produced by fat cells and which interacts with neurons in the brain and thereby influences weight. It was then discovered that in mice leptin is also antiosteogenic, and it was speculated that increased bone mass in obese people may result from resistance to leptin's anti-osteogenic activity.

R. Bartl, C. Bartl, *Bone Disorders*, DOI 10.1007/978-3-319-29182-6_111

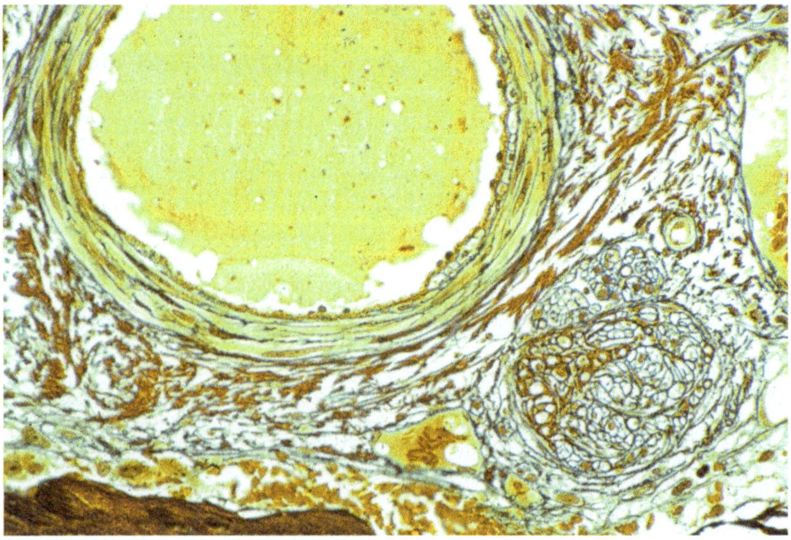

Fig. 111.1 Large blood vessel accompanied by nerve (*lower right*). Gomori staining

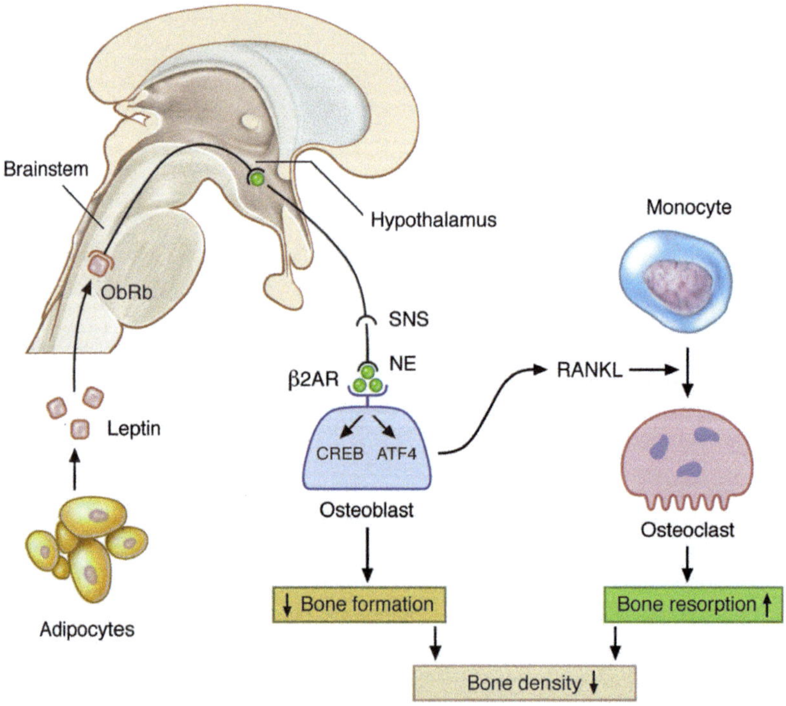

Fig. 111.2 Bone remodelling under the control of the brain stem and hypothalamic serotonergic neurons. Sympathetic nerve signals activate bone resorption and inhibits bone formation (Modified from F. Elefteriou and G. Karsenty. *Primer on the metabolic bone disorders and disorders of mineral metabolism*, 2013)

Leptin is a peptide hormone that is synthesised by fat cells (adipocytes). It stimulates activity of the sympathetic nervous system, causing a decrease in bone mass through an adrenergic receptor in osteoblasts.

The amount of leptin released into the bloodstream is proportional to the amount of body fat. Leptin regulates the body's energy balance as well as the bone mass by binding to certain receptor proteins of specific neurons in the hypothalamus, and these in turn activate sympathetic nerves. The nerves extend into the bones, where they stimulate release of the neurotransmitter noradrenaline, which then activates beta-2-adrenergic receptors on osteoblasts, inhibiting osteoblastic activity. Leptin thus prevents bone formation through its action on already differentiated osteoblasts; it has no overt effect on osteoclast differentiation or function. These results seem to suggest that the millions of patients who have been treated with "beta-blockers" such as propranolol for hypertension should have increased bone mass – an argument for reassessing these clinical studies with respect to changes in bone density. Extreme changes in body weight and bone mass are also partly mediated by leptin, as well as the sex hormones. The identification of leptin as a powerful inhibitor of bone formation definitely has potential therapeutic implications in the future.

To summarise briefly: Leptin has a circadian pattern of secretion with peak levels at midnight; it reflects total-body adipose tissue mass. Many effects of leptin on energy metabolism are mediated by interaction with insulin. Leptin impacts skeletal metabolism, and it is also involved in pathological conditions such as obesity, atherosclerosis, oxidative stress and malignancies. Other neuropeptides such as neuromedin U are also involved in control of bone remodelling, as are the endocannabinoids, synthesised by both osteoclasts and osteoblasts. Receptors for these substances are present in the sympathetic nerve terminals located near the bone cells and constitute a signalling pathway between brain and bone. The endocannabinoid receptors are also involved in the regulation of bone mass, and osteoclast function, as for example, enhancement of bone loss in ovariectomised animals. The endocannabinoids are involved in food intake and energy metabolism. These systems influence pathways from insulin signalling in the pancreas to oxidative processes in skeletal muscles. In summary, it should be stressed that the skeleton is equipped with numerous nerve fibres which participate in the regulation of skeletal metabolism by the CNS. More than ten neuropeptides have already been identified in bone, including substance P (SP). Receptors for SP are located on osteoclasts and SP stimulates resorption.

111.3 Neuropsychiatric Diseases with Changes in Bone Mass

Neuropsychiatric disorders are mental disorders caused by nervous system pathology, mainly brain pathology. It is now well established that some of these disorders, mainly depressive disorders, anorexia nervosa and traumatic brain injury, are associated with bone loss and bone marrow changes (e.g. bone marrow oedema). Recent studies have shown that also schizophrenia and Alzheimer's disease are accompanied by bone loss.

State of depression: Depression by itself is most probably not a main cause of secondary osteoporosis, but the accompanying circumstances are. Studies have shown that women with severe long-standing depression have 6% less bone mass than matched controls without depression. The main contributory factors linking depression, low BMD and fracture risk are:

- High levels of stress hormones
- Low levels of gonadal steroids
- Various antidepressant drugs
- Lack of appetite and inadequate nutrition
- Increased alcohol abuse
- Comorbid medical conditions
- Reduced physical activity

- Lack of motivation
- Alterations in serotonergic and adrenergic transmission of central systems

Anorexia nervosa is an eating disorder triggered by an overwhelming fear of weight gain. It affects young women and disrupts the menstrual cycle, lowers oestrogen levels, lowers muscle mass and so inhibits a normal peak bone mass. As many as 50 % of patients with anorexia nervosa have low bone density in their lower spine (osteoporosis) and increased bone resorption. Patients with anorexia nervosa have the highest mortality rate of all psychiatric disorders. The only possibility to improve the skeletal changes is rescue of weight loss and menstrual function.

112 Bone and Immune System

112.1 Osteoimmunology

For many years, it was known that osteoblasts regulate the differentiation of the osteoclast precursors (OPG) and the activation of osteoclasts (OC). It was also recognised that inflammatory and infectious diseases affect the skeleton by means of inflammatory cytokines and produce localised bone lesions or generalised osteoporosis. However, the molecular mechanisms and the connection between the immune cells and bone cells that produce bone destruction were unknown. It has now been well established that osteoclasts are derived from the haematopoietic stem cells that also give rise to immune cells. In the 1980s, it was shown that the RANK/RANKL/OPG system plays a crucial role in the osteoclastogenesis. It was also demonstrated that calcitonin and some inflammatory mediators such as PGE2 and interferon-γ inhibit the osteoclastic bone resorption. Osteoclasts are positively regulated by TRANCE-TRANCE-R signalling and negatively by OPG. Studies show that activated T-cells my induce osteoclastogenesis through expression of TRANCE (TNF-related activation cytokine, a member of the TNF family) (Fig. 112.1). But activated T-cells can also produce interferon-γ and via this pathway suppress osteoclastic activity. This suggests that activated T-cells may both positively and negatively regulate osteoclastic bone resorption. This balance may be influenced by local and systemic factors, including infections, nutrition, metabolism, mechanical factors, hormones and cytokines (TNFs and interleukins).

> Since the discovery of the RANKL system, many other factors and mechanisms are known that regulate the interactions between immune cells, mesenchymal stem cells (MSCs) and haematopoietic stem cells (HSCs) under normal and pathological conditions. The bone tissue is not only controlled and regulated by the central nervous system, but also by the immune system.

Again the RANKL system is the crucial link in the function between immune and bone cells. B- and T-lymphocytes may also express RANKL, cooperate with the osteoblasts in order to stimulate osteoclasts and produce inflammatory cytokines such as tumour necrosis factor (TNF), interleukin-1 (IL-1) and interleukin-6 (IL-6). TNF especially directly activates the differentiation and activity of the osteoclasts. Correspondingly, TNF-blocking biologicals increase bone mass in many inflammatory diseases, including rheumatoid arthritis, ankylosing spondylitis and Crohn's disease. Furthermore, IL-17 and Th17 T-cells activate osteoclastic bone resorption, together with stromal cells and osteoblasts. T-cells produce growth factors for bone

R. Bartl, C. Bartl, *Bone Disorders*, DOI 10.1007/978-3-319-29182-6_112

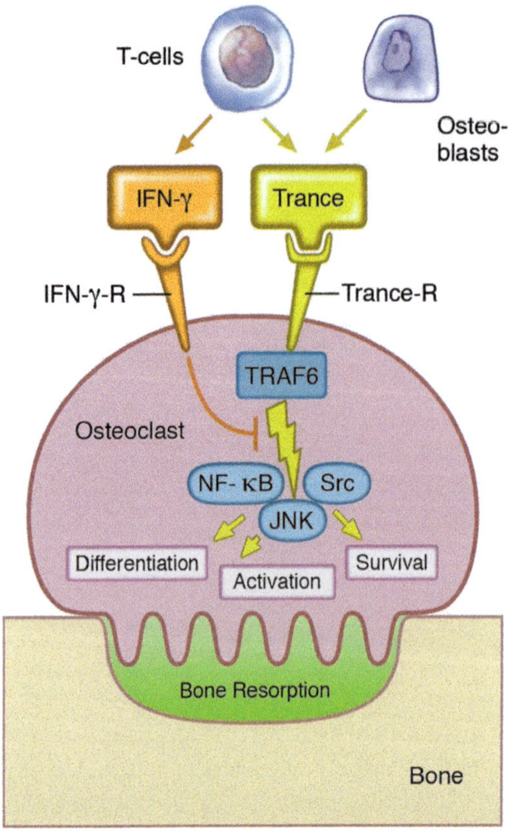

Fig. 112.1 Complex role of activated T-cells and osteoblasts in osteoclastic activation (Modified from Rho et al. *Mol. Cells.* **17**:1–9 2004)

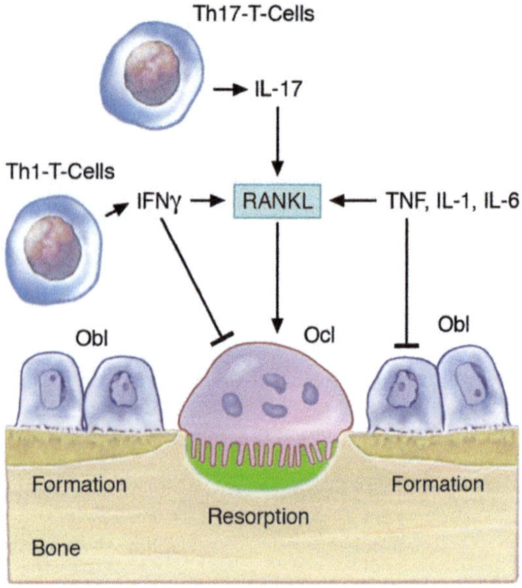

Fig. 112.2 T-lymphocytes and cytokine network regulating osteoclastic bone resorption and triggering bone loss in autoimmune disorders

formation. B-cells are also an important source for RANKL and play an important role in the pathogenesis of postmenopausal osteoporosis (Fig. 112.2).

> Inflammation is known to increase osteoclastic activity. T-cell-derived TRANCE plays a central role in inflammatory bone loss.

112.2 Osteomyelitis and the Immune System

Many inflammatory processes affect the skeleton and may produce a localised or a generalised bone resorption.

> Inflammatory cells and cytokine network in inflammatory bone loss:
>
> *Inflammatory cells:* T-cells (Th1, Th2, Th17), B-cell, macrophage, osteoclast, monocyte, dendritic cell, fibroblast, endothelial cell
>
> *Cytokines:* IL1, IL6, IL17, IL21, IL33, TNF-α

Common examples include acute and chronic bacterial osteomyelitis and rheumatoid arthritis (RA). In RA, above all, a group of T-cells (Th and Treg cells), B-cells, plasma cells and macrophages play an important role and are found in the synovial fluid of the affected joints. Inflamed synoviocytes and activated T-cells secrete RANKL and cause the inflammation-associated bone destruction in RA. Plasma cells secrete antibodies in chronic inflammation and may also produce autoantibodies in autoimmune diseases.

> There are close interactions between immune cells, osteoblasts and osteoclasts that influence bone mass in inflammatory disorders. Further study of osteoimmunology will lead to the development of new drugs to treat disorders that affect both the bone and the immune system.

In inflammatory disorders of other organs, various cell types can produce RANKL and cause systemic bone loss. For example, RANKL is expressed from cells of the gastrointestinal tract, from cells of atherosclerotic plaques in the arteries as a result of cardiovascular disorder and from cells of bone metastases (Fig. 112.3).

> Summarising, T-cells play a major role in osteoclastic differentiation, activation and survival through signalling cross-talk between IFNs and TRANCE in bone remodelling.

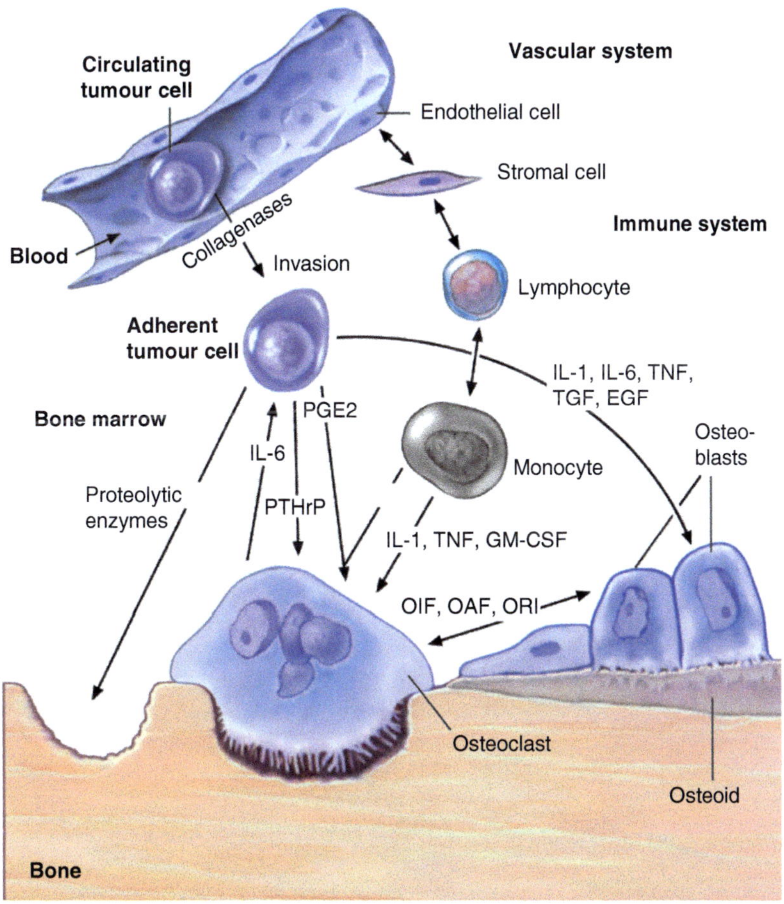

Fig. 112.3 Demonstration of interactions between the immune system and tumour cells, blood vessels, bone, bone marrow and stroma

113 Bone and Teeth

113.1 Oral Bone Mass in Old Age

The bone structure of the upper and lower jaw resembles that of the total skeleton. It is therefore assumed that these skeletal components are subject to a similar ageing process of bone loss, thus reduction of the trabecular bone, thinning of the cortical bone and increased porosity. Since the 1960s, it has also been known that the upper and lower jaws are subject to age-related atrophy of the bone. An additional regression of bone mass is observed in the form of tooth loss (Fig. 16.1). Absorptiometric studies have shown that oral bone mass also correlates significantly with the entire calcium mass of the body and with the bone density of the forearm and vertebrae.

> The loss of the alveolar bone is part of the osteoporotic syndrome.

Direct measurements of the bone density of the lower jaw using DXA or CT show that the mandibular bone mass decreases annually in older women by 1.5 % and in older men by 0.9 % and correlates well with the bone density values in the region of the forearm.

113.2 Tooth Loss and Osteoporosis

The relationship between tooth loss and osteoporosis is more difficult to provide, as many other causal factors should also be considered. Nevertheless, most studies have shown that a lower bone density correlates with a lower number of teeth. Tooth loss was more common in patients with osteoporosis. Other studies have shown that tooth loss correlates strikingly with significantly lower mandibular and vertebral bone mass, as well as the incidence of vertebral fractures. The concept to be able to assess the extent of generalised bone loss according to the criteria of dental health has, in practice, proved unreliable, as it is not clear what criteria can be categorised as reliable. The prediction of fracture risk through tooth loss proved to be too unreliable, because too many other causes are taken into account.

113.3 Osteoporosis Therapy and Oral Bone Health

Several smaller studies have shown the positive effect of *vitamin D* on the health of the dental apparatus. Thus, patients who had one year of calcium and vitamin D supplements had

R. Bartl, C. Bartl, *Bone Disorders*, DOI 10.1007/978-3-319-29182-6_113

significantly healthier teeth compared to patients without supplements. *Oestrogen deficiency* also correlated with a lower density of the alveolar bones.

Accordingly, oestrogen replacement has a positive effect on oral as well as systemic bone health. Modern bisphosphonates (BP) – potent inhibitors of bone resorption – should in theory protect against both systemic and alveolar bone loss, as both processes are fundamentally similar. Studies with oral and local application of alendronate show an increase of oral bone mass and a positive effect on the teeth. The inhibiting effect of BP on collagenases (metalloproteinases) was shown, in smaller studies, to be successful for the treatment of *periodontitis* (periodontal disease).

A recent study in *JAMA* has, for the first time, shown a direct connection between periodontal disease and atherosclerosis. With successful treatment of the dental disease, the calcification of the arteries was slowed down for three years. This observation which shows the distribution of locally secreted inflammatory mediators into the bloodstream is comparable to the situation in rheumatoid arthritis.

But these positive effects on dental health are overshadowed by the well-known associations of BP and jaw necrosis, which are discussed elsewhere in the book. This serious complication is observed almost exclusively with certain BP, when administered as long-term or high-dose treatment of infection-prone tumour patients (especially multiple myeloma and metastatic breast cancer). In our practice, no jaw necrosis was observed in the treatment of osteoporosis, with much lower doses of BP and with careful exclusion of risk factors.

113.4 Other Osteopathies and Oral Bone Health

Up to 17 % of patients with *Paget's* disease show an infestation of the lower and upper jaw. Expansions of the facial skeleton, hypercementosis of the tooth roots and tooth ankylosis and on the other hand tooth loss in the osteolytic phase are typical changes of the oral bone. There is little information about the effect of a systemic BP therapy for Paget's disease with oral localisation. A case description of a 6-month therapy with alendronate could show no negative influence on dental implants in a patient with Paget's disease. Some manifestations in the oral bone area have also been described in the case of *primary hyperparathyroidism* and the *renal osteodystrophy*: loss of the lamina dura, bone loss with subperiosteal bone resorption in the area of the alveolar bone up to a "brown tumour" in an advanced stage.

Literature

The most relevant and useful books and reviews are given at the end of the text. The books listed contain comprehensive summaries and reviews of the different aspects of bone disorders published during the past 10 years or so. They also contain extensive and exhaustive reference lists.

In addition to the other books recently published (not listed here), an astronomical number of articles on all aspects of bone disorders, has appeared in the international literature. These are readily available through the internet. For example the key words "disorders of bone" yielded over 200,000 citations!

1. Avioli, L., Krane, S.: Metabolic Bone Disease and Clinically Related Disorders. Academic, San Diego (1997)
2. Barlow, D., Francis, R., Miles, A.: The Effective Management of Osteoporosis. Aesculapius Medical Press, London/San Francisco/Sydney (2001)
3. Bartl, R.: Klinische Osteologie. Thieme Verlag, Stuttgart (2014)
4. Bartl, R., Frisch, B., von Tresckow, E., Bartl, C.: Bisphosphonates in Medical Practice. Springer, Heidelberg (2007)
5. Bartl, R., Frisch, B.: Biopsy of Bone in Internal Medicine – An Atlas and Sourcebook. Kluwer Academic Publishers, Boston/London/Dordrecht (1993)
6. Bartl, R., Frisch, B.: Bisphosphonates for Bones: Guidelines for Treatment in All Medical Disciplines. Blackwell, Berlin (2002)
7. Bartl, R., Frisch, B.: Osteoporosis, Prevention, Diagnosis, Therapy, 2nd edn. Springer, Heidelberg (2009)
8. Baur-Melnyk, A.: Magnetic Resonance Imaging of the Bone Marrow. Springer, Heidelberg (2013)
9. Bilezikian, J., Raisz, L., Rodan, G.: Principles of Bone Biology. Academic, San Diego (1996)
10. Browner, B., Jupiter, J., Lewine, A., Trafton, P., Krettek, C.: Skeletal Trauma. Basic Science, Management, and Reconstruction, 4th edn. Elsevier, Philadelphia (2009)
11. Bucholz, R., Heckman, J., Court-Brown, C., Tornetta, P.: Rockwood and Green's Fractures in Adults, 7th edn. Wolters Kluwer, Philadelphia (2010)
12. Campbell, G., Compston, J., Crisp, A.: The Management of Common Metabolic Bone Disorders. Cambridge University Press, Cambridge (1993)
13. Clunie, G., Keen, R.: Osteoporosis. Oxford University Press, Oxford (2008)
14. Cooper, C., Woolf, A.: Osteoporosis: Best Practice & Research Compendium. Elsevier, Edinburgh (2006)
15. Cummings, S., Cosman, F., Jamal, S.: Osteoporosis: An Evidence-Based Guide to Prevention and Therapy. American College of Physicians, Philadelphia (2002)
16. Davies, A., Sundaram, M., James, S.: Imaging of Bone Tumors and Tumor-Like Lesions. Springer, Heidelberg (2009)

R. Bartl, C. Bartl, *Bone Disorders*, DOI 10.1007/978-3-319-29182-6

17. Duque, G., Kiel, D. (eds.): Osteoporosis in Older Persons. Springer, London (2008)
18. Eastell, R., Baumann, M., Hoyle, N., Wieczorek, L. (eds.): Bone Markers, Biochemical and Clinical Perspectives. Martin Dunitz, London (2001)
19. Favus, M.J. (ed.): Primer on the Metabolic Bone Diseases and Disorders of Mineral Metabolism. Lippincott, Philadelphia (1999)
20. Fleisch, H.: Bisphosphonates in Bone Disease, 4th edn. Academic, San Diego (2000)
21. Freyschmidt, J., Freyschmidt, G.: SKIBO-Diseases: Disorders Affecting the Skin and Bones. Springer, Heidelberg (1999)
22. Frisch, B., Bartl, R.: Biopsy Interpretation of Bone and Bone Marrow. Arnold, London (1998)
23. Geusens, P. (ed.): Osteoporosis in Clinical Practice. Springer, Heidelberg (2004)
24. Goldman, L., Schafer, A.: Goldman's Cecil Medicine, 24th edn. Elsevier, Philadelphia (2012)
25. Grampp, S.: Radiology of Osteoporosis. Springer, Heidelberg (2003)
26. Gueldner, S., Grabo, T., Newman, E., Cooper, D.: Osteoporosis, Clinical Guidelines for Prevention, Diagnosis, and Management. Springer Publishing Company, New York (2008)
27. Henderson, J.E., Goltzman, D. (eds.): The Osteoporosis Primer. Cambridge University Press, Cambridge (2000)
28. Heuck, F.: Allgemeine Radiologie und Morphologie der Knochenkrankheiten. In: Diethelm, L. (ed.) Diseases oft the Skeletal System (Roentgen Diagnosis) Part 1, pp. 3–267. Springer, Berlin/Heidelberg/New York (1976)
29. Heuck, A.: Radiologie der Knochen- und Gelenkerkrankungen. Thieme, Stuttgart (1997)
30. Hodgson, S.: Mayo Clinic on Osteoporosis. Mayo Clinic, Rochester (2003)
31. Hochberg, M., Silman, A., Smolen, J., Weinblatt, M., Weisman, M. (eds.): Rheumatology, 4th edn. Mosby Elsevier, Philadelphia (2007)
32. Hosking, D., Ringe, J.: Treatment of Metabolic Bone Disease – Management Strategy and Drug Therapy. Martin Dunitz, London (2000)
33. Jaffe, H.: Metabolic, Degenerative, and Inflammatory Diseases of Bones and Joints. Lea & Febiger, Philadelphia (1972)
34. Järvinen, T., et al.: Osteoporosis: The Emperor Has No Clothes. Key Symposium. J. Intern. Med. **277**, 662–673 (2015)
35. Kleerekoper, M., Siris, E., McClung, M. (eds.): The Bone and Mineral Manual. Academic, London (1999)
36. Kleerekoper, M.: Drug Therapy for Osteoporosis. Taylor & Francis, London (2005)
37. Khurana, J., McCarthy, E., Zhang, P.: Essentials in Bone and Soft-Tissue pathology. Springer, New York (2010)
38. Kuhlencordt, F., Bartelheimer, H.: Klinische Osteologie A und B, Handbuch der Inneren Medizin, Band 6. Springer, Berlin/Heidelberg/New York (1980)
39. Lanham-New, S., O'Neill, T., Morris, R., et al.: Managing Osteoporosis. Clinical Publishing, Oxford (2007)
40. Marcus, R., Feldman, D., Nelson, D., Rosen, C. (eds.): Fundamentals of Osteoporosis. Academic, San Diego (2010)
41. Marcus, R., Feldman, D., Nelson, D., Rosen, C. (eds.): Osteoporosis. Academic, San Diego (2008)
42. Marcus, R.: Osteoporosis. Academic, San Diego (2008)
43. Martin, B., Burr, D., Sharkey, N. (eds.): Skeletal Tissue Mechanics. Springer, New York (1998)
44. Martin, B., Burr, D., Sharkey, N.: Skeletal Tissue Mechanics. Springer, New York (1998)
45. McCarthy, E.: Pathology of Bone and Joint Disorders, with Clinical and Radiographic Correlation, 2nd edn. Cambridge University Press, Cambridge (2015)
46. McDermott, M., Zapalowski, C., Miller, P. (eds.): Osteoporosis. Hanley & Belfus, St. Louis (2004)
47. McIlwain, H., Bruce, D.: The Osteoporosis Cure. Avon Books, New York (1999)

48. Meunier, P.J.: Osteoporosis: Diagnosis and Management. Martin Dunitz, London (1998)
49. Mundy, G.: Bone Remodelling and Its Disorders, 2nd edn. Martin Dunitz, London (1999)
50. Notelovitz, M.: Osteoporosis: Prevention, Diagnosis and Management. Professional Communications, Caddo (1999)
51. Orwoll, E. (ed.): Atlas of Osteoporosis, 3rd edn. Springer, Philadelphia (2009)
52. Orwoll, E. (ed.): Osteoporosis in Men. Academic, San Diego (1999)
53. Otto, S.: Medication-Related Osteonecrosis of the Jaws. Springer, Heidelberg (2015)
54. Reid, I.R.: Efficacy, Effectiveness and Side Effects of Medications Used to Prevent Fractures. Key Symposium. J. Intern. Med. **277**, 690–706 (2014)
55. Remagen, W., Morscher, E., Rösli, A.: Primäre und sekundäre Tumoren der Knochen und Gelenke. In: Kuhlencordt, F., Bartelheimer, H. (eds.) Klinische Osteologie A und B, Handbuch der Inneren Medizin, Band 6, pp. 1317–1475. Springer, Berlin/Heidelberg/New York (1980)
56. Rosen, C. (ed.): Primer on the Metabolic Bone Diseases and Disorders of Mineral Metabolism, 8th edn. Wiley-Blackwell, Ames (2013)
57. Rubens, R., Mundy, G. (eds.): Cancer and the Skeleton. Martin Dunitz, London (2000)
58. Schajowicz, F.: Tumors and Tumor-like Lesions of Bone, 2nd edn. Springer, Berlin (1994)
59. Stovall, D. (ed.): Osteoporosis, Diagnosis and Management. Wiley Blackwell, Chichester (2013)
60. Wolff, J.: The Law of Bone Remodelling. Springer, Heidelberg (1986)
61. Woolf, A., Akesson, K.: Osteoporosis. An Atlas of Investigation and Management. Clinical Publishing, Oxford (2008)

Added Literature

62. Bartl, C., Stengel, D., Bruckner, T., Gebhard, F., and the ORCHID Study Group: The treatment of displaced intra-articular distal radius fractures in elderly patients. Dtsch Arztebl Int. **111**, (46): 779–787 (2014)
63. Black, D.M., Rosen, C.J.: Clinical practice. Postmenopausal osteoporosis. N Engl J Med. **374**, (3): 254–262 (2016)
64. Abrahamsen, B., Eiken, P., Prieto-Alhambra, D., Eastell, R.: Risk of hip, subtrochanteric, and femoral shaft fractures among mid and long term users of alendronate: nationwide cohort and nested case-control study. BMJ. **353**, 3365–3376 (2016)

Index

R. Bartl, C. Bartl, *Bone Disorders*, DOI 10.1007/978-3-319-29182-6

Administration is requesting $151.3 million in new funding across the Federal government to strengthen efforts to detect, and prevent and treat illicit drug use in our communities and break the cycle of illicit drug use, crime, and incarceration.

In: U.S. National Drug Control Strategy
Editor: Benjamin F. Turner
ISBN: 978-1-61470-629-8

Chapter 1

REAUTHORIZING THE OFFICE OF NATIONAL DRUG CONTROL POLICY: ISSUES FOR CONSIDERATION*

Kristin M. Finklea

SUMMARY

The Office of National Drug Control Policy (ONDCP) has the responsibility for creating policies, priorities, and objectives for the federal Drug Control Program. This national program is aimed at reducing the use, manufacturing, and trafficking of illicit drugs and the reduction of drug-related crime and violence and of drug-related health consequences. The Director of ONDCP has primary responsibilities of (1) developing a comprehensive National Drug Control Strategy (Strategy) to direct the nation's anti-drug efforts; (2) developing a National Drug Control Budget (Budget) to implement the National Drug Control Strategy, including determining the adequacy of the drug control budgets submitted by contributing Drug Control Program agencies; and (3) evaluating the effectiveness of the National Drug Control Strategy implementation by the various agencies contributing to the Drug Control Program. Authorization for ONDCP expired at the end of FY2010, but it has continued to receive appropriations. Congress, while continuously charged with ONDCP's oversight, is now faced with its possible reauthorization.

In May 2009, Director R. Gil Kerlikowske called for an end to use of the term "war on drugs." This is in part because while drug use was previously considered a law enforcement or criminal justice problem, it has transitioned to being viewed more as a public health problem. Indeed, the Obama Administration has indicated that a comprehensive strategy should include a range of prevention, treatment, and law enforcement elements. The 2010 National Drug Control Strategy outlines seven specific objectives—ranging from reducing the prevalence of youth engaged in illegal drug use to reducing the number of drug-related deaths—aimed at reducing both illicit drug use and its consequences.

---

* This is an edited, reformatted and augmented version of a Congressional Research Service publication, CRS Report for Congress R41535, from www.crs.gov, dated December 10, 2010.

In creating the National Drug Control Strategy, ONDCP consults with the various federal Drug Control Program agencies. ONDCP then reviews their respective drug budgets and incorporates them into the National Drug Control Budget, which is submitted to Congress as part of the annual appropriations process. In the FY2011 Budget, there are five priorities for which resources are requested across agencies: substance abuse prevention and substance abuse treatment (both of which are considered demand-reduction areas), and drug interdiction, domestic law enforcement, and international partnerships (the three of which are considered supply-reduction areas). The FY2011 request proposes to use 64.0% of the funds ($9.952 billion) for supply-side functions and 36.0% of the funds ($5.600 billion) for demand-side functions. There is currently a continuing resolution (P.L. 111-290) funding federal drug control activities at the FY2010 enacted level of almost $15.032 billion.

In considering ONDCP's reauthorization, there are several issues that policymakers may deliberate. Congress may consider whether to authorize specific supply-reduction or demand-reduction programs. Congress may also exercise oversight regarding ONDCP's implementation of evidenced-based activities. Another issue up for debate is whether the Budget captures the full scope of the nation's anti-drug activities. Further, ONDCP is creating a new Performance Reporting System (PRS) to evaluate annual progress toward each of the Drug Control Program's strategic goals. Congress may exercise oversight regarding the new PRS.

INTRODUCTION

The Office of National Drug Control Policy (ONDCP) has the responsibility for creating policies, priorities, and objectives for the federal Drug Control Program. This national program is aimed at reducing the use, manufacturing, and trafficking of illicit drugs and the reduction of drug-related crime and violence and of drug-related health consequences.[1] ONDCP is located in the Executive Office of the President. It was initially created by the Anti-Drug Abuse Act of 1988[2] and most recently reauthorized in the Office of National Drug Control Policy Reauthorization Act of 2006.[3] ONDCP was authorized to receive "such sums as may be necessary for each of fiscal years 2006 through 2010."[4] Authorization for ONDCP expired at the end of FY2010, but it has continued to receive appropriations. Congress, while continuously charged with ONDCP's oversight, is now faced with its possible reauthorization.

The Director of ONDCP, often referred to as the "Drug Czar," has numerous responsibilities, of which the primary three are

- developing a comprehensive National Drug Control Strategy to direct the nation's anti-drug efforts;
- developing a National Drug Control Budget to implement the National Drug Control Strategy, including determining the adequacy of the drug control budgets submitted by contributing Drug Control Program agencies (listed below); and
- evaluating the effectiveness of the National Drug Control Strategy implementation by the various agencies contributing to the Drug Control Program.[5]

In carrying out these responsibilities, Director R. Gil Kerlikowske has put an end to the use of the term "war on drugs"[6] and has stated that the Obama Administration views a

comprehensive drug control strategy as including a range of prevention, treatment, and law enforcement elements.[7] The Director is reported to favor a more balanced strategy[8] that shifts more resources toward treatment and further away from enforcement and incarceration—where the vast majority of federal efforts have been focused to date—as a means to control the United States' drug issues. And the American public does indeed view these issues as a significant challenge facing the nation. According to a 2009 Gallup survey, 35% of survey participants indicated that drug problems pose an "extremely serious" problem for the United States. Thirty-three percent indicated that drugs were a "very serious" problem, and 26% found them to be a "moderately serious" problem.[9]

This report provides a discussion of the National Drug Control Strategy, the National Drug Control Budget, and ONDCP's evaluation of the National Drug Control Strategy implementation. It then provides an analysis of selected legislative and oversight issues that Congress may consider when debating the reauthorization of ONDCP. Policymakers may question the status of the war on drugs, whether drug use should be seen as more of a law enforcement issue or a public health issue, and whether drug control resources are more effective when directed toward prevention and treatment or toward law enforcement. Another issue for consideration is whether the National Drug Control Budget—as currently conceived—represents a comprehensive view of federal drug control activities in the United States. Further, Congress may exercise oversight over ONDCP's means of evaluating the nation's federal drug control programs.

NATIONAL DRUG CONTROL STRATEGY

Congress has specified that the purpose of the National Drug Control Strategy (Strategy) is to outline a plan to reduce (1) illicit drug consumption in the United States and (2) the consequences of such use.[10] In creating the Strategy, ONDCP consults with the 34 contributing federal Drug Control Program agencies as well as Congress; state, local, and tribal officials; foreign government representatives; and private sector representatives with expertise in both supply and demand reduction.

In the 2010 Strategy, ONDCP outlines seven specific objectives—to be accomplished by 2015— aimed at reducing both illicit drug use and its consequences.[11] These objectives include reducing the following:

- The prevalence of 12–17 year olds who report having used any illicit drugs in the past 30 days (by 15%). According to the 2009 National Survey on Drug Use and Health (NSDUH),[12] 10.0% of youth in this age range report being "current" (in the past month) users of illicit drugs.[13]
- The prevalence of 8th graders who report having used any alcohol, tobacco, or illicit drugs in their lifetimes (by 15%). According to the 2009 Monitoring the Future (MTF) study,[14] 19.9% of 8th graders report having used some form of illicit drug in their lifetimes.[15]
- The prevalence of 18–25 year olds who report having used any illicit drugs in the past 30 days (by 10%). In 2009, 21.2% of adults in this age range reported being current illicit drug users.[16]

- The number of chronic drug users (by 15%). For instance, the 2009 NSDUH suggests that about 4 million individuals used marijuana on a daily or near-daily basis in the previous year.[17]
- The number of drug-induced deaths (by 15%). In 2007, there were a reported 38,371 drug-induced deaths in the United States.[18]
- Drug-related morbidity (by 15%). In 2008, the rate (per 100,000) of drug-related emergency department visits was estimated at 326.7.[19]
- The prevalence of drugged driving (by 10%). In 2009, an estimated 4.2% of the 12-and-older population drove under the influence of an illicit drug.[20]

In order to attain these goals, the Strategy proposes initiatives to bolster community-based drug prevention efforts; expand health care opportunities, both for early drug and substance abuse intervention as well as for treatment and recovery; improve the handling of substance abuse within the criminal justice systems; disrupt domestic drug production and trafficking; strengthen international law enforcement, intelligence, and civic partnerships; and enhance the use of science to inform program evaluation and policymaking.

National Drug Control Budget

In creating the National Drug Control Strategy, ONDCP consults with the various federal Drug Control Program agencies; ONDCP then reviews their respective drug budgets and incorporates them into the National Drug Control Budget (Budget), which is submitted to Congress as part of the annual appropriations process. ONDCP has acknowledged that it is difficult to get a full picture of federal resources allocated to drug control. This is, in part, because the activities of many contributing agencies are multi-faceted, and it is difficult to determine precisely what portion of their resources are dedicated to drug control and related activities.[21]

Another factor that presents a challenge in determining the full scope of federal drug control resources is the disparity between those agencies contributing to the Strategy and those included in the Budget. Of note, while ONDCP consults with 34 National Drug Control Program agencies to create the *Strategy,* not all of these agencies are included in the *Budget.* Under the current Budget formulization, only those agencies whose missions directly support the Strategy are included in the Budget. Those agencies "whose primary mission does not include drug control, nor have readily identifiable drug control line items" are not currently included in the Budget.[22] For instance, the Drug Enforcement Administration (DEA)—whose primary mission includes enforcing the federal controlled substance laws and regulations—is included in the Budget. However, the U.S. Attorneys—whose primary mission includes prosecuting *all* criminal cases brought by the federal government, not only drug-related cases—is not included in the Budget.

Federal departments, agencies, and programs receiving funding directly under the National Drug Control Budget currently include

- Department of Defense
- Department of Education

- Department of Health and Human Services
    - Centers for Medicare and Medicaid Services
    - Substance Abuse and Mental Health Services Administration
    - National Institutes of Health—National Institute on Drug Abuse
    - Indian Health Service
- Department of Homeland Security
    - U.S. Customs and Border Protection
    - U.S. Immigration and Customs Enforcement
    - U.S. Coast Guard
    - Office of Counternarcotics Enforcement
- Department of the Interior
    - Bureau of Indian Affairs
- Department of Justice
    - Federal Bureau of Prisons
    - U.S. Drug Enforcement Administration
    - Organized Crime Drug Enforcement Task Force Program
    - Office of Justice Programs
    - National Drug Intelligence Center
- Office of National Drug Control Policy
    - Counterdrug Technology Assessment Center
    - High Intensity Drug Trafficking Areas Program
    - Other Federal Drug Control Programs
- Department of State
    - Bureau of International Narcotics and Law Enforcement Affairs
- U.S. Agency for International Development
- Department of Transportation
    - National Highway Traffic Safety Administration
- Department of the Treasury
    - Internal Revenue Service
- Department of Veterans Affairs
    - Veterans Health Administration
- Small Business Administration[23]

In the FY2011 Budget, there are five priorities for which resources are requested across agencies: substance abuse prevention, substance abuse treatment, drug interdiction, domestic law enforcement, and international partnerships.[24] The FY2011 request includes over $15.5 billion for these priorities, an increase of $521.0 million over the FY2010 enacted amount of over $15.0 billion.[25] There is currently a continuing resolution (P.L. 111-290) funding federal drug control activities at the FY2010 enacted level.

ONDCP manages three primary program accounts: the Counterdrug Technology Assessment Center (CTAC), the High Intensity Drug Trafficking Area (HIDTA) Program, and the Other Federal Drug Control Programs.

Counterdrug Technology Assessment Center (CTAC)

The CTAC was given statutory authority in the Office of National Drug Control Policy Reauthorization Act of 2006 (P.L. 109-469).[26] It serves two primary functions: (1)

counterdrug technology research and development and (2) technology transfer. Funds under this account may be transferred from ONDCP to other federal departments and agencies. ONDCP has proposed that this account be discontinued starting in FY2011, as its roles have been taken on by various federal Drug Control Program agencies.

High Intensity Drug Trafficking Area (HIDTA) Program

The HIDTA program, originally authorized by the Anti-Drug Abuse Act of 1988 (P.L. 100-690),[27] provides assistance to federal, state, and local law enforcement operating in areas deemed as most-impacted by drug trafficking. The ONDCP Director has the authority to designate areas within the United States that are centers of illegal drug production, manufacturing, importation, or distribution as HIDTAs—of which there are currently 28. Four main criteria are considered when designating an area as a HIDTA:

> (1) the extent to which the area is a significant center of illegal drug production, manufacturing, importation, or distribution; (2) the extent to which State, local, and tribal law enforcement agencies have committed resources to respond to the drug trafficking problem in the area, thereby indicating a determination to respond aggressively to the problem; (3) the extent to which drug-related activities in the area are having a significant harmful impact in the area, and in other areas of the country; and (4) the extent to which a significant increase in allocation of Federal resources is necessary to respond adequately to drug related activities in the area.[28]

Other Federal Drug Control Programs

The Other Federal Drug Control Programs account is administered by ONDCP, and its funds support high-priority drug control programs. The FY2011 Budget request includes monies for the National Youth Anti-Drug Media Campaign, the Drug-Free Communities Program, Performance Measures Development, Anti-Doping Activities, U.S. Membership Dues to the World Anti-Doping Agency (WADA), the National Drug Court Institute, and the National Alliance for Model State Drug Laws.[29]

Evaluation of the Strategy

The Office of National Drug Control Policy Reauthorization Act of 1998 (Title VII of P.L. 105- 277) made it a requirement for ONDCP to submit to Congress—along with the National Drug Control Strategy—a report on a national drug control performance measurement system.[30] In essence, the report is aimed at evaluating the effectiveness of the Strategy. The performance measurement system report is to contain two- and five-year performance measures (along with descriptions of information and data that will be used for each measure) and targets for each of the Strategy's goals and objectives for reducing drug use, drug availability, and the consequences of drug use. It should also identify federal programs and activities that support the Strategy and evaluate the contribution of both demand- and supply-reduction activities. The evaluation should also ensure that each contributing federal drug control agency's goals and budgets are consistent with the Strategy. In addition, it is to assess existing national instruments and techniques to measure drug use, supply- and demand-reduction activities, and the effectiveness of substance abuse treatment in reducing illicit drug use and criminal behavior—both during and after treatment.

Currently, ONDCP is in the process of developing an updated Performance Reporting System that will aid in carrying out these evaluation responsibilities. It has indicated that the evaluation, while not submitted with the 2010 Strategy, will be included in the 2011 Strategy.[31] To date, ONDCP has relied on data from multiple sources in its evaluation of individual drug control agencies. It has used not only national research and indicators—such as the National Survey on Drug Use and Health and the Monitoring the Future study—but records maintained by individual agencies.[32] ONDCP encourages agencies to improve performance by linking performance to the certification of agency budgets. In the process of creating the National Drug Control Budget, ONDCP certifies each agency budget. It remains to be seen how the reformulated Performance Reporting System will impact ONDCP's ability to evaluate the contribution of each National Drug Control agency and program to the overall Strategy.

Selected Reauthorization Issues

Status of the War on Drugs

The term "war on drugs," popularized by former President Richard Nixon, was commonly used for nearly 40 years. In May 2009, ONDCP Director Kerlikowske called for an end to use of the term "war on drugs."[33] He noted that using this term is misleading because the United States is not at war with the individuals consuming drugs, but rather with the illegal drugs and their effects. He also described a gradual shift in societal thoughts on drug use and abuse. The Director notes that while drug use was previously considered a law enforcement or criminal justice problem, it transitioned to being viewed as a combination of criminal justice, social policy, and public health problems. He contends that recently, drug use has been seen more as a public health problem.[34]

Drug Use: A Public Health Issue

According to the National Survey on Drug Use and Health, in 2009 about 21.8 million Americans aged 12 and older were current (in the past month) illegal drug users, representing 8.7% of this population.[35] This also represents the largest proportion in the past decade of people aged 12 and older being identified as current illegal drug users. Further, the abuse of alcohol and illicit drugs contribute to over 100,000 deaths in the United States annually.[36]

The elevated proportion of drug users in 2009 was accompanied by an estimated 1,663,582 arrests for drug abuse violations.[37] Further, of the total number of federal cases in which offenders were sentenced in 2009 (N = 81,372), 25,164 (or 34.4% of all cases with available sentencing information) were sentenced for federal drug violations.[38] This is a decrease—both in number as well as in proportion—from the number of drug offenders sentenced at the federal level in 2008. In 2008, of the 76,478 federal cases in which offenders were sentenced, 25,500 (or 36.2% of cases with available sentencing information) were sentenced for federal drug violations (e.g., drug trafficking, simple possession, or participation in a continuing criminal enterprise).[39] While there was a decrease in federal offenders sentenced for drug crimes between 2008 and 2009, two years of data is insufficient for analysts to determine whether there is a relationship between this drop and any shift in

Administration policies toward viewing drug use/abuse as a public health issue. With additional years of sentencing and drug use data, analysts will be better positioned to evaluate such a relationship.

Budget Priorities

The FY2011 Budget request includes almost $15.553 billion across both supply- and demand-related programs.[40] This is an increase of $521.1 million over the FY2010 enacted amount of nearly $15.032 billion. In the FY2011 request, the Administration proposes to use 64.0% of the funds ($9.952 billion) for supply-side functions and 36.0% of the funds ($5.600 billion) for demand-side functions. Supply reduction includes funding for domestic law enforcement ($3.917 billion), interdiction ($3.727 billion), and international support ($2.308 billion), while demand reduction focuses on treatment (almost $3.883 billion) and prevention (nearly $1.718 billion).[41] The Administration proposes five new demand reduction priority areas for which $151.3 million of FY2011 funds would be used. These priority areas include

- creating a nationwide community-based drug prevention system targeting adolescents;
- training primary healthcare givers to intervene in developing drug abuse cases;
- expanding and improving specialty addiction care;
- developing safe, effective means to manage drug-related offenders; and
- creating a permanent drug monitoring system.[42]

Policymakers have questioned whether the National Drug Control Budget aims funding toward the most effective, evidence-based strategies to reduce illicit drug use and abuse. Currently, the Budget can be thought of as funding two broad categories of demand-reduction and supply-reduction activities. Further, the funding allocated for each contributing Drug Control Program agency is deemed as either supply-related or demand-related in its entirety. This approach cannot accurately measure the true breakdown of Drug Control Program funds dedicated to either supply or demand reduction because contributing agencies may have programs that target both supply and demand reduction. For instance, the Drug Enforcement Administration (DEA) uses funds for intelligence, investigations, state and local assistance, international support, and prevention[43]—a mix of both supply- and demand-reduction activities—but for classification purposes, the funds that DEA receives are considered to be supply-reduction funds. As a result of this current classification structure, ONDCP has suggested a restructuring of the way funding is captured and presented in future Budgets and Strategies.[44]

Critics of the current—and previous—Budget's focus on supply reduction activities may argue that research on prevention and treatment programs has suggested that such demand-reduction programs may be effective at reducing drug use. Research on supply-reduction, enforcement programs have not yielded the same results.[45] In addition to considering *outcome effectiveness*, policymakers have questioned the *cost effectiveness* of supply- and demand-reduction activities.

Director Kerlikowske has indicated that the most cost effective elements of the Strategy and Budget are in prevention and treatment[46]—the two components of demand reduction. Research has indicated, for instance, that drug treatment for high-risk populations, such as criminal offenders, can reduce societal costs.[47] Expert analysis of drug enforcement programs,

on the other hand, indicates that while enforcement may produce short-term drug market disruption, the effects are not lasting.[48] In considering ONDCP's reauthorization, policymakers may deliberate on whether to authorize specific supply-reduction or demand-reduction programs. Congress may also exercise oversight regarding ONDCP's implementation of evidenced-based activities.

SCOPE OF THE NATIONAL DRUG CONTROL BUDGET

Policymakers and industry experts alike have questioned whether the National Drug Control Budget captures the full scope of the nation's anti-drug activities. For instance, the Budget does not currently include costs for prosecuting and incarcerating drug offenders. In fact, the proportion of costs incurred by the U.S. Attorneys related to prosecuting drug-related crimes is not included in the current Budget. The U.S. Attorneys prosecute the entire spectrum of federal crimes; while some cases may be entirely drug-related, others may only have a drug component, while still others may not be related to drugs at all. For instance, in FY2009 the U.S. Attorneys reported 67,864 cases filed against 89,633 defendants. Of these, 15,321 narcotics cases were filed against 28,790 defendants.[49] There may still be other cases with a drug component that were not necessarily classified as narcotics cases. If the costs for prosecuting drug-related crimes were included in the Budget, ONDCP, with relevant drug control agencies, may need to determine whether to include costs related only to those cases that are entirely drug-related and classified as narcotics cases or whether to include costs for prosecuting all cases with a drug component. Additionally, there would need to be a system in place for the U.S. Attorneys to record monetary and personnel resources allocated for the prosecution of these cases.

A similar story holds true for the Federal Bureau of Prisons (BOP). BOP is responsible for housing federal inmates—not solely those incarcerated for drug crimes. While BOP is included in the current Budget, the resources accounted for are only those for inmate treatment programs. The Budget does not include funds for the housing of inmates incarcerated for drug-related crimes. As of October 30, 2010, BOP reported a total inmate population of 210,148.[50] Of those inmates whose offense information was available, 51.4% (100,439) were incarcerated for drug offenses. Additionally, the most recent statistics indicate that the cost of incarcerating someone in a BOP facility in FY2009 was $74.66 per day ($27,251.50 annually), and the cost for incarceration in a community correction center was $67.83 per day ($24,758.22 annually).[51] One challenge in including incarceration costs in the Budget would be determining whether to include costs for housing only those inmates incarcerated for drug crimes or costs for housing all inmates who are determined to have drug abuse issues, regardless of whether drugs are related to the crime(s) for which they are sentenced.

While experts have expressed concern about drug control policy elements *omitted* from the Budget, some have also questioned whether some elements *included* in the current Budget may be overly broad and may not directly tackle the nation's drug problems. For instance, some have argued that policies such as those assisting the Afghan government in combating the drug trade and those funding Colombian rule of law programs do not directly reduce the supply of drugs to the United States.[52] On the other hand, some may argue that these programs impacting drug source countries can, in turn, reduce the availability of illicit drugs

at home. Thus, policymakers may also debate whether the current Budget elements, such as those under the international supply-reduction strategy, are directly related to the National Drug Control Strategy and should be maintained as part of the Budget.

PERFORMANCE MEASUREMENT FOR FEDERAL DRUG CONTROL PROGRAMS

When Congress reauthorized ONDCP in 1998 (Title VII of P.L. 105-277), policymakers made it a requirement for ONDCP to create and report on a national drug control performance measurement system, as discussed above.[53] To date, ONDCP has measured performance by using data from individual agencies—data collected as required by the Government Performance and Results Act (P.L. 103-62)—and from national research.[54] Critics of this measurement system have argued that while it allows ONDCP to evaluate individual programs and agencies, the current system does not allow ONDCP to holistically assess whether the Strategy's goals and objectives are truly being accomplished.[55] ONDCP has indicated that the forthcoming Performance Reporting System (PRS) will address this concern. Director Kerlikowske described the new PRS as being able to evaluate annual progress toward each of the Drug Control Program's strategic goals. The new PRS is also expected to be adaptable to changing metrics as new drug control threats emerge.[56] When debating issues surrounding ONDCP's reauthorization, Congress may exercise oversight regarding the new PRS and whether this system will indeed allow for evaluation of individual programs and agencies as well as programmatic goals.

END NOTES

[1] For more information on ONDCP and its mission, see http://www.whitehousedrugpolicy.gov/index.html.

[2] P.L. 100-690, Title I, Subtitle A, National Narcotics Leadership Act of 1988, November 18, 1988, 102 Stat. 4181.

[3] P.L. 109-469. For detailed information on the 2006 reauthorization as well as background on ONDCP, see archived CRS Report RL32352, *War on Drugs: Reauthorization and Oversight of the Office of National Drug Control Policy*, by Mark Eddy.

[4] P.L. 109-469, Title VI, Section 601.

[5] Executive Office of the President, Office of National Drug Control Policy, *Fiscal Year 2011 Congressional Budget Submission*, p. 3.

[6] Gary Fields, "White House Czar Calls for End to 'War on Drugs'," *The Wall Street Journal*, May 14, 2009, http://online.wsj.com/article/SB124225891527617397.html.

[7] Testimony by ONDCP Director Kerlikowske before the U.S. Congress, House Committee on Oversight and Government Reform, Subcommittee on Domestic Policy, *ONDCP's Fiscal Year 2011 National Drug Control Budget: Are We Still Funding a War on Drugs?*, 111th Cong., 2nd sess., April 14, 2010.

[8] Executive Office of the President, Office of National Drug Control Policy, *National Drug Control Strategy, A New Balanced Approach, Highlights 2010*, http://www.whitehousedrugpolicy.gov/strategy/highlight_brochure.pdf.

[9] For more information, see Gallup at http://www.gallup.com/poll/1657/Illegal-drugs

[10] 21 U.S.C. § 1705(a)(1).

[11] Executive Office of the President, Office of National Drug Control Policy, *2010 National Drug Control Strategy*, p. 6.

[12] The NSDUH is an annual survey of approximately 67,500 people, including residents of households, non-institutionalized group quarters, and civilians living on military bases. The survey is administered by the Substance Abuse and Mental Health Services Administration of the U.S. Department of Health and Human Services and is available at http://www.oas.samhsa.gov/nsduhLatest.htm.

[13] U.S. Department of Health and Human Services, Substance Abuse and Mental Health Services Administration, Office of Applied Studies, *Results from the 2009 National Survey on Drug Use and Health: Volume I. Summary of National Findings*, September 2010, p. 1, http://oas.samhsa.gov/NSDUH/2k9NSDUH/2k9ResultsP.pdf (hereafter, *2009 NSDUH*).

[14] Monitoring the Future is an annual survey of about 50,000 8th, 10th, and 12th grade students. It is used to assess behaviors, attitudes, and values of these students, and conducts follow-up assessments after graduation. Research is conducted at the University of Michigan, Institute for Social Research. For more information, see http://monitoringthefuture.org/.

[15] Lloyd D. Johnston, Patrick M. O'Malley, and Jerald G. Bachman, et al., The University of Michigan Institute for Social Research, *Monitoring the Future, National Results on Adolescent Drug Use: Overview of Key Findings 2009*, U.S. Department of Health and Human Services, National Institute on Drug Abuse, National Institutes of Health, NIH Publication No. 10-7583, May 2010, p. 50, http://monitoringthefuture.org/pubs/monographs/overview2009.pdf (hereafter, *MTF 2009*).

[16] *2009 NSDUH*, p. 2.

[17] Ibid., p. 27.

[18] Jiaquan Xu, Kenneth D. Kochanek, and Sherry L. Murphy, et al., *National Vital Statistics Reports, Deaths: Final Data for 2007*, U.S. Centers for Disease Control and Prevention, Volume 58, Number 19, May 20, 2010, p. 93, http://www.cdc.gov/nchs/data/nvsr/nvsr58/nvsr58_19.pdf.

[19] U.S. Department of Health and Human Services, Substance Abuse and Mental Health Services Administration, Office of Applied Studies, *Drug Abuse Warning Network, 2008: Selected Tables of National Estimates of Drug-Related Emergency Department Visits*, 2009.

[20] *2009 NSDUH*, p. 28.

[21] Executive Office of the President, Office of National Drug Control Policy, *2010 National Drug Control Strategy*, p. 99.

[22] Executive Office of the President, Office of National Drug Control Policy, *Fiscal Year 2011 Congressional Budget Submission*, p. 4.

[23] Executive Office of the President, Office of National Drug Control Policy, *2010 National Drug Control Strategy*, p. 111.

[24] Testimony by ONDCP Director Kerlikowske before the U.S. Congress, House Committee on Oversight and Government Reform, Subcommittee on Domestic Policy, *ONDCP's Fiscal Year 2011 National Drug Control Budget: Are We Still Funding a War on Drugs?*, 111th Cong., 2nd sess., April 14, 2010.

[25] Ibid.

[26] 21 U.S.C. § 1707.

[27] 21 U.S.C. § 1706.

[28] Office of National Drug Control Policy, *The High-Intensity Drug Trafficking Area Program: An Overview*, http://whitehousedrugpolicy.gov/hidta/overview.html.

[29] Executive Office of the President, Office of National Drug Control Policy, *National Drug Control Strategy, FY2011 Budget Summary*, 2010, p. 157, http://www.whitehousedrugpolicy.gov/publications/policy/fy11budget.pdf

[30] 22 U.S.C. § 1705(c).

[31] Executive Office of the President, Office of National Drug Control Policy, *Fiscal Year 2011 Congressional Budget Submission*, p. 5.

[32] Executive Office of the President, Office of National Drug Control Policy, *2009 National Drug Control Strategy*, pp. 37–38.

[33] Gary Fields, "White House Czar Calls for End to 'War on Drugs'," *The Wall Street Journal*, May 14, 2009, http://online.wsj.com/article/SB124225891527617397.html.

[34] Ibid. See the full interview with *The Wall Street Journal* at http://online.wsj.com/article/SB124233331735120871.html.

[35] *2009 NSDUH*, p. 1.

[36] National Institutes of Health, National Institute on Drug Abuse, *Drugs, Brains, and Behavior—The Science of Addiction*, NIH Pub No. 10-5605, August 2010, http://www.nida.nih.gov/scienceofaddiction/sciofaddiction.pdf.

[37] Sourcebook of Criminal Justice Statistics Online, Table 4.1.2009, http://www.albany.edu/sourcebook/pdf/t412009.pdf. Data estimations are based on the Federal Bureau of Investigation (FBI) Uniform Crime Report (UCR) program data. The UCR program compiles data from monthly reports transmitted directly to the FBI from approximately 17,000 local police departments or state agencies.

[38] U.S. Sentencing Commission, *Sourcebook of Federal Sentencing Statistics*, http://www.ussc.gov/ANNRPT/2009/figi.pdf.

[39] U.S. Sentencing Commission, *Sourcebook of Federal Sentencing Statistics*, http://www.ussc.gov/ANNRPT/2008/figi.pdf.

[40] Ibid., p. 109.

[41] As mentioned, a continuing resolution (P.L. 111-290) is currently funding federal drug control activities at the FY2010 enacted level of more than $15.0 billion.

[42] Executive Office of the President, Office of National Drug Control Policy, *National Drug Control Strategy, FY2011 Budget Summary*, 2010, pp. 1-2, http://www.whitehousedrugpolicy.gov/publications/policy

[43] Ibid., p. 121.

[44] Executive Office of the President, Office of National Drug Control Policy, *2009 National Drug Control Strategy*, p. 99.

[45] Rosalie Liccardo Pacula, *An Assessment of the Scientific Support Underlying the FY2011 Budget Priorities of the Office of National Drug Control Policy*, RAND Corporation, CT-344, April 2010, http://www.rand.org/pubs/testimonies/2010/RAND_CT344.pdf.

[46] Testimony by ONDCP Director Kerlikowske before the U.S. Congress, House Committee on Oversight and Government Reform, Subcommittee on Domestic Policy, *ONDCP's Fiscal Year 2011 National Drug Control Budget: Are We Still Funding a War on Drugs?*, 111th Cong., 2nd sess., April 14, 2010.

[47] Kathryn E. McCollister, Michael T. French, and Michael Prendergast, et al., "Is In-Prison Treatment Enough? A Cost-Effective Analysis of Prison-Based Treatment and Aftercare Services for Substance-Abusing Offenders," *Law & Policy*, vol. 25, no. 1 (2003).

[48] Rosalie Liccardo Pacula, *An Assessment of the Scientific Support Underlying the FY2011 Budget Priorities of the Office of National Drug Control Policy*, RAND Corporation, CT-344, April 2010, http://www.rand.org/pubs/testimonies/2010/RAND_CT344.pdf.

[49] U.S. Department of Justice, Executive Office for U.S. Attorneys, *United States Attorneys' Annual Statistical Report, Fiscal Year 2009*, p. 5, http://www.justice.gov/usao/reading_room/reports/asr2009/09statrpt.pdf*.com*. If drug cases from the Government Regulatory/Money Laundering Program category are included, there were 15,388 narcotics cases filed against 28,909 defendants.

[50] U.S. Department of Justice, Federal Bureau of Prisons, *Quick Facts About the Bureau of Prisons*, http://www.bop.gov/about/facts.jsp.

[51] Information provided to CRS by the Administrative Office of the U.S. Courts.

[52] Rosalie Liccardo Pacula, *An Assessment of the Scientific Support Underlying the FY2011 Budget Priorities of the Office of National Drug Control Policy*, RAND Corporation, CT-344, April 2010, http://www.rand.org/pubs/testimonies/2010/RAND_CT344.pdf.

[53] 22 U.S.C. § 1705(c).

[54] Executive Office of the President, Office of National Drug Control Policy, *2009 National Drug Control Strategy*, pp. 37-38.

[55] See the written statement of John T. Carnevale, Ph.D., President, Carnevale Associates, LLC, before the U.S. Congress, House Committee on Oversight and Government Reform, Subcommittee on Domestic Policy, *ONDCP's Fiscal Year 2010 National Drug Control Budget and the Policy Priorities of the Office of National Drug Control Policy under the New Administration*, 111th Cong., 1st sess., May 19, 2009, p. 12.

[56] See the written statement of ONDCP Director Kerlikowske before the U.S. Congress, House Committee on Oversight and Government Reform, Subcommittee on Domestic Policy, *ONDCP's Fiscal Year 2011 National Drug Control Budget: Are We Still Funding a War on Drugs?*, 111th Cong., 2nd sess., April 14, 2010, pp. 14-15.

In: U.S. National Drug Control Strategy
Editor: Benjamin F. Turner
ISBN: 978-1-61470-629-8

Chapter 2

NATIONAL DRUG CONTROL STRATEGY – FY 2011 BUDGET SUMMARY*

Office of the President

I. EXECUTIVE SUMMARY

The President's Fiscal Year (FY) 2011 National Drug Control Budget requests $15.5 billion to reduce drug use and its consequences in the United States. This represents an increase of $521.1 million (3.5 percent) over the FY 2010 enacted level of $15.0 billion. These resources are categorized around five major functions: (1) Substance Abuse Prevention, (2) Substance Abuse Treatment, (3) Domestic Law Enforcement, (4) Interdiction, and (5) International Support. Figure 1 details funding by function.

Substance abuse takes a terrible toll on the public health, public safety and financial resources of the United States. The Administration's national drug control policy seeks to reduce Americans' drug use and its related health, social and criminal problems. To help meet this goal, the Administration has developed five demand reduction priority areas. The Administration is requesting $151.3 million in new funding across the Federal government to strengthen efforts to detect, and prevent and treat illicit drug use in our communities and break the cycle of illicit drug use, crime, and incarceration.

These priorities are to:

1) Create a National, Community-Based Prevention System to Protect our Adolescents ($22.6 million)
2) Train and Engage Primary Healthcare to Intervene in Emerging Cases of Drug Abuse ($7.2 million)
3) Expand and Improve Specialty Addiction Care for Addiction ($44.9 million)
4) Develop Safe and Efficient Ways to Manage Drug-Related Offenders ($34.0 million)
5) Create a Permanent Drug Monitoring System ($42.6 million)

---

* This is an edited, reformatted and augmented version of an Office of the President publication, dated 2010.

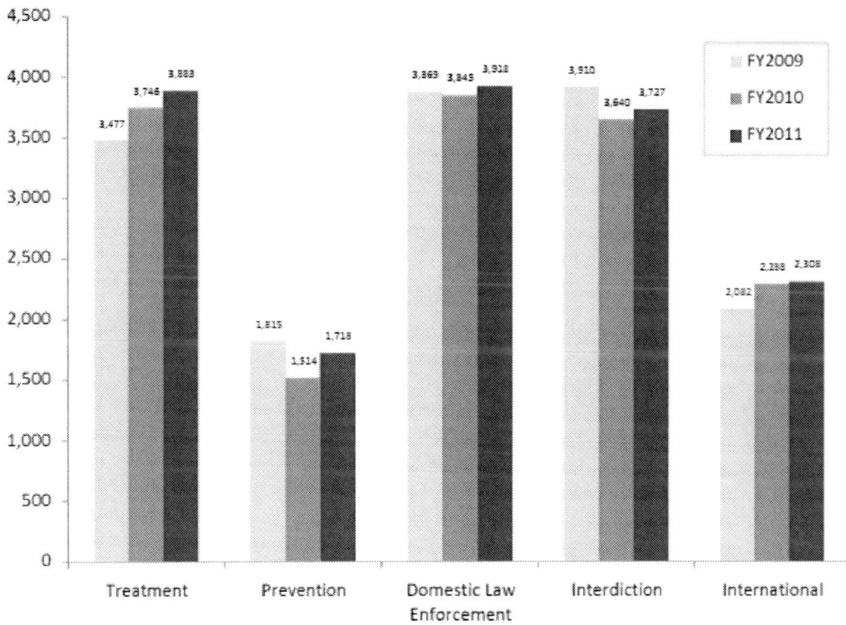

Figure 1. National Drug Control Funding by Function (Funding in Millions).

HIGHLIGHTS OF THE FY 2011 BUDGET

Prevention

Federal resources totaling $1.7 billion support a variety of education and outreach programs aimed at preventing the initiation of drug use. This represents a 13.4 percent increase over the FY 2010 enacted level; the major changes are highlighted below:

Substance Abuse and Mental Health Services Administration: Prevention Programs of Regional and National Significance

Department of Health and Human Services: $254.2 Million
(Reflects $29.6 Million Increase over FY 2010)

In support of the first priority to create a national, community based prevention system to protect our adolescents, the budget includes:

- Prevention Prepared Communities: The FY 2011 request includes $15.0 million to fund an interagency pilot program for a national network of "prevention prepared communities" intended to offer a continuous system of evidence based prevention interventions throughout the full course of adolescence.
- Enhancing State Capacity to Develop/Support Communities: This proposal also includes $5.6 million to fund community prevention specialists within States to facilitate development of prevention prepared communities and increase collaboration among State agencies in achieving these goals. Specific activities include establishing and maintaining a State level drug abuse surveillance monitoring system,

providing intensive technical assistance, and developing a Statewide support network to promote coaching and mentoring.

- Evaluations: The FY 2011 request includes $2.0 million to fund an evaluation of the Prevention Prepared Communities demonstration pilot program. The evaluation design will be created in partnership with ONDCP and NIH.

Drug Free Communities (DFC)

Office of National Drug Control Policy: $85.5 Million
(Reflects $9.5 Million Decrease from FY 2010)

DFC funding supports the development of community drug free coalitions throughout the United States. The program provides up to $125,000 per year, for a total of up to 10 years, in grant funding to local drug free community coalitions; the funding must be matched at a minimum 1:1 ratio by local communities. Community coalitions strive to increase community involvement and effectiveness in carrying out a wide array of drug prevention strategies, initiatives, and activities.

Successful, Safe, and Healthy Students Grant Program

Department of Education: $283.1 Million
(Reflects $107.3 Million Increase over FY 2010)

This new program would support student achievement and help ensure that students are mentally and physically healthy and ready to learn. The objective is creation of an improved school climate that reduces drug use, violence, and harassment and improves school safety and students' physical and mental wellbeing. Within the program, the Department would use $144.6 million to award grants to assist State educational agencies and local educational agencies (LEAs) to develop and implement programs and activities that create safe environments; $77.8 million would provide grant awards under the "Safe Schools/Healthy Students" initiative. Safe Schools/Healthy Students supports LEAs and communities in developing and implementing a comprehensive set of programs and services designed to prevent youth drug use and violence, support early childhood development activities, and provide needed student mental health services. Education funds this initiative jointly with the Department of Health and Human Services (HHS) and administers it in collaboration with both HHS and the Department of Justice.

National Youth Anti-Drug Media Campaign

Office of National Drug Control Policy:
$66.5 Million (Reflects $21.5 Million Increase over FY 2010)

The Campaign uses media channels such as paid advertising, interactive media, and public information to educate and motivate youth to develop antidrug beliefs and behaviors, and encourage adults to play a more effective role in keeping youth drug free. Funding (providing for television, radio, newspaper, Internet, and nontraditional advertising) enables the Media Campaign to address emerging drug issues among youth, such as prescription and over the counter drug abuse.

Consolidated Tribal Grant

Department of Justice: $111.6 Million (Reflects $111.6 Million Increase over FY 2010)

The Department of Justice has set aside 7% of the Office of Justice Program's (OJP) discretionary funding for grants or reimbursement programs under a new tribal criminal justice assistance program which consolidates previous OJP tribal funding streams and increases funding available for Indian Country public safety. In addition to funding grants to improve public safety outcomes in Indian Country, these grants will support training and technical assistance to improve tribal criminal justice outcomes, including drug and alcohol related issues. (This program has been scored evenly between Prevention efforts and Domestic Law Enforcement efforts.)

Drug Impaired Driving Program

Department of Transportation: $2.7 Million (Reflects No Change from FY 2010)

The National Highway Traffic Safety Administration's (NHTSA) FY 2011 request supports the Drug Impaired Driving Program, which will provide public information and outreach efforts, as well as improved law enforcement training in the area of drug impaired driving. Funding will also support data collection efforts to better develop programs and countermeasures to address the problem.

Arrestee Drug Abuse Monitoring II Program (ADAM)

Department of Justice: $10.0 Million (Reflects $10.0 Million Increase over FY 2010)

In support of the fifth priority to create a permanent performance monitoring system, the FY 2011 request includes $10 million for Justice to expand and enhance the Arrestee Drug Abuse Monitoring II program (ADAM), which collects data on booked arrestees in ten U.S. counties on their drug abuse and related behavior.

Treatment

The FY 2011 Budget dedicates nearly $3.9 billion in Federal funds for early intervention and treatment services for individuals with drug problems. This represents a 3.7% increase over the FY 2010 funding level. The major changes are highlighted below:

Substance Abuse and Mental Health Services Administration: Treatment Programs of Regional and National Significance

Department of Health and Human Services: $635.4 Million
(Reflects $101.2 Million Increase over FY 2010)

In support of three priorities, train and engage primary healthcare to intervene in emerging cases of drug abuse, expand and improve specialty addiction care for addiction, and develop safe and efficient paradigms to manage drug related offenders in community corrections, the FY 2011 Budget includes $86.2 million for a wide array of new and expanded programs. These programs include:

- Training and Equipping Mainstream Healthcare Establish an SBIRT Code Monitoring System: The FY 2011 request includes $0.5 million to monitor and

encourage Statewide Screening, Brief Intervention and Referral to Treatment (SBIRT) code adoption and implementation. SAMHSA will collaborate with the Centers for Medicare & Medicaid Services on the design, collection, and reporting of data for this initiative.

- Training and Equipping Mainstream Healthcare Expand SBIRT Code Adoption Through Technical Assistance Initiative: The FY 2011 request also includes $0.7 million to enhance and expand the Center for Substance Abuse Treatment's state financing academies, promote statewide adoption of SBIRT via code adoption, and secure inclusion of SBIRT into health care credentialing policies.
- Expanding Identification and Management of Substance Use Disorders by Physicians: The FY 2011 request includes $3.0 million to establish a pilot project based on its Physician Clinical Support System model to train generalist physicians and other health care providers in SBIRT and general drug use treatment clinical decisionmaking. The pilot will be assessed to determine whether there has been an increase in knowledge and applied practice by clinicians.
- Performance Contracting Pilot Project: The FY 2011 request includes $6.0 million for a performance contracting pilot project for competitive grants to State or Tribal authorities. Grant funding will be used to enhance overall drug treatment quality by incentivizing treatment providers to achieve specific performance targets. Examples could include payment supplements for treatment providers who are able to connect higher proportions of detoxified patients with continuing recoveryoriented treatment, or for outpatient providers who are able to successfully retain greater proportions of patients in active treatment participation for longer time periods.
- Enhancing Substance Abuse Care in Federal Health Care Systems: The FY 2011 request includes $25.0 million to add qualified and trained behavioral health counselors and other addiction specialists in HRSAsupported community health centers. HRSA will collaborate with the Department of Veterans Affairs and the Substance Abuse and Mental Health Services Administration by utilizing each agency's technical assistance expertise. This initiative will include training on performing Screening, Brief Intervention and Referral to Treatment (SBIRT) for the health counselors and other addiction specialists. (Note: As HRSA is not a drug control agency, for display purposes only these resources are being shown as part of the SAMHSA drug control budget.)
- Expanding ATR Grants: The FY 2011 request includes $9.9 million to expand the Access to Recovery Program (ATR), a recoveryoriented system of care approach to service delivery that uses electronic vouchers and client choice. Funds will support up to four new ATR grants.
- Enhance Community Corrections Programs by DrugInvolved Offenders: This proposal includes an increase of more than $10.0 million to provide continuation funding for adult and juvenile treatment drug courts, and will support continuation of all the new treatment drug courts jointly funded with DOJ elements in FY 2010.
- Adult Exoffender ReEntry Court Program: The FY 2011 request includes $5.0 million to expand the integration of the proven practices of drug courts into the management of drugrelated offenders being released from incarceration back into the community. These grants provide screening, assessment and comprehensive treatment and recovery support services.

- Creating Mechanisms to Collect/Use Community Level Information: The FY 2011 President's Budget request from SAMHSA includes an additional $13.6 million to design, develop and field test a community level early warning and monitoring system to detect the emergence of new drug threats and to assist in identifying the public health and public safety consequences of drug use. The proposed system does not currently exist and thus will require substantial scientific input combined with practical considerations to achieve the system's intended purpose. Thus, SAMHSA is expected to work closely and collaboratively with NIDA, NIAAA, and ONDCP on all aspects of system development and deployment. (Note: This program has been scored as 80 percent ($10.9 million) treatment and 20 percent ($2.7 million) prevention.)
- Preserving National Strategic Data Resources: The FY 2011 President's Budget request includes $19.0 million to expand and enhance the Drug Abuse Warning Network, which provides national and local area estimates of drug related emergency department visits and mortality; and improve the National Survey on Drug Use and Health by enhancing its ability to gather information such as that related to the chronic heavy drug using population. (Note: This program has been scored as 80 percent ($15.2 million) treatment and 20 percent ($3.8 million) prevention.)

Substance Abuse Prevention and Treatment (SAPT) Block Grant

Department of Health and Human Services: $1,799.0 Million
(Reflects No Change from FY 2010)

The goal of the SAPT Block Grant is to support and expand substance abuse prevention and treatment services, while providing maximum flexibility to states. States may provide SAPT Block Grant funds to community and faith based organizations to provide services. Of the amounts appropriated for the SAPT Block Grant, 95 percent are distributed to states through a formula prescribed by the authorizing legislation. The SAPT Block Grant program in FY 2011 is funded at the same level as FY 2010, and will provide support to the current 60 jurisdictions (states, territories, the District of Columbia, and the Red Lake Band of Chippewa Indians in Minnesota) for a similar level of prevention and treatment services. These resources will support approximately 2 million treatment episodes. (Note: A minimum of 20% of the SAPT Block Grant is set aside for the prevention activities.)

Additional Substance Abuse Treatment at the Indian Health Service

Department of Health and Human Services: $83.9 Million
(Reflects $6.7 Million Increase over FY 2010)

In support of the priority to expand and improve specialty addiction care, the FY 2011 Budget includes $4.0 million to add qualified and trained behavioral health counselors and other addiction specialists in IHS funded facilities. IHS, in partnership with Indian Communities, will continue to collaborate with the Department of Veterans Affairs and the Department of Health and Human Services' Substance Abuse and Mental Health Services Administration by utilizing each agency's technical assistance expertise. IHS will also continue efforts to expand screening and brief intervention training for Indian health providers.

Second Chance Act

Department of Justice: $50.0 Million (Reflects $20.0 Million Increase over FY 2010)

In support of the priority to develop safe and efficient paradigms to manage drug related offenders in community corrections, the budget includes the following initiatives:

- Prosecution led Drug Treatment Alternatives to Prison: The FY 2011 request includes $10.0 million to provide full funding of this activity authorized under Section 112 of the Second Chance Act. Funds will allow the Attorney General to make grants to State, Tribal, and local prosecutors to improve the infrastructure, knowledge, and systems needed to operate the judicial aspects of alternative to prison initiatives.
- Adult Re Entry Court Initiative: The FY 2011 request includes $5.0 million to integrate the proven practices of drug courts into the management of drug related offenders being released from incarceration back into the community. Funds will be issued through a competitive bidding process and will be used to support training of probation officers and judges, creation of needed data systems, and expansion of drug testing capabilities.
- Innovative Diversion/Re Entry Programs for Juvenile Drug Offenders: The FY 2011 request includes $4.0 million to provide support to develop and test innovative strategies for serving juvenile offenders with co occurring substance abuse problems. Funds will be issued via a competitive bidding process.

VA Treatment

Department of Veterans Affairs: $418.0 Million
(Reflects $13.0 Million Increase over FY 2010)

The Department of Veterans Affairs, through its Veterans Health Administration (VHA), operates a national network of substance abuse treatment programs located in the Department's medical centers, residential rehabilitation facilities, and outpatient clinics. The goal of VHA's Office of Mental Health Services is to provide effective, safe, efficient, recovery oriented, and compassionate care for veterans with substance use disorders and mental illness, for those who are vulnerable to substance use disorders, and for those who are in continuing care to sustain recovery.

Residential Substance Abuse Treatment

Department of Justice: $30.0 Million (Reflects No Change from FY 2010)

The Residential Substance Abuse Treatment program for state prisoners was established to help states and local governments develop, implement, and improve residential substance abuse treatment programs in correctional facilities, and establish and maintain community based aftercare services for probationers and parolees. Ultimately, the program goal is to help offenders become drug free and learn the skills needed to sustain themselves upon return to the community.

Domestic Law Enforcement

Over $3.9 billion in Federal resources support domestic law enforcement efforts, an increase of $73.8 million (1.9%) over the FY 2010 level. The Departments of Justice, Homeland Security, and Treasury, with support from the Department of Defense's National Guard, provide key domestic law enforcement support; the major changes are highlighted below.

Organized Crime Drug Enforcement Task Force

Department of Justice: $579.3 Million (Reflects $50.8 Million Increase over FY 2010)

The Organized Crime Drug Enforcement Task Force (OCDETF) Program is a partnership of federal law enforcement agencies and prosecutors, with assistance from state and local police departments, to identify, dismantle and disrupt sophisticated national and international drug trafficking and money laundering organizations. The FY2011 Budget Request adds funding for additional agents, analysts and attorneys performing investigative, intelligence, and prosecutorial work focused on the U.S. southwest border.

DEA Diversion Control Efforts

Department of Justice: $291.8 Million (Reflects $40.0 Million Increase over FY 2010)

DEA's Diversion Control Program (DCP) enforces the Controlled Substances Act and its regulations pertaining to pharmaceutical controlled substances and listed chemicals. The DCP actively monitors more than 1 million individuals and companies that are registered with DEA to handle controlled substances or listed chemicals through a system of scheduling, quotas, recordkeeping, reporting, and security requirements. The FY 2011 request includes funding for 174 new positions for pharmaceutical and chemical diversion control activities. These resources will support regulatory and enforcement efforts, including an expansion of Tactical Diversion Squads, intelligence support, and Internet investigations. The budget request also supports for the priority to train and engage primary healthcare to intervene in emerging cases of drug abuse, with a $3.0 million enhancement for the Prescription Drug Monitoring Program, which will initiate a program to establish a well functioning standardized prescription drug monitoring program in every State to reduce prevalence of overdose deaths, drug interactions, diversion of prescribed medications, and early identification of patients at risk for addiction.

High Intensity Drug Trafficking Areas (HIDTA) Program

Office of National Drug Control Policy: $210.0 Million
(Reflects $29.0 Million Decrease from FY 2010)

The HIDTA program was established by the Anti-Drug Abuse Act of 1988 to provide assistance to federal, state and local law enforcement entities operating in areas most adversely affected by drug trafficking. A central feature of the HIDTA program is the discretion granted to HIDTA Executive Boards to design a strategy to respond to the specific drug trafficking threats found in each HIDTA region and to develop initiatives to implement the strategy.

National Guard Counterdrug Support

Department of Defense: $177.7 Million (Reflects $43.4 Million Decrease from FY 2010)

The National Guard, through the Governor's State Plans, provides counterdrug support to federal, state, and local law enforcement agencies (LEAs), Community Based Organizations (CBOs), and educational and government organizations that request assistance. Types of National Guard provided military unique support include linguistics, communications, transportation, logistics, intelligence, engineering, and reconnaissance.

Interdiction

With an increase of $86.9 million (2.4%) over the FY 2010 level, $3.7 billion supports Federal interdiction efforts. The Departments of Homeland Security, Defense, and State perform activities designed to interrupt the trafficking of illicit drugs into the United States by targeting the transportation link; major changes are highlighted below.

U.S. Coast Guard Interdiction

Department of Homeland Security: $1,208.1 Million
(Reflects $45.9 Million Increase over FY 2010)

As part of the United States Coast Guard's maritime security strategic goal, its drug interdiction objective is to reduce the flow of illegal drugs entering the United States by denying smugglers access to maritime routes. The President's Budget seeks funding for recapitalization of increasingly outdated and unreliable assets (e.g., cutters, aircraft, boats, and C4ISR) and infrastructure that supports this mission. Recapitalization is vital to preserving future surface, air, and shore asset capability, and is an essential investment for the Nation.

Caribbean Basin Security Initiative

Department of State: $31.2 Million
(Reflects $31.2 Million Increase over FY 2010)

The Caribbean Basin Security Initiative will curtail the flow of illegal drugs into the region by strengthening the region's capacity to detect and interdict drug shipments, bring traffickers and other criminals to trial, and attack money laundering and associated corruption. FY 2011 drug control funding will support both bilateral and regional counternarcotics initiatives, including support for Sovereign Skies, interdiction, eradication, law enforcement reform and development, and demand reduction.

Western Hemisphere Regional Program

Department of State: $37.5 Million
(Reflects $31.3 Million Increase over FY 2010)

To encourage the region's elected leaders' use of democratic processes and free market economies to improve the lives of their citizens, the Western Hemisphere Regional program strengthens democratic institutions; promotes prosperity; protects the democratic state; and invests in people. These pillars not only frame U.S. foreign policy priorities for the region, but also are used to build multilateral consensus.

Customs and Border Patrol: Border Security and Trade Facilitation at Ports of Entry

Department of Homeland Security: $805.9 Million
(Reflects $5.8 Million Increase over FY 2010)

Customs and Border Patrol (CBP) uses its resources to support aggressive border enforcement strategies that are designed to interdict and disrupt the flow of narcotics and ill gotten gains across our Nation's borders and dismantle the related smuggling organizations. CBP narcotics interdiction strategies are designed to be flexible so that they can successfully counter the constantly shifting narcotics threat at the ports of entry. CBP's overall budget requests an adjustment to base of $46.9 million and 389 FTEs for an increase to Customs and Border Protection Officers (CBPOs) in the Office of Field Operations (based on CBP's drug budget methodology, $5.8 million of this adjustment to base would be drug related). The proposed adjustment will allow CBP to maintain staffing for critical positions.

Joint Interagency Task Force South

Department of Defense: $50.5 Million (Reflects $5.3 Million Decrease from FY 2010)

Joint Interagency Task Force South (JIATFS), under the Department of Defense's U.S. Southern Command, conducts counterdrug operations, intelligence fusion and multi sensor correlation operation to detect, monitor, and interdict the South to North flow of illicit drugs and other narcoterrorist threats to the security of the U.S. Specific tasks include: detection, monitoring, tracking and hand off of suspect targets to appropriate U. S. and participating nation law enforcement authorities; providing intelligence fusion support to law enforcement agencies and country teams; providing planning assistance for counternarcotics operations; and support to counternarcotics initiatives of U.S. Country Teams and partner nations.

International

The Budget requests over $2.3 billion to provide international support, an increase of $20.1 million (0.9%) over the FY 2010 level. The Departments of Defense, Justice and State perform a wide range of drug control activities primarily focused on or conducted in areas outside of the United States, focusing on the disruption or dismantlement of the most significant international drug organizations, and increasing the drug enforcement capability of partner nations. Major changes are highlighted below.

DoD CN Support in Central Asia

Department of Defense: $501.5 Million (Reflects $121.4 Million Increase over FY 2010)

In Afghanistan and Central Asia, the role of the Department of Defense (DoD) is to provide military assistance, with a focus on building the Afghan government's capacity to address the drug trade and to coordinate those efforts with Coalition Partners. DoD takes a regional approach, focusing on Afghanistan as the source zone and Pakistan and Central Asian States as the transit zone. DoD bolsters regional partners' border security and CN efforts to stem the flow of drugs from Afghanistan and stop precursor chemicals from entering Afghanistan. In FY2011, a greater focus will be on interdiction than in previous

years, as DoD has built the initial capacity of the Afghan CN vetted units that are now capable of conducting combined interdiction operations with DEA and U.S. military forces.

DEA International Enforcement

Department of Justice: $435.3 Million (Reflects $26.1 Million Increase over FY 2010)
The major focus of DEA's International Enforcement program is the disruption or dismantlement of the most significant international drug and chemical trafficking organizations. The FY 2011 request includes $10.8 million in non personnel funding to provide permanent funding for the expanded Sensitive Investigative Unit (SIU) program in Mexico, which is a key tool in the effort to disrupt and dismantle Mexican Drug Cartels. DEA's SIU program recruits, selects, and trains foreign police officers to work cooperatively with DEA in major case development and the exchange of intelligence.

Africa

Department of State: $13.2 Million
(Reflects $10.0 Million Increase over FY 2010)
The FY 2011 request of $13.2 million will be used for counternarcotics projects in West Africa, including Benin, Cape Verde, Ghana, Guinea, Guinea Bissau, Nigeria, Senegal, Sierra Leone, The Gambia, and Togo. Programs will develop strong law enforcement investigative abilities and justice sectors capable of prosecuting and convicting narco traffickers. While the majority of the cocaine transiting West Africa flows to Europe, the primary USG concern is the destabilizing effect this trafficking will have on the region and the potential it represents for corroding good governance.

Colombia

Department of State: $178.6 Million
(Reflects $26.6 Million Decrease from FY 2010)
The FY 2011 request continues a transparent and predictable glide path in transferring financial and management responsibility for counternarcotics and security activities to the Government of Colombia, while increasing funding for alternative development, rule of law, and humanitarian assistance. Decreases will be taken from INCLE funded eradication and interdiction, counternarcotics, stabilization operations and transnational crime programs.

CHANGES TO THE NATIONAL DRUG CONTROL BUDGET

The National Drug Control Budget structure includes two changes in this submission.

- A portion of the Department of Justice's new Flexible Tribal Grants Program (a seven percent set aside from all discretionary OJP programs, which consolidates previous OJP tribal funding streams and increases funding available for Indian Country public safety issues, including drug and alcohol related issues) has been scored as drug related.

- The drug control budget includes for the first time funding for the Health Resources and Services Administration (HRSA), which will provide qualified and trained behavioral health counselors and other addiction specialists in HRSAsupported community health centers. As HRSA is not currently a drugcontrol agency, for display purposes only these resources are being shown as part of the SAMHSA drug control budget.

Other Related Drug Control Program (ORDCP) Agencies and the Coming Review

Included in the appendix of this volume are ORDCP agencies that receive federal funds for drug control activities, but their primary mission does not include drug control, nor have readily identifiable drug control line items in the Budget of the President.

ONDCP coordinates and certifies the drug control budgets of federal departments and advises the President on what resources are necessary to implement the Administration's Drug Control Strategy. Parallel to the development of the President's Annual National Drug Control Strategy, ONDCP gathers and incorporates the various departments' planned -drug control spending into the National Drug Control Budget, displayed in this annual Budget Summary.

Currently, it is difficult to fully determine what activities are drug control related because of the multi-faceted nature of each department and the complex structure of the federal budget. To establish an accurate and reliable accounting of federal resources that are being spent on the drug control mission, ONDCP will undertake a thorough review of the Federal Budget during this calendar year. This review will include two parts: first, a review of how funding in the budget is categorized and characterized, and second, an examination of programs to determine their suitability for inclusion in the Federal Drug Control Budget.

At the present time, an agency's drug control spending is characterized as either "supply" or "demand." This categorization may present an incomplete picture of what some agency programs actually do, as some may be engaged in both demand and supply activities simultaneously. ONDCP is exploring appropriate ways to precisely capture how drug control activities are actually performed in the field. As the Administration develops the FY 2012 Budget Submission, ONDCP will, in consultation with stakeholders, consider other possible ways to display federal drug control funding.

The second part of the review will focus on the agencies and programs that should constitute the National Drug Control Budget. Working with the interagency and the Congress to fully examine this structure, ONDCP will consult with a group of interagency experts to review and recommend any required changes to the structure. This review will define what criteria should be used when determining if an agency should remain or be added to the federal drug control budget and what portion of that agency activities may be fairly counted toward drug control activities.

Once the review is complete, the FY 2012 Budget Summary will reflect the any revisions to the budget structure and framework as may be necessary.

PERFORMANCE MEASUREMENT

The National Drug Control Strategy is a guide to our country on how to address the myriad of serious challenges posed by illicit drugs and by the illegal use of alcohol and tobacco. ONDCP's mission is to coordinate Federal drug control agencies to achieve the goals outlined in this *Strategy* and to oversee agency activities towards this end. This entails assessing the *Strategy* and its supporting programs and activities. Additionally, ONDCP is required to submit annual progress reports to Congress.

Under the current paradigm, ONDCP evaluates the annual performance of Federal Drug Control Agencies by drawing on existing agency data systems required by the Government Performance and Results Act (GPRA) and national studies and surveys such as Monitoring the Future and the National Survey on Drug Use and Health to inform the assessment of Federal drug control agencies., Additional information is also employed from budget justifications, program assessments, and internal management documents.

ONDCP continues to work with the Federal drug control agencies to develop tailored performance metrics that reflect their contributions to the Strategy. Because the measures focus on the unique contributions of each agency, the measures cover a wide range of activities and data.

ONDCP is currently establishing a Performance Reporting System (PRS) that will provide the agency timely and accurate data on the Federal drug control budget agencies and will help to inform policymaking, planning, resource allocation, and program effectiveness. ONDCP will report on progress towards achieving these goals in the 2011 and subsequent strategies and reports. The design and implementation of the PRS has commenced and will continue in FY 2011. The first step is to establish the PRS and subsequently to add new interagency measures, the lack of which was a shortcoming of the previous measurement system. This comprehensive system focuses not only on programs but also on Federal policies and activities.

An ambitious set of five year goals has been established in the *Strategy*. The PRS will identify second-tier performance measures and targets that support these overarching *Strategy* goals. The PRS will also identify agencies that contribute to each performance target. The system will establish with partner agencies, a process for collecting data and monitoring annual progress toward the outcomes that the Strategy is intends to achieve by 2015.

The system will be supported by a database that enables efficient reporting, analysis, and reporting of performance information in the PRS. This database will shorten the time required for agencies to provide information for documents such as the PRS Report and the Budget Summary. The PRS system will be assessed and refined as needed in fiscal years 2012 and 2013 – refinements include incorporating interagency performance targets for which data sources do not currently exist, identifying and rectifying gaps, and recalibrating metrics in response to new and emerging drug control threats.

II. Drug Control Funding Tables

Table 1. Federal Drug Control Spending by Function FY 2009 - FY 2011 (Budget Authority in Millions)

				10-11 Change	
	FY 2009 Final	FY 2010 Enacted	FY 2011 Request	Dollars	Percent
Function					
Treatment	3,561.9	3,745.5	3,882.5	136.9	3.7%
Percent	23.3%	24.9%	25.0%		
Prevention	1,854.7	1,514.3	1,717.7	203.3	13.4%
Percent	12.1%	10.1%	11.0%		
Domestic Law	3,869.4	3,843.5	3,917.3	73.8	1.9%
Percent	25.3%	25.6%	25.2%		
Interdiction	3,910.2	3,640.1	3,727.0	86.9	2.4%
Percent	25.6%	24.2%	24.0%		
International	2,082.2	2,288.0	2,308.1	20.1	0.9%
Percent	13.6%	15.2%	14.8%		
Total	$15,278.4	$15,031.5	$15,552.5	$521.1	3.5%
Supply/Demand					
Demand Reduction	5,416.6	5,259.9	5,600.2	340.3	6.5%
Percent	35.5%	35.0%	36.0%		
Supply Reduction	9,861.8	9,771.6	9,952.4	180.8	1.9%
Percent	64.5%	65.0%	64.0%		
Total	$15,278.4	$15,031.5	$15,552.5	$521.1	3.5%

Note: Detail may not add due to rounding.

Table 2. Federal Drug Control Spending by Agency (Budget Authority in Millions)

	FY2009 Final	**FY2010 Enacted**	**FY2011 Request**
Department of Defense	1,405.1	1,598.8	1,588.5
Department of Education	429.8	175.8	283.1
Department of Health and Human Services			
Centers of Medicare and Medicaid Services	215.0	430.0	400.0
Substance Abuse and Mental Health Services	2,494.1	2,557.4	2,688.2
National Institutes of Health - National Institute on Drug Abuse	1,293.6	1,059.4	1,094.1
Indian Health Service	91.5	96.0	103.1
Total, Health and Human Services	**4,094.2**	**4,142.8**	**4,285.4**

	FY2009 Final	FY2010 Enacted	FY2011 Request
Department of Homeland Security			
Customs and Border Protection	2,101.0	2,108.6	2,086.1
Immigration and Customs Enforcement	437.1	477.7	499.8
United States Coast Guard	1,096.9	1,162.3	1,208.1
Office of Counternarcotics Enforcement	3.7	3.6	3.9
Total, Homeland Security	**3,638.7**	**3,752.2**	**3,797.9**
Department of the Interior Bureau of Indian Affairs	6.3	10.0	10.0
Department of Justice			
Bureau of Prisons	79.2	87.6	93.5
Drug Enforcement Administration	2,203.5	2,271.5	2,421.9
Organized Crime Drug Enforcement Task Force Program	515.0	528.6	579.3
Office of Justice Programs	397.5	288.4	307.6
National Drug Intelligence Center	44.0	44.0	44.6
Total, Justice	**3,239.2**	**3,220.1**	**3,446.9**
Office of National Drug Control Policy			
Counterdrug Technology Assessment Center	3.0	5.0	0.0
High Intensity Drug Trafficking Areas	234.0	239.0	210.0
Other Federal Drug Control Programs	174.7	154.4	165.3
Salaries and Expenses	27.2	29.6	26.2
Total, Office of National Drug Control Policy	**438.9**	**428.0**	**401.4**
Department of State			
Bureau of International Narcotics and Law Enforcement Affairs	1,150.4	870.7	892.0
United States Agency for International Development	418.6	365.1	365.1
Total, State	**1,569.0**	**1,235.9**	**1,257.1**
Department of Transportation National Highway Traffic Safety Administration	2.7	2.7	2.7
Department of the Treasury Internal Revenue Service	60.6	59.2	60.3
Department of Veterans Affairs Veterans Health Administration	392.8	405.0	418.0
Small Business Administration	1.0	1.0	1.0
	15,278.4	**15,031.5**	**15,552.5**

Note: Detail may not add due to rounding.

Table 3. Historical Drug Control Funding by Function
FY 2002 –FY 2010
(Budget Authority in Millions)

FUNCTIONS	FY 2002 Final	FY 2003 Final	FY 2004 Final	FY 2005 Final	FY 2006 Final	FY 2007 Final	FY 2008 Final	FY 2009 Final	FY 2010 Enacted	FY 2011 Requested
Demand Reduction										
Drug Abuse Treatment	2,358.3	2,387.7	2,545.5	2,556.9	2,470.4	2,465.1	2,647.2	2,747.3	3,092.3	3,208.3
Treatment Research	547.8	611.4	607.2	621.2	600.3	600.8	608.0	814.7	653.2	674.2
Total Treatment	2,906.1	2,999.1	3,152.7	3,178.1	3,070.7	3,065.9	3,255.2	3,561.9	3,745.5	3,882.5
Drug Abuse Prevention	1,642.5	1,567.2	1,557.3	1,544.0	1,465.4	1,423.4	1,334.7	1,358.0	1,090.2	1,279.8
Prevention Research	367.4	382.9	412.4	422.0	411.5	413.4	415.6	496.7	424.1	437.9
Total Prevention	2,009.9	1,950.1	1,969.7	1,966.0	1,876.9	1,836.8	1,750.3	1,854.7	1,514.3	1,717.7
Total Demand Reduction	4,916.0	4,949.2	5,122.4	5,144.1	4,947.6	4,902.7	5,005.5	5,416.6	5,259.9	5,600.2
Percentage	45.6%	44.1%	42.7%	40.2%	37.6%	35.4%	37.7%	35.5%	35.0%	36.0%
Supply Reduction										
Domestic Law Enforcement	2,867.2	3,018.3	3,189.8	3,318.1	3,475.0	3,715.3	3,544.8	3,869.4	3,843.5	3,917.3
Interdiction	1,913.7	2,147.5	2,534.1	2,928.7	3,287.0	3,175.9	2,901.4	3,910.2	3,640.1	3,727.0
International	1,084.5	1,105.1	1,159.3	1,393.3	1,434.5	2,050.2	1,824.6	2,082.2	2,288.0	2,308.1
Total Supply Reduction	5,865.4	6,270.9	6,883.2	7,640.1	8,196.5	8,941.4	8,270.8	9,861.8	9,771.6	9,952.4
Percentage	54.4%	55.9%	57.3%	59.8%	62.4%	64.6%	62.3%	64.5%	65.0%	64.0%
TOTALS	10,781.4	11,220.1	12,005.6	12,784.2	13,144.1	13,844.1	13,276.3	15,278.4	15,031.5	15,552.5
Detail may not add due to rounding.										

III. Agency Budget Summaries

Department of Defense

Drug Interdiction and Counterdrug Activities

Resource Summary

	Budget Authority (in Millions)		
	FY 2009	FY 2010	FY 2011
Drug Resources by Function			
Intelligence	$195.780	$253.755	$272.092
Interdiction	388.618	327.621	329.227
International	417.489	647.500	656.145
Investigations	51.434	51.685	45.721
Prevention	135.024	134.610	132.567
Research & Development	54.442	25.728	28.338
State and Local Assistance	152.554	150.358	116.807
Treatment	9.800	7.572	7.454
Total Drug Resources by Function	**$1,405.141**	**$1,598.829**	**$1,588.351**
Drug Resources by Decision Unit			
Counternarcotics Central Transfer Account	$1,096.743	$1,158.226	$1,131.241
Supplemental/Overseas Contingency Operations	308.398	440.603	457.110
Total Drug Resources by Decision Unit	**$1,405.141**	**$1,598.829**	**$1,588.351**
Drug Resources Personnel Summary			
Total FTEs (direct only)	1,528	1,691	1,708
Drug Resources as a Percent of Budget			
Total Agency Budget (in Billions)	$659.0	$693.4	$708.3
Drug Resources Percentage	0.21%	0.23%	0.22%

Program Summary

Mission

The Department of Defense's Drug Interdiction and Counterdrug Activities authorities and resources provide a useful and flexible way to achieve national security goals. The threat to US national security posed by illicit drugs extends beyond traditional challenges to public health and safety. The drug trade is a powerful corrosive that weakens the rule of law in affected countries, preventing governments from effectively reducing or containing other transnational hazards, such as terrorism, insurgency, organized crime, weapons trafficking, money laundering, human trafficking, and piracy.

For the Department of Defense (DoD), the clear linkages between international narcotics trafficking and international terrorism constitute a threat to the national security interests of the United States. The global and regional terrorists who threaten United States interests can finance their activities with the proceeds from narcotics trafficking. The Department's

counternarcotics-funded resources and operations can detect, monitor and support the interdiction, disruption or curtailment of emerging narcotics-related threats to our national security. Counternarcotics resources and authorities are an effective combination that supports overseas contingency operations efforts.

Therefore, in accordance with its statutory authorities, DoD uses its counternarcotics resources and authorities as effectively and efficiently as possible to achieve national and Departmental counternarcotics priorities, focusing on two primary missions:

- Maintaining DoD readiness through drug demand reduction programs.
- Helping local, state, federal and foreign agencies address the drug trade and narcoterrorism, by detecting and monitoring drug trafficking, sharing information and helping countries to build their capacity and to control their ungoverned spaces.

The Office of Counternarcotics and Global Threats, with oversight from the Under Secretary of Defense for Policy, is the single focal point for DoD's counterdrug activities, and it ensures that DoD develops and implements a focused counternarcotics program with clear priorities and measured results. Consistent with applicable laws, authorities, regulations, and funding/resource availability, DoD will ensure that sufficient forces and resources are allocated to the counternarcotics mission to achieve high-impact results.

Budget

In FY 2011, the Department of Defense requests $1,588.4 million, which is a decrease of $10.5 million from the FY 2010 enacted level of $1,598.8 million.

Counternarcotics Central Transfer Account

Total FY 2011 Request: $1,588.4 Million
(Reflects $10.5 Million Decrease from FY 2010)

The Department of Defense resources are initially appropriated into the Central Transfer Account and later identified by program and project in order to be transferred out to the DoD service most appropriate for carrying out the prescribed mission. With this flexibility, the DoD counternarcotics program can address the ever-changing patterns in the narcotrafficking threats by shifting counterdrug resources where they will be most effectively used. Within the $1,588.4 million request is a FY 2011 Overseas Contingency Operations (OCO) request of $457.1 million.

The Department of Defense defines four mission areas that encompass the scope of their counternarcotics program. These mission areas are, (1) Demand Reduction; (2) Domestic Support; (3) Intelligence and Technology; and (4) International Support.

Demand Reduction

FY 2011 Request: $140.0 Million
(Reflects $2.2 Million Decrease from FY 2010)

The Department places emphasis on demand reduction through its random drug testing, anti-drug education and treatment programs. DoD has policies in place like drug testing for active duty military, National Guard and Reserve personnel and civilian personnel. The focus is to deter drug use by way of costeffective means, such as drug testing. The Department invests its demand reduction resources in critical areas like drug abuse prevention programs for military and civilian personnel as well as their dependents. An example of the DoD's commitment to demand reduction is evident in programs like the National Guard State Plans, which supports community based activities where National Guard volunteers assist community groups in providing drug prevention information and education.

FY 2011 Total Changes (-$2.2 Million)

This change from the prior year is largely a result of Congressional adjustments to the President's request for National Guard State Plans Outreach programs in FY 2010.

Domestic Support

FY 2011 Request: $213.8 Million
(Reflects $46.0 Million Decrease from FY 2010)

The FY 2010 enacted resources of $259.8 million finance DoD's domestic support operations. In FY 2011, the requested resources will fund National Guard State Plans that provide Federal, State and local law enforcement agencies' counternarcotics support with project management, communications, translation skills and counternarcotics related training. The Department will provide domestic operational support to both Domestic Drug Law Enforcement Agencies (DLEAs) and designated High Intensity Drug Trafficking Areas detection and monitoring activities conducted by the US Northern Command and with the Department's Title 10 counternarcotics authority provide critical support to lead Federal agencies to reduce the flow of drugs into the arrival zone.

DoD will continue to provide robust support along the southern border of the U.S. The Tethered Aerostat Program will provide dedicated radar surveillance capability for continued detection and monitoring of the U.S. Southwestern Border.

FY 2011 Total Changes ($46.0 million)

This decrease primarily reflects Congressional adjustments to the National Guard State Plans supply reduction and CN Schools programs in FY 2010.

Intelligence and Technology

FY 2011 Request: $237.4 Million
(Reflects $49.2 Million Increase from FY 2010)

The requested resources will provide for critical intelligence support to national policies designed to dismantle narcotics trafficking and international terrorist organizations benefiting from drug trafficking. The use of new technology continues to be instrumental in combating

narcoterrorist activities. Resources will allow DoD to continue to test, evaluate, develop and deploy technologies that are used to collect and survey suspect narcoterrorist smuggling operations in air, land, and sea. This request will provide for counternarcoterrorism intelligence support and analysis, as well as signal intelligence (SIGINT) collection and processing.

FY 2011 Total Changes (+$49.2 million)

This increase primarily reflects baseline and supplemental/OCO funding increases for intelligence operations in support of U.S. government CN efforts in Afghanistan.

International Support

FY 2011 Request: $997.1 Million
(Reflects $11.5 Million Decrease from FY 2010)

In FY 2011, DoD will continue with its counternarcotics mission to include targeting terrorist groups in regions where they benefit from illicit drug revenue or use drug smuggling systems. Resources will fund counternarcotics operations in these Areas of Responsibility (AOR), which includes training, regional planning assistance, operational planning support to partner nations and interagency partners, and equipment support. The requested resources will sustain detection and monitoring platforms and assets, and support AOR Command and Control support.

FY 2011 Total Changes ($11.5 million)

This decrease is primarily a result of the Congressional adjustment to support to Mexico in FY 2010. The FY 2011 budget will support the Central America Regional Initiative, a new initiative that includes an emphasis on Mexico's vulnerable southern drug "arrival zone", as well as continue to support CN efforts in Afghanistan.

Performance

Introduction

This section on the FY 2009 performance of the Department of Defense program is based on agency GPRA documents, and OMB review, and other agency information. The table includes performance measures, targets, and achievements for the latest year for which data are available. The Department is in the process of establishing performance measures for every major activity within the counternarcotics program.

In FY 2009, the Department of Defense continued to provide significant support to U.S. and partner nation drug law enforcement agencies in the areas of training, communications support, infrastructure, intelligence, transportation, equipment, command and control, and detection and monitoring. Additionally, the Department is committed to keeping drug use low among its active duty and civilian personnel. Selected examples of performance measures used to monitor its activities are provided in the following table.

In FY 2010 and FY 2011, the Department of Defense is working to refine the architecture of the performance metrics program so that it offers a basis for measurement along the dimensions of efficiency, capability and effectiveness. This architecture will provide an

understanding of how the counterdrug resources are supporting Federal, State, local, and tribal partner nation law enforcement entities to execute drug interdiction activities.

Department of Defense			
Selected Measures of Performance		FY 2009 Target	FY 2009 Achieved
Demand Reduction			
» Percentof active duty military personnel testing positive for drug use		under 2%	0.99%
Building Partner Capacity			
» Colombia: Number of basic rotary pilots trained and graduated		132	124
» Colombia: Number of COLAR helicopter mechanics trained and graduated		42	41
» Operational Readiness rate for COLAR rotary wing UH-60 FMF aircraft		75%	71%
» Operational Readiness rate for COLAF C-130 FMF aircraft		75%	33%
» Afghanistan/Central Asia: Number of persons trained		*	9,085
» Andean Ridge/Central America/Carribbean: Number of personnel trained		*	5,769
» Mexico: Number of personnel trained		*	441
» Pacific Region: Number of personnel trained		*	1,586
African Region: Number of personnel trained		*	1,632
» European Region: Number of personnel trained		*	342
Detection and Monitoring and Interdiction Support			
» Pounds of heroin seized with National Guard support		*	1,699
» Pounds marijuana seized with National Guard support		*	1,087,335
» Number of marijuana plants seized with National Guard support		*	9,115,748
» Pounds cocaine seized with National Guard support		*	537,904
» Number of tablets of ecstasy seized with National Guard support		*	2,169,894
» AWACS/E-3C (AEW)	Number of sorties	*	279
	Number of operational hours	*	2,771
» ROTHR	Number of tracks declared suspect	*	230
	Number of pounds seized	*	20,189
» E-2C (MPA,AEW/MPA)	Number of sorties	*	121
	Number of operational hours	*	491
	Number of pounds seized	*	23,074
» P-3C and P-3 CDU	Number of sorties	*	78
	Number of operational hours	*	703

Note: Defense has not established targets for support external to Defense.

Discussion

Demand Reduction

Defense is on track to keep the illicit drug positive rate below 2 percent. The actual active duty percent positive test rate for FY 2009 was .99 percent. Defense policy is to ensure 100 percent random urine drug testing for all active, reserve, National Guard, and civilians.

Sharing Information

DoD shares critical information and intelligence with U.S. Government Agencies, U.S. Law Enforcement and partner nations' forces in order to dismantle narcotics trafficking and international terrorist organizations benefiting from drug trafficking. Most of the collection and analysis is critical, unique and essential to the national and international efforts.

Building Partner Capacity

DoD provides training and equipment to partner nations worldwide to increase their capacity to conduct and sustain operations against narcotics trafficking, and related international terrorist organizations. Three prime examples are Afghanistan, Mexico and Colombia.

In ***Afghanistan***, the Department directly supports law enforcement interdiction efforts to build a sustainable Afghan capacity to deal with narcotics traffickers which threaten the establishment of stable Afghan institutions. This support includes specialized unit training and equipping of counternarcotics forces, providing training and operational bases and facilities, an organic aviation capacity and capability, and providing the linguist, information and analysis required for both interdiction operations and prosecutions.

In ***Mexico***, DoD's contribution has been in building the Mexican and Central American capacity to detect, monitor and interdict the drug threat before it arrives at the border. A significant effort has been providing flight training on Initial Entry Wing Helicopters.

In ***Colombia***, the Department of Defense continues to transition major programs of record to the Colombians. For example, the Ground Based Radars continue to provide critical aerial domain awareness for the Colombian Air Force. These systems coupled with their command and control tools and aircraft have curtailed aerial trafficking within Colombia. The Midnight Express boats provide an important interdiction capability for go-fast boats departing both the northern and western coasts of Colombia.

The Logistics Command and Control System will integrate Colombian National Police supply, maintenance, and communications networks used to defeat drug trafficking. JIATF-South continues to integrate the Colombian Military into all counterdrug operations within the departure zone of Colombia. Additionally, DoD funded Technical Assistance Field Training Teams (TAFT) continue their assistance in the training and readiness of both COLAR and COLAF helicopters and crews.

Within the United States, the National Guard supports the maintenance and management of four regional counternarcotics training centers. These training centers provide training for US regional law enforcement agencies.

Detection & Monitoring and Interdiction Support

Defense provides air and maritime assets in support of multi-agency counternarcotics detection and monitoring operations. These assets include aircraft, helicopters, naval ships,

patrol boats, and radars employed in concert with other assets from the U.S. Coast Guard (USCG) and Immigration and Customs Enforcement (ICE). Defense assets usually have USCG law enforcement detachments that actually conduct the lawful search and seizure of suspect narcotrafficking vessels. Defense also provides intelligence, analysis and communications support plus command and control for JIATFs South and West. In addition to the drug seizure results depicted in the table, National Guard support to law enforcement resulted in the confiscation of over 26,369 weapons, 35,383 vehicles, and $693.7 million of currency from illicit drug traffickers.

DEPARTMENT OF EDUCATION
OFFICE OF SAFE AND DRUG-FREE SCHOOLS

Resource Summary

	Budget Authority (in Millions)		
	FY 2009 Final	**FY 2010 Enacted**	**FY 2011 Request**
Drug Resources by Function			
Prevention	$429.837	$175.841	$283.095
Total Drug Resources by Function	**$429.837**	**$175.841**	**$283.095**
Drug Resources by Decision Unit			
Successful, Safe, and Healthy Students	0.000	0.000	283.095
State and Local Grants (non-add)	0.000	0.000	144.560
Safe Schools/Healthy Students (non-add)	0.000	0.000	77.816
Safe and Drug-Free Schools and Communities			
National Programs	135.078	175.841	0.000
Improving the Climate for Learning (non-add)	0.000	32.000	0.000
Safe Schools/Healthy Students (non-add)	77.816	77.816	0.000
Alcohol Abuse Reduction (non-add)	32.088	32.712	0.000
State Grant Program	294.759	0.000	0.000
Total Drug Resources by Decision Unit	**$429.837**	**$175.841**	**$283.095**
Drug Resources Personnel Summary			
Total FTEs (direct only)	0	0	0
Drug Resources as a Percent of Budget			
Total Agency Budget (in Billions)	$45.4	$46.2	$49.7
Drug Resources Percentage	0.95%	0.38%	0.57%

Note: Total agency budget reflects discretionary funds only, and for comparability across years excludes funds for Pell Grants, which were discretionary funds in FYs 2009 and 2010 and are proposed to be mandatory in FY 2011.

Program Summary

Mission

The Department of Education (Education) administers programs to help ensure that all students can meet challenging standards and to improve elementary and secondary education; special education and early intervention programs for children with disabilities; English language acquisition for limited English proficient and immigrant children; career, technical, and adult education; and higher education. In addition, Education carries out research, data collection, and civil rights enforcement activities. The programs funded under the Safe and Drug-Free Schools and Communities (SDFSC) Act and the proposed *Successful, Safe, and Healthy Students* program comprise the only Education operations included in the drug control budget.

The SDFSC program supports grants and discretionary activities to foster a safe, secure, and drug-free learning environment, facilitate emergency management and preparedness, and prevent student drug use and violence at all educational levels. The *Successful, Safe, and Healthy Students* program would consolidate several existing, narrowly targeted programs that seek to provide the environment that students need to succeed (including safe and drug-free schools, access to counseling and mental health services, and fostering a physically fit and healthy lifestyle). The SDFSC program supports (and the *Successful, Safe, and Healthy Students* program once enacted and funded would support) the prevention mission of the *National Drug Control Strategy.*

Budget

In FY 2011, Education requests $283.1 million for drug control activities, which is an increase of $107.3 million over the FY 2010 level, due primarily to the new *Successful, Safe, and Healthy Students* State and Local Grants.

Successful, Safe, and Healthy Students

Total FY 2011 Request: $283.1 Million
(Reflects $107.3 Million Increase from FY 2010)

This new program would support student achievement to high standards and help ensure that students are mentally and physically healthy and ready to learn, by strengthening efforts to: improve school climate by reducing drug use, violence, and harassment and by improving school safety; improve students' physical health and wellbeing through the use of, or provision of access to, comprehensive services that improve student nutrition, physical activity, and fitness; and improve students' mental health and well-being through the use of or provision of access to comprehensive services, such as counseling, health, and mental health services, social services, and innovative family engagement programs or supports. Excluded from the drug control budget are the following activities that have no clear drug control nexus: (1) school and college emergency preparedness initiatives; (2) Project SERV (School Emergency Response to Violence); and (3) continuation costs that would be subsumed under the proposed Successful, Safe, and Healthy Students program for projects originally funded under the Physical Education program and the Elementary and Secondary School Counseling program.

Successful, Safe, and Healthy Students State and Local Grants

FY 2011 Request: $144.6 Million
(Reflects $144.6 Million Increase from FY 2010)

Within the budget request for the Successful, Safe, and Healthy Students program, the Department would use $144.6 million to award grants to assist State educational agencies (SEAs), local educational agencies (LEAs), and partnerships between LEAs and nonprofit organizations or local governmental entities to develop and implement programs and activities that increase the extent to which schools are safe environments that support student achievement to high standards and help ensure that students are mentally and physically healthy and ready to learn.

FY 2011 Total Changes (+$144.6 Million)

The new program would increase the capacity of States, districts, and schools to create safe, healthy, and drug free environments in a comprehensive manner, so that students are able to focus on learning and teachers on teaching. Further, it would provide increased flexibility for States and districts to design strategies that best reflect the needs of their students and communities.

Successful, Safe, and Healthy Students: Safe Schools/Healthy Students

FY 2011 Request: $77.8 Million (Reflects No Change from FY 2010)

Within the budget request for the Successful, Safe, and Healthy Students program, $77.8 million is included for grant awards under the "Safe Schools/Healthy Students" initiative to support LEAs and communities in developing and implementing a comprehensive set of programs and services designed to prevent youth drug use and violence, support early childhood development activities, and provide needed student mental health services. Education funds this initiative jointly with the Department of Health and Human Services (HHS), and administers it in collaboration with both HHS and the Department of Justice To be eligible for Safe Schools/Healthy Students funding, an LEA must demonstrate agreement in the form of a partnership among the major community systems serving students – schools, the local public mental health authority, law enforcement, and juvenile justice – to work collaboratively in assessing needs and providing programs and services in the following five areas: (1) safe school environments and violence prevention; (2) alcohol, tobacco, and other drug prevention; (3) student behavioral, social, and emotional supports; (4) mental health services; and (5) early childhood social and emotional learning programs.

Successful, Safe, and Healthy Students: Other

FY 2011 Request: $60.6 Million
(Reflects $37.3 Million Decrease from FY 2010)

The budget request for the *Successful, Safe, and Healthy Students* program also includes funding for the following National Activities:

- $ 7.9 million to help institutions of higher education address such problems as under age, binge, and high risk drinking by students.
- $16.1 million for other activities that promote safe and healthy students such as research and development, developing and implementing school climate measurement systems and programs to improve school climate, data collection, dissemination, outreach, and other forms of technical and financial assistance to States, LEAs, community based organizations, and IHEs.
- $36.6 million for other continuation costs for grants originally awarded under the Safe and Drug Free Schools and Communities Program. Within the budget request for the *Successful, Safe, and Healthy Students* program, the Department would pay continuation awards for multi year grants for drug prevention projects funded originally under the Safe and Drug Free Schools and Communities program, as follows:
    - o $30.1 million for grants for projects to address and improve school climate,
    - o $6.5 million for grants to LEAs to develop and implement innovative and effective programs to reduce alcohol abuse in secondary schools.

Performance

Introduction

This section on the FY 2009 performance of the SDFSC program is based largely on agency GPRA documents and other information. The table includes performance measures, targets, and achievements for the latest year for which data are available.

Department of Education			
Selected Measures of Performance (National Grants)		FY 2009 Target	FY 2009 Achieved
Alcohol Abuse Reduction			
» Percentage of Alcohol Abuse Reduction grantees whose target students show measurable decrease in binge drinking	2007 cohort	76.9	47
	2008 cohort	61.5	50.7
» Percentage of Alcohol Abuse Reduction grantees showing measurable increase in percent of target students who believe alcohol abuse is harmful to their health	2007 cohort	86.5	76.5
	2008 cohort	69.2	58.6
» Percentage of Alcohol Abuse Reduction grantees that show measurable increase in percent of target students who disapprove of alcohol abuse	2007 cohort	86.5	47
	2008 cohort	69.2	49.3
Safe Schools/Healthy Students			
» Percentage of Safe Schools/Healthy Students grant sites that experience decrease in substance use during the 3-year grant period	2006 cohort	76.67	1
	2005 cohort	86.25	1
» Percentage of Safe Schools/Healthy Students grant sites that report a decrease in the percentage of their students who report current (30-day) marijuana use	2007 cohort	2	1
	2008 cohort	2	1
» Percentage of Safe Schools/Healthy Students grant sites that report a decrease in the percentage of their students who report current (30-day) alcohol use	2007 cohort	2	1
	2008 cohort	2	1

Department of Education			
Selected Measures of Performance (National Grants)		FY 2009 Target	FY 2009 Achieved
Student Drug Testing			
» Percentage of Student Drug Testing grantees experiencing 5% annual reduction in past-year drug use by student in target population served by grants » Percentage of Student Drug Testing grantees experiencing 5% annual reduction in past-month drug use by students in target population served by grants	2006 cohort	70	13
	2007 cohort	50	42
	2008 cohort	33	49
	2006 cohort	60	13
	2007 cohort	50	33
	2008 cohort	33	58

[1] 2009 data expected in mid-2010

[2] Target not established since two years of performance data are needed to establish the baseline for this cohort.

Discussion

For the SDFSC National Programs grant competitions, the Department has identified outcome measures and targets; however, 2009 grantee data have not yet been compiled for all of the measures.

Data are based primarily on analysis of grantee performance reports. It is difficult to pinpoint why performance results for the 2006 and 2007 cohorts fell short of their established targets. Possible explanations include turnover in leadership at the grantee level, variances in project design, and differences in cohort size and composition. Also, targets may have reflected baseline data from grantees most able to report results effectively and accurately.

The ***Safe Schools/Healthy Students*** initiative provides support to Local Educational Agencies (LEAs) for implementation of a comprehensive plan to create safe, disciplined, and drug-free environments that provide needed mental health services and support healthy development. Grantees collect and report data concerning rates of student drug use as one of the initiative's GPRA measures. Nearly 80 percent of sites in the 2006 grant cohort reported 2008 data for this GPRA measure and of those, two-thirds reported a reduction in student drug use.

The first evaluation of this program focused on the fiscal year 1999, 2000, and 2001 cohorts supported under the initiative, a total of 97 sites. Data from this evaluation identified statistically significant improvements in student outcomes related to alcohol, tobacco, and other drug use. For example, student self-report data for high school students reflected decreases in 30- day alcohol and tobacco use and cigarette sales on school property; those data also reflected increases in perceived disapproval of peer substance use. Current alcohol use was down 10 percent, and current tobacco use declined 13 percent. A second evaluation, focusing on fiscal year 2005 - 2007 cohorts, is expected to provide data later in 2010.

The ***School-Based Student Drug Testing*** program provides grants to local educational agencies and other entities to support development, implementation, or expansion of school-based student drug testing programs. The drug testing funded by these grants must be part of a comprehensive drug prevention program in the schools served by the grant and must provide for the referral to treatment or counseling of students identified as drug users. The

projects supported must also be consistent with recent Supreme Court decisions regarding student drug testing and ensure the confidentiality of testing results. GPRA data for the 2008 cohort of grantees indicate that during school year 2008-2009, 49 percent of grantees achieved a reduction of at least 5 percent in past-month drug use by students and that, during this same period, more than half of grantees (58 percent) reported they achieved a reduction of at least 5 percent in past-year drug use by students.

Some individual sites posted even more significant improvements in reported drug use in this timeframe after the student drug testing program was implemented. For example, 11 sites in the FY 2008 cohort reported reductions in past-month drug of 50 percent or greater. Twelve sites from this cohort also reported reducing past-year drug use rates by one-third or more.

The ***Grants to Reduce Alcohol Abuse*** program provides funds to LEAs to support the implementation of proven strategies designed to reduce the use and abuse of alcohol by secondary school students. Results for the 2008 cohort of grantees reported in 2009 annual performance reports reflect some successes during the first year of project implementation. About 50 percent of grantees cite measurable decreases in student binge drinking after one year of project implementation. Also among the 2008 cohort, an increased number of students in about 59 percent of grant sites believed that alcohol abuse was harmful to their health, while an increased number of students in nearly 50 percent of sites disapproved of alcohol abuse.

Some individual sites achieved particularly meaningful improvements. For example, the Gadsden City, Alabama Board of Education site reported cutting rates of binge drinking significantly (from about 38 percent down to about 15 percent, a 61 percent reduction), as well as increases of about 20 percent in the percentage of students who disapproved of alcohol abuse and 11 percent in the percentage of students who believed that alcohol abuse is harmful to their health.

The ***Grants to Prevent High-Risk Drinking among College Students*** competition provides funds to institutions of higher education or other eligible entities to prevent binge drinking by college students. The Department established as the GPRA measure for these grants, the percentage of grantees operating for two years that report a 5 percent decrease in high-risk drinking among students served. Grantees from the FY 2005 cohort have completed their projects and reported baseline and project-end data to the Department indicating that 81 percent of grantees experienced a 5 percent decrease in high-risk drinking.

In FY 2011, with the consolidation of programs into the newly proposed Successful, Safe, and Healthy Students, later this year the Department will be developing performance measures for the new program.

Department of Health and Human Services
Center for Medicaid and Medicare Management Services

Resource Summary

	Budget Authority (in Millions)		
	FY 2009 Estimate	FY 2010 Estimate	FY 2011 Estimate
Drug Resources by Function Treatment	215.000	430.000	400.000
Total Drug Resources by Function	$215.000	$430.000	$400.000
Total Drug Resources by Function	$215.000	$430.000	$400.000
Drug Resources by Decision Unit Grants to States for Medicaid[1]	215.000	430.000	400.000
Total Drug Resources by Decision Unit	$215.000	$430.000	$400.000
Total Drug Resources by Decision Unit	$215.000	$430.000	$400.000
Drug Resources Personnel Summary Total FTEs (direct only)	0	0	0
Drug Resources as a Percent of Budget Total Agency Budget (in Billions)	$657.1	$696.1	$763.3
Drug Resources Percentage	0.03%	0.06%	0.05%

[1] Only includes the estimated federal cost for certain screening and brief intervention services. Does not include Medicaid costs for the reimbursement of substance abuse treatment.

Program Summary

Mission

The Centers for Medicare & Medicaid Services' (CMS) mission is to ensure effective, up to-date health care coverage and to promote quality care for beneficiaries. Through its coverage of drug treatment services in the Medicaid programs, CMS helps support the goals of the Office of National Drug Control Policy (ONDCP) by continuing to meet the challenges of providing drug abuse treatment care to eligible Medicaid patients.

Methodology

CMS was designated as a National Drug Control Program Agency in 2007. As part of their responsibility, CMS must report the Federal contribution to Medicaid and in support of Substance abuse treatment. As an entitlement program run by the States, CMS reimburses States on their medical assistance expenditures. The above estimate is an actuarial estimate of the cost to the federal government of certain Substance abuse Medicaid reimbursable services. CMS has established two Healthcare Common Procedure Coding System (HCPCS) codes for alcohol and drug screening and brief intervention (SBI).

CMS provided estimates of Federal costs to support the HCPCS service codes when implemented by State Medicaid programs. Some States began to implement and provide Medicaid coverage for the new HCPCS codes during FY 2008. The amount of spending that would be captured by the use of these codes is dependent on the number and relative size of States which opt to cover these services. These actuarial cost estimates assume that approximately 17 States have elected to implement and provide coverage for these SBI reporting codes. State Medicaid programs determine their own reimbursement cost schedule.

- 10 percent effective participation rate;
- An average cost of $21.00 per each screening of a beneficiary;
- An average cost of $61.50 per each brief intervention; and
- 15 percent probability that a given screening will lead to an intervention.

Budget

In FY 2011, the CMS estimate is $400.0 million, which is a decrease of $30.0 million from the FY 2010 estimate.

Healthcare Common Procedure Coding System (HCPCS) Codes

Total FY 2011 Request: $400.0 Million
(Reflects $30.0 Million Decrease from FY 2010)

Medicaid is a means-tested health care entitlement programs with costs shared by both States and the Federal government. States have considerable flexibility in structuring their Medicaid programs. At the request of ONDCP, CMS introduced two new Healthcare Common Procedure Coding System (HCPCS) codes on January 1, 2007 that facilitate Medicaid payment for screening and brief intervention services. This supports national public health initiatives, including the Screening, Brief Intervention and Referral to Treatment (SBIRT) Initiative, targeting those with nondependent substance use and provides effective strategies for intervention prior to the need for more extensive or specialized treatment. These codes are available for health care providers and States to use, though there is no requirement to do so.

The first code, H0049, is for alcohol and/or drug screening, a preventative service. It is generally accomplished using a brief questionnaire concerning a patient's alcohol or drug use and can be carried out in various settings, e.g., a physician's office or a hospital emergency room. The second code, H0050, covers a brief intervention that generally occurs right after the screening. It is a 15- to 30-minute brief counseling session with a health professional intended to help motivate the beneficiary to develop a plan to moderate their alcohol or drug use.

FY 2011 Total Changes (-$30.0 million): The estimated decrease in FY 2011 is primarily due to the December 2010 expiration of the temporary Federal Assistance Percentage (FMAP) increase that enacted in the American Recovery and Reinvestment Act of 2009 (ARRA). ARRA authorized an estimated $85.4 billion in additional federal funding for States, in the form of a temporary increase in the share of expenditures the Federal government contributes toward Medicaid and Title IV-E programs. This increase has the effect of increasing the federal budget estimates for Medicaid reimbursement of certain drug

screening services in FY 2009 and 2010, However, since the temporary increase in the federal share of expenditures expires in December 2010, this results in a decrease in the estimate in FY 2011.

Performance

ONDCP will be working with CMS regarding performance measurement requirements as part of the development of the Performance Reporting System required by the ONDCP reauthorization.

DEPARTMENT OF HEALTH AND HUMAN SERVICES

Substance Abuse and Mental Health Services Administration

Resource Summary

Budget Authority (in Millions)			
	FY 2009 Final	FY 2010 Enacted	FY 2011 Request
Drug Resources by Function			
Prevention	$578.747	$584.316	$613.932
Treatment	$1,915.320	$1,973.060	$2,074.308
Total Drug Resources by Function	$2,494.067	$2,557.376	$2,688.240
Drug Resources by Decision Unit and Function:[1]			
Programs of Regional and National Significance			
Prevention	$201.003	$202.209	$225.075
SPF-SIG (non-add)	(110.374)	(111.777)	(103.511)
Prevention Prepared Communities (non-add)	(0.000)	(0.000)	(22.600)
Treatment	$412.342	$452.629	$501.878
ATR (non-add)[2]	(98.954)	(98.954)	(108.854)
SBIRT (non-add)	(28.972)	(29.106)	(41.106)
Treatment Drug Courts (non-add)	(23.925)	(43.882)	(56.438)
Ex-Offender Re-Entry (non-add)	(10.092)	(18.200)	(23.200)
Treatment Systems for Homeless (non-add)	(42.879)	(42.750)	(58.556)
Prescription Drug Monitoring Program (NASPER)	$2.000	$2.000	$2.000
HRSA Behavioral Health Grants/Federal Health Care Systems[3]	$0.000	$0.000	$25.000
Substance Abuse Prevention and Treatment Block Grant [4]	$1,778.591	$1,798.591	$1,798.591
Program Management [5]	$100.131	$101.947	$135.696
Total Drug Resources by Decision Unit	$2,494.067	$2,557.376	$2,688.240
Drug Resources Personnel Summary			
Total FTEs (direct only)	528	549	553

(Continued).

Budget Authority (in Millions)			
	FY 2009 Final	FY 2010 Enacted	FY 2011 Request
Drug Resources as a Percent of Budget			
Total Agency Budget (in Billions)	$3.5	$3.6	$3.7
Drug Resources Percentage	71.9%	71.8%	73.2%

[1] Includes both Budget Authority and PHS Evaluation funds. PHS Evaluation Fund levels are as follows: $110.5 million in FY 2009 Actual; $110.5 million in FY 2010 Enacted; and $111.2 million in the FY 2011 Request.

[2] Includes PHS evaluation funds for ATR in the amount of $1.4 million in FY 2009.

[3] The $25 million in HRSA funding is included in the SAMHSA table because HRSA is not yet designated as a National Drug Control Agency.

[4] Consistent with ONDCP guidance, the entire Substance Abuse Block Grant, including funds expended for activities related to alcohol, is included in the Drug Budget. The Block Grant is distributed 20% to prevention and 80% to treatment.

[5] Consistent with ONDCP guidance, all SAMHSA Program Management funding is included. Program Management is distributed 20% to prevention and 80% to treatment.

Program Summary

Mission

The Substance Abuse and Mental Health Services Administration's (SAMHSA) mission is to build resilience and facilitate recovery for people with, or at risk for, substance abuse and mental illness. SAMHSA supports the *President's National Drug Control Strategy* through a broad range of programs focusing on prevention and treatment of drug use. Major programs include the Substance Abuse Prevention and Treatment (SAPT) Block Grant, competitive grant Programs of Regional and National Significance (PRNS), and a Prescription Drug Monitoring program (NASPER). These programs are administered through SAMHSA's Center's for Substance Abuse Prevention (CSAP) and Substance Abuse Treatment (CSAT).

Methodology

SAMHSA distributes drug control funding into two functions, prevention and treatment. Included in prevention are SAMHSA/CSAP funds supporting Programs of Regional and National Significance (PRNS), 20% of the Substance Abuse Prevention and Treatment Block Grant (SAPTBG) funds, and 20% of SAMHSA Program Management funds. Included in treatment are SAMHSA/CSAT funds supporting Programs of Regional and National Significance (PRNS), 80% of the Substance Abuse Prevention and Treatment Block Grant (SAPTBG) funds, 80% of SAMHSA Program Management funds, and all funding that supports the Prescription Drug Monitoring Program (NASPER). In addition, in FY 2011, $25.0 million in Health Resources and Services Administration (HRSA) funding has been included in the SAMHSA Drug Budget display because HRSA is not designated as a national drug control agency.

Budget

In FY 2011, SAMHSA requests a total of $2,688.2 million for drug control activities, which is an increase of $130.9 million over the FY 2010 level. The Budget directs resources to activities that have demonstrated improved health outcomes and that increase service capacity. SAMHSA has five major drug-related decision units: Substance Abuse Prevention PRNS, Substance Abuse Treatment PRNS, Prescription Drug Monitoring, the Substance Abuse Prevention and Treatment Block Grant, and Program Management. Each decision unit is discussed below:

Programs of Regional and National Significance – Prevention

Total FY 2011 Request: $225.1 Million
(Reflects $22.9 Million Increase from FY 2010)

CSAP PRNS programs are organized into two categories: 1) Capacity, and 2) Science and Service. Several important drug-related programs within these categories are detailed below.

Prevention Capacity Activities

Capacity activities include service programs, which provide funding to implement service improvement using proven evidence-based approaches, and infrastructure programs, which identify and implement needed systems changes. A major drug-related program included in this category is the Strategic Prevention Framework (formerly named Strategic Prevention Framework State Incentive Grants).

Strategic Prevention Framework (SPF)

FY 2011 Request: $103.5 Million
(Reflects $8.3 Million Decrease from FY 2010)

The FY 2010 resources of $111.8 million for SPF will support 51 Strategic Prevention Framework-State Incentive Grants (SPF SIG) to states, tribes, and territories; 5 Partnerships for Success grants (State and Community Performance Initiative); 1 CADCA Leadership grant; and several contracts. CSAP's SPF SIG uses a public health approach that supports the delivery of effective programs, policies and practices to prevent substance use disorders. It is an approach that can be embraced by multiple agencies and levels of government that share common goals. It emphasizes developing community coalitions; assessing problems, resources, risk and protective factors; developing capacity in states and communities; implementing evidencedbased programs with fidelity; and monitoring, evaluating, and sustaining those programs. The Partnerships for Success program builds on the success of the SPF SIG program and adds an incentive for grantees that meet state-wide substance abuse prevention targets. The decreased funding in the FY 2011 Budget will still allow continued funding of 35 SPF SIGs (16 will come to a natural end) as well as 5 continuation and 10 new Partnership for Success grants.

Prevention Prepared Communities

FY 2011 Request: $22.6 Million (Reflects $22.6 Million Increase from FY 2010)

The Prevention Prepared Communities program will assist communities in developing community prevention systems offering evidence-based prevention of substance abuse and mental illness across the course of childhood and adolescence in multiple community venues. The program builds on scientific evidence that a) a common set of risk factors is predictive of a range of negative outcomes, such as academic failure (including school dropout), aggression, violence, delinquency, and substance use; b) mental, emotional, and behavioral problems tend to co-occur; c) some experiences early in development are highly predictive of later positive and negative outcomes; d) intervening early and throughout childhood and adolescence can reduce risk factors and change children's trajectories in a positive fashion; and e) shared community environments can play an influential role in supporting healthy behaviors. The FY 2011 President's Budget request is $22.6 million, all of which is new for FY 2011. Of the total amount, $15 million will support approximately 30 grants to communities, $5.6 million will support a contract to enhance State capacity to develop and support communities through community prevention specialists, and $2.0 million will support a contract for evaluation.

Other Prevention Capacity Programs

FY 2011 Request: $60.9 Million
(Reflects $2.9 Million Decrease from FY 2010)

The FY 2010 Budget includes resources of $63.8 million for existing Mandatory Drug Testing programs, the Center for Substance Abuse Prevention/Minority AIDS grants (SAP/MAI), STOP Act, Performance Management (formerly named Data Coordination and Consolidation Center), and Congressional projects. The FY 2011 level would maintain current contracts, supports 123 HIV/AIDS prevention grants as well as 101 continuation and 20 new STOP Act grants. The reduced funding level reflects discontinuation of one-time Congressional projects.

Prevention Science and Service Activities

Science and Service Activities promote the identification and increase the availability of practices thought to have the potential for broad service improvement. A major drug-related program included in this category is the National Registry of Evidence-based Programs and Practices.

National Registry of Evidence-based Programs and Practices

FY 2011 Request: $0.7 Million (Reflects No Change from FY 2010)

The FY 2010 resources of $0.7 million will support the National Registry of Evidence-based Programs and Practices (NREPP). This includes both prevention and treatment. NREPP is a system designed to support informed decision making and to disseminate timely and reliable information about interventions that prevent and/or treat mental and substance use disorders. The NREPP system allows users to access descriptive information about interventions, as well as peer-reviewed ratings of outcome-specific evidence across several

dimensions. NREPP provides information to a range of audiences, including service providers, policy makers, program planners, purchasers, consumers, and researchers. The NREPP website provides an array of descriptive information on all reviewed interventions, as well as quantitative ratings (on zero to four scales) for two important dimensions strength of evidence, and readiness for dissemination. In addition, the website also has the capacity to generate customized searches on one or multiple factors including specific types of outcomes, types of research designs, intervention costs, populations and/or settings, as well as the two quantitative dimensions (strength of evidence and readiness for dissemination).

Other Prevention Science and Service Programs

FY 2011 Request: $25.7 Million
(Reflects $0.2 Million Decrease from FY 2010)

The FY 2010 Budget provides resources of $25.9 million in support of the Fetal Alcohol Spectrum Disorder program; the Center for the Application of Prevention Technologies; the SAMHSA Health Information Network; Science and Service Program Coordination (formerly named Best Practices Program Coordination); and Minority Fellowship program. The FY 2011 budget continues all of these programs.

Programs of Regional and National Significance – Treatment

Total FY 2011 Request: $501.9 Million
(Reflects $49.2 Million Increase from FY 2010)

CSAT PRNS programs are also organized into two categories: 1) Capacity, and 2) Science and Service. Several important drug related programs within these categories are detailed below.

Treatment Capacity Activities

As stated above, capacity activities include services programs, which provide funding to implement service improvement using proven evidence based approaches, and infrastructure programs, which identify and implement needed systems changes. Key activities included in this category are: Access to Recovery (ATR); Screening, Brief Intervention, Referral, and Treatment (SBIRT) activities; Treatment Drug Courts; Ex Offender Re Entry program; and Treatment Systems for Homeless.

Access to Recovery

FY 2011 Request: $108.9 Million
(Reflects $9.9 Million Increase from FY 2010)

FY 2010 resources for ATR reflect $99.0 million to support a new Request for Applications (RFA) for a third cohort (approximately 30 new grants). The new RFA expanded ATR to a 4 year program. ATR is designed to: (1) allow recovery to be pursued through personal choice and many pathways; (2) require grantees to manage performance based outcomes that demonstrate client successes; and, (3) expand capacity by increasing the number and types of providers who deliver clinical treatment and/or recovery support services. The program is administered through State Governor's Offices, recognized Tribal Organizations, or through the Single State Authority overseeing substance abuse activities.

ATR uses vouchers, coupled with state flexibility and executive discretion, to offer an opportunity to create positive change in substance abuse treatment and recovery service delivery across the Nation. FY 2011 funding will fully support the second year of the third cohort of grantees and will provide funding to support the award of 4 new ATR grants.

Screening, Brief Intervention and Referral to Treatment Activities

FY 2011 Request: $41.1 Million
(Reflects $12.0 Million Increase from FY 2010)

Substance abuse is one of our Nation's most significant public health challenges, and the SBIRT approach can intervene early in the disease process before individuals become dependent and/or addicted, and can motivate the addicted to pursue a referral to treatment. Since the beginning of this program, almost one million individuals have been screened, and of those screened, 23% required a brief intervention, brief treatment, or referral to a specialty substance abuse treatment program. The FY 2010 resources of $29.1 million, supported continuation of eight State SBIRT grants, and continuation of eleven grants supporting SBIRT training in selected Medical Residency programs. The FY 2011 Budget will fully fund continuation of four State grants (four State grants end in FY 2010) and the eleven Medical Residency programs. In addition, in FY 2011, CSAT will fund a new $15.0 million initiative that adds a mental health screening component to a new cohort of SBIRT grantees. Also in FY 2011, $3.0 million will be used to develop a pilot project based on the Physician Clinical Support System model to extend SBIRT training and general substance abuse treatment information and clinical decision making support to physicians and other healthcare professionals.

Treatment Drug Courts

FY 2011 Request: $56.4 Million
(Reflects $12.6 Million Increase from FY 2010)

Drug courts are problem solving courts which help reduce recidivism and substance abuse among offenders and increase an offender's likelihood of successful rehabilitation through early, continuous, and intense judicially supervised treatment, mandatory periodic drug testing, community supervision, and appropriate sanctions and other habilitation services. FY 2010 resources of $43.9 million will provide continuation funding for 64 adult drug courts and 3 juvenile drug courts, and funding for new awards that are anticipated in FY 2010 for 8 adult treatment drug courts, 8 juvenile treatment drug courts, and 13 family dependency treatment drug courts which will focus on children who are victims of substance abuse/methamphetamine use in families that may also have concurrent involvement in the criminal justice system. In addition, a new collaborative effort in FY 2010 between SAMHSA/CSAT and the Department of Justice will result in funding approximately 31 new adult treatment drug court grants jointly with the DOJ/Office of Justice Programs/Bureau of Justice Assistance (OJP/BJA), and 3 new juvenile treatment drug court grants jointly with DOJ/Office of Juvenile Justice and Delinquency Prevention. The FY 2011 Budget will provide continuation funding for 44 adult treatment drug courts (20 adult drug courts end in FY 2010), 3 juvenile treatment drug courts, and will support continuation of all the new treatment drug courts jointly funded with DOJ elements in FY 2010. Also, the FY 2011

Budget will provide sufficient increased funding for award of approximately 45 new treatment drug courts; however, the split among adult/juvenile/family courts has not yet been determined.

Ex Offender ReEntry Program

FY 2011 Request: $23.2 Million
(Reflects $5.0 Million Increase from FY 2010)

SAMHSA recognizes the need to continue efforts to return and reintegrate offenders back into the community by providing substance abuse treatment and other related re entry services while also ensuring public safety for the community and family. The ex offender re entry grants provide screening, assessment and comprehensive treatment and recovery support services to offenders reentering the community, as well as offenders who are currently on or being released from probation or parole. The FY 2010 Budget of $18.2 million supports continuation of 24 grants and award of approximately 20 grants for a new ex offender re entry cohort. To further address this population in FY 2011, an increase of $5.0 million will support a new (third) cohort of ex offender reentry grants that will provide substance abuse treatment and recovery support services to adult and juvenile offenders returning to society from incarceration. Approximately 12 new grants are expected to be awarded.

Treatment Systems for Homeless Programs

FY 2011 Request: $58.6 Million
(Reflects $15.8 Million Increase from FY 2010)

SAMHSA/CSAT manages two grant portfolios under its Grants for the Benefit of Homeless Individuals (GBHI) program, both of which provide focused services to individuals with a substance use disorder or who have co occurring disorders. Through a recovery and public health oriented system of care, grantees are encouraged to address gender, age, race, ethnicity, sexual orientation, disability status, veteran's status, and criminal justice status as these issues relate to both substance use disorder services and co occurring disorder services for homeless individuals. The FY 2010 Budget reflects resources of $42.8 million to support continuation of 72 grants and for a new cohort of approximately 23 new grants. The FY 2010 GBHI portfolio includes services in supportive housing (SSH) grants that seek to expand and strengthen treatment services for clients already in housing that is permanent, affordable, and linked to health, employment, and other support services. This approach combines long term, community based housing assistance with intensive individualized treatment and recovery support services. In FY 2011, in addition to continuing a robust portfolio of GBHI/SSH grants, a new $8.4 million Homeless Initiative Program will be announced. The Homeless Initiative Program is a robust collaboration with the Department of Housing and Urban Development. This collaboration will combine health, behavioral health, and other support services to move and maintain chronically homeless individuals with mental and substance us disorders into permanent housing.

Other Treatment Capacity Programs

FY 2011 Request: $187.6 Million
(Reflects $5.2 Million Decrease from FY 2010)

The FY 2010 Budget includes resources of $192.8 million for several other Treatment Capacity programs including: the Minority AIDS Initiative; Opioid Treatment Programs and Regulatory Activities; Children and Families; Pregnant and PostPartum Women; Services Accountability; and TCEGeneral, as well as others. The FY 2011 Budget includes funds for continuing grants and contracts in the various programs, reflects discontinuation of onetime Congressional projects, and includes $6.0 million in funds for a new Performance Contracting Program, funded within the TCEGeneral program line, which will enable SAMHSA to offer competitive grants to State or Tribal authorities. Grant funding will be used to enhance overall drug treatment quality by incentivizing treatment providers to achieve specific performance targets. Examples of grant awards could include supplements for treatment providers who are able to connect higher proportions of detoxified patients with continuing recovery oriented treatment; or for outpatient providers who are able to successfully retain greater proportions of patients in active treatment participation for longer time periods.

Treatment Science and Service Activities

As stated in the Prevention section above, Science and Service Activities promote the identification and increase the availability of practices thought to have the potential for broad service improvement. A major drug related program included in this category is the Addiction Technology Transfer Centers (ATTCs).

Treatment Science and Service

FY 2011 Request: $26.1 Million (Reflects $0.9 Decrease from FY 2010)

The FY 2010 Budget includes resources of $27.0 million for Treatment Science and Service programs including: the National Registry of EvidenceBased Programs and Practices (as described in the Prevention section); the SAMHSA Health Information Network (a jointly funded effort by all SAMHSA Centers); and the Addiction Technology Transfer Center (ATTC) initiative (a network of fourteen regional activities and a National ATTC Office that support training and technology transfer activities and promotion of workforce development in the addiction treatment field), among others. The FY 2011 budget continues all of these programs at the same funding level as FY 2010.

Prescription Drug Monitoring Program

Total FY 2011 Request: $2.0 Million (Reflects No Change from FY 2010)

Although the latest SAMHSA survey reported a reduction in prescription drug abuse, it continues to be a significant public health problem, with 6.2 million people over the age of 12 indicating current nonmedical use of pain relievers, tranquilizers, sedatives, and stimulants (National Survey on Drug Use and Health, 2008). Under provisions of the National All Schedules Prescription Electronic Reporting Act of 2005 ("NASPER" P.L. 109 60), SAMHSA/CSAT was provided $2.0 million in FY 2010 to award formula grants to eligible States to foster establishment or enhancement of State administered controlled substance

monitoring systems, ensuring that health care providers and law enforcement officials have access to accurate, timely prescription history information. (In FY 2009, the first year funding was appropriated for this program, the thirteen States that applied were all awarded NASPER grants.) The expansion and establishment of prescription monitoring systems has the potential for assisting in early identification of patients at risk for addiction, and early identification will lead to enhanced substance abuse treatment interventions. The FY 2011 Budget continues NASPER at the same level as FY 2010.

Enhancing Substance Abuse Care in Federal Health Care Systems

Total FY 2011 Request: $25.0 Million
(Reflects $25.0 Million Increase from FY 2010)

The FY 2011 request includes $25 million to expand the integration of behavioral health into existing primary health care systems, which will enhance the availability and quality of addiction care provided by Health Centers. This will be accomplished by adding qualified and trained behavioral health counselors and other addiction specialists in HRSA supported Health Centers. HRSA will collaborate with the Department of Veterans Affairs and the Substance Abuse Mental Health Services Administration by utilizing each respective agency's technical assistance expertise. This initiative will include training on performing Screening, Brief Intervention and Referral to Treatment (SBIRT) to the health counselors and other addiction specialists.

Substance Abuse Prevention and Treatment (SAPT) Block Grant

Total FY 2011 Request: $1,798.6 Million (Reflects No Change from FY 2010)

The overall goal of the SAPT Block Grant is to support and expand substance abuse prevention and treatment services, while providing maximum flexibility to states. States and territories may expend their funds only for the purpose of planning, carrying out, and evaluating activities related to these services. States may provide SAPT Block Grant funds to community and faith-based organizations to provide services. Of the amounts appropriated for the SAPT Block Grant, 95 percent are distributed to states through a formula prescribed by the authorizing legislation. Factors used to calculate the allotments include total personal income; state population data by age groups (total population data for territories); total taxable resources; and a cost of services index factor. Remaining funds are used for data collection, technical assistance, and program evaluation, which are retained by SAMHSA for these purposes. The set-aside is distributed among CSAP, CSAT, and the SAMHSA Office of Applied Studies for purposes of carrying out the functions prescribed by the SAPT Block Grant legislation. The FY 2010 resources of $1.799 billion will provide grant awards to 60 jurisdictions: states, territories, the District of Columbia, and the Red Lake Band of Chippewa Indians in Minnesota. These resources will support approximately 2 million treatment episodes. The SAPT Block Grant program in FY 2011 is funded at the same level as FY 2010, and will provide support to the current 60 jurisdictions for a similar level of prevention and treatment services.

Program Management

Total FY 2011 Request: $135.7 Million
(Reflects $33.7 Million Increase from FY 2010)

The FY 2010 resources of $102.0 million support staffing and activities to administer SAMHSA programs. Program Management supports the majority of SAMHSA staff who plan, direct, and administer agency programs and who provide technical assistance and program guidance to states, mental health and substance abuse professionals, clients, and the general public. In addition, Program Management includes funding for a portion of the survey activities conducted by the SAMHSA Office of Applied Studies (OAS). Agency staffing represents a critical component of the budget. There are currently 57 members of the SAMHSA staff who provide direct state technical assistance and are funded through the 5% Block Grant set-asides. Program Management also includes: contracts for block grant investigations (monitoring); support for the Unified Financial Management System (UFMS); administrative activities such as Human Resources, Information Technology, and centralized services provided by the Program Support Center and the Department of Health and Human Services. The FY 2011 Budget reflects increased funding for current OAS National Surveys and for a new OAS initiative to design, develop, and field-test a community-level early warning system to detect emergence of new drug threats and to assist in identifying the public health and public safety consequences of drug abuse. SAMHSA/OAS will be working closely and collaboratively with NIDA, NIAAA, and ONDCP on all development and deployment aspects of this system.

Performance

Introduction

This section on the FY 2009 performance of SAMHSA programs is based on agency GPRA documents, OMB assessments, and other agency information. The tables include performance measures, targets, and achievements for the latest year for which data are available.

The Substance Abuse Treatment Programs of Regional and National Significance (PRNS) were reviewed in 2002 with a rating of “Adequate.” In 2003, the Substance Abuse Prevention and Treatment Block Grant Program was given a rating of “Ineffective.” The Substance Abuse Prevention PRNS was rated “Moderately Effective” in 2004 as was the Access to Recovery Program in 2007 and Adult and Juvenile Drug Courts in 2008.

Over the past several years, SAMHSA, in collaboration with the states, has identified a set of standardized National Outcome Measures (NOMs) that are monitored across all SAMHSA programs. The NOMs have been identified for both treatment and prevention programs, as have common methodologies for data collection and analysis.

SAMHSA continues to implement online data collection and reporting systems for mental health, substance abuse prevention and treatment programs, and has assisted states in developing their data infrastructures. Efficiency measures have also been implemented for all programs.

SUBSTANCE ABUSE PREVENTION AND TREATMENT BLOCK GRANT (SAPTBG)

SAPT Block Grant - Treatment Activities		
Selected Measures of Performance	FY 2009 Target	FY 2009 Achieved
Percent clients reporting abstinence from drug use at discharge	69.3%	TBR -- Nov. 2010
Number of admissions to substance abuse treatment programs receiving public funding	1,881,515	TBR -- Nov. 2011

Discussion

SAMHSA has established a data-driven block grant mechanism which monitors the National Outcome Measures (NOMs) and improves data collection, analysis, and utilization. Data for the treatment NOMs are drawn from a combination of sources, including the Web Block Grant Application System (WEBBGAS). A major milestone was reached when the reporting of NOMs was made mandatory in the FY 2008 SAPT Block Grant Application..

In 2005, the CSAT and CSAP funded an Independent Evaluation of the Substance Abuse Prevention and Treatment Block Grant (SAPT BG) Program. The evaluation was completed in December of 2008. The purpose of the evaluation was to assess the extent to which the SAPT BG Program is effective, functioning as intended, and achieving desired outcomes.

The evaluation resulted in a number of key findings, which include: a demonstrated positive effect on the health and lives of substance abuse treatment clients; the SAPTBG as a major impetus for improving State prevention and treatment systems' infrastructure and capacity; States' ability to leverage SAPTBG requirements, resources, and Federal guidance to sustain and improve their systems; demonstration of effective federal and state management of the program; and a contribution to the development and maintenance of successful State collaborations with other agencies and stakeholders concerned with preventing and treating substance abuse.

Data on FY 2009 achievements are not yet available. For FY 2008, the Block Grant program exceeded the target (1,881,515) for the number of clients served: a total of 2,272,250 clients. At discharge, 78.2% of clients had abstained from alcohol, 73.7% had abstained from drug use (exceeding the 2008 target of 69%), 37.2% were employed, and 92% reported having no involvement with the criminal justice system.

SAPT Block Grant - 20% Prevention Set-Aside		
Selected Measures of Performance	FY 2009 Target	FY 2009 Achieved
» Percent of States showing an increase in State level estimates of survey respondents who rate the risk of substance abuse as moderate or great	45.1%	TBR August 2010
» Percent of States showing a decrease in State level estimates of survey respondents who report 30 day use of alcohol (age 12 20)[1]	51%	TBR August 2010
» Percent of States showing a decrease in State level estimates of survey respondents who report 30 day use of illicit drugs (age 12 17)[2]	52.9%	TBR August 2010

[1] Percent, ages 12 – 20, who report they have used alcohol in the last 30 days.

[2] Percent, ages 12 – 17, who report they have used illicit drugs in the last 30 days Note: SAPT state applications vary in years these data are collected.

Discussion

In previous years, populationbased measures taken from the National Survey on Drug Use and Health (NSDUH) have been used as proxy measures for the 20% setaside. Since they do not reflect change at a grantee level, they have been retired and replaced with separate measures reflecting the percentage of States improving, based on Statelevel estimates from the NSDUH. Baseline data for FY 2007 have been identified for these new measures and targets set for FY 20082012. The data used to determine the percent of States improving on each measure come from the NSDUH state estimates.

In 2009, the latest state estimates were found in the 2007 State estimates report. These data represent change from 2005/2006 and 2006/2007. Additionally, SAMHSA has changed its data reporting time periods. Previously, data were reported as a result for the following year. For example, results for 2008 reflected data collected in 2007. In order to achieve consistency across SAMHSA, reporting has been revised so that results reflect data actually collected in that year.

States are placing an increased emphasis on applying the strategic prevention framework (SPF) to the use of SAPT funds. For example, 58 States and Territories now require that their SAPT funded programs use the SPF or the equivalent for conducting needs assessments, 57 for building State capacity, 59 for planning, 45 for program implementation, and 42 for evaluation efforts. The strategic plans developed by local SAPT funded communities implementing the SPF model ensures that they will identify populations with the greatest need for evidencebased prevention programs, practices and policies, that resources are maximized and targeted where most needed, and that outcomes will be achieved through a datadriven process. This SPF provides States with the necessary tools to better monitor the statewide performance of their local SAPT funded programs.

States are providing details about how SPF implementations are enhancing their infrastructure. In Nebraska, the Federation of Families for Children's Mental Health sponsors events to increase awareness of children/adolescents experiencing mental health challenges. Using a behavioral health approach, these familyaffiliated peer support nonprofit organizations have expanded their role in preventing substance abuse with the youth and families they serve. In order to support parental sobriety, increase family stability and provide prevention/intervention activities and resources to parents and their children, they offer family peer support through State and local contracts mainly to substance abusing parents whose children are in the Welfare system.

Data on FY 2009 achievements are not yet available. For FY 2008, the 20% Prevention SetAside program exceeded the target (17,482,060) for the number of participants reached/served by prevention programs, practices and strategies for a total of 70,647,674. It is important to note that many prevention approaches are population rather than individualbased and include duplicate counts.

The percent of States showing an increase in Statelevel estimates of survey respondents who rate the risk of substance abuse as moderate or great (age 1217) was 47.1%; the percentage of states that reported a decrease in 30day use of alcohol (age 1220) was 52.9%; and 64.7% of states reported a decrease in 30day use of other illicit drugs (age 1217).

Programs of Regional and National Significance (PRNS)

Treatment PRNS		
Selected Measures of Performance	FY 2009 Target	FY 2009 Achieved
» Percent of adult clients currently employed/engaged in productive activities	50%	44%
» Percent of adult clients with a permanent place to live	49%	44%
» Percent of adult clients with no involvement in the criminal justice system	94%	96%
» Percent of adult clients with no/reduced alcohol or illegal drug-related health, behavioral, or social consequences	65%	86%
» Percent adult clients with no past-month substance abuse	61%	66%
» Number of clients served[1]	31,659	32,939

[1] Total of all SAMHSA's CSAT Capacity programs excluding Access to Recovery and the Screening, Brief Intervention, Referral, and Treatment program.

Discussion

The Treatment PRNS provides funding to implement service improvements, using proven evidence-based approaches, system changes, and programs to promote identification and increase the availability of practices with potential for broad service improvement. The PRNS enables SAMHSA's CSAT to address emerging issues in the field. CSAT integrates data and performance into program and management decisions via, a real-time data reporting system. Staff routinely monitor grantees' progress to ensure that program goals and objectives are being met. In 2009, the PRNS programs exceeded their target (31,659) for the number of clients served – total number served was 32,939. The programs achieved an abstinence level of 66%, an employment level of 44%, a housing level of 44%, and a level of 96% for clients having no involvement with the criminal justice system at six-month follow-up.

Among the PRNS programs is the Screening, Brief Intervention, and Referral to Treatment program (SBIRT), implemented in 2003. In FY 2009, SBIRT provided over 180,000 substance abuse screenings in primary care and generalist settings.

The Access to Recovery program, implemented in 2005, is described below.

Discussion

The Access to Recovery (ATR) program provides grants to States, Tribes, and Tribal organizations to undertake voucher programs that expand substance abuse treatment capacity and promote choice among clinical treatment and recovery support providers.

In 2009, the ATR program substantially exceeded its target for the number of clients served: 89,595 clients as compared to the target of 65,000. In total, over 316,000 clients have been served since inception. Moreover, the program's achievements include a number of positive developments measured at the time of discharge: an abstinence level of 81%, an employment level of 49%, an improved social support level of 91%, and a level of 96% of clients having no involvement with the criminal justice system.

Access to Recovery		
Selected Measures of Performance	FY 2009 Target	FY 2009 Achieved
» Percentage of individuals receiving services who had no past month substance use	81%	81%
» Percentage of individuals receiving services who had improved family and living conditions	52%	47%
» Percentage of individuals receiving services who had no involvement with the criminal justice system	96%	96%
» Percentage of adults receiving services who had improved social support	90%	91%
» Percentage of individuals receiving services who are currently employed or engaged in productive	53%	49%
» Average cost per client through ATR	$1,588	$1,071
» Number of clients gaining access to treatment	65,000	89,595

Substance Abuse Drug Courts

Introduction

The data for the treatment completion measure is collected from clients upon discharge from the program. The other two measures are collected at 6 month follow-up. SAMHSA grantees are required to have an 80% followup rate at 6 months. As a result from time to time, data is reportable from one, but not the other.

Substance Abuse Drug Courts		
Selected Measures of Performance	FY 2009 Target	FY 2009 Achieved
» Percentage of juvenile clients receiving services who had a permanent place to live in the community	82%	79%
» Percentage of juvenile clients that complete treatment	75%	N/A[1]
» Percentage of juvenile clients receiving services who had no involvement with the criminal justice system	93%	92%

[1] The treatment completion measure for juveniles is collected upon discharge from treatment. Due to the small number of grantees during the FY 2009, this measure could not be calculated with any reliability.

Discussion

The Treatment Drug Court program provides funding to address the treatment needs of substance-using individuals involved in a Drug Court. The Program is designed to provide holistic treatment and wrap-around services to criminally-involved substance-using

individuals in order to assist them in achieving and maintaining abstinence from substance use along with improving their overall quality of life.

The Juvenile Drug Court Program demonstrated successful results in 2009, meeting or exceeding targets related to substance use, health and social consequences, employment, and criminal justice involvement. The Juvenile Drug Court Program did not meet its target for housing; however, SAMHSA considers this to be within acceptable range of the target set.

The Adult Drug Court Program is discussed in the Department of Justice – Office of Justice Programs section of the FY 2010 Budget Summary.

Prevention PRNS

Prevention PRNS		
Selected Measures of Performance	FY 2009 Target	FY 2009 Achieved
» Percent SPF SIG States with decrease in 30-day use of illicit drugs (age 12 -17)[1]	59.8%	TBR August 2010
» Percent SPF SIG States with increase in perception of risk from substance abuse (age 12 -17)	78.7%	TBR August 2010
» HIV: Percent of participants who rate the risk of substance abuse as moderate or great	76.6%	TBR August 2010
» HIV: Percent of participants who used illicit drugs at pre-test who report a decrease in 30-day use at post-test (age 18 and up)	70.6%	TBR August 2010

[1] SPF SIGs are Strategic Prevention Framework State Incentive Grants.

Discussion

The Prevention PRNS programs primarily focus on the Strategic Prevention Framework State Incentive Grants (SPF SIG) and the Minority Substance Abuse/HIV Prevention Initiative.

The SPF SIG takes a public health approach for the prevention of substance abuse by requiring a systematic, comprehensive, prevention process, first at the State and then at the community level. This State and community infrastructure and capacity building is expected to have stronger and longer lasting effects over time. SPF SIG grantees are required to go through multiple stages of the SPF process before they begin implementing services. These initial steps lead to a lag between the time the grants are awarded and community change is observable. State level percentages of use and non use are also affected by numerous factors external to prevention programs, such as state level demographic and socioeconomic changes.

Additionally, as in the SAPT, there is lag time in the availability of NSDUH data used to populate these measures. The data used to determine the percent of States improving on each measure come from the NSDUH state estimates. In 2009, the latest state estimates were found in the 2007 State estimates report. These data represent change from 2005/2006 and 2006/2007.

The goal of the HIV 6 cohort program is to increase the capacity of communities serving the target populations to deliver evidence based substance abuse prevention, HIV and hepatitis prevention services. This program was redesigned in FY 2007 to incorporate the Strategic Prevention Framework model.

Given these substantial program changes, we have established baselines for new measures, including pre/post 30 day use data on participants who have participated in

prevention interventions lasting at least 30 days. Each participant is followed up from program entry to program exit and to 3 to 6 months thereafter. FY 2009 actuals will be reported in August 2010 following the complete online submission of grantee data and review, correction, and analysis of data.

Data on FY 2009 achievements are not yet available. For FY 2008, the percent of SPF SIG states with a decrease in 30day use of illicit drugs (age 1217) was 67.6% (target: 61.5%), while 47.1% of States had an increase in the perception of risk from substance abuse (age 12 17) (target: 80.9%). In the HIV program, 90.1% of participants rated the risk of substance abuse as moderate or great (age 1217) (target: 75.8%), whilst 59.1% of the participants who used illicit drugs at pre-test reported a decrease in 30day use at posttest (age 18 and up) (target: 69.2%).

SAMHSA has changed its data reporting time periods. Previously, data were reported as a result for the following year. For example, results for 2008 reflected data collected in 2007. In order to achieve consistency across SAMHSA, reporting has been revised so that results reflect data actually collected in that year.

DEPARTMENT OF HEALTH AND HUMAN SERVICES

National Institute on Drug Abuse

Resource Summary

	Budget Authority (in Millions)		
	FY 2009 Final	FY 2010 Enacted	FY 2011 Request
Drug Resources by Function			
Prevention	493.984	421.428	435.204
Treatment	799.629	638.018	658.874
Total Drug Resources by Function	$1,293.613	$1,059.446	$1,094.078
Drug Resources by Decision Unit			
National Institute On Drug Abuse	1032.457	1059.446	1094.078
American Recovery and Reinvestment Act	261.156	0.000	0.000
Total Drug Resources by Decision Unit	$1,293.613	$1,059.446	$1,094.078
Drug Resources Personnel Summary			
Total FTEs (direct only)	394	392	410
Drug Resources as a Percent of Budget			
Total Agency Budget (in Billions)	$1,293.6	$1,059.4	$1,094.1
Drug Resources Percentage	100.00%	100.00%	100.00%

Program Summary

Mission

Over the past three decades, NIDAsupported research has revolutionized our understanding of addiction as a chronic, relapsing brain disease—knowledge that is helping to correctly situate addiction as a serious public health issue and to frame how we ultimately treat this disease. By supporting research that reveals how drugs affect the brain and behavior and how multiple factors influence drug abuse and its consequences, including HIV, NIDA is advancing effective strategies to prevent people from ever using drugs and to treat them when they cannot stop.

NIDA continues to carry out its mission "to lead the Nation in bringing the power of science to bear on drug abuse and addiction," which includes rapidly disseminating the results of our research to better prevent and treat this disease and its consequences.

Budget

In FY 2011, NIDA requests $1,094.1 million, which is an increase of $34.6 million from the FY 2010 enacted. NIDA's accelerating rate of discovery is beginning to spur the advent of better medications and behavioral interventions to counteract drug.induced changes in brain function. Among the strategies NIDA supports for medications development are those to: counter stress responses, which frequently trigger relapse to drug use; strengthen executive function and inhibitory control so that drug abusers can better control their urge to take drugs; and interfere with drug.conditioned memories to prevent relapse when drug abusers are exposed to environments or cues they associate with drug use.

Other research includes development of vaccines, or antibody.based approaches, which can block both illicit and licit drugs (e.g., nicotine) from ever reaching the brain, thereby inhibiting their rewarding effects. In the context of nicotine addiction, this approach may help prevent smokers from escalating to addiction and/or facilitate abstinence in those who seek to quit. It also complements ongoing efforts to discover new, more effective medications through conducting screens of novel compounds and chemical libraries and applying promising findings to help people achieve abstinence from tobacco and other addictive substances.

A steady flow of genetic discoveries is uncovering previously unsuspected genes whose products may be involved in the addiction process and therefore present good candidates for medications development. Such discoveries also herald the advent of more personalized interventions based on a patient's genetic profile. And, because genes influence both vulnerability and resilience to substance abuse and other mental disorders, genetic data will further our understanding of the basic mechanisms underlying the disease of addiction, as well as its frequently associated comorbid conditions.

But genes do not act in isolation; rather, they work in tandem with developmental and environmental factors to determine a person's drug abuse vulnerability. Therefore, NIDA is encouraging more research to understand how genes might mitigate or amplify social influences that affect individual choices and behaviors related to substance abuse. Conversely, environmental elements, such as parenting quality, home conditions, stress, diet, pollutants, and, of course, exposure to drugs of abuse, can regulate gene expression. Uncovering the mechanisms behind these so called *epigenetic* effects, offers a path to

alleviate and perhaps even override a genetic predisposition by adjusting environmental variables.

NIDA's HIV/AIDS research strategy addresses the critical need for improved treatment for drug abusers with HIV and for research designed to uncover the complex medical consequences of this disease, such as neuroAIDS. Initiatives in this area will help elucidate the effects of genetic variations on disease progression, and on how drugs of abuse and medications (for drug addiction and HIV) interact with both host and viral genes.

National Institute on Drug Abuse

Total FY 2010 Request: $1,094.4 Million (Reflects $34.6 Million Increase from FY 2010)

Basic and Clinical Neuroscience Research

FY 2011 Request: $519.5 Million
(Reflects $15.9 Million Increase from FY 2010)

Basic and Clinical neuroscience represent two programs in NIDA that work together to enlarge understanding of the neurobiological, genetic/epigenetic, and behavioral factors underlying drug abuse and addiction. Specifically, they examine the factors affecting increased risk and/or resilience to drug abuse, addiction, and drug.related disorders; the mechanisms of addiction; and the effects of drugs on the brain and behavior. Collectively, this research provides the fundamental information to develop and communicate prevention and treatment interventions for drug abuse and addiction.

FY 2011 Total Changes (+$15.9 million): In FY 2010, NIDA will pursue opportunities in line with our mission to study drug abuse and its consequences across the lifespan, from birth to youth to old age. Because adolescents are a key population of interest, an FY 2010 Request For Applications will award grants that integrate findings from research on brain development, cognition, and neuroscience into the creation of innovative and effective, drug abuse treatments targeted for youth. Results should enhance our understanding of adolescent neurodevelopment, including normal cognitive growth, executive function impairments stemming from drug abuse, and the specific thinking capacities that are necessary for treatments to be efficacious, thereby improving our ability to tailor treatments to individual needs and capabilities. Another RFA will support studies proposing to use deep sequencing technologies to identify the specific genetic variants that affect addiction risk in well. characterized drug abusing population samples. Genomewide association studies (GWAS) have identified genomic regions associated with addiction phenotypes, providing opportunities for further refinement using this deep sequencing approach.

Epidemiology, Services and Prevention Research

FY 2011 Request: $260.5 Million
(Reflects $8.0 Million Increase from FY 2010)

This major program area seeks to promote integrated approaches to understand and address the interactions between individuals and environments that contribute to the continuum of drug abuse.related problems. This NIDA division supports research and major data collection systems, as well as surveillance networks. Program efforts help identify

PREFACE

Substance abuse takes a terrible toll on the public health, public safety and financial resources of the United States. The Administration's national drug control policy seeks to reduce Americans' drug use and its related health, social and criminal problems. To help meet this goal, the Administration has developed five demand reduction priority areas. The Administration is requesting $151.3 million in new funding across the Federal government to strengthen efforts to detect and prevent and treat illicit drug use in our communities and break the cycle of illicit drug use, crime, and incarceration. This book provides an overview of the National Drug Control Strategy for fiscal year 2011 and an examination of issues for consideration in reauthorizing the Office of National Drug Control Policy.

Chapter 1- The Office of National Drug Control Policy (ONDCP) has the responsibility for creating policies, priorities, and objectives for the federal Drug Control Program. This national program is aimed at reducing the use, manufacturing, and trafficking of illicit drugs and the reduction of drug-related crime and violence and of drug-related health consequences. The Director of ONDCP has primary responsibilities of (1) developing a comprehensive National Drug Control Strategy (Strategy) to direct the nation's anti-drug efforts; (2) developing a National Drug Control Budget (Budget) to implement the National Drug Control Strategy, including determining the adequacy of the drug control budgets submitted by contributing Drug Control Program agencies; and (3) evaluating the effectiveness of the National Drug Control Strategy implementation by the various agencies contributing to the Drug Control Program. Authorization for ONDCP expired at the end of FY2010, but it has continued to receive appropriations. Congress, while continuously charged with ONDCP's oversight, is now faced with its possible reauthorization.

Chapter 2- The President's Fiscal Year (FY) 2011 National Drug Control Budget requests $15.5 billion to reduce drug use and its consequences in the United States. This represents an increase of $521.1 million (3.5 percent) over the FY 2010 enacted level of $15.0 billion. These resources are categorized around five major functions: (1) Substance Abuse Prevention, (2) Substance Abuse Treatment, (3) Domestic Law Enforcement, (4) Interdiction, and (5) International Support. Figure 1 details funding by function.

Substance abuse takes a terrible toll on the public health, public safety and financial resources of the United States. The Administration's national drug control policy seeks to reduce Americans' drug use and its related health, social and criminal problems. To help meet this goal, the Administration has developed five demand reduction priority areas. The

CONTENTS

For permission to use material from this book please contact us:
Telephone 631-231-7269; Fax 631-231-8175
Web Site: http://www.novapublishers.com

Library of Congress Cataloging-in-Publication Data

U.S. national drug control strategy / Editor, Benjamin F. Turner. p. cm..

Includes index. ISBN 978-1-61470-629-8 (hardcover) 1. United States. Office of National Drug Control Policy. 2. Drug control --United States. 3. Drug abuse - Government policy --United States. 4. Drug abuse --United States --Prevention. I. Turner, Benjamin F. HV5825 .U3 2011

362.29/15610973

2011025576

Published by Nova Science Publishers, Inc. † New York

DRUG TRANSIT AND DISTRIBUTION, INTERCEPTION AND CONTROL

U.S. NATIONAL DRUG CONTROL STRATEGY

Benjamin F. Turner
EDITOR

Nova Science Publishers, Inc.
New York

DRUG TRANSIT AND DISTRIBUTION, INTERCEPTION AND CONTROL

Additional books in this series can be found on Nova's website under the Series tab.

Additional E-books in this series can be found on Nova's website under the E-book tab.

U.S. NATIONAL DRUG CONTROL STRATEGY

Prevention – SRO-3.5

NIDA also contributes to NIH's scientific research goal of identifying and characterizing human candidate genes that influence risk for substance use disorders and risk of psychiatric disorders. NIDA researchers used genome wide analysis techniques in clinical and non clinical samples to identify or verify several genetic variants associated with nicotine dependence, including variants in the dopamine system. Separately, researchers identified or verified genetic markers that impact the efficacy of smoking cessation treatments. This includes linking a genotype that corresponds to slow metabolism of nicotine to light smoking behavior and higher smoking quit rates among African Americans.

NIDA Priorities for the American Recovery and Reinvestment Act (ARRA)

In FY 2009, NIDA received about $261million under the Recovery Act to speed the pace of research, provide jobs, and advance the science needed to address addiction and its related health consequences. NIDA has designated three Signature Areas as key subsets of this research: (i) eradicate tobacco addiction, (ii) genetic influence on the development and structure of the human brain, and (iii) research and development of anti-drug vaccines.

To address two of our signature areas, NIDA used ARRA funds to award a grant for development of a nicotine vaccine and move it closer to final FDA approval. The grantee has entered an agreement with another company to provide an additional $40 million to exclusively in license NicVAX on a worldwide basis and develop follow on, next generation nicotine vaccines.

The following highlight some key achievements in FY 2009:

Gene x environment research is unraveling the interwoven factors affecting addiction risk. A trio of recent studies on genetic vulnerabilities and environmental influences related to risk for behavioral problems, including substance abuse resulted in the following findings:

- prenatal tobacco exposure combined with a specific genetic variant places children at increased risk for antisocial behavior;
- family centered skill building curricula countered a genetic vulnerability to risk behaviors in preadolescence—the first time a rigorous prevention program has demonstrated this capability;
- parental monitoring, along with analyses of externalizing behaviors, show that high levels of the former could diminish the latter in those prone to these behaviors—who were also more likely to carry the genotype previously associated with increased risk of adult alcohol dependence.

Such studies further our understanding of how genetic influences interact with the environment and a host of other factors, such as gender and developmental stage.

NIDA is using the Web to broaden the delivery of effective treatments. Delivery of evidence based psychosocial interventions for drug abuse and HIV prevention via the web or other computer based media has the potential to increase cost effectiveness and provide a means for broader dissemination of proven treatments. Two recent studies demonstrate the feasibility and efficacy of this approach. One employed computer based training to reduce drug use by means of cognitive behavioral therapy (CBT)—an approach that teaches people to cope with stressful situations and anticipate and avoid triggers of maladaptive behaviors. The computer based CBT training had both short term and enduring effects in reducing drug use, an improvement over treatment as usual.

Positive Choice, a computer based intervention, was tested in HIV positive patients as a means of reducing risky behaviors that lead to HIV spread. While patients waited to see their provider, they were exposed to a "video doctor" that conducted a risk assessment and risk reduction counseling. This intervention was successful and sharply reduced sexual and drug risk behaviors in HIV positive patients. These delivery methods may increase the cost effectiveness of interventions, provide fidelity in treatment delivery, and lead to more widespread adoption of evidence based approaches.

Methadone treatment begun in prison decreases subsequent drug use and crime. NIDA supported a randomized clinical trial to examine the effectiveness of methadone maintenance treatment (MMT) provided to prisoners with pre incarceration heroin addiction. This trial demonstrated that, at 12 months following release, those who received MMT in prison were significantly more likely to enter and remain in community based treatment, and had fewer days of heroin use and criminal activity than participants who received counseling only.

NIDA is changing drug abuse research and practice in the U.S. NIDA's National Drug Abuse Clinical Trials Network (CTN) has fueled a cultural shift toward research based care for substance abuse treatment. For example, studies on buprenorphine, demonstrating its effectiveness in detoxification and maintenance treatment, have resulted in its greater acceptance and wider use by community treatment providers once skeptical of the use of a partial opiate agonist medication to treat opiate abuse. Studies showing the effectiveness of contingency management—providing low cost incentives for verified abstinence or continued treatment attendance—garnered acceptance from providers who previously did not accept a treatment model they viewed as rewarding people for what they should be doing anyway.

Finally, a 2009 study is dispelling the myth that substance abuse must be treated *before* providers can address a patient's posttraumatic stress disorder (PTSD). In fact, a study of women receiving an intervention for PTSD (Seeking Safety or health education control intervention) found that patients whose PTSD symptoms improved with treatment also showed subsequent improvements in substance use disorder symptoms. These findings provide needed data for programs addressing this common comorbidity, and suggest that abstinence from alcohol or drug use is not critical before trauma work can commence.

Program Summary

Mission

The Indian Health Service (IHS), an agency within the Department of Health and Human Services, is responsible for providing federal health services to American Indians and Alaska Natives. IHS supports substance abuse treatment and prevention services as part of this mission.

DEPARTMENT OF HEALTH AND HUMAN SERVICES

Indian Health Service

Resource Summary

Budget Authority (in Millions)			
	FY 2009 Final	FY 2010 Enacted	FY 2011 Request
Drug Resources by Function			
Prevention	18.139	18.771	19.208
Treatment	73.379	77.246	83.921
Budget Authority (in Millions)			
	FY 2009 Final	FY 2010 Enacted	FY 2011 Request
Total Drug Resources by Function	$91.518	$96.017	$103.130
Drug Resources by Decision Unit			
Alcohol and Substance Abuse	87.162	91.661	98.774
Urban Indian Health Program	4.356	4.356	4.356
Total Drug Resources by Decision Unit	$91.518	$96.017	$103.130
Drug Resources Personnel Summary			
Total FTEs (direct only)	168	171	174
Drug Resources as a Percent of Budget			
Total Agency Budget (in Billions)	$ 4.5	$ 5.0	$5.4
Drug Resources Percentage	2.03%	1.92%	1.93%

Methodology

The Indian Health Service (IHS) includes the appropriation for Alcohol and Substance Abuse (excluding the amount designated as Adult Alcohol Treatment) and the portion of Urban Indian Health Program (UIHP) funds for National Institute on Alcohol Abuse and Alcoholism programs transferred to the HIS under the UIHP budget.

Budget

In FY 2011, IHS requests $103.1 million for its drug control activities. This is $7.1 million above the FY 2010 Enacted level.

Alcohol and Substance Abuse

Total FY 2011 Request: $98.8 Million (Reflects $7.1 Million Increase from FY 2010)

In FY 2011, IHS will continue to serve American Indian and Alaska Natives impacted by methamphetamine abuse through its Youth Regional Treatment Centers and other federal and Tribally operated substance abuse treatment and prevention programs. IHS, through the Methamphetamine and Suicide Prevention Initiative (MSPI), provides Area allocations funding for pilot projects and federal grant awards 114 Area Tribal awardees, 11 Urban grantees, 3 Tribal Youth grantees, and one federally operated Youth Regional Treatment Center (YRTC) program award to establish evidence based or practice based methamphetamine and suicide prevention and intervention pilot projects. The award and grant recipients will participate on regular conference calls on methamphetamine and suicide prevention initiative. The goal of the group conference calls is to share evidence based and promising practices in methamphetamine and suicide prevention programs in American

Indian/Alaska Native communities. In addition, an annual meeting on methamphetamine and suicide interventions will be held to share evidence-based and practice based models.

FY 2011 Total Changes (+$7.1 million): The FY 2011 request includes $4.0 million to add qualified and trained behavioral health counselors and other addiction specialists in IHS supported facilities. IHS, in partnership with Indian Communities, will continue to collaborate with the Department of Veterans Affairs and the Department of Health and Human Services' Substance Abuse and Mental Health Services Administration by utilizing each agency's technical assistance expertise. IHS will also continue efforts to expand screening and brief intervention training for Indian health providers. The program will target sites with the greatest need for substance abuse services. The main goal of the grant program will be to enable I/T/Us to hire additional staff to provide evidence based and practice based culturally competent treatment services. All grant recipients will be required to report on appropriate performance measures, including mandatory reporting of the number of addicted patients that received services.

Urban Indian Health ProgramAlcohol and Substance Abuse Title V Grants

Total FY 2011 Request: $4.5 million (Reflects no change from FY 2010)

The FY 2011 budget estimate includes funds for the Urban Indian Health Program, a portion of which is provided in the form of federal grants to 34 urban Indian 501(c) 3 non profit organizations to carry out alcohol and substance abuse prevention and treatment activities in the communities served. All urban programs have active partnerships with their local Veteran's Health Administration programs and several have identified joint program alcohol and substance abuse initiatives.

FY 2011 Total Changes (no change): In FY 2011, IHS will continue to serve urban American Indians and Alaskan Natives impacted by alcohol and substance abuse through the Title V grant program, Alcohol and Substance Abuse Prevention and Treatment. Substance abuse prevention and education programs services address alcohol/drugs, suicide, selfesteem, injury control, domestic violence, and sexual abuse.

PERFORMANCE

Introduction

This section on the FY 2009 performance of the drug control portion of the IHS Alcohol and Substance Abuse Program is based on agency GPRA documents. The IHS Alcohol and Substance Abuse Program undertakes anti-drug abuse activities to raise community awareness and target high-risk groups in addition to educating staff on issues and skills related to substance abuse. In 2007, IHS' Tribally-Operated Health Program (TOHPs) including its drug control activities, were assessed in FY 2005 and received an assessment rating of "Adequate."

IHS Alcohol and Substance Abuse Program		
Selected Measures of Performance	FY 2009 Target	FY 2009 Achieved
» Alcohol-use screening among appropriate female patients	47%	52%
» Accreditation rate for Youth Regional Treatment Centers*	100%	91%

* In operation 18 months or more.

Discussion

The measures reported in the table indicate results from both Tribally-Operated Health Programs and Federally-Administered Health Programs. Currently, Tribally-Operated Health Programs have 17 measures, including alcohol- and health-related performance indicators.

The percent of appropriate female patients screened for alcohol-use (Fetal Alcohol Syndrome prevention) at Federally-operated facilities increased from 47% in FY 2008 to 52% in FY 2009, which is 5% over the target of 47%.

The accreditation measure – "Accreditation rate for Youth Regional Treatment Centers" – was not met in FY 2009. The FY 2010 and FY 2011 performance target will remain at 100% and the agency is confident that the target will be met.

DEPARTMENT OF HOMELAND SECURITY

U.S. Customs and Border Protection

Resource Summary

	Budget Authority (in Millions)		
	FY 2009 Actual	FY 2010 Enacted	FY 2011 Request
Drug Resources by Function			
Intelligence	$298.434	$335.702	$329.771
Interdiction	1,612.258	1,772.856	1,756.354
Total Drug Resources by Function	1,910.692	2,108.558	2,086.125
Drug Resources by Decision Unit			
Salaries & Expenses	$1,490.895	$1,640.715	$1,633.199
Border Security and Trade Facilitation at POEs (non-add)	[746.023]	[800.164]	[805.933]
Border Security and Control between POEs (non-add)	[399.617]	[449.830]	[456.888]
HQ Management and Administration (non-add)	[105.605]	[112.055]	[101.881]
Air & Marine Operations -Salaries (non-add)	[239.650]	[278.666]	[268.497]
Air & Marine Operations	419.797	467.843	452.926
Total Drug Resources by Decision Unit	$1,910.692	$2,108.558	$2,086.125
Drug Resources Personnel Summary			
Total FTEs (direct only)	8,407	10,315	10,268
Drug Resources as a Percent of Budget			
Total Agency Budget (in Billions)	$10.3	$10.1	$9.9
Drug Resources Percentage	18.62%	20.82%	21.05%

Program Summary

Mission

Titles 18 U.S.C. and 19 U.S.C. authorize U.S. Customs and Border Protection (CBP) to regulate the movement of carriers, persons, and commodities between the U.S. and other nations. It is through this statutory authority that CBP plays a key role in the overall anti-drug effort at the border. CBP's jurisdiction is triggered by the illegal movement of criminal funds, services, or merchandise across our national borders and is applied pursuant to the authority of the Bank Secrecy Act, "USA PATRIOT Act," Money Laundering Control Act, and other laws.

Methodology

Customs and Border Protection (CBP) is a multi-mission bureau, and calculates obligations, by budget decision unit and function, pursuant to an approved drug methodology. On the basis of past practice, five organizations within CBP, the Offices of: Border Patrol; Field Operations; Information Technology; Training and Development; and Air and Marine were provided with guidance on preparing estimates for the reporting of drug control funds. These offices were asked to estimate on the basis of their expert opinion; what portion of their activities is related to drug enforcement. All five organizations identified resources in their financial plans that support the drug enforcement mission of the agency. The Office of Information Technology, Office of Field Operations, and the Office of Air and Marine attribute their resources to both intelligence and interdiction functions; while the Office of Training and Development and the Office of Border Patrol attribute their resources solely to interdiction.

Office of Field Operations

The Office of Cargo Conveyance and Security/Non-Intrusive Inspection Division of the Office of Field Operations estimates that for FY 2011 there will be 3,941 CBP officer positions related to drug enforcement on Anti-Terrorism Contraband Enforcement Teams (A-TCET). CBP established these teams in 2003, uniting the former Contraband Enforcement Teams (CET), Manifest Review Units (MRU), Non-Intrusive Inspection, Canine, and Outbound teams to form a single A-TCET enforcement team. The A-TCET also works closely with the Passenger Enforcement Rover Team (PERT) and Passenger Analytical Unit (PAU) teams to coordinate all enforcement activities. Although the primary mission of A-TCET teams is anti-terrorism, they also focus on all types of contraband, including narcotics. CBP estimates that 69 percent of the A-TCET is devoted to drug enforcement. The smuggling methodologies and their indicators are similar for both narcotics and anti-terrorism activities.

Also for FY 2011, OFO estimates there will be a total of 448 Canine Enforcement Officers with assigned dogs. Among the dogs paired with an officer, 208 were Narcotics Detection Teams, 32 Currency Firearms Detection Teams and 208 Narcotics/Human Smuggling Detection Teams that were nearly 100 percent devoted to smuggling interdiction. Finally, in FY 2011 OFO expects to have an additional 16,226 CBP officers, who in addition to the interdiction of contraband and illegal drugs, enforce hundreds of laws and regulations of many other Federal government agencies. The other Federal Agencies include, for example, the U.S. Fish and Wildlife Service, the Bureau of Alcohol, Tobacco, Firearms and Explosives, and the Bureau of Export Administration among many others. CBP subject matter experts estimate that roughly 30 percent of these officers' time is devoted to drug related activities.

Office of Border Patrol

The Office of Border Patrol is responsible for controlling almost 6,000 miles of land borders between ports of entry with Canada and Mexico and nearly 2,700 miles of coastal waters surrounding the Florida Peninsula and Puerto Rico. There were 20,187 Border Patrol agents as of December 19, 2009, assigned to the mission of detecting and apprehending illegal entrants between the portsofentry. These illegal entries include aliens and drug smugglers, potential terrorists, wanted criminals, and persons seeking to avoid inspection at the designated ports of entry due to their undocumented status, thus preventing their illegal entry. It has been determined that 15 percent of the total agent time nationwide is related to drug activities. Of the 15% related to drug interdiction, 3.5% of these efforts are related to intelligence and 96.5% is related to drug interdiction. These activities include staffing 34 permanent border traffic checkpoints nationwide including 755 canine units trained in the detection of humans and certain illegal drugs that are concealed within cargo containers, truck trailers, passenger vehicles and boats. In addition, agents perform line watch functions in targeted border areas that are frequent entry points for the smuggling of drugs and people into the United States.

Office of Information Technology OIT

The Office of Information Technology (OIT) supports the drug enforcement mission through the acquisition, and support and maintenance of technology, such as nonintrusive inspection systems and mission critical targeting software systems. Of OIT's spending, 30 percent of base of the Enforcement Technology Center; 25 percent of Automated Targeting Systems (Passenger, Narcotics, and Anti-Terrorism) systems software costs, 50 percent of the TECS; and 10 percent of data center operations costs are estimated in support of the drug mission. OIT reduced their ONDCP resources by 10 percent cut due to the reductions they received to their base resources in the FY 2011 Presidents budget.

Office of Training Development

Office of Training Development (OTD) has revised its methodology for calculating the portion of their budget attributable to drug control funding. OTD issued a data call for all FY 2010 training courses to reassess if any items were related to drug enforcement material and activities, which are funded via the National Training Plan (NTP). The curriculum of each course was reviewed and subject matter experts determined course hours delivered related to drug enforcement for this tasking. If specific courses offered through the NTP contained drug enforcement related material, a specific percentage for that course was defined (hours related to drug enforcement training was divided by the total number of course hours). Specific training programs identified include the canine training programs and basic, specialized, and advanced training for CBP Officers. OTD's daytoday operational resources were attributed to drug enforcement activities at a rate of 20 percent. OTD evaluated each offices mission statement and training development/delivery functions to determine the total weighted percentage of its drug enforcement activities. In light of recent restructuring of OTD's programs such as anti-terrorism, development of national programs, career development, leadership, new course design/development, and succession management for the workforce;

there was an overall reduction of the percentage of operational budget related to drug enforcement FY 2009 to FY 2010 from 31 percent to 20 percent.

Office of Air & Marine

CBP Air and Marine's core competencies are air and marine interdiction, air and marine law enforcement, and air domain security. In this capacity, the Office of Air and Marine (OAM) targets the conveyances that illegally transport narcotics, arms, and aliens across our borders and in the Source, Transit and Arrival Zones. In support of source and transit zone interdiction operations, the Air and Marine P3 Program continues to program a minimum of 7,200 hours a year in support of Joint Interagency Task Force – South (JIATF S). Although OAM's P3 fleet continued its Service Life Extension Program (SLEP) and wing replacement program in FY 2009, the P3's flew over 7,700 flight hours. CBP OAM P3 is expected to meet flight hour commitments to JIATF South during FY 2011 and provide additional surveillance support along the northern border. Successful completion of the SLEP program will add 15,000 flight hours to the service life of the CBP OAM P3 fleet. The first set of wings was delivered in November 2009. Installation will begin immediately and the aircraft will be returned to service the 3rd quarter of 2010. The P3 fleet will continue to play a significant role in interdiction, law enforcement, and air domain security in source, transit and arrival zones through FY 2027.

Although 90 percent of the resources that support CBP Air and Marine are considered to be drug related, since September 11, 2001, Air and Marine has steadily increased its support to counterterrorism by developing a more cohesive and integrated response to national security needs as well as more emphasis on illegal immigration. Currently, Air and Marine is dedicating significant assets and personnel in support of Operation HALCON – a US/Mexico interdiction initiative, and support to the Office of Border Patrol in Southwest Border illegal alien intervention.

Budget

In FY 2011 the President's Budget requests $2,086.1 million in drug related resources, which is a decrease of $22.4 million from the FY 2010 enacted level. These resources support CBP as America's frontline border agency. CBP employs over 58,000 (48,000 from direct appropriations) highly trained personnel to not only prevent terrorists and terrorist weapons from entering the United States, but also to perform its missions, which include stemming the flow of illegal drugs and other contraband. CBP is determined to improve security at and between our ports of entry (POEs) along the entire length of land and maritime borders, and extend the zone of security beyond the physical borders.

Salaries and Expenses

Total FY 2011 Request: $1,633.2 Million
(Reflects $7.5 Million Decrease from FY 2010)

Salaries and Expenses funds CBP's primary field occupations including CBP officers, Border Patrol agents, pilots, marine officers, import and entry specialists, and agricultural specialists. The agency's field organization is comprised of 20 Border Patrol Sectors with 34 permanent border and 69 tactical checkpoints between the ports of entry; 142 stations and substations; and, 20 Field Operations Offices and 327 associated ports of entry, of which 15 are preclearance stations. Field personnel use a mix of air and marine assets, nonintrusive technology such as largescale xrays and radiation portal monitors, targeting systems, and automation to ensure the identification and apprehension of highrisk travelers and trade.

Border Security and Trade Facilitation at POEs

FY 2011 Request: $805.9 Million
(Reflects $5.8 Million Increase from FY 2010)

The FY 2011 drug budget resources of $805.9 million represents an overall increase of $5.8 million in drug enforcement funds from the FY 2010 Enacted Budget and will fund border security and trade facilitation at the ports of entry (POEs). CBP will use its resources to support aggressive border enforcement strategies that are designed to interdict and disrupt the flow of narcotics and ill-gotten gains across our Nation's borders and dismantle the related smuggling organizations. CBP narcotics interdiction strategies are designed to be flexible so that they can successfully counter the constantly shifting narcotics threat at, and between, the ports of entry.

CBP is intent on using resources to develop and implement security programs that safeguard legitimate trade from being used to smuggle the implements of terror and other contraband, including narcotics into the U.S. Under Customs-Trade Partnership Against Terrorism (C-TPAT), CBP works closely with importers, carriers, brokers, freight forwarders, and other industry sectors to develop a seamless, security-conscious trade environment resistant to the threat of international terrorism. CTPAT provides the business community and government a venue to exchange ideas, information, and best practices in an ongoing effort to create a secure supply chain, from the factory floor to U.S. ports of entry. Under C-TPAT, Americas Counter Smuggling Initiative (ACSI), the Carrier Initiative Program (CIP), and the Business Anti-Smuggling Coalition (BASC), partnership programs remain instrumental in expanding CBP's anti-narcotics security programs with trade groups and governments throughout the Caribbean, Central and South America and Mexico.

CBP has implemented a Field Operations Intelligence Program, which provides support to CBP inspection and border enforcement personnel in disrupting the flow of drugs through the collection and analysis of all source information and dissemination of intelligence to the appropriate components. In addition, CBP interdicts undeclared and bulk currency under 31 USC 5317 and 31 USC 5332, respectively, cutting off funds that fuel terrorism, narcotics trafficking, and criminal activities worldwide. CBP officers perform

Buckstop Operations, which involve screening outbound travelers and their personal effects. CBP also supports Cashnet Operations that focus on interdicting bulk currency exported in cargo shipments. CBP uses mobile X-ray vans and specially trained currency canine teams to target individuals, personal effects, conveyances and cargo acting as vehicles for the illicit export of undeclared currency.

FY 2011 Total Changes (+$5.8 million): CBP requests a total adjustment to base of $46.9 million and 389 FTEs for an increase to Customs and Border Protection Officers (CBPOs) in the Office of Field Operations. The adjustment to base will fund 318 CBPOs and 71 support positions. The proposed adjustment will allow CBP to maintain staffing for critical positions that had been funded from fee revenue supporting CBP's mission to protect the U.S. at its Ports of Entry from the infiltration of terrorists and other criminal elements into the country as well as efforts to address the illegal smuggling of drugs, money instruments, and aliens across our borders. Based on OFO's drug budget methodology, OFO estimates that 30% or $5.8 million of this adjustment to base would be drug related.

Border Security and Control between the POEs

FY 2011 Request: $ 456.9 Million
(Reflects $7.1 Million Increase from FY 2010)

The FY 2011 President's Budget request of $456.9 million fund border security and control between the POE's. The Border Patrol has primary responsibility for drug interdiction between the land ports-ofentry. In pursuit of drugs, Border Patrol agents engage in surveillance activities supported by computer-monitored electronic ground sensors. Traffic check operations are also conducted along major routes of travel to restrict access to the interior by drug and alien smugglers. Transportation centers are placed under surveillance for the same reason.

In addition, the Border Patrol canine program was implemented in 1986 in response to escalating alien and drug smuggling activities along the Mexican and Canadian borders. The canines are trained at the Border Patrol National Canine Facility in El Paso, Texas, to locate hidden persons, marijuana, heroin and cocaine. The canines are used in nearly every enforcement activity of the Border Patrol including line watch, traffic check operations, and train and bus checks. The canine program is responsible each year for the detection of record numbers of smuggled aliens and large narcotic loads, including the arrest of the criminals involved in smuggling activities.

The Border Patrol also participates in numerous interagency drug task force operations with other federal, state and local law enforcement agencies through Operation Alliance along the southern border. The Border Patrol is also an active participant in the southwest border HIDTA in Texas, New Mexico, Arizona and California. To further assist the Border Patrol in this endeavor, all Border Patrol agents receive Drug Enforcement Administration Title 21 cross-designated authority as part of their basic training.

FY 2011 Total Changes (+$7.1 million): The FY 2011 President's Budget request proposes a $7.1 million increase in the drug-related resources associated with border security and control between the POE's. The increase is the net of reductions to travel, premium pay and Border Patrol Agents amidst increasing the adjustment to base for the Journeyman pay level. Specifically, funding will largely be used to fund the increased salary and benefit requirements associated with the implementation of raising the journeyman grade level for the frontline Border Patrol Agents (BPAs) within CBP. The journeyman increase from the GS-11 to the GS-12 level will bring these agents on par with other federal law enforcement officers including other CBP law enforcement positions. The net increase from the journeymen pay raise was impacted by reduced employee travel costs, a reduction to premium pay as a result of a proposed change to the management of premium pay policy, and a reduction to Border Patrol agent staffing by 181 Border Patrol agents in FY 2011.

Headquarters Management and Administration

FY 2011 Request: $101.9 Million
(Reflects $10.2 Million Decrease from FY 2010)

The FY President's Budget 2011 request of $101.9 million provides critical policy and operational direction, mission support, and technical expertise to CBP mission operations. Headquarter and Management includes drug control budget dollars from the Office of Training and Development (OTD) and the Office of Information Technology (OIT). These programs are essential in carrying out CBP's dual mission of protecting our homeland while facilitating legitimate trade and travel.

FY 2011 Total Changes (-$10.2 million): The FY 2011 President's Budget requests a decrease of $10.2 million over FY 2010 Enacted level associated with Headquarters Management and Administration in support of in support of the OIT change in methodology to include a 10 percent decrease to their ONDCP resources due to the reductions they received to their base resources in the FY 2011 Presidents budget. OIT reduced the amount of funding available for contract support in a number of areas. The reductions will result in less direct support to the field and more centralized IT Help Desk support. OIT plans to mitigate the impacts by standardizing desktops servers and storage; consolidate and centralize management of desktops; virtualize services/workstations and circuit/bandwidth optimization. The Office of Training and Development service contracts and the National Training plan (NTP) will be reduced. The NTP reduction is a result of identified savings and a projected decrease in training requirements for basic students. This reduction is based on three areas of savings: (1) reduction in TDY instructors; (2) new development costs as this function is brought in-house; and (3) savings for student travel based on past spending trends. The reductions to OTD will be mitigated by the need for fewer classes for new Border Patrol agents, since there will not be the increased growth as there had been during previous years.

Air and Marine Operations Salaries

FY 2011 Request: $268.5 Million
(Reflects $10.2 Million Decrease from FY 2010)

CBP Air and Marine secures the borders against terrorists, acts of terrorism, drug smuggling and other illegal activity by operating air and marine branches at strategic locations along the borders. Multi-mission aircraft with advanced sensors and communications equipment provide powerful interdiction and mobility capabilities directly in support of detecting, identifying and interdicting suspect conveyances, and apprehending suspect terrorists and smugglers. CBP Air and Marine partners with numerous stakeholders in performing its missions throughout the continental United States and the Western Hemisphere. This includes domestic operations at the borders, source, transit and arrival zone operations, interior law enforcement support and support to other agencies. In fulfilling the priority mission of CBP to protect the borders, CBP Air and Marine's geographical Area's of Responsibility (AOR) are the southwest, northern and southeast/coastal border of the United States also to include the Caribbean regions.

FY 2011 Total Changes (-$10.2 million): The FY 2011 President's Budget requests a $10.2 million decrease in the drug-related resources associated with CBP's Air and Marine - Salaries. The programmatic decrease to Air and Marine Salaries is the result of not sustaining a FY 2010 Air personnel enhancement. OAM will not sustain approximately 120 positions received in FY 2010. OAM had planned to utilize those resources to continue the expansion of its aviation (including P-3 and UAS) capabilities across the southwest, northern and coastal borders and place heavy emphasis on the maritime requirements along the southeast/Caribbean borders. OAM maximizes the capabilities of air and marine assets through a cohesive joint air operations model for centralized command and control and a responsive and integrated control system for decentralized execution. OAM partners with numerous stakeholders in performing its missions throughout the continental United States and the Western Hemisphere. This includes domestic operations at the borders, source, transit and arrival zone operations, interior law enforcement support, and support to other agencies.

Air and Marine

Total FY 2011 Request: $452.9 Million
(Reflects $14.9 Million Decrease from FY 2010)

CBP Air and Marine's interdiction assets are deployed throughout the Western Hemisphere. The Air and Marine Operations Center in Riverside, California, provides command, control, communications, and intelligence for those assets by assimilating information from a wide array of sensors.

The President has authorized the Department of State (DOS) to continue assistance to Colombia in carrying out an "Airbridge Denial Program" against civil aircraft suspected of trafficking in illicit drugs. CBP Air and Marine P-3 aircraft supplement Department of Defense (DOD) aircraft to fly in and over Colombia in support of this Presidential Determination and Directive. The P-3 Airborne Early Warning (AEW) and slick aircraft are critical to interdiction operations in the source and transit zones because they provide vital radar coverage in regions where mountainous terrain, expansive jungles and large bodies of water limit the effectiveness of ground-based radar. Because the P-3 AEW is the only Detection and Monitoring (D&M) asset solely dedicated to the counter-drug mission, it is a critical component of the National Drug Control Strategy (NDCS).

In the Transit Zone, CBP Air and Marine crews work in conjunction with the law enforcement agencies and military forces of other nations in support of their counter-narcotic programs. CBP is prepared to support counterdrug missions in the Source Zone following a new Presidential Decision Directive granting authorization and completion of training with South American partner nation law enforcement agencies and military forces. Counterdrug missions include detection and monitoring, interceptor support, and coordinated training with military and other law enforcement personnel.

CBP Air and Marine aviation assets include: sensor-equipped, detection and monitoring jet interceptors, long-range trackers, and maritime patrol aircraft; high performance helicopters; and single/multi-engine support aircraft. CBP Air and Marine's range of maritime assets includes interceptor, utility and blue water-type vessels.

FY 2011 Total Changes (-$14.9 million): The President's Budget request includes a decrease of $14.9 million for Air and Marine Interdiction, Operations, Maintenance, and Procurement. The FY 2010 enacted level was $467.8 million and the FY 2011 President's Budget request is $452.9 million. The FY 2011 budget request includes a planned decrease of $17.3 million for P-3 SLEP which brings the total funding level to $47.7 million. These funds will continue the procurement of the new wing/tail assembly, the wing/tail refurbishment kits for aircraft that do not need new wings/tails, continue the special structural inspections (SSI) and extended special structural inspections (ESSI), and induct an additional P-3 platform into the SLEP program. From within base resources, OAM will continue the acquisition of up to eight AS-350 (Light Enforcement Helicopters). By the end of FY 2011, OAM will have acquired 39 of the 50 AS-350's under contract. Funding is provided for 1 MQ9 Maritime Variant (Guardian) Unmanned Aircraft System and for P-3 Sensor Upgrades, specifically 3 additional SeaVue maritime radars. The resources will allow CBP to convert one UH-60 Medium Lift Helicopter from an A (alpha) to L (lima) model and one UH-1 to UH-2 Utility Helicopter. Funding is also provided for various marine vessels, to include up to 6 additional coastal interceptors and additional riverine vessels.

PERFORMANCE

Introduction

This section on the U.S. Customs and Border Protection's (CBP) drug control program is based on agency GPRA documents, an OMB assessment, and other agency information.

The table includes performance measures, targets, and achievements for the latest year for which data are available.

The Office of Field Operations' (OFO) drug control efforts were included as part of 2005 OMB assessment of Border Security, Inspections, and Trade Facilitation (BSITF) at the Ports of Entry program. The program received an overall rating of "Effective." OFO drug control efforts were not separately assessed.

CBP Air and Marine (CBP A&M) drug efforts were also included as part of the FY 2006 OMB assessment of CBP Air and Marine program. The program received an overall rating of "Moderately Effective".

The Office of Border Patrol (OBP) drug efforts were included as part of the FY 2007 OMB of Border Security and Control between the Ports of Entry program. The program received an overall rating of "Moderately Effective."

The data below reflect the joint FY 2009 achievements of OFO, CBP A&M, and OPB.

Customs and Border Protection		
Selected Measures of Performance	FY 2009 Target	FY 2009 Achieved
» Inspection Narcotics Seizures - Cocaine (thousands of pounds)	NA	135,949
» Inspection Narcotics Seizures - Marijuana (thousands of pounds)	NA	4,330,327
»Inspection Narcotics Seizures - Heroin (thousands of pounds)	NA	2,011

Discussion

CBP is the largest uniformed, federal law enforcement agency in the country, with over 20,000 Border Patrol Agents between the ports of entry and more than 20,000 CBP officers stationed at air, land, and sea ports nationwide. These forces are supplemented with 1,165 Air and Marine agents, and 2,388 agricultural specialists and other professionals. FY 2009 was a record year for CBP, with data showing a significant increase in drug seizures. CBP seized more than 4 million pounds of drugs. Outbound currency seizures nationwide also increased 74 percent, surpassing $57.9 million. CBP's Office of Field Operations (OFO) completed its most successful drug enforcement year in the past five fiscal years, seizing nearly 1.5 million pounds of drugs at ports of entry – an increase of 53 percent for cocaine, 19 percent for marijuana and 11 percent for ephedrine.

Since the establishment of the Southwest Border Initiative, DHS has intensified its efforts with federal, state, local, and tribal authorities and the Government of Mexico to secure the southwest border. Results include a dramatic increase in outbound currency and inbound drug seizures. From late March to November 2009, CBP seized $22.1 million in outbound currency at land border ports of entry —an increase of 299 percent from the $5.5 million seized during the same period last year. In addition, CBP and the U.S. Immigration and Customs Enforcement (ICE) jointly seized 911,800 kilos of narcotics along the southwest border—an increase of 36 percent from the 670,800 kilos seized during the same period last year.

The table indicates the amounts of cocaine, marijuana, and heroin seized by Border Patrol Agents, CBP Officers, and CBP Air Interdiction Agents. These statistics were compiled using the CBP BorderStat system. The BorderStat system was developed and is maintained by the Office of Intelligence and Operations Coordination (OIOC). The system aggregates enforcement and operational statistical data from a wide-range of CBP component reporting systems, e.g. ENFORCE and SEACTS, and serves as the single statistical reporting mechanism for CBP. The ability to generate statistical reporting from disparate sources via a single user interface ensures consistency and enhances CBP operational/enforcement analytical efforts at all levels of the agency. The BorderStat system has accurate data for all operational offices for FY 2009.

In FY 2009, CBP seized a total of 135,949 pounds of cocaine, which is a 24% decrease from FY 2008; 4,330,327 pounds of marijuana, a 75% increase from FY 2008; and 2,011 pounds of heroin, which is an 8% decrease from FY 2008.

CBP is currently exploring counterdrug performance measures in addition to or in lieu of drug seizure statistics for FY2010 that would adequately reflect CBP's drug control activities.

DEPARTMENT OF HOMELAND SECURITY

Immigration and Customs Enforcement

Resource Summary

	Budget Authority (in Millions)		
	FY 2009 Final	FY 2010 Enacted	FY 2011 Request
Drug Resources by Function			
Intelligence	$6.286	$8.276	$8.426
International	4.687	4.289	4.320
Investigations	426.122	465.173	487.025
Total Drug Resources by Function	$437.095	$477.738	$499.771
Drug Resources by Decision Unit			
Immigration Enforcement	$437.095	$477.738	$499.771
Interagency Crime and Drug Enforcement [non-add]	[46.852]	[47.833]	[48.936]
Total Drug Resources by Decision Unit	$437.095	$477.738	$499.771
Drug Resources Personnel Summary			
Total FTEs (direct only)	2,282	2,480	2,592
Drug Resources as a Percent of Budget			
Total Agency Budget (in Billions)	$5.6	$5.5	$5.5
Drug Resources Percentage	7.8%	8.7%	9.1%

PROGRAM SUMMARY

Mission

U.S. Immigration and Customs Enforcement (ICE) uses aggressive border enforcement strategies to investigate and disrupt the flow of narcotics and ill.gotten gains across the Nation's borders, and dismantle related smuggling organizations. ICE achieves these objectives by maintaining an aggressive cadre of Title 21 cross.designated Special Agents and a multi.disciplined money laundering control program to investigate financial crimes and interdict bulk currency shipments exported out of the United States.

Methodology

ICE is a multi.mission bureau, and budget authority is reported pursuant to an approved drug methodology. ICE's methodology is based on investigative case hours recorded in the agency's automated Case Management System TECS (formerly known as Treasury Enforcement Communication System). ICE agents record the type of work they perform in this system. Following the close of the fiscal year, a report is run showing investigative case hours that are coded as general drug cases and money laundering drug cases. A second report is run showing all investigative case hours logged.

Separate calculations exist for ICE's three drug related components: Office of Investigations (OI), Office of International Affairs (OIA), and Office of Intelligence (Intelligence). OI and Intelligence derive a percentage by dividing the number of investigative case hours linked to drug control activities by the total number of investigative case hours. OIA represents the investigative hours recorded in TECS as full time equivalent (FTE) agents. OIA derives a percentage by dividing the number of FTE agents by the total number of overseas agents. In FY 2009, 28.2 percent of case hours were drug related for OI, 3.8 percent for OIA, and 11.85 percent for Intelligence.

The Intelligence Requirement Intake System IRIS tracks requests for intelligence work by customer. Requests originating from the Office of International Affairs are classified as inherently international and all other customer requests are classified as inherently domestic. In FY 2009, 5 percent of IRIS requests were international in nature.

Budget

The total drug control request for ICE for FY 2011 is $499.7 million, a net increase of $22.0 million from the FY 2010 enacted level. This level includes $22.0 million for three additional Border Enforcement Security Task forces (BEST) facilities and additional law enforcement investigative mission support staff. This initiative is intended to increase national security by expanding activities to control our borders.

Salaries and Expenses

Total FY 2011 Request: $499.8 Million
(Reflects $22.0 Million Increase from FY 2010)

The Salaries and Expenses account contribute to the ICE mission of bringing a unified and coordinated focus to the enforcement of Federal immigration and customs laws. Salaries and Expenses resources are used to address terrorism and illegal immigration through the investigation, detention, and prosecution of criminal and non criminal aliens, and domestic gangs. These activities protect the infrastructure and persons within the United States.

Investigative Activities

FY 2011 Request: $487.0 Million
(Reflects $21.9 Million Increase from FY 2010)

The FY 2011 request for the Office of Investigation's (OI) drug-related activities is $487.0 million. The requested resources will support investigative efforts; coordination with other Federal, State, local, and foreign law enforcement agencies; and through participation in task forces, such as the Organized Crime Drug Enforcement Task Force (OCDETF), the High Intensity Drug Trafficking Areas (HIDTA), Drug Enforcement Administration's (DEA) Special Operations Division (SOD) and Border Enforcement Security Task Force (BEST) initiative.

As a member of OCDETF, ICE has access to interagency information available through the OCDETF Fusion Center. This collaboration with other Fusion Center agencies, including the Federal Bureau of Investigation (FBI), the DEA and the Bureau of Alcohol, Tobacco, Firearms and Explosives (ATF), will enhance ICE's ability to develop target profiles and actionable investigative leads to disrupt and dismantle significant drug traffickers.

In further support of interagency collaboration, ICE will remain an active participant in the DEA-led SOD, an interagency coordination unit consisting of representatives from several federal agencies that include DEA, FBI, and the Internal Revenue Service. During ICE field investigations, ICE targets the command and control communication devices employed by criminal organizations operating across jurisdictional boundaries on a regional, national, and international level and coordinates this information among law enforcement agencies, foreign and domestic, to maximize efforts to disrupt and dismantle targeted organizations.

Implemented in FY 2006, the BEST initiative developed a comprehensive approach that identifies, disrupts, and dismantles criminal organizations posing significant threats to border security. The BEST teams incorporate personnel from ICE; U.S. Customs and Border Protection (CBP); DEA; ATF; FBI; the U.S. Coast Guard; and the U.S. Attorney's Office along with other key Federal, State, local and foreign law enforcement agencies.

As part of its investigative authorities, ICE will utilize the requested resources to fund operations that target the systems used by international criminal organizations to launder the proceeds of their criminal activities, such as the Cornerstone Initiative. Other examples of ICE's financial investigations are the Trade Transparency Unit (TTU) and Money Laundering Coordination Center, which provide the analytical infrastructure to support financial and trade investigations. The TTU provides the capability to identify and analyze complex trade-based money laundering systems and has the unique ability to analyze domestic trade and financial data in addition to the trade and financial data of foreign cooperating partners.

FY 2011 Total Changes (+$22.0 million): The OI FY 2011 request provides for the expansion of existing facilities and the creation of two new BEST facilities. These new teams will focus on all aspects of the enforcement process, from interdiction to prosecution and removal. The goal of the expansion is to strengthen the program's ability to dismantle the leadership and supporting infrastructure of the criminal organizations responsible for perpetrating violence and illegal activity along our borders and in the Nation's interior. The BEST program is a critical cornerstone of the Secure Border Initiative program. The request also funds an increase of investigative mission support staff in field offices nationwide to assist Special Agents performing criminal investigations.

Intelligence Activities

FY 2011 Request: $8.4 Million
(Reflects $0.1 Million Increase from FY 2010)

The FY 2011 request of $8.4 million will fund the Office of Intelligence (Intelligence) drug related operations. Intelligence collects, analyzes and shares strategic and tactical data with Federal, State, local and tribal law enforcement partners in an effort to disrupt the flow of drugs by collecting and analyzing all source information and disseminating strategic intelligence to the appropriate partner. ICE estimates that approximately 5 percent of Intelligence activities will be international in nature.

FY 2011 Total Changes (+$0.15 million): The FY 2011 request provides for additional analysis and support of DHS components' requests for strategic intelligence information and reports.

International Affairs Activities

FY 2011 Request: $4.3 Million (Reflects No Change from FY2010)

The FY 2011 resources of $4.3 million support the Office of International Affairs (OIA) drug-related operations. As the primary component of DHS international law enforcement operations, OIA is responsible for enhancing national security by conducting and coordinating international investigations involving transnational criminal organizations and serving as ICE's liaison to counterparts in local government and law enforcement. Based on a memorandum of understanding, all foreign narcotics investigations are coordinated with the Drug Enforcement Administration.

A part of the Strategy is to attack the vulnerabilities of drug trafficking organizations and disrupt key business sectors and weaken the economic basis of the drug trade. The illegal drug market in the U.S. is based on illegal narcotics grown or manufactured in foreign countries and smuggled across our nation's borders. ICE agents enforce a wide range of criminal statutes including Title 18 and Title 19 of the U.S. Code. These statutes address general smuggling issues as well as customs violations. ICE also enforces Title 21, which covers the importation, distribution, manufacture and possession of illegal narcotics.

FY 2011 Total Changes (no change): ICE will continue to conduct and coordinate international investigations involving transnational criminal organizations.

PERFORMANCE

Introduction

This section on the FY 2009 performance of the drug control mission of Immigration and Customs Enforcement (ICE) is based on agency GPRA documents and other agency information.

The ICE mandate to detect, disrupt and dismantle smuggling organizations supports ONDCP initiatives and U.S. drug control policy. Within their respective spheres of operation, the Investigations, International Affairs, and Intelligence divisions contribute to the Strategy's counterdrug efforts. Specifically, ICE efforts contribute to disrupting the market for illicit drugs and creating secure borders.

Immigration and Customs Enforcement		
Selected Measures of Performance	FY 2009 Target	FY 2009 Achieved
» Number of counterintelligence requests satisfied	86	1,969
» Percent of closed drug smuggling investigations that have an enforcement consequence (arrest, conviction, seizure, fine or penalty)	75.0%	74.3%

Discussion

As the primary investigative agency within the Department of Homeland Security (DHS), ICE's enforcement efforts directly impact DHS' ability to secure our borders, enforce immigration law, and stem illegal trafficking and related transnational crime. ICE targets its investigative resources on the illicit drug trade networks that exploit our nation's borders.

Dismantling criminal organizations that exploit vulnerabilities at our borders is a critical step to preventing organizations from leveraging criminal networks to weaken America's national security.

ICE participates in and dedicates resources to the Organized Crime Drug Enforcement Task Forces (OCDETF) investigations that target major drug smuggling organizations. For instance, ICE participates with DEA and FBI on Operation Panama Express (PANEX). PANEX is an OCDETF investigation targeting Colombian narcotrafficking organizations. These Colombian trafficking organizations are responsible for the importation to and distribution within the U.S. as well as Canada.

In FY 2009, the percentage of closed drug smuggling investigations that resulted in an enforcement consequence was 74.3%. An enforcement consequence includes arrests, indictments, convictions, seizures, fines and/or penalties. Investigations that result in an enforcement consequence increase deterrence and contribute to the elimination of vulnerabilities in various aspects of trade and immigration. ICE has broad authority to investigate international financial crime and money laundering. The dollar value of real or other property seized from drug operations was $94.2 million in FY 2009. In addition, ICE seized $155.3 million of currency and monetary instruments from drug operations. The seizure of currency and monetary instruments reduces the financial incentives for criminals.

In FY 2009, 1,969 counter-narcotics intelligence requests were satisfied out of 2,669 that were received. Examples of intelligence services include assessing drug trafficking patterns, identifying trends, and detecting methods employed by drug traffickers and organizations. Satisfying customer requirements allows customers to make informed decisions about executing law enforcement actions. The FY 2009 target was 86 counternarcotics requests satisfied. Since the baseline for this measure was established in the previous fiscal year, the Office of Intelligence is currently realigning the target for the annual number of intelligence requests satisfied. Consequently, the Office of Intelligence reset the target for FY 2010 at 1,200 for counternarcotics intelligence requests satisfied.

DEPARTMENT OF HOMELAND SECURITY

United States Coast Guard

Resource Summary

Budget Authority (in Millions)			
	FY 2009 Final	FY 2010 Enacted	FY 2011 Request
Drug Resources by Function			
Interdiction	$1,094.788	$1,157.852	$1,205.446
Research and Development	2.078	4.403	2.678
Total Drug Resources by Function	$1,096.866	$1,162.255	$1,208.124
Drug Resources by Decision Unit			
Acquisition, Construction and Improvements	$332.048	$365.473	$398.835

(Continued).

Budget Authority (in Millions)			
	FY 2009 Final	FY 2010 Enacted	FY 2011 Request
American Recovery and Reinvestment Act of 2009 [non-add] [1]	[12.778]	[0.000]	[0.000]
Operating Expenses	747.085	776.569	790.486
Research and Development	2.078	4.403	2.678
Reserve Training	15.655	15.810	16.125
Total Drug Resources by Decision Unit	$1,096.866	$1,162.255	$1,208.124
Drug Resources Personnel Summary			
Total FTEs (direct only)	5,967	6,099	6,119
Drug Resources as a Percent of Budget			
Total Agency Budget (in Billions)	$ 10.1	$ 10.4	$ 10.1
Drug Resources Percentage	10.87%	11.16%	11.99%

[1] Reflects the drug control funding appropriated in P.L. 111-5, *The American Recovery and Reinvestment Act of 2009*, within the Acquisition, Construction and Improvements decision unit.

Program Summary

Mission

The United States Coast Guard is America's lead maritime safety, security, and stewardship agency enforcing all applicable federal laws and international conventions on, under and over the high seas and waters subject to the jurisdiction of the United States. This includes U.S. territorial seas, the contiguous zone, and the Exclusive Economic Zone. As part of its maritime security strategic goal, the Coast Guard's drug interdiction objective is to reduce the flow of illegal drugs entering the United States by denying smugglers access to maritime routes.

The Coast Guard developed a counterdrug strategy called STEEL WEB, which is a comprehensive approach to maritime counterdrug law enforcement in the transit and arrival zones. The cornerstones of this plan are: (1) maintain a strong interdiction presence to deny smugglers access to maritime routes and deter trafficking activity; (2) strengthen ties with source and transit zone nations to increase their willingness and ability to reduce the production and trafficking of illicit drugs within their sovereign boundaries, including territorial seas; and (3) support interagency and international efforts to stem drug smuggling through increased cooperation and coordination.

The Coast Guard primarily conducts counterdrug operations in the transit and arrival zones. In the six million square mile transit zone (Caribbean and Eastern Pacific), although difficult to locate, drugs are in their most concentrated form and trafficking activities are highly vulnerable once detected. The Drug Trafficking Organizations (DTOs) leverage diverse trafficking means, presenting a formidable challenge to the limited United States Government resources whose purpose is to stop them. The Coast Guard continues to enhance its effective presence in both the Caribbean and Eastern Pacific portions of the transit zone by increasing overall efficiency, reducing cutter days lost during post-seizure operations, and strengthening relationships with transit and source zone countries through combined operations and bilateral/multilateral agreements, including International Maritime Interdiction Support.

DTOs continue to modify their trafficking tactics to evade maritime interdiction modes and routes, for example, in part due to the Coast Guard's increased effectiveness stopping go-fast and fishing vessels laden with cocaine bound to the United States, DTOs have employed Self-Propelled Semi-Submersible (SPSS) vessels to transport large quantities of cocaine via the maritime transit zone. SPSS vessels are designed to evade law enforcement detection and to easily scuttle (intentionally sink) when intercepted by law enforcement assets for the purpose of destroying the contraband and avoiding prosecution.

The ability to smuggle large loads of cocaine in an inconspicuous manner continues to make SPSSs an attractive smuggling asset, accounting for approximately one-third of all non-commercial maritime cocaine flow in metric tons destined for the U.S. However, the Drug Trafficking and Vessel Interdiction Act of 2008 continues to provide an effective prosecution tool by outlawing the operation of stateless SPSSs in international waters with the intent to evade detection. This new law has already resulted in the effective prosecution of smugglers embarked on SPSSs in the absence of recovered contraband. Despite the increased use of SPSSs in recent years, the go fast vessel remains the smuggling vessel of choice due to its availability, speed, maneuverability, and characteristics that allow it to blend easily with legitimate traffic, particularly along the littorals.

In FY 2011, the Coast Guard will continue to leverage partnerships to employ a holistic strategy to thwart the illegal maritime drug flow. For example, the Coast Guard will continue to utilize over 30 bilateral agreements with source and transit zone nations to enlist the international cooperation essential to denying the use of territorial waters for drug smuggling activity and to ensure successful prosecution of drug smugglers.

Methodology

The Coast Guard does not have a specific appropriation for drug interdiction activities. All Coast Guard operations, capital improvements and acquisitions, reserve training, and research and development activities targeted toward drug interdiction are funded out of the associated appropriations specified herein.

Reflecting the multimission nature of Coast Guard units, the accounting system is keyed to operating and support facilities, rather than to specific missions. Consistent with that approach, personnel and other costs are administered and tracked along operational and support capability lines requiring detailed cost accounting techniques.

The Coast Guard uses a Mission Cost Model (MCM) methodology to compute its drug attribution. The MCM allocates funding across Coast Guard missions in the Performance Based Budget (PBB) presentation. The MCM allocates all direct and support costs to mission performing units (e.g., a 378 foot cutter). Established baselines of operational activity are used to further allocate those costs to the various missions.

Operating Expenses (OE)

OE funds are used to operate facilities, maintain capital equipment, improve management effectiveness, and recruit, train, and sustain all active duty military and civilian personnel. Budget presentations for current and future years use the most recent OE asset cost data. The MCM systematically allocates all OE costs in the following way:

- **Direct Costs:** Applied directly to the operating assets (major cutters, HC 130 aircraft, 41 foot utility boat) that perform missions;
- **Support Costs:** Applied to assets for which cost variability can be specifically linked to operating assets (based on carefully developed allocation criteria); and,
- **Overhead Costs:** Applied to assets based on proportion of labor dollars spent where cost variability cannot be specifically linked to operating assets. This is a standard industry approach to overhead allocation.

Once all Operating Expense costs are fully loaded on mission performing assets, those costs are further allocated to Coast Guard missions (Drug Enforcement, Search and Rescue, etc.) using actual or baseline projections for operational employment hours.

Acquisition, Construction & Improvements (AC&I)

The MCM is used to develop an allocation of costs by mission areas for proposed AC&I projects based on the typical employment of assets germane to the project. For example, if a new asset is being proposed for commissioning through an AC&I project, costs would be applied to missions using the operational profile of a comparable existing asset. The Coast Guard uses a zero based budget approach in developing its request for AC&I funding. Program changes in the AC&I account may vary significantly from year to year depending on the specific platforms or construction projects supported. AC&I funding finances the acquisition of new capital assets, construction of new facilities and physical improvements to existing facilities and assets. The funds cover Coast Guard owned and operated vessels, shore facilities and other equipment, such as computer systems.

Research, Development, Test & Evaluation (RDT&E)

The MCM is used to develop an allocation of costs by mission areas for proposed Research, Development, Test and Evaluation projects. Allocation of drug interdiction funding is accomplished within the zero based RDT&E appropriation by evaluating each project's anticipated contribution to drug interdiction efforts based on subject matter expert professional judgment.

Reserve Training (RT)

RT funds are used to support Selected Reserve personnel who in turn support and operate facilities, maintain capital equipment, improve management effectiveness, and assist in sustaining all operations. Allocation of RT funding to the Coast Guard's drug interdiction mission is done using the same methodology used for the OE appropriation.

Budget

In FY 2011, the Coast Guard requests $1,208.1 million to fund drug control operations including AC&I, OE, RDT&E, and RT. This level represents a $45.9 million increase from the FY 2010 enacted level.

In FY 2011, the Coast Guard's highest priority budget initiative is to continue to recapitalize its aging assets and infrastructure. Robust recapitalization is key to ensuring long-term achievement of ONDCP and Coast Guard counternarcotics strategies.

To account for a potential short-term performance loss associated with decommissioning legacy cutters and aircraft, the Coast Guard reduced target drug removal rate levels in FY

2011 from 18% to 15.5%. However, any performance impact will be mitigated through the timely delivery of new replacement assets. In the long-term, continued timely replacement of aging assets will significantly increase the Coast Guard's overall performance to the Nation.

Acquisition, Construction and Improvements

Total FY 2011 Request: $398.8 Million
(Reflects $33.4 Million Increase from FY 2010)

The FY 2011 President's Budget provides funding to continue replacement or refurbishment of increasingly outdated and unreliable assets used today to prevent the flow of illegal drugs into the U.S.

These assets include the National Security Cutters (NSC), Fast Response Cutters (FRC), and the Maritime Patrol Aircraft (MPA). The timely replacement of aging 378 foot High Endurance Cutters (HECs) through the 418 foot National Security Cutter (NSC) program is the Coast Guard's top recapitalization priority. Specifically, FY 2011 recapitalization priorities include funding for the production of NSC #5. Other replacements include the HC 144A MPA for the 26 year old HU 25 Falcon aircraft, and the 150' FRC for the 110' Island Class Patrol Boat. All of the assets being replaced have reached the end of their service lives.

FY 2011 Total Changes (+$33.4 million): The FY 2011 President's Budget provides funding to operate these newly acquired assets and also funds the critical logistics and C4&IT investments needed to support them.

Operating Expenses

Total FY 2011 Request: $790.5 Million
(Reflects $13.9 Million Increase from FY 2010)

The FY 2011 President's Budget supports the operation and maintenance of Coast Guard capability, including personnel pay and allowances, training and recruiting, operating funds for newly acquired assets delivered through Coast Guard recapitalization programs, and unit and depot level maintenance. It also includes a targeted deployable law enforcement capability enhancement to mitigate emergent terrorism and border security risks, including the illegal flow of drugs.

The FY 2011 President's Budget enhances deployable Law Enforcement Detachment team (LEDET) capacity to mitigate emergent terrorism and border security risks. LEDETs embark on naval assets to primarily support the Drug Interdiction and National Defense Readiness missions. In FY 2009, the deployment of Coast Guard LEDETs aboard U.S. Navy and partner nation warships accounted for over 50% of total cocaine removals. The President's Budget will bring 18 teams to full operational capacity. The Coast Guard will continue to work closely with the Department of Defense and international partners to provide platforms to leverage the full benefit of enhanced LEDET capacity.

The Budget also annualizes new funding provided by Congress in FY 2010 for counterdrug operations and new watchstanders and also provides funds to operate and maintain newly acquired assets delivered through Coast Guard recapitalization programs.

FY 2011 Total Changes (+$13.9 million): The $13.9 million increase in Operating Expenses consists primarily of pay, annualization of prior year funding and operating funds for newly acquired assets delivered through Coast Guard recapitalization programs, and unit and depot level maintenance.

Research and Development

Total FY 2011 Request: $2.7 Million
(Reflects $1.7 Million Decrease from FY 2010)

Research, Development, Test and Evaluation (RDT&E) funding allows the Coast Guard to sustain critical missions by the Department of Homeland Security.

FY 2011 Total Changes ($1.7 million): FY 2011 resources will continue to support the development of technologies to improve detection of hidden contraband; improve tactical communications systems to improve interagency coordination, command and control; and develop technologies that give operational commanders a wider range of options to stop fleeing vessels.

Reserve Training

Total FY 2011 Request: $16.1 Million (Reflects $0.3 Million Increase from FY 2010)

Reserve Training (RT) budget funding assumes a drug control allocation equivalent to that of the OE program costs since RT personnel augment OE program functions. RT funds are used to support Selected Reserve personnel who in turn support and operate facilities, maintain capital equipment, improve management effectiveness, and assist in sustaining all operations.

FY 2011 Total Changes (+$0.3 million): The Budget includes an increase of $0.3 million for drug-related Reserve Training. RT funds are used to support Selected Reserve personnel who in turn support and operate facilities, maintain capital equipment, improve management effectiveness, and assist in sustaining all operations. In the RT budget, allocating a share of budget authority using the same methodology used for OE derives the amount allocated to the drug control mission area.

PERFORMANCE

Introduction

This section on the FY 2009 performance of the USCG program is based on agency GPRA documents and Coast Guard data. The Coast Guard did not complete any independent program evaluation or assessments of its drug interdiction in FY 2009. The last independent program evaluation was completed by the Center of Naval Analyses (CNA); the Coast Guard changed the methodology for measuring its primary outcome in FY 2009, thus successfully implementing one of the recommendations from the CNA report.

US Coast Guard		
Selected Measures of Performance	FY 2009 Target	FY 2009 Actual
» Removal Rate for Cocaine from Non-commercial Vessels in Maritime Transit Zone	15.7%	15.0%
» Metric tons of cocaine removed	≥ 134	160.1

Discussion

In FY 2009 the CG revised its methodology for measuring its drug interdiction performance. The Coast Guard started using the Consolidated Counter Drug Database (CCDB) as its source for tracking cocaine movement estimates in lieu of the Interagency Assessment for Cocaine Movement (IACM). Adopting the CCDB quarterly, event-based estimates, which are historically more than 60% higher than the annual production and consumption based IACM estimates, results in a perceived drop in Coast Guard's measured performance from FY 2008.

In FY 2009, the Coast Guard removed 160.1 MT (352,862 lbs) of cocaine, 71,234 lbs of marijuana; seized 58 vessels, and detained 322 suspected smugglers.

The first national security cutter, Coast Guard Cutter BERTHOLF disrupted a multi-vessel drug transfer in the eastern Pacific while on its first operational patrol in July 2009. While operating as part of the Joint Interagency Task Force- South (JIATF-S), Coast Guard Cutter BERTHOLF intercepted two go-fast vessels with maritime patrol aircraft support. BERTHOLF deployed an Airborne Use of Force (AUF) capable CG helicopter and both of its small boats simultaneously to effect a successful interdiction. The case resulted in removing more than two metric tons of cocaine bound for the United States. BERTHOLF"s improved technological capabilities and onboard Command, Control, Communications, Computers, Intelligence, Surveillance, Reconnaissance (C4ISR) technology played a key role in a successful "endgame".

The Coast Guard directly contributed in disrupting 123 illicit drug movements with 42 of these events involving the Coast Guard's Airborne Use of Force (AUF) capability deployed aboard Coast Guard cutters and U.S. Naval warships (USN). Coast Guard AUF aircraft and precision marksmen deployed on USN warships assisted in confiscating 24% of total cocaine removed in FY 2009. The AUF capability remains indispensible for interdicting the littoral go-fast threat.

Deployment of Coast Guard Law Enforcement Detachments (LEDETs) aboard USN and partner nation warships accounted for over 50% of total fiscal year cocaine removals. In FY 2009, LEDETs deployed aboard USN and partner nation warships removed over 187,737 lbs of cocaine, 4,035 lbs of marijuana, detained 128 suspected smugglers, and seized 16 vessels.

The Coast Guard successfully exercised bilateral agreements and operational procedures to interdict 36 foreign flagged vessels involved in drug smuggling. This led to the removal of over 40 MT (88,000 lbs) of cocaine and 21,000 lbs of marijuana in the transit zone.

On April 8, 2009, defendants from the above case were the first to be prosecuted under the Drug Trafficking Vessel Interdiction Act of 2008 (DTVIA), pleading guilty in a federal court in Tampa, Florida. DTVIA makes it a felony offense to operate a stateless SPSS vessel in international waters with the intent to evade detection. This law enables the U.S. Government to prosecute drug traffickers without having to risk the safety of law enforcement personnel to try to recover contraband from a scuttled vessel. In FY 2009, the Coast Guard interdicted 11 SPSS vessels traveling from Colombia via Eastern Pacific routes.

On December 31, 2008, a Coast Guard LEDET embarked aboard the USS RODNEY M. DAVIS responded to a Self-Propelled Semi-Submersible (SPSS) vessel sighting by a maritime patrol aircraft (MPA) in the Eastern Pacific Ocean. The MPA monitored the SPSS vessel and vectored RODNEY M. DAVIS to the location. Once in range, the ship launched its helicopter to monitor the SPSS. Upon counter-detecting the helicopter, the SPSS crewmembers donned life jackets and scuttled the vessel. The LEDET arrived in a small boat and safely embarked the four crewmembers from the SPSS vessel just prior to its sinking. An interagency group that convenes every quarter in support of the CCDB later estimated over 5.5 MT (12,122 lbs) of cocaine aboard the scuttled SPSS vessel.

DEPARTMENT OF HOMELAND SECURITY

Office of Counternarcotics Enforcement

Resource Summary

Budget Authority (in Millions)			
	FY 2009 Final	FY 2010 Enacted	FY 2011 Request
Drug Resources by Function			
Intelligence	$0.339	$0.326	$0.350
Interdiction	2.956	2.858	3.063
International	0.005	0.005	0.005
Investigations	0.416	0.421	0.451
Research & Development	0.002	0.002	0.003
Total Drug Resources by Function	$3.718	$3.612	$3.872
Drug Resources by Decision Unit			
Salaries and Expenses	$3.718	$3.612	$3.872
Total Drug Resources by Decision Unit	$3.718	$3.612	$3.872
Drug Resources Personnel Summary			
Total FTEs (direct only)	13	15	15
Drug Resources as a Percent of Budget			
Total Agency Budget (in Billions)	$ 0.004	$ 0.004	$ 0.004
Drug Resources Percentage	100.00%	100.00%	100.00%

PROGRAM SUMMARY

Mission

A primary mission of the Department of Homeland Security (DHS) is to monitor connections between illegal drug trafficking and terrorism, coordinate efforts to sever such connections, and otherwise contribute to efforts to interdict illegal drug trafficking [6 U.S.C. 111 (b) (1) (H)].

The Office of Counternarcotics Enforcement (CNE) is statutorily charged with supporting this mission by (1) coordinating policy and operations within the Department, between the Department and other Federal departments and agencies, and between the Department and State and local agencies with respect to stopping the entry of illegal drugs into the United States; (2) ensuring the adequacy of resources within the Department for stopping the entry of illegal drugs into the United States; (3) recommending the appropriate financial and personnel resources necessary to help the Department better fulfill its responsibility to stop the entry of illegal drugs into the United States; (4) within the Joint Terrorism Task Force construct tracking and severing connections between illegal drug trafficking and terrorism; and (5) serving as a representative of the Department on all task forces, committees, or other entities whose purpose is to coordinate the counternarcotics enforcement activities of the Department.

Budget

In FY 2011, CNE requests current services funding of $3.9 million, a net increase of $0.3 million from the FY 2010 enacted level.

Office of Counternarcotics Enforcement

Total FY 2011 Request: $3.9 Million
(Reflects $0.3 Million Increase from FY 2010)

As the principal advisor to the Secretary on counterdrug matters, the CNE Director reviews and evaluates all DHS counterdrug activities. CNE's Policy Division works closely with DHS components and other Federal departments to develop and coordinate counternarcotics policies and operations. In FY 2009, the CNE Policy Division drafted "DHS Counternarcotics Doctrine," a document that reflects the best practices and fundamental operating principles of the Department's counternarcotics enterprise. In 2010, CNE Policy will conclude the coordination process for this document through the Department, and will ensure that it is suitable for promulgation by the Secretary. To further enhance coordination of the DHS counternarcotics effort, in FY 2010 CNE's Policy Division will plan and facilitate quarterly meetings of the Counternarcotics Coordinating Council (CCC), an advisory body made up of decisionmakers representing the DHS counternarcotics components. As a result of the first FY 2010 meeting of the CCC, the DHS Policy Division has undertaken the task of reviewing intraDHS counternarcoticsrelated memoranda of agreement (MOAs) and memoranda of understanding (MOUs). The DHS Policy Division will complete this effort by the end of FY 2010. In FY 2010, the CNE Policy Division will also undertake the task of analyzing the performance measures used by the DHS counternarcotics components, and identifying ways of improving these measures. In FY 2010, the Policy Division will continue to coordinate the National Southwest Counternarcotics Border Strategy and lay out the foundations for the FY 2011 update to the National Southwest Border Counternarcotics Strategy.

The DrugTerror Nexus (DTX) Division works closely with DHS intelligence and law enforcement entities to assist in tracking and severing connections between drugs and terrorism. CNE works within the Joint Terrorism Task Force (JTTF) construct in support of its DTX mission. Further, CNE is producing a Situation Report that will assess drugterror activity in the TriBorder Area, located in South America. This Situation Report will provide a state of play and overview of crimeterror activities that exist in the TriBorder Area and will provide recommendations that may be used to address identified areas of concern in support of homeland security. CNE will work closely with intelligence and law enforcement entities within the DHS enterprise to implement recommendations that will address identified vulnerabilities. CNE will also promote interagency collaboration and advocate knowledge and information sharing between law enforcement and intelligence as it relates to the connection between illegal drug trafficking and terrorism, and other related transnational criminal activity that may contribute to the drugterror threat.

FY 2011 Total Changes (+$0.3 million): The $0.3 million increase reflects technical adjustments to the base for current services.

DEPARTMENT OF THE INTERIOR

Bureau of Indian Affairs

Resource Summary

	Budget Authority (in Millions)		
	FY 2009 Final	FY 2010 Enacted	FY 2011 Request
Drug Resources by Function			
Investigations	$6.338	$10.000	$10.000
Total Drug Resources by Function	$6.338	$10.000	$10.000
Drug Resources by Decision Unit			
Drug Initiative	$6.338	$10.000	$10.000
Total Drug Resources by Decision Unit	$6.338	$10.000	$10.000
Drug Resources Personnel Summary			
Total FTEs (direct only)	15	51	85
Drug Resources as a Percent of Budget			
Total Agency Budget (in Billions)	$2.4	$2.6	$2.6
Drug Resources Percentage	0.27%	0.38%	0.39%

Program Summary

Mission

The Mission of the Bureau of Indian Affairs (BIA) is to fulfill its trust responsibilities and promote self determination on behalf of Tribal Governments, American Indians and Alaska Natives.

Budget

The FY 2011 Budget requests $10.0 million for BIA, which is the same as the FY 2010 enacted level. Budget funding for the Bureau of Indian Affairs' Office of Justice Services will continue to focus resources on providing additional officers for both law enforcement agencies and detention programs, specialized drug training for existing BIA and tribal officers, continued drug public awareness campaigns for Indian country, drug investigation equipment and tools, and resource officers to address drug and gang issues with students.

Substance Abuse – Drug Initiative

Total FY 2011 Request: $10.0 Million (Reflects No Change from FY 2010)

The FY 2011 funding will address the highly visible drug crime and trafficking crisis that Indian country is faced with through the expansion of the drug program and training for Bureau and tribal officers in an effort to reduce the health and economic impact on Indian communities. The BIA is actively recruiting for newly authorized drug enforcement positions, increasing the staffing from 15 FTE in 2009 to a total of 85 authorized FTE by 2011. Indian country law enforcement agencies experience a number of challenges in regards to filling these vacancies. While the initial cost of training and equipment for most positions will be purchased with 2010 funds, an estimated 34 vacant positions will not be filled until late 2010 or early 2011. The program will continue to provide instrumental training in the efforts against drug trafficking that includes vehicle interdiction and Spanish immersion. With an increased focus on training, awareness, and the hiring of additional fulltime drug enforcement agents, the program will be better prepared to perform full investigations and projects, increase the number of drug seizures, and contribute to a substantial reduction in drug trafficking.

Border Interdiction Teams will be cooperatively engaged with Immigration and Customs Enforcement (ICE) to interdict drug trafficking coming into the United States through Indian Country. Various methods of investigation will be utilized such as human tracking, traffic/vehicle interdiction and border security. This team will be comprised of police officers and special agents trained in these methods.

Drug Enforcement Officers (DEOs) will be responsible for managing investigations and implementing interdiction programs necessary to reduce the effects of drugs and drug related crime in Indian country. The DEOs will perform activities that include the eradication of marijuana cultivations, conducting criminal investigations, infiltrating drug trafficking networks, developing and implementing undercover techniques, executing search warrants, confiscating illegal drug supplies, collecting and processing evidence, writing highly detailed technical reports, giving sworn testimony in court, developing evidence to seize financial assets gained from the proceeds of drug trafficking, and establishing and maintaining cooperative relationships with other Federal, state, local, and tribal law enforcement organizations.

Intelligence gathering, reporting and investigation support, which is needed in all parts of Indian country for assistance in drug investigations, will still be provided. With this component, national, regional, and local threat assessments can be established and presented to law enforcement agencies working on or near Indian country. We have not had these services in the past and investigators have had to incorporate and gather intelligence piecemeal during an investigation, validating and disseminating the information as part of their investigation. This program will allow the production of real time data on trends, threats, and analysis of drug trafficking and distribution throughout most of Indian country, thus allowing investigators to have advanced information and to focus on law enforcement issues.

Cooperating witnesses, victims of drug crimes, and tribal court systems are major issues when drug investigations are conducted. The Victim/Witness Services (VWS) provides needed support for victims/witnesses during drug investigations. Additionally, VWS staff also provides guidance to tribes developing their own VWS programs. VWS will also include an effort to assess existing victim/witness programs and expand this program to all BIA law enforcement districts.

PERFORMANCE

Introduction

This section on the FY 2009 performance of BIA's program is based on agency GPRA documents, agency records, an OMB assessment, and other agency information. The Law Enforcement Program was rated favorably through the OMB review process. Individual components, such as the drug control functions, were not reviewed separately. The table includes performance measures, targets, and achievements for the latest year for which data are available.

Bureau of Indian Affairs		
Selected Measures of Performance	FY 2009 Target	FY 2009 Achieved
» Number of patrol officers trained as certified drug officers	200	270
» Number of drug cases worked	830 Cases	600 Cases
» Amount of drugs seized (new baseline in 2008)		
Meth (ICE)	0.5kg	6.2kg
Meth (powder)	0.1kg	2.0kg
Cocaine (crack)	0.6kg	0.3kg
Cocaine (powder)	1.3kg	80.7kg
Prescription drugs	1.1kg	6.2kg
Heroin	0.6kg	0.2kg
Marijuana (processed)	6.0kg	34.8kg
Marijuana (plants)	<0.1kg	<0.1kg
MDMA	2g	12g

Discussion

In FY 2009, the BIA trained 270 patrol officers in basic drug training so they could assist Drug Enforcement Officers in drug-related investigations and arrests. Drug Enforcement Offiicers are responsible for managing investigations and implementing the interdiction programs necessary to reduce the effects of drugs and drug-related crime in Indian country. In October 2007, there were only five BIA drug agents investigating issues related to narcotics throughout Indian country. This Drug Unit increased from five to 30 agents, strategically placed within or near other task force units in order to address the narcotics epidemic in Indian country. This was very beneficial to the drug enforcement unit, which led to six Title III drug investigations and six Organized Crime Drug Enforcement Task Force (OCDETF) cases within Indian country. This led to a 1412% increase of drug arrests since 2007.

Working together with the Department of Justice-Office of Victim's of Crime (OVC), has opened the door for the funding of four victim/witness advocate positions for the BIA. This, along with additional base funding, has provided 11 positions throughout Indian country.

The BIA continues to share resources with various other entities that gather intelligence-related information, providing a solid network for tribal, Federal, state and local law enforcement to work collaboratively on information-sharing and personnel resources related to illegal drug activities or other law violations. For example, an Intelligence Analyst position is currently assigned to the El Paso Intelligence Center, southwest border intelligence workgroup to assist tribes throughout the United States in providing intelligence information threats and analytical assistance. BIA is seeking to expand this capacity through the hiring of additional analysts. This exchange of information increases knowledge of Indian communities, various governing laws, procedures and jurisdictional matters related to drug enforcement, and other related law enforcement issues on Tribal lands.

A Tribal Equipment Loan program continues to loan tribes expensive, updated drug enforcement equipment to Tribal law enforcement programs. In exchange, the tribes are required to supply the BIA with the data gathered from using this equipment. In FY 2009, drug surveillance equipment was provided to seven tribes under the pilot phase of the equipment exchange program. This equipment was provided to Tribal Law Enforcement Agencies and Police Departments operating under P.L. 93-638 contract or Self-Governance compact in Indian Country with high rates of drug use and crime within their community. The tribes receiving the equipment must either have a specific drug task force in place and/or personnel dedicated to the investigation of drug crimes. The surveillance equipment contributed to higher rates of drug seizures and arrests for drug crimes.

DEPARTMENT OF JUSTICE

Bureau of Prisons

Resource Summary

Budget Authority (in Millions)			
	FY 2009 Final	FY 2010 Enacted	FY 2011 Request
Drug Resources by Function			
Treatment	$79.200	$87.646	$93.508
Total Drug Resources by Function	$79.200	$87.646	$93.508
Drug Resources by Decision Unit			
Inmate Programs	$79.200	$87.646	$93.508
Total Drug Resources by Decision Unit	$79.200	$87.646	$93.508
Drug Resources Personnel Summary			
Total FTEs (direct only)	576	600	600
Drug Resources as a Percent of Budget			
Total Agency Budget (in Billions)	$6.2	$6.2	$6.7
Drug Resources Percentage	1.282%	1.417%	1.404%

PROGRAM SUMMARY

Mission

The mission of the Bureau of Prisons (BOP), an agency of the Department of Justice (DOJ), is to protect society by confining offenders in the controlled environments of prisons and community based facilities that are safe, humane, cost efficient, and appropriately secure, and that provide work and other self improvement opportunities to assist offenders in becoming law abiding citizens.

The BOP's mission statement has two equally important parts: the first part addresses our obligation to help protect public safety through the secure and safe confinement of inmates. The second part addresses our obligation to help inmates prepare to return to their communities and to remain crime free. Post release success is as important to public safety as is inmates' secure incarceration.

Preparing inmates for eventual release to the community has been one of BOP's key objectives. The BOP's drug treatment program facilitates the successful reintegration of inmates into society, consistent with community expectations and standards. Treatment Programs assist the inmates in identifying, confronting, and altering the attitudes, values, and thinking patterns that led to criminal behavior and drug use.

Budget

In FY 2011, the BOP requests $93.5 million for drug treatment programs. This is an increase of $5.9 million from the FY 2010 enacted level primarily for population adjustment, pay increases and other inflationary adjustments.

Inmate Care and Programs

Total FY 2011 Request: $93.5 Million (Reflects $5.9 Million Increase from FY 2010)

The Violent Crime Control and Law Enforcement Act (VCCLEA) of 1994 requires the BOP (subject to the availability of funds) to provide residential substance abuse treatment to all eligible inmates. There is enormous demand for these services in part because of the potential for some nonviolent offenders to earn a reduction in sentence following the successful completion of the program. The treatment strategy often begins with drug abuse education and can end with the strong community transition component. The objective is to reduce the likelihood of inmates relapsing to drug use and criminal activity.

The FY 2011 resources of $93.5 million will support BOP's drug treatment programs. Approximately 40 percent of new inmates entering BOP custody have a diagnosis of a drug use disorder. Accordingly, BOP continues to develop a strong and comprehensive drug abuse treatment strategy consisting of screening and assessment; drug abuse education; non residential drug abuse treatment services; residential drug abuse treatment programming; and community transitional drug abuse treatment.

Drug Program Screening and Assessment

Upon entry into a BOP facility, an inmate's records are assessed to determine whether there is evidence in the pre sentence investigation that alcohol or other drug use contributed to the commission of the offenses, the inmate received a judicial recommendation to participate in a drug treatment program, or the inmate violated his or her community supervision as a result of alcohol or other drug use. If an inmate's record reveals any of these elements, the inmate must participate in a Drug Abuse Education course, available at every BOP institution. In addition, as part of the initial psychological screening, inmates are interviewed concerning their past drug use to determine their need for BOP drug abuse treatment options.

Drug Abuse Education

Participants in the Drug Abuse Education course receive factual information on alcohol and drugs and the physical, social, and psychological impact of these substances. Participants assess the impact of substance use on their lives, the lives of their family, and on their community. Drug abuse education participants are also informed of program options available to them and are encouraged to volunteer for appropriate programs. In FY 2011, BOP estimates that 23,400 inmates will participate in the Drug Abuse Education program.

Residential Drug Abuse Treatment Program (RDAP)

RDAP provides intensive drug abuse treatment to inmates diagnosed with a drug use disorder. At present, 59 BOP institutions and one contract facility offer RDAP programming. The programs are staffed by a doctoral level psychologist (the Drug Program Coordinator) who supervises the treatment staff. The average ratio of drug abuse treatment staff to inmates is 1 to 24. Inmates in the residential program are housed in a treatment unit that is set apart from the general population. Treatment is provided for a minimum of 500 hours over a 9 12 month period.

The BOP's RDAP program adheres to a cognitive behavior therapy treatment model. This treatment model targets the major criminal drug using risk factors, especially anti-social and pro criminal attitudes, values, beliefs, and behaviors. Using evidence based practices, the BOP targets these behaviors by reducing antisocial peer associations; promoting positive relationships; increasing self control, self management, and problem solving skills; and ending drug use. In FY 2011, the BOP estimates that over 18,000 inmates will participate in the Residential Drug Abuse Treatment Program.

Non-Residential Drug Abuse Treatment

Non residential treatment is designed to provide maximum flexibility to meet the needs of the offenders, particularly those individuals who have relatively minor or low level substance abuse impairment. These offenders do not require the intensive level of treatment needed by individuals with moderate to severe addictive behavioral problems. Unlike residential programs, inmates are not housed together in a separate unit; rather, they are housed in and with the general inmate population.

A second purpose of the program is to provide those offenders who have a moderate to severe drug abuse problem with supportive program opportunities during the time they are waiting to enter RDAP, or for those who have little time remaining on their sentence and are preparing to return to the community. In FY 2011, the BOP estimates that it will provide Non Residential Drug Abuse Treatment to over 14,500 inmates.

Non-Residential Follow-up Treatment

Follow up treatment is required of inmates who complete RDAP and return to the general population. This program reviews all the key concepts of RDAP and lasts for a minimum of one year.

Community Transition Drug Abuse Treatment

Community Transitional Drug Abuse Treatment (TDAT) is the final component of the BOP's RDAP. In order to successfully complete all components of RDAP, the inmate must be transferred to a Residential Reentry Center (RRC), also known as a Community Corrections Center or Halfway House, and participate in community based drug treatment. In addition, offenders who did not have an opportunity to participate in RDAP may be referred to TDAT by community corrections staff. In FY 2011, 15,400 inmates are projected to participate in this program.

FY 2011 Total Changes (+$5.9 million): The FY 2011 request includes adjustments for these programs totaling $5.9 million. The BOP will continue to provide a drug treatment program that facilitates the successful reintegration of inmates into society, consistent with community expectations and standards.

PERFORMANCE

Introduction

This section on the FY 2009 performance of BOP's program is based on agency GPRA documents, an OMB Assessment, and other agency information. The table below includes performance measures, targets and achievements.

Bureau of Prisons		
Selected Measures of Performance	FY 2009 Target	FY 2009 Achieved
» Number of inmates participating in Residential Drug Abuse Treatment	17,500	18,732
» Number of inmates participating in Non-Residential Drug Abuse Treatment	14,500	14,613

Discussion

In response to the rapid growth of federal inmates with a diagnosis of a drug use disorder (40 percent of inmates entering the Bureau), the BOP continues to develop evidence based treatment practices to manage and treat inmates with drug use disorders. The BOP's strategy includes early identification through psychology screening, drug education, non-residential drug abuse treatment, intensive residential drug abuse treatment and community transition treatment.

The Violent Crime Control and Law Enforcement Act (VCCLEA) of 1994 requires the BOP, subject to the availability of appropriations, to provide appropriate substance abuse treatment for 100 percent of inmates who have a diagnosis for substance abuse or dependence, and who volunteer for treatment.

In FY 2009, 59 BOP institutions operated a Residential Drug Abuse Treatment Program (RDAP). In addition, one facility under contract with the BOP also provided the RDAP program. The Bureau provided Residential Drug Abuse Treatment to 18,732 inmates, and 14,613 inmates participated in the Non-Residential Drug Treatment program.

In FY 2009, the BOP provided RDAP to 100 percent of the Federal inmate population that was eligible for treatment. In the previous year, RDAP treated 93 percent of eligible inmates before their release from custody. The increase in the treatment rate to 100 percent in

FY 2009 is due in part to an in-house expansion of drug programming and more than 3,000 early releases related to the change in the U.S. Sentencing Commission sentencing guidelines to retroactively shorten sentences of inmates convicted of crack cocaine offenses.

BOP also introduced blended mental health treatment and drug abuse treatment for offenders with co-occurring disorders. In addition, inmates with behavioral disorders who also have co-occurring substance use disorders received transitional community treatment, combining supervision with continued drug abuse treatment while residing in Residential Re-entry Centers.

Finally, in March of 2009, the Bureau released a new policy on all Psychology Treatment Programs calling for all institutions to follow "evidence-based" treatment practices. This policy works to ensure all Bureau psychology programs are effective in positively changing inmate behavior.

The principal goal of treatment is to equip the inmates with the cognitive, emotional, and behavioral skills necessary to choose and maintain a drug-free and crime-free lifestyle following release from prison. To measure the effectiveness of BOP's treatment program, the BOP will assess the recidivism rates for RDAP inmates. The data will be available by the end of next year.

DEPARTMENT OF JUSTICE

Drug Enforcement Administration

Resource Summary

	Budget Authority (in Millions)		
	FY 2009 Final	FY 2010 Enacted	FY 2011 Request
Drug Resources by Function			
Intelligence	$130.077	$134.430	$180.605
International	390.000	390.732	415.659
Investigations	1,675.743	1,738.443	1,817.666
Prevention	1.206	1.253	1.286
State and Local Assistance	6.508	6.614	6.733
Total Drug Resources by Function	$2,203.534	$2,271.472	$2,421.949
Drug Resources by Decision Unit			
Diversion Control Fee Account	$244.450	$251.790	$291.832
Construction	$0.000	$0.000	$41.941
Salaries & Expenses			
Domestic Enforcement	1,544.160	1,603.885	1,646.156
International Enforcement	408.416	409.183	435.287
State and Local Assistance	6.508	6.614	6.733
Total Drug Resources by Decision Unit	$2,203.534	$2,271.472	$2,421.949

(Continued).

	Budget Authority (in Millions)		
	FY 2009 Final	FY 2010 Enacted	FY 2011 Request
Drug Resources Personnel Summary Total FTEs (direct only)	9,293	9,432	9,597
Drug Resources as a Percent of Budget Total Agency Budget (in Billions)	$ 2.2	$ 2.3	$ 2.4

PROGRAM SUMMARY

Mission

DEA's mission is to enforce the controlled substances laws and regulations of the United States and bring to the criminal and civil justice system of the United States, or any other competent jurisdiction, those organizations and principal members of organizations involved in the growing, manufacturing, or distribution of controlled substances appearing in or destined for illicit traffic in the United States, including organizations that use drug trafficking proceeds to finance terror; and to recommend and support programs aimed at reducing the availability of and demand for illicit controlled substances on the domestic and international markets.

Budget

The FY 2011 President's Budget requests $2,421.9 million for DEA's Salaries and Expenses Account, Construction Account, and Diversion Control Fee Account (DCFA), which is an increase of $150.5 million over the FY 2010 enacted level. Additional resources support Southwest Border enforcement, including intelligence sharing initiatives and efforts to disrupt and dismantle violent Mexican drug cartels.

Salaries & Expenses (S&E)

Total FY 2011 Request: $2,088.2 Million
(Reflects $68.5 Million Increase from FY 2010)

DEA's resources are divided into four strategic focus areas to achieve the maximum impact against the full spectrum of drug trafficking activities. These focus areas are: *International Enforcement, Domestic Enforcement, State and Local Assistance and Diversion Control*. These areas, with the exception of Diversion Control, comprise the Salaries & Expenses Account. A portion of DEA's FY 2011 request is also funded in its Construction Account.

Domestic Enforcement

FY 2011 Request: $1,646.2 Million
(Reflects $42.3 Million Increase from FY 2010)

The Domestic Enforcement decision unit comprises the majority of DEA's investigative and support resources, including domestic enforcement groups, state and local task forces, other federal and local task forces, intelligence groups, and all the support functions, including labs, essential to accomplishing their mission.

DEA's Priority Targeting Program identifies, targets, investigates and disrupts or dismantles those international, national, regional, and local impact drug trafficking and/or money laundering organizations having a significant impact on drug availability within the United States. Through this program, DEA disrupts and dismantles Priority Target Organizations (PTOs), including those PTOs with a direct connection to DOJ's Consolidated Priority Organization Targets (CPOTs), which includes the most significant international command and control organizations threatening the United States as identified by OCDETF member agencies.

The Southwest Border (SWB) is a major focus of DEA's Drug Flow Attack Strategy. The Drug Flow Attack Strategy is an innovative, multi-agency strategy, designed to significantly disrupt the flow of drugs, money, and chemicals between the source zones and the United States by attacking vulnerabilities in the supply, transportation systems, and financial infrastructure of major drug trafficking organizations. Mexico is home to over one-third of the United States' "Most Wanted" drug trafficking and money laundering organizations—of the 55 criminal targets on the FY 2009 Consolidated Priority Organization Target (CPOT) list, 21 (38 percent) were based in Mexico. The SWB is also the primary arrival zone for most illicit drugs smuggled into our country. It is estimated that 80 percent of the methamphetamine consumed in the United States comes from Mexican drug trafficking organizations and approximately 90 percent of the cocaine destined for the United States transits the Mexico/Central America corridor. Additionally, large quantities of Mexican-produced marijuana and heroin enter the United States by way of the SWB.

FY 2011 Total Changes (+$42.3 million): The FY 2011 request includes base adjustments of $36.7 million for the 2011 pay raise and the annualization of the 2010 pay raise. It also funds inflationary adjustments for costs such as benefits and GSA rent. DEA requests $1.5 million to fund servers and software licenses to increase the capacity of the El Paso Intelligence Center's (EPIC) System Portal (ESP) infrastructure since the current system capacity is insufficient to accommodate the estimated growth of users. The requested funding will increase user capacity while ensuring that system performance is maintained. The additional users will include Federal, State, local and tribal law enforcement personnel and the enhancement will provide them with full access to all applications within the ESP. Users access the ESP to report seizure incidents, query EPIC's databases, obtain various reports in support of their investigations, share intelligence, and submit queries to and obtain results from the EPIC Watch Operations Section. DEA requests $4.9 million in support of DEA's Speedway program which synthesizes data to produce valuable, timely intelligence regarding international and national communication structures used by major drug trafficking organizations, as well as drug-related financial and/or terrorist organizations and makes it available to all agencies that participate at the Special Operations Division (SOD). As part of a Director of National Intelligence initiative, DEA is requesting $0.3 for infrastructure upgrades that will allow DEA to better share information within the Intelligence Community through the Intelligence Community Information Sharing Initiative. In FY 2011, DOJ is focusing on travel as an area in which savings can be achieved. For DEA, travel or other management efficiencies will result in offsets of $2.1 million.

International Enforcement

FY 2011 Request: $435.3 Million
(Reflects $26.1 Million Increase from FY 2010)

The main focus of DEA's International Enforcement program is the disruption or dismantlement of the most significant international drug and chemical trafficking organizations, or PTOs, including those with a direct connection to DOJ's CPOTs. Recently, the International Narco-Terrorism Provisions in the USA PATRIOT Improvement and Reauthorization Act of 2005 (USA PATRIOT Act) enhanced DEA's investigative authority overseas. DEA now has the authority to pursue drug traffickers who are terrorists or provide funding to terrorists even if the drugs are not destined for the U.S. In addition, the USA PATRIOT Act makes it a Federal crime to engage in drug trafficking to benefit terrorists. To attack the vulnerabilities of major international drug and chemical trafficking organizations, DEA is working to strengthen partnerships with its international law enforcement counterparts worldwide.

DEA coordinates all programs involving drug law enforcement in foreign countries. DEA also provides intelligence to assist the interagency community in determining future trends in drug trafficking and evaluating these trends to determine their long-term impact on drug trafficking. DEA works closely with the United Nations, Interpol, and other organizations on matters relating to international drug and chemical control programs.

FY 2011 Total Changes (+$26.1 million): The FY 2011 request includes base adjustments of $16.2 million for the 2011 pay raise and the annualization of the 2010 pay raise. It also funds inflationary adjustments for costs such as benefits, rent, and State Department charges for DEA positions stationed in foreign locations. The FY 2011 request includes $10.8 million in non-personnel funding to provide permanent funding for the expanded Sensitive Investigative Unit (SIU) program in Mexico, which is a key tool in the effort to disrupt and dismantle Mexican Drug Cartels. In response to the escalating drug violence, DEA has assessed the challenges faced by its Mexican law enforcement counterparts and made strategic and operational changes to the SIU program in Mexico. DEA's SIU program recruits, selects, and trains foreign police officers to work cooperatively with DEA in major case development and the exchange of intelligence.

State & Local Assistance

FY 2011 Request: $6.7 Million
(Reflects $0.1 Million Increase from FY 2010)

As the nation's drug law enforcement organization, DEA has the responsibility to respond to clandestine laboratory training requirements, hazardous waste cleanup, and cannabis eradication/suppression needs of the U.S. law enforcement community. DEA supports State and local law enforcement with methamphetaminerelated assistance and training, which allows State and local agencies to better address the methamphetamine threat in their communities and reduce the impact that methamphetamine has on the quality of life for America's citizens.

FY 2011 Total Changes (+$0.1 million): The FY 2011 request includes base adjustments of $0.1 million for the 2010 pay raise and the annualization of the 2009 pay raise. It also funds inflationary adjustments for costs such as benefits and GSA rent.

Diversion Control Fee Account

Total FY 2011 Request: $291.8 Million
(Reflects $40.0 Million Increase from FY 2010)

DEA's Diversion Control Program (DCP) enforces the Controlled Substances Act and its regulations pertaining to pharmaceutical controlled substances and listed chemicals. The DCP actively monitors more than 1 million individuals and companies that are registered with DEA to handle controlled substances or listed chemicals through a system of scheduling, quotas, recordkeeping, reporting, and security requirements.

FY 2011 Total Changes (+$40.0 million): The FY 2011 request includes base adjustments of $3.5 million for the 2011 pay raise and the annualization of the 2010 pay raise. It also funds inflationary adjustments for benefits, GSA rent, and costs related to employees stationed in foreign locations. The FY 2011 request also includes $36.5 million and 174 new positions (including 62 special agents and 60 diversion investigators) for pharmaceutical and chemical diversion control activities. These resources will support regulatory and enforcement efforts, including an expansion of Tactical Diversion Squads, intelligence support, and Internet investigations. Included in the $36.5 million request is $3.0 million to support the Administration's Prescription Drug Monitoring Program (PDMP), which will initiate establishing a well functioning standardized prescription drug monitoring program in every State to reduce prevalence of overdose deaths, drug drug interactions, diversion of prescribed medications, and early identification of patients at risk for addiction.

Construction

Total FY 2011 Request: $41.9 Million
(Reflects $41.9 Million Increase from FY 2010)

EPIC currently houses employees from 22 federal, state and local agencies. Construction funding for expansion and renovation will enable EPIC to absorb this additional support and allow further development of interagency partnerships.

FY 2011 Total Changes (+$41.9 million): The FY 2011 request includes $41.9 in no year construction funding for an expansion and renovation project to enlarge the existing EPIC facility.

PERFORMANCE

Introduction

This section on the FY 2009 performance of the DEA program is based on agency GPRA documents, an OMB Assessment, and other agency information. The table below includes performance measures, targets and achievements for the latest year for which data are available. The 2003 OMB Assessment concluded with a favorable rating.

DEA accomplishes its primary goal of reducing drug availability by disrupting or dismantling Priority Target Organizations (PTOs) including organizations linked to the Attorney General's FY 2009 Consolidated Priority Organization Target (CPOT) list – the "Most Wanted" drug trafficking and money laundering organizations believed to be primarily responsible for the Nation's illicit drug supply. During FY 2009, DEA disrupted or dismantled 2,362 PTOs, of which 364 were linked to CPOT targets, and 1,998 were not linked to CPOT targets.

Drug Enforcement Administration		
Selected Measures of Performance	FY 2009 Target	FY 2009 Achieved
» Contribution to DOJ's Goal to reduce the availability of drugs in the U.S.	N/A	Indicator to be developed
» Number of active International and Domestic Priority Targets linked to CPOT targets disrupted or dismantled1	355	364
» Number of active International and Domestic Priority Targets not linked to CPOT targets disrupted or dismantled1	2,020	1,998

[1] Includes disruptions pending dismantlement.

Discussion

DEA's ultimate objective is to dismantle PTOs, ensuring that these criminal organizations cannot re-establish themselves. In FY 2009, DEA fell short of its overall target for the number of PTO investigations not linked to CPOT targets disrupted or dismantled by less than one percent. DEA exceeded its FY 2009 target for the disruption or dismantlement of PTO investigations linked to CPOT organizations. Additionally, the FY 2009 CPOT-linked dismantlements increased by 43 percent over FY 2008 actual performance. As of September 30, 2009, 53 of the 55 targets on the FY 2009 CPOT list (96 percent) had active PTO investigations directed at or linked to them.

Attacking the financial infrastructure of major drug trafficking organizations and members of the financial community who facilitate the laundering of their proceeds, through DEA's Financial Attack Strategy is a vital component of DEA's overall strategy. In FY 2009, DEA denied drug traffickers over $3.4 billion in revenue through asset and drug seizures, a 14 % increase over the agency's FY 2009 goal of $3 billion.

During FY 2009, DEA maintained 21 money laundering investigative groups to support this Financial Attack Strategy. The 2009 National Drug Threat Assessment stated that Mexican and Columbian drug trafficking organizations annually generate, remove, and launder between $18 billion and $39 billion in wholesale drug proceeds that are largely smuggled in bulk out of the U.S via the Southwest Border. As of September 2009, DEA's total cash seizures were $736.3 million.

DEA implemented several national initiatives focused on targeting bulk cash derived from drug proceeds, such as the Money Trail Initiative. The Money Trail Initiative, targets the financing of the illegal drug trade. This initiative focuses on identifying and disrupting the flow of money back to the sources of drug supply. As of September 9, 2009, the Money Trail Initiative has been responsible for the seizure of $298.6 million, 44,637 kilograms of cocaine,

3,699 pounds of methamphetamine, 281,308 pounds of marijuana, 24 million marijuana plants, 844 vehicles, and 1,443 weapons. Additionally, 2,607 individuals have been arrested.

In addition, Operation All-Inclusive, the centerpiece of DEA's Drug Flow Attack Strategy, has caused major disruptions in the flow of drugs, money, and chemicals between source zones and the U.S. by attacking trafficker vulnerabilities in the areas of financial, maritime, land, and air smuggling. From December 2008 through September 2009, DEA conducted the fifth international initiative under Operation All-Inclusive. As of September 30, 2009, this initiative has resulted in the seizure of over 91 metric tons of cocaine, 1,396 kilograms of methamphetamine, 645 kilograms of heroin, 132 metric tons of marijuana, 415 metric tons of precursor chemicals, $368 million, and 867 weapons.

Additionally, 1,332 arrests occurred.

DEA directed Organized Crime Drug Enforcement Task Force (OCDETF) investigations that resulted in the August 2009 indictments of eight CPOTs (Arturo Beltran Leyva, Joaquin Guzman Loera, Ismael Zambada Garcia, Vicente Carrillo Fuentes, Ignacio Coronel Villarreal, Esteban and Luis Rodriguez Olivera, and Tirso Martinez Sanchez) and two other cartel leaders (Hector Beltran Leyva and Jesus Zambada Garcia). The charges involve continuing criminal enterprises and/or participating in international drug trafficking conspiracies.

Through a combination of DEA-led operations such as the Drug Flow Attack Strategy, international partnerships with Mexico and Columbia, the Financial Attack Strategy, and foreign and domestic enforcement operations, DEA has significantly weakened a host of major drug trafficking organizations. One indicator of the overall effectiveness of these efforts is the price and purity of drugs. According to DEA's System to Retrieve Information on Drug Evidence (STRIDE) data for all domestic cocaine purchases from January 2007 through June 2009, the price per pure gram of cocaine increased 77.1 percent, from $99.48 to $176.14, while the purity decreased 27.4 percent, from 67 percent to 49 percent. The results for heroin price and purity are also favorable. For the same time period, the price per pure gram of heroin increased 12.1 percent, from $679.75 to $761.69, while the purity remained stable.

Department of Justice

Interagency Crime and Drug Enforcement

Resource Summary

	Budget Authority (in Millions)		
	FY 2009 Final	FY 2010 Enacted	FY 2011 Request
Drug Resources by Function			
Investigations	$325.411	$334.851	$362.651
Prosecutions	145.653	149.027	168.349
Intelligence	43.936	44.691	48.319
Total Drug Resources by Function	$515.000	$528.569	$579.319
Drug Resources by Decision Unit DEPARTMENT OF JUSTICE			

(Continued).

	Budget Authority (in Millions)		
	FY 2009 Final	FY 2010 Enacted	FY 2011 Request
Bureau of Alcohol, Tobacco, Firearms, and Interagency Crime and Drug Enforcement			
Explosives (ATF)	$11.500	$11.813	$14.513
Drug Enforcement Administration (DEA)	199.292	205.43	220.22
Federal Bureau of Investigations (FBI)	138.237	141.743	149.233
U.S. Marshals Service (USMS)	8.542	8.780	12.844
OCDETF Fusion Center	11.776	11.776	14.160
Criminal Division	2.877	2.897	3.021
Threat Response Unit	0.000	0.331	2.765
Tax Division	0.331	0.000	0.000
U.S. Attorneys	142.445	145.799	162.563
Total Drug Resources by Decision Unit	$515.000	$528.569	$579.319
Drug Resources Personnel Summary Total FTEs (direct only)	3,376	3,277	3,358
Drug Resources as a Percent of Budget			
Total Agency Budget (in Billions)	$0.5	$0.5	$0.6
Drug Resources Percentage	100.00%	100.00%	100.00%

PROGRAM SUMMARY

Mission

The Organized Crime Drug Enforcement Task Force (OCDETF) Program was established in 1982 as a multiagency partnership of federal law enforcement agencies and prosecutors, with assistance from state and local police departments, to identify, dismantle and disrupt sophisticated national and international drug trafficking and money laundering organizations. OCDETF's attack on all the related components of major drug trafficking and money laundering organizations disrupts the drug market, resulting in a reduction in the drug supply and money laundering, and bolsters law enforcement efforts.

Budget

For FY 2011, OCDETF requests $579.3 million, which is an increase of $50.8 million above the FY 2010 Enacted Level. The majority of OCDETF's funding goes to payroll costs for agents, analysts and attorneys performing investigative, intelligence, and prosecutorial work.

OCDETF's major priority is the Consolidated Priority Organization Target (CPOT) List - a unified agency list of the top drug trafficking and money laundering targets. OCDETF Regional Coordination Groups also target and identify Regional Priority Organization Targets (RPOTs), which represent the most significant drug and money laundering organizations threatening the regions. In addition, OCDETF requires that all cases include a financial investigation to enable the identification and destruction of the financial systems supporting drug organizations.

The Southwest Border Enforcement Initiative will strengthen OCDETF's efforts to stem the flow of illicit drugs, guns, and drug proceeds along the Southwest Border of the United States by attacking the operations of the most significant Mexico-based drug trafficking organizations, along with the affiliated organizations involved in weapons trafficking and bulk cash smuggling. OCDETF is seeking $37.3 million to support these efforts across the Southwest Border. This enhancement will allow OCDETF to target those organizations having a significant impact on the U.S. drug supply and those contributing to the escalating violence along the Southwest Border. OCDETF formulated this request in coordination with its Justice partners, which include DEA, FBI, USMS, ATF, the Criminal Division, and the United States Attorneys' Offices, to ensure OCDETF resources sought herein align and do not duplicate our partners' FY 2010 and FY 2011 requests to support Southwest Border investigative and prosecution resource requirements.

Investigations/Intelligence

Total FY 2011 Request: $411.0 Million
(Reflects $31.4 Million Increase from FY 2010)

Investigations include the reimbursable resources that support investigative activities of the following participating agencies: ATF, DEA, FBI, and the USMS (Investigative activities for ICE, Coast Guard, and IRS in support of the OCDETF Program are funded out of the direct appropriations of the Departments of Homeland Security and Treasury). Reimbursable resources that support the intelligence activities of OCDETF's member agencies and the OCDETF Fusion Center are also included.

Bureau of Alcohol, Tobacco, Firearms, and Explosives

FY 2011 Request: $14.5 Million
(Reflects $2.7 Million Increase from FY 2010)

The FY 2011 resources of $14.5 million support ATF's investigative activities as a member of the OCDETF Program. ATF agents focus on major drug traffickers who have violated laws related to the illegal trafficking and misuse of firearms, arson, and explosives. Firearms often serve as a form of payment for drugs and, together with explosives and arson, are used as tools by drug organizations in order to intimidate, enforce, and retaliate against their own members, rival organizations, or the community.

FY 2011 Total Changes (+$2.7 million): The Budget proposes a program enhancement of $2.2 million and adjustments of $0.5 million for a pay raise and other inflationary increases. The program enhancement provides 11 new positions, including 7 agents to support the OCDETF initiatives for intelligence exploitation and coordination and OCDETF Co-located Strike Forces to targeted Southwest Border investigations and prosecutions.

Drug Enforcement Administration

FY 2011 Request: $220.2 Million
(Reflects $14.8 Million Increase from FY 2010)

The FY 2011 resources of $220.2 million support DEA's involvement in OCDETF investigations. DEA is the most active agency involved in the OCDETF Program with a participation rate in investigations that exceeds 80 percent. DEA's knowledge of international drug rings, its relationship with foreign law enforcement entities, and its working relationships with state and local authorities have made it an essential partner.

FY 2011 Total Changes (+$14.8 million): The Budget proposes a program enhancement of $10.8 million and adjustments of $4.0 million for a pay raise and other inflationary increases. The program enhancement provides for the operational costs necessary to DEA participation in the OCDETF initiative to targeted Southwest Border investigations and prosecutions by the OCDETF Co-located Strike Forces.

Federal Bureau of Investigation

FY 2011 Request: $149.2 Million
(Reflects $7.5 Million Increase from FY 2010)

The FY 2011 resources of $149.2 million support the FBI's involvement in OCDETF investigations. FBI brings to OCDETF its expertise in the investigation of traditional organized crime and white collar/financial crimes. The FBI also has developed relationships with foreign, state, and local law enforcement. The FBI uses its skills to gather and analyze intelligence data and to undertake sophisticated electronic surveillance. The FBI is committed to the OCDETF program and to the goal of targeting major drug trafficking organizations and their financial infrastructure.

FY 2011 Total Changes (+$7.5 million): The Budget proposes a program enhancement of $4.7 million and adjustments of $2.8 million for a pay raise and other inflationary increases. The program enhancement provides 22 new positions, including 14 agents to support the OCDETF initiative to targeted Southwest Border investigations and prosecutions by the OCDETF Co-located Strike Forces.

U.S. Marshals Service

FY 2011 Request: $12.8 Million
(Reflects $4.1 Million Increase from FY 2010)

The FY 2011 resources of $12.8 million support USMS's involvement in OCDETF investigations. USMS is the agency responsible for the apprehension of OCDETF fugitives. Fugitives are typically repeat offenders who flee apprehension only to continue their criminal enterprise elsewhere. The USMS is responsible for apprehension of approximately 90 percent of all OCDETF fugitives.

FY 2011 Total Changes (+$4.1 million): The Budget proposes a program enhancement of $3.7 million and adjustments of $0.4 million for a pay raise and other inflationary increases. The program enhancement provides 11 new positions, including 8 new deputies to support the OCDETF initiatives for Mexican and Colombian fugitive apprehension and to targeted Southwest Border investigations and prosecutions by the OCDETF Co-located Strike Forces.

OCDETF Fusion Center

FY 2011 Request: $14.2 Million
(Reflects $2.4 Million Increase from FY 2010)

The FY 2011 resources of $14.2 million will support operations at the OFC, a comprehensive data center containing all drug and related financial intelligence information from the seven OCDETF member investigative agencies, the Financial Crimes Enforcement Network, the National Drug Intelligence Center, and others. The OFC conducts cross-agency integration and analysis of drug and related financial data to create comprehensive intelligence pictures of targeted organizations, including those identified as CPOTs and RPOTs, and to pass actionable leads through the multi-agency SOD to OCDETF participants in the field. These leads ultimately result in the development of better-coordinated, more comprehensive, multi-jurisdictional OCDETF investigations of the most significant drug trafficking and money laundering networks.

FY 2011 Total Changes (+$2.4 million): The Budget proposes a program enhancement of $2.3 million and adjustments of $0.1 million for a pay raise and other inflationary increases. The program enhancement will allow the OFC to expand its support to the field and acquire necessary physical space.

Prosecution

Total FY 2011 Request: $168.4 Million
(Reflects $19.3 Million Increase from FY 2010)

Prosecution includes reimbursable resources for the 94 U.S. Attorneys Offices around the country (executed through the Executive Office for U.S. Attorneys) and the Criminal Division of the Department of Justice.

Criminal Division

FY 2011 Request: $3.0 Million
(Reflects $0.1 Million Increase from FY 2010)

The FY 2011 resources of $3.0 million aid the OEO in providing direct operational support to U.S. Attorneys offices as it reviews all applications for electronic surveillance and assists agents and attorneys by providing guidance on the justification for and development of such applications. With the increasing complexity and scope of OCDETF cases, senior attorneys are called upon with greater frequency to assist in the supervision and prosecution of OCDETF cases. OCDETF funded NDDS attorneys assigned to SOD play a critical role in supporting and coordinating nationwide investigations.

FY 2011 Total Changes (+$0.1 million): The Budget proposes adjustments of $0.1 million for pay raises and other inflationary increases.

Threat Response Unit

FY 2011 Request: $2.8 Million
(Reflects $2.4 Million Increase from FY 2010)

The FY 2011 resources of $2.8 million support the OCDETF Executive Office in hiring new personnel to be detailed to OEO to enhance its support of OCDETF Southwest Border-related wiretap applications and requests for approval to employ sensitive investigative techniques; and to OIA to support the high priority extraditions related to OCDETF prosecutions of Mexican Cartels. Base funds represent a realignment of funds previously provided to the Tax Division.

FY 2011 Total Changes (+$2.4 million): The Budget proposes increased funding of $2.4 million to support 11 attorneys and 3 support positions to enhance the efforts of the OIA and OEO.

U.S. Attorneys

FY 2011 Request: $162.6 Million
(Reflects $16.8 Million Increase from FY 2010)

The FY 2011 resources of $162.6 million support the United States Attorneys' involvement in the development of case strategy for OCDETF investigations and prosecutions. OCDETF attorneys are able to coordinate investigative efforts more efficiently and minimize the risk of legal challenges because of their familiarity with the intricacies of drug trafficking investigations. Their involvement ensures that the prosecutions are well prepared, comprehensively charged, and expertly handled.

FY 2011 Total Changes (+$16.8 million): The Budget proposes a program enhancement of $11.3 million and adjustments of $5.5 million for a pay raise, Administratively Determined (AD) pay plan and other inflationary increases. The program enhancement provides 100 new positions including 47 new Assistant US Attorneys (AUSAs) to support the OCDETF Strike Forces and pursue the growing number of OCDETF prosecutions along the Southwest Border.

PERFORMANCE

Introduction

This section on the FY 2009 performance of the Interagency Crime and Drug Enforcement (OCDETF) program is based on agency GPRA documents and other agency information. The table includes performance measures, targets and achievements for the latest year for which data are available.

OCDETF monitors performance in two program areas: investigations and prosecutions. For investigations, OCDETF tracks the percent of active investigations linked to the Attorney General's Consolidated Priority Organization Target CPOT list and the number of CPOT-linked organizations dismantled or disrupted. For prosecutions, OCDETF tracks leadership convictions and financial convictions.

Organized Crime Drug Enforcement Task Force (OCDETF)		
Selected Measures of Performance	FY 2009 Target	FY 2009 Achieved
» Percent of aggregate domestic supply related to dismantled/disrupted CPOT-linked organizations	1	1
» Percent of OCDETF investigations resulting in conviction of a leader	75%	77%
» Percent of OCDETF investigations resulting in financial convictions	27%	23%
» Percent of OCDETF investigations resulting in assets forfeited or restrained	80%	74%
» Percent of OCDETF investigations resulting in disruption/dismantlement of targeted organization[2]	78%	83%
» Number of CPOT-linked trafficking organizations:		
Disrupted	189	162
Dismantled	90	99

[1] This measure is to be determined. The establishment of meaningful baselines for the supply of drugs available for consumption in the United States must first be established.

[2] Data based on information reported in OCDETF Final Reports. Due to the lag in reporting, activity may have occurred in the prior year.

Discussion

The goal of the OCDETF Program is to identify, investigate, and prosecute the most significant drug trafficking and money laundering organizations and related enterprises, and to disrupt and dismantle their operations in order to reduce the drug supply in the United States. By dismantling and disrupting trafficking organizations that are CPOT-linked, OCDETF is focusing enforcement efforts against organizations that include heads of narcotic and/or money laundering organizations, poly-drug traffickers, clandestine manufacturers and producers, and major drug transporters, all of whom are primarily responsible for the domestic drug supply. Additionally, OCDETF's financial investigations focus on eliminating the entire infrastructure of CPOT-linked organizations and permanently removing their profits.

It should be noted that in FY 2009, OCDETF made important gains against both CPOT-linked organizations and CPOTs including significant successes against the leaders of the Autodefensas Unidas de Colombia/The United Self-Defense Groups of Colombia, the Norte Valle Cartel, and the Tijuana Cartel, a violent and feared Mexican organization. Sixteen percent of OCDETF investigations are linked to CPOT targets.

OCDETF has dismantled 99 (81 DEA and 18 FBI) CPOT-linked organizations in FY 2009, thus exceeding its target. This is a 43 percent increase over the 69 that were dismantled in FY 2008. OCDETF has disrupted 162 (130 DEA and 32 FBI) CPOTlinked organizations in FY 2009, falling short of its target for disruptions. However, the dismantling of 99 CPOT-linked trafficking organizations in FY 2009 made up for some of the below-target number of disruptions. These numbers do not include FBI and DEA direct funded disruptions and dismantlements as reflected in the FY 2010 Performance and Accountability Report (PAR).

On the whole, OCDETF investigations have resulted in the disruption or dismantlement of 83% of targeted organizations. Assets seized from OCDETF investigations totaled more than $514 million in FY 2009. Seventy-seven percent of OCDETF investigations resulted in the conviction of a leader, 23% in finance-related convictions, and 74% in the forfeiture or restraining of assets. Although the actual is slightly lower than the estimated target for the measure pertaining to the percent of OCDETF investigations resulting in financial convictions, significant progress was made in accomplishing the goal. Two Supreme Court decisions, Santos and Cuellar, impacted OCDETF's ability to file money laundering charges and caused dismissals of charges in some cases.

The target for the performance measure pertaining to the percent of OCDETF investigations resulting in assets forfeited and restrained applies to the performance of all OCDETF agencies, including non-DOJ federal, state and local law enforcement. However, forfeiture proceedings take a long time, often creating a lag in reporting for this measure. OCDETF's reporting is often closed before forfeiture data can be reported. Additionally, the two aforementioned Supreme Court decisions impacted OCDETF's ability to file money laundering charges and caused dismissals that may have impacted forfeitures in some investigations.

Some of U.S. law enforcement's hardest blows against the major Mexican drug cartels have been struck by agents and prosecutors in OCDETF Strike Forces. For example, Strike Forces were integral participants in two recent successful operations, "Operation Xcellerator" and "Project Reckoning." These multi-agency, multi-national efforts have resulted in more than 1,350 arrests and the seizure of more than $137 million in currency, 32,000 kilograms of cocaine, thousands of pounds of methamphetamine, thousands of pounds of marijuana, approximately 1.3 million Ecstasy pills, hundreds of weapons, three aircraft and three maritime vessels.

DEPARTMENT OF JUSTICE

Office of Justice Programs

Resource Summary

	Budget Authority (in Millions)		
Drug Resources by Function	FY 2009 Final	FY 2010 Enacted	FY 2011 Request
Prevention	27.000	27.000	69.793
State and Local Assistance	303.500	144.385	100.793
Treatment	67.000	117.000	137.000
Total Drug Resources by Function	397.500	288.385	307.586
Drug Resources by Decision Unit			
Regional Information Sharing System	45.000	45.000	9.000
Enforcing Underage Drinking Laws	25.000	25.000	0.000
Prescription Drug Monitoring	7.000	7.000	0.000
Residential Substance Abuse Treatment	10.000	30.000	30.000
Southwest Border Prosecution	31.000	31.000	0.000
Consolidated Tribal Grant	0.000	0.000	111.586
Northern Border Prosecution	3.000	3.000	0.000
Second Chance Act[1]	7.000	30.000	50.000

	Budget Authority (in Millions)		
Drug Resources by Function	FY 2009 Final	FY 2010 Enacted	FY 2011 Request
Byrne Criminal Justice Innovation Program[2]	25.000	20.000	40.000
Arrestee Drug Abuse Monitoring	0.000	0.000	10.000
Methamphetamine Enforcement and Clean Up	39.500	40.385	0.000
Drug, Mental Health, and Problem Solving Courts[3]	50.000	57.000	57.000
Combating Criminal Narcotics Activity Stemming from the [4]	30.000	0.000	0.000
Rural Law Enforcement to Combat Drugs and Crime[4]	125.000	0.000	0.000
Total Drug Resources by Decision Unit	397.500	288.385	307.586
Drug Resources Personnel Summary			
Total FTEs (direct only)	60	67	67
Drug Resources as a Percent of Budget			
Total Agency Budget (in Billions)[5]	$ 2.5	$ 2.4	$ 2.2
Drug Resources Percentage	16.06%	12.10%	13.82%

[1] In FY 2011, amount reported for the Second Chance Act decision unit reflects 50% of total funding, as directed by the Office of Management and Budget and Office of National Drug Control Policy. In FY 2010, amount represents 30% of total funding of Second Chance Act.

[2] In FY 2011, the Byrne Criminal Justice Innovation Program replaces the Weed and Seed Program.

[3] In FY 2011, the Drug, Mental Health, and Problem Solving Courts Program replaces Drug Courts.

[4] Funding for this program was provided through the American Recovery and Reinvestment Act of 2009.

[5] Agency Budget total is less OJP's Crime Victims Fund and Public Safety Officers Benefits mandatory accounts, as well as reimbursement dollars.

PROGRAM SUMMARY

Mission

The Justice Assistance Act of 1984 established the Office of Justice Programs (OJP), whose mission is to provide federal leadership in developing the nation's capacity to prevent and control crime, administer justice, and assist crime victims. As such, OJP resources are primarily targeted to providing assistance to state, local, and tribal governments. In executing its mission, OJP dedicates specific resources in support of the *National Drug Control Strategy* that focus on breaking the cycle of drug abuse and crime including: drug testing and treatment, provision of graduated sanctions, drug prevention and education, and research and statistics.

Budget

The total drug control request for OJP in FY 2011 is $307.6 million, a net increase of $19.2 million above the FY 2010 enacted level of $288.4 million.

Residential Substance Abuse Treatment

Total FY 2011 Request: $30.0 Million (Reflects No Change rom FY 2010)

The Residential Substance Abuse Treatment (RSAT) program for state prisoners was established to help states and units of local governments develop, implement, and improve residential substance abuse treatment programs in correctional facilities, and establish and maintain community-based aftercare services for probationers and parolees. Ultimately, the program goal is to help offenders become drug-free and learn the skills needed to sustain themselves upon return to the community.

FY 2011 Total Changes (no change): The Budget will continue to fund treatment services to prisoners.

Drug, Mental Health, and Problem Solving Courts

Total FY 2011 Request: $57.0 Million (Reflects No Change from FY 2010)

This program consolidates separate funding streams for the Drug Court Program and Mental Health Problem Solving Courts. This consolidation will provide OJP the flexibility to continue providing grants to state, local, and tribal criminal justice agencies to help plan, implement, and improve drug court programs; and assist state, local, and tribal criminal justice agencies in working with mental health, substance abuse, housing, and related systems to decrease recidivism of mentally ill offenders, thus improving public safety and public health.

FY 2011 Total Changes (no change): The program will continue to assist state, local, and tribal governments in developing and implementing problem solving court strategies to address their jurisdiction's unique needs.

Second Chance Act

Total FY 2011 Request: $50.0 Million
(Reflects $20.0 Million Increase from FY 2010)

The Second Chance Act Program builds on the success of OJP's past reentry initiatives by providing grants to establish and expand adult and juvenile offender reentry programs. This program authorizes various grants to government agencies and nonprofit groups to provide employment assistance, substance abuse treatment, housing, family programming, mentoring, victims support, and other services that can help reduce re-offending and violations of probation and parole.

FY 2011 Total Changes (+$20.0 million): The Budget proposes an increase of $20.0 million to further expand the program. Funded with Second Chance are 3 IWG programs:

- Prosecution led Drug Treatment Alternatives to Prison: $10 million to allow the Attorney General to make grants to State, Tribal, and local prosecutors to improve the infrastructure, knowledge, and systems needed to operate the judicial aspects of alternative to prison initiatives.
- Adult Re Entry Court Initiative: $5 million to extend the proven practices of drug courts into the management of drug related offenders being released from incarceration back into the community. Funds will support training of probation

officers and judges, creation of needed data systems, and expansion of drug testing capabilities.

- Innovative Diversion/ReEntry Programs for Juvenile Drug Offenders: $4 million to provide support to develop and test innovative strategies for use with juvenile offender populations having cooccurring substance abuse problems.

Byrne Criminal Justice Innovation Program

Total FY 2011 Request: $40.0 Million
(Reflects $20.0 Million Increase from FY 2010)

Recent research findings in areas such as community violence prevention and community policing have demonstrated that law enforcement or crime prevention efforts tailored to address particular problems in a defined area often achieve much better results than more general efforts targeting broader areas.

FY 2011 Total Changes (+$20.0 million): The Byrne Criminal Justice Innovation Program, successor to the Weed and Seed Program, will build on these findings by encouraging state, local, and tribal governments to develop and implement innovative public safety initiatives using evidence-based program strategies in order to develop new programs that can be replicated in other locations.

Arrestee Drug Abuse Monitoring (ADAM) Program

Total FY 2011 Request: $10.0 Million
(Reflects $10.0 Million Increase from FY 2010)

The Arrestee Drug Abuse Monitoring (ADAM) Program is a survey to collect data on drug use by arrestees to help inform policy decisions about evolving trends in the types of drugs used by offenders and their relationship to the crimes being committed. In conjunction, this survey provides a wealth of information on the characteristics of arrestees not available from administrative record systems, including their demographic, educational, employment and economic characteristics, as well as their prior involvement with the criminal justice system. ADAM also provides unique detailed information about illicit drug markets and the nature of illicit drug transactions not available from any other source.

FY 2011 Total Changes (+$10.0 million): The FY 2011 request includes $10.0 million to expand and enhance ADAM, which collects arrestee-reported data on drug use and related behaviors.

Consolidated Tribal Grants

Total FY 2011 Request: $111.6 Million
(Reflects $111.6 Million Increase from FY 2010)

The Department of Justice has set aside 7% of the Office of Justice Program's (OJP) discretionary funding for grants or reimbursement programs under a new tribal criminal justice assistance program which consolidates previous OJP tribal funding streams and increases funding available for Indian Country public safety.

FY 2011 Total Changes (+$111.6 million): In addition to funding grants to improve public safety outcomes in Indian Country, these grants will support training and technical assistance to improve tribal criminal justice outcomes, including drug and alcohol-related issues.

Prescription Drug Monitoring Program

Total FY 2011 Request: $0.0
(Reflects $7.0 Million Decrease from FY 2010)

The purpose of the Prescription Drug Monitoring Program (PDMP) is to enhance the capacity of regulatory and law enforcement agencies to collect and analyze controlled substance prescription data. In coordination with the Department of Health and Human Services, the program aims to assist states that want to establish a PDMP. Objectives of the program include building a data collection and analysis system at the state level, enhancing existing programs' ability to analyze and use collected data, facilitating the exchange of collected prescription data between states, and assessing the efficiency and effectiveness of the programs funded under this initiative.

FY 2011 Total Changes (-$7.0 million): The Budget proposes a decrease of $7.0 million. The PDMP program is now funded through the Drug Enforcement Administration's Diversion Control program.

Regional Information Sharing System

Total FY 2011 Request: $9.0 Million
(Reflects $36.0 Million Decrease from FY 2010)

RISS is the only national criminal intelligence system operated by and for state and local law enforcement agencies.

FY 2011 Total Changes (-$36.0 million): The Budget proposes a decrease of $36.0 million in order to fund other priority initiatives.

Enforcing Underage Drinking Laws

Total FY 2011 Request: $0.0
(Reflects $25.0 Million Decrease from FY 2010)

The Enforcing Underage Drinking Laws (EUDL) program supported and enhanced efforts by states and local jurisdictions to prohibit the purchase and consumption of alcoholic beverages by minors. Minors are defined as individuals under 21 years of age.

FY 2011 Total Changes (-$25.0 million): The Budget proposes a decrease of $25.0 million in order to fund other priority initiatives.

Southwest Border Prosecution

Total FY 2011 Request: $0.0
(Reflects $31.0 Million Decrease from FY 2010)

This program provided funding for local prosecutor offices in the four Southwest Border states of California, New Mexico, Arizona, and Texas for the costs of processing, detaining, and prosecuting drug and other cases referred from Federal arrests or Federal investigations.

FY 2011 Total Changes (-$31.0 million): The Budget proposes a decrease of $31.0 million in order to fund other priority initiatives.

Northern Border Prosecution

Total FY 2011 Request: $0.0
(Reflects $3.0 Million Decrease from FY 2010)

This program provided reimbursement of some expenses to state and local law enforcement agencies (including prosecutors, probation officers courts, and detention facilities) along the northern border with the handling and processing of drug and alien cases referred from Federal arrests.

FY 2011 Total Changes ($3.0 million): The Budget proposes a decrease of $3.0 million in order to fund other priority initiatives.

Methamphetamine Enforcement and Lab Cleanup

Total FY 2011 Request: $0.0
(Reflects $40.4 Million Decrease from FY 2010)

The Methamphetamine Enforcement and Lab Cleanup Grants provided assistance to state, local and tribal law enforcement agencies in support of programs designed to address methamphetamine production and distribution, as well as target "hot spots" characterized by high levels of drug production or distribution.

FY 2011 Total Changes (-$40.4 million): The Budget proposes a decrease of $40.4 million in order to fund other priority initiatives.

PERFORMANCE

Introduction

This section on the FY 2009 performance of the OJP program is based on agency GPRA documents, the OMB Assessment, and other agency information. The tables below include performance measures, targets and achievements for the latest year for which data are available.

The Drug Court program was rated favorably in the 2008 OMB Assessment. In 2004, the Weed and Seed program was rated favorably, reflecting its monitoring of homicides and its efforts towards sustainability.

Drug Courts		
Selected Measures of Performance	FY 2009 Target	FY 2009 Achieved
» Percent of drug court participants who graduate from the drug court program	69%	57%
» Percent of drug court participants who exhibit a reduction in substance use while in the drug court program »	87%	79%

Discussion

OJP has gradually shifted its program emphasis from establishing new drug courts to building and enhancing existing drug court capacity through training and technical assistance, management information system enhancements, evaluations, increased services to drug court clients, and information dissemination.

In FY 2008 OJP developed new outcome measures to monitor the percent of participants who exhibit a reduction in substance use while in the program, and the percent of participants who re-offend one year post program completion. In addition, several actions are being taken to improve the performance of the program.

OJP is working to improve program design and implementation by focusing on coordination, both internal and with other agencies. Although OJP and the Substance Abuse and Mental Health Services Administration (SAMHSA) do not duplicate what they fund or emphasize (OJP provides grants for new and existing drug courts, while SAMHSA focuses on building treatment capacity), OJP has begun coordinating with SAMHSA. Representatives from SAMHSA and BJA met in June 2009 to discuss coordinated solicitation timing, performance measures, and the possibility of conducting joint trainings and/or peer reviews. OJP and SAMHSA's Center for Substance Abuse Treatment are issuing a jointly-funded drug court enhancement solicitation in FY 2010.

OJP is conducting a comprehensive needs assessment to determine how future funding should be allocated (geographically and by type of drug court: adult, family, and juvenile). OJP reviewed drug court performance measures, and will complete the needs assessment by August 2010.

OJP is conducting a Multi-site Adult Drug Court Evaluation to examine the influence of offender, court, and community characteristics on offender motivation, service access, compliance, relapse, recidivism, and employment. The evaluation will utilize data for 1,800 probationers from multiple interviews, treatment/recidivism records, drug tests; site staff interviews/observations; and detailed budget information for cost studies.

OJP anticipates final evaluation results in the spring of 2010, which coincides with the National Association of Drug Court Professionals conference.

RSAT		
Selected Measures of Performance	CY 2008[1] Target	CY 2008 Achieved
» Ofth e offenders that complete the progam, the number who have remained arrest free for 1 year following release from aftercare	1,800	2,808
» Number of participants in RSAT	20,000	28,308

[1] Reporting due dates are on a calendar year (CY) basis. The data for CY 2008 data are reported in the table. CY 2009 data will be available in October 2010.

Discussion

RSAT, created by the Violent Crime Control and Law Enforcement Act of 1994 (Public Law 103-322), assists state and local governments in developing and implementing residential substance abuse treatment programs (individual and group treatment activities) in correctional and detention facilities. The RSAT program must be provided in residential treatment facilities set apart from the general correctional population; be focused on the inmate's substance abuse problems; and develop the inmate's cognitive, behavioral, social, vocational, and other skills to solve the substance abuse and related problems.

Several actions are being taken to improve the performance of the program. OJP reduced the reporting burden on RSAT grantees by enabling electronic reporting for performance measurement. In FY 2008, BJA added RSAT performance measure data collection to its Performance Measurement Tool (PMT) (currently being used to collect performance metrics data for other BJA programs, including the Drug Court program). Grantees began reporting via the PMT in January 2009.

OJP drafted new performance measures, field-tested them with grantees and analyzed the resulting data before adding the new measures to the PMT. OJP has made performance data publicly available at http://www.ojp.usdoj.gov/BJA/grant/RSATPM 0609.pdf.

Weed and Seed		
Selected Measures of Performance	CY 2008[1] Target	CY 2008 Achieved
» Percent reduction in homicides per site funded under the Weed and Seed program	1.2%	7.5%
» Number of homicides per site (average for sites reporting)	3.9	3.5

[1] Program runs on a calendar year basis. CY 2008 data are being reported in the table. CY 2009 data will be available in October 2010.

Discussion

The Weed and Seed Program provides assistance to address violent crimes and gang-related activities in adversely-impacted neighborhoods. The Community Capacity Development Office (CCDO), which assists over 270 communities with coordination of law enforcement efforts while developing their capacity to implement crime prevention programs such as Safe Havens, after-school enrichment activities, and substance use treatment options.

During CY 2009, 90% of reporting Weed and Seed sites included Anti-Drug activities as a component of their weeding strategy. Active participation in the Drug Education for Youth (DEFY) program, a major partnership between CCDO and the Department of the Navy, was reported by 22% of the sites.

Several actions have been taken to improve the performance of the program. OJP selected an evaluator to conduct a rigorous national evaluation to assess the impact of the Weed and Seed program and its component strategies in sites across the nation. A web-based survey instrument was launched in December 2008. All data gathered (site visits, resident surveys and stakeholder surveys) have been coded, and initial analyses have begun. The new data are now being compared with GPRA data to develop a complete process and impact analysis. The final evaluation report is due in February 2010.

CCDO improved the automation of performance data collection and handling to better track how the program is performing. Starting in CY 2007, CCDO provided GPRA forms and instructions electronically in PDF file format and distributed these forms to all sites. As a result, in CY 2007, 66% of the GPRA forms were received through this submission method. CCDO then reassessed the process and made improvements to the form's layout and the submission process, resulting in an 88% electronic transmittal rate in CY 2008 and a 90%

electronic transmittal rate in CY 2009. The electronic forms' capability also improved data entry accuracy.

DEPARTMENT OF JUSTICE

National Drug Intelligence Center

Resource Summary

Budget Authority (in Millions)			
	FY 2009 Final	FY 2010 Enacted	FY 2011 Request
Drug Resources by Function			
Intelligence	$44.000	$44.023	$44.580
Total Drug Resources by Function	$44.000	$44.023	$44.580
Drug Resources by Decision Unit			
Salaries and Expenses	$44.000	$44.023	$44.580
Total Drug Resources by Decision Unit	$44.000	$44.023	$44.580
Drug Resources Personnel Summary			
Total FTEs (direct only)	239	239	274
Drug Resources as a Percent of Budget			
Total Agency Budget (in Billions)	$0.4	$0.4	$0.4
Drug Resources Percentage	100%	100%	100%

PROGRAM SUMMARY

Mission

The National Drug Intelligence Center (NDIC) mission is to provide domestic strategic drug.related intelligence support to the drug control, public health, law enforcement, and intelligence communities of the United States in order to reduce the adverse effects of drug trafficking, drug abuse, and other drug.related criminal activity.

Budget

In FY 2011, the budget request is $44.6 million, a net increase of $0.6 million over the Fiscal Year 2010 enacted level. The funding will allow NDIC to provide domestic strategic counterdrug analysis in support of policymakers and resource planners and also provide support to law enforcement authorities and the intelligence community by conducting document and media exploitation of materials collected in federal, state, and local law enforcement activity associated with counterdrug, counterterrorism, and national security investigations and operations.

Salaries and Expenses (S&E)

Total FY 2011 Request: $44.6 Million (Reflects $0.6 Million Increase from FY 2010)

NDIC prepares strategic analytical studies on the trafficking of illegal drugs and on related illegal activities that pose a threat to the national security of the United States. NDIC intelligence reports provide reports of the threat posed by illicit drugs in the United States. NDIC also provides real-time support to the law enforcement and intelligence communities by conducting document and media exploitation of materials associated with counterdrug and counterterrorism investigations. In addition to intelligence products and document exploitation, NDIC provides counterdrug training to the law enforcement and intelligence communities.

NDIC partners with the Department of Homeland Security Office of Counternarcotics Enforcement to provide critical intelligence to identify, track, and sever the nexus between drug trafficking and terrorism. NDIC also produces strategic money laundering reports that help implement anti-money laundering initiatives. NDIC reports address the methods wholesale-level traffickers use to launder drug proceeds. NDIC supports the National Money Laundering Threat Assessment and the National Money Laundering Strategy--interagency projects that enhance the nation's ability to counter international money laundering.

NDIC has 274 direct authorized positions for FY 2011, an adjustment of 35 positions intended to account for existing positions at NDIC that were not captured within the FY 2010 President's Budget. Specifically, these positions are existing U.S. Air Force personnel at NDIC which are reimbursably funded by NDIC.

FY 2011 Total Changes (+$0.6 million): The FY 2011 increase is an adjustment to base over the FY 2010 enacted level for 2010 pay raises and the annualization of the 2009 pay raise.

OFFICE OF NATIONAL DRUG CONTROL POLICY

Counterdrug Technology Assessment Center

Resource Summary

Budget Authority (in Millions)			
	FY 2009 Final	FY 2010 Enacted	FY 2011 Request
Drug Resources by Function			
Research & Development	$3.000	$5.000	$0.000
Total Drug Resources by Function	$3.000	$5.000	$0.000
Drug Resources by Decision Unit			
Research & Development	$3.000	$5.000	$0.000
Total Drug Resources by Decision Unit	$3.000	$5.000	$0.000
Drug Resources Personnel Summary			
Total FTEs (direct only)	0	0	0
Drug Resources as a Percent of Budget			
Total Agency Budget (in Billions)	$0.003	$0.005	$0.000
Drug Resources Percentage	100.00%	100.00%	N/A

PROGRAM SUMMARY

Mission

The Counterdrug Technology Assessment Center's (CTAC) mission was to serve as the central counterdrug technology research and development organization of the Federal Government. The CTAC program has been discontinued beginning in FY 2011 as its program activities are either being addressed by other Federal Drug Control Program agencies or represent one, among many contributors to various projects.

Budget

The CTAC program is being proposed for deletion in order for ONDCP to focus on higher drug control priorities.

PERFORMANCE

Introduction

This section on the FY 2009 performance of the CTAC Research & Development program is based on agency GPRA documents, OMB reviews, and other agency documents. The tables include performance measures, targets and achievements for the latest year for which data are available.

Counterdrug Technology Assessment Center		
Selected Measures of Performance	FY 2009 Target	FY 2009 Achieved
» Number of research projects initiated to expand understanding of demand-and supply-side of illegal drug markets	2	8
» Percentage of research projects that form the basis of or contribute to policy or program direction	50%	50%

Discussion

In 2009, CTAC approved the following eight projects:

Expand the re-engineered national vital statistics system (RENVSS). This project will contribute to the enhancement of the Government's ability to track drug overdose deaths and improve the timeliness of the reporting;

Develop a mortality coding tracking component for the RENVSS. This project is closely related to the prior project and will improve the process of collecting the cause of death data (including drug overdose deaths) and improve the timeliness of the reporting;

Enhance Magnetic Resonance Imaging (MRI). This project continues to build upon prior CTAC support for MRI research by enhancing the imaging resolution capability of those machines at much less cost than purchasing new machines with improved resolution;

Develop tunnel detection and activity monitoring for the U.S. southwest border. This project will contribute to the development of sensor technology and deployment in existing public infrastructure (e.g., storm drains) along the southwest border to suppress its use for drug trafficking and other forms of smuggling;

Improve and standardize prescription drug monitoring programs (PDMPs). This project will assist in identifying best practices among existing PDMPs and develop software to automate those practices which will be provided to existing and developing PDMPs to improve their efficiency and timeliness;

Develop communications internet intercept capability (working with the Drug Enforcement Administration). This project contribute to the development of mobile technology to permit law enforcement agencies to intercept internet communications among drug traffickers;

Leverage remote sensing technologies to improve detection of cannabis cultivation sites on public lands. This project will assist in developing technology to enable remote sensing of outdoor marijuana grows early in the production cycle; and

Convene CTAC-hosted conferences. This project will help support the convening of two technology conferences to bring together the world's leading drug supply and demand researchers to discuss their latest advancements.

Six of these 8 projects are being conducted jointly with interagency partners. Interagency Agreements are either in process or have been signed between ONDCP and the relevant agency. The projects will be implemented over the coming year.

Office of National Drug Control Policy

High Intensity Drug Trafficking Areas

Resource Summary

Budget Authority (in Millions)			
	FY 2009 Final	FY 2010 Enacted	FY 2011 Request
Drug Resources by Function			
Intelligence	$60.198	$61.376	53.600
Interdiction	21.667	22.091	19.292
Investigations	134.474	137.104	119.736
Prevention	2.728	2.728	2.728
Prosecution	8.565	8.733	7.626
Research & Development	2.100	2.700	2.700
Treatment	4.268	4.268	4.268
Total Drug Resources by Function	$234.000	$239.000	$209.950
Drug Resources by Decision Unit			
High Intensity Drug Trafficking Areas	$234.000	$239.000	209.950
Total Drug Resources by Decision Unit	$234.000	$239.000	$209.950
Drug Resources Personnel Summary Total FTEs (direct only)	0	0	0
Drug Resources as a Percent of Budget Total Agency Budget (in Billions)	$0.2	$0.2	$0.2
Drug Resources Percentage	100.00%	100.00%	100.00%

Program Summary

Mission

The HIDTA program was established by the Anti-Drug Abuse Act of 1988 to provide assistance to federal, state and local law enforcement entities operating in areas most adversely affected by drug trafficking. HIDTA was reauthorized in the Office of National Drug Control Policy Reauthorization Act of 2006 (P.L. 109-469). The mission of the HIDTA Program is to disrupt the market for illegal drugs in the United States by assisting federal, state, local and tribal law enforcement entities to dismantle and disrupt drug trafficking organizations, with particular emphasis on drug trafficking regions that have harmful effects on other parts of the United States.

Budget

In FY 2011, ONDCP requests $210.0 million, which is a decrease of $29.0 million from the FY 2010 level.

High Intensity Drug Trafficking Areas Program

Total FY 2011 Request: $210.0 Million
(Reflects $29.0 Million Decrease from FY 2010)

A central feature of the HIDTA program is the discretion granted to HIDTA Executive Boards to design a strategy to respond to the specific drug trafficking threats found in each HIDTA region and to develop initiatives to implement that strategy. This discretion ensures that each HIDTA Executive Board can tailor its strategy and initiatives closely to local conditions and can respond quickly to changes in those conditions. In FY 2009, these locally-designed strategies used 67 percent of HIDTA funds for multi-agency investigative task forces and interdiction initiatives and 26 percent for intelligence and information sharing initiatives. Smaller amounts were used for prosecution (3 percent), prevention and treatment (3 percent) and research and development (1 percent).

FY 2011 Total Changes (-$29.0 million): The FY 2011 budget reflects a $29.0 million reduction, which will be spread based upon ONDCP performance assessments for the HIDTA initiatives.

Performance

Introduction

This section on the performance of the HIDTA program is based on agency GPRA documents and other program information. The table includes performance measures, targets, and achievements.

Discussion

For FY 2008, the most recent year for which complete data is available, annual reports indicate that there were almost 670 HIDTA initiatives in the 28 HIDTAs and five U.S. southwest border regions. These initiatives were staffed by more than 6,300 Federal agents and analysts and nearly 16,000 state and local officers, analysts, and other representatives.

HIDTA initiatives identified more than 8,200 DTOs operating in their areas, of which they expected to disrupt or dismantle 2,935. Data from the Performance Management Process (PMP) show that many of the DTOs identified (34%) trafficked in more than one illegal substance. Of those identified as trafficking in a specific drug, approximately 22% trafficked cocaine, about 17% were reported to traffic in marijuana, 12% methamphetamine, and 5% heroin. Prescription drugs accounted for less than 3% of drugs trafficked.

Selected Measures of Performance	FY 2008 Target	FY 2008 Achieved
»Number of DTOs disrupted or dismantled	2,317	3,171
»Cumulative Number of DTOs disrupted or dismantled	8,997	10,613
»Number of multi-state or international DTOs disrupted or dismantled	1,463	2,009
»Cumulative Number of multi-state or international DTOs disrupted or dismantled	5,684	6,738
»Value of drugs, cash, and other assests seized	$10.4B	$33.9B
»Cumulative value of drugs, cash, and other assests seized	$40.4B	$87.5B
»Number of CPOT-related DTOs disrupted or dismantled	208	107
»Cost per DTO disrupted or dismantled	$75,400	$51,981

HIDTAs reported disrupting or dismantling 3,171 (108%) of the DTOs they expected to disrupt or dismantle in FY 2008. More than half (63%) of the disrupted and dismantled DTOs were identified as part of a multistate or international operation. In the process, HIDTA initiatives removed drugs with a wholesale value of more than $33 billion from the market, and seized $572 million in cash and $203 million in non-cash assets from drug traffickers. PMP data further indicate that 81% of HIDTAs achieved the targets established in the PMP for seizing drugs and 50% achieved PMP targets for the average cost per DTO disrupted or dismantled. In addition, 84% of HIDTAs achieved the desired PMP return on investment (ROI) targets for the wholesale value of drugs taken off the market and cash and non-cash assets seized.

In FY 2009, ONDCP provided $3,023,323 in discretionary funding to the Domestic Marijuana Eradication and Investigation Project (DMEIP), which contributed to record eradication of domestic marijuana by Federal, state, and local law enforcement. Such resources help coordinate eradication efforts by the Drug Enforcement Administration, the Department of the Interior, the Department of Agriculture, the National Guard, and the M7 states which, in 2008, resulted in 7.7 million plants being eradicated, an increase of more than 2,000,000 plants from 2007. The HIDTA funding was used for officer overtime, aviation flying hours, special equipment purchases, and other investigative costs.

In FY 2009, ONDCP awarded $200,000 in discretionary funding and $500,000 in baseline funding to the National Methamphetamine and Pharmaceuticals Initiative (NMPI). The purpose of the NMPI is to counter the production, distribution and consumption of methamphetamine and precursor chemicals in the United States through training; information sharing; assisting in targeting criminal enterprises involved in these activities; and investigative support. In FY 2009, the NMPI continued to sponsor and manage conferences between U.S. Federal, state, and local law enforcement and certain international partners such as China and Canada. As a result of added responsibilities regarding pharmaceuticals, the

NMPI further monitors programs or legislation that impact diversion control of legal substances that could be or have been abused.

In FY 2009, ONDCP released the second National Southwest Border Counternarcotics Strategy. The HIDTA Program, specifically the five regions of the Southwest Border (SWB) HIDTA, plays a major role with the implementation of that strategy. The SWB HIDTA has as its primary goal the disruption of the flow of illicit drugs from Mexico, and has expanded its mission to include the movement of cash, assets, and weapons from the U.S. into Mexico. While it continued to participate in various initiatives along the entire border and in the Domestic Highway Enforcement (DHE) Program, the SWB HIDTA increased its focus on initiatives in support of the Southwest Border Counternarcotics Strategy. Improved and enhanced cooperation, communications, and coordination are an integral part of the SWB HIDTA as it assists in the implementation of the Strategy.

OFFICE OF NATIONAL DRUG CONTROL POLICY

Other Federal Drug Control Programs

Resource Summary

Budget Authority (in Millions)			
	FY 2009 Final	FY 2010 Enacted	FY 2011 Request
Drug Resources by Function			
Prevention	$160.000	$140.000	$152.000
Research & Development	13.450	13.400	12.350
Treatment	1.250	1.000	0.950
Total Drug Resources by Function	$174.700	$154.400	$165.300
Drug Resources by Decision Unit			
National Youth Anti-Drug Media Campaign	70.000	45.000	66.500
Drug-Free Communities	90.000	95.000	85.500
National Drug Court Institute	1.250	1.000	0.950
Anti-Doping Activities	9.800	10.000	9.025
Performance Measures Development	0.500	0.250	0.237
National Alliance of Model State Drug Laws	1.250	1.250	1.188
World Anti-Doping Agency Dues	1.900	1.900	1.900
Total Drug Resources by Decision Unit	$174.700	$154.400	$165.300
Drug Resources Personnel Summary			
Total FTEs (direct only)	1	1	1
Drug Resources as a Percent of Budget			
Total Agency Budget (in Billions)	$0.2	$0.2	$0.2
Drug Resources Percentage	100.00%	100.00%	100.00%

PROGRAM SUMMARY

Mission

The Anti-Drug Abuse Act of 1988, as amended, and the Office of National Drug Control Policy (ONDCP) Reauthorization Act of 2006, established this account to be administered by the Director of ONDCP. The funds appropriated to the program support high-priority drug control programs and may be transferred to drug control agencies.

Budget

In FY 2011, ONDCP requests $165.3 million for the Other Federal Drug Control Programs (OFDCP), which is an increase of $10.9 million above the FY 2010 level. OFDCP has seven decision units: National Youth Anti-Drug Media Campaign; Drug-Free Communities (DFC); National Drug Court Institute (NDCI); Anti-Doping Activities; Performance Measures Development (PMD); the National Alliance of Model State Drug Laws (NAMSDL); and World Anti Doping Agency (WADA).

National Youth Anti-Drug Media Campaign

Total FY 2011 Request: $66.5 Million
(Reflects $21.5 Million Increase from FY 2010)

The FY 2010 resources of $45 million will enable the Media Campaign to begin implementing a new two-tiered strategy, including a pilot program targeting at-risk communities or populations. Tier one includes a fully integrated effort that combines TV, radio, print, and interactive media with public communications outreach to reach youth, providing a broad prevention base nationally. This tier will include more emphasis on the use of online media to increase teen engagement and participation. Messages will largely focus on educating young people on the negative health, social, academic and financial consequences of using substances and persuading them to remain "Above the Influence." The second tier will involve more targeted efforts focusing on populations or communities at risk of drug use. This includes an emphasis on addressing methamphetamine in the specific states with high usage rates as well as a specific initiative targeting American Indian youth. In addition, the Campaign will begin to develop and test small-scale, pilot projects designed to reach at-risk youth at the community level, which might include the youth who are particularly impacted by the negative consequences of substance abuse (e.g., African American, Hispanic, American Indian youth, inner city youth or rural youth who may not have ready access to digital media). The Media Campaign will continue to develop popular, science-based materials in order to fulfill public and constituent requests received by national clearinghouses and through the Media Campaign's web sites. At this funding level, the parent paid advertising and online efforts will be discontinued.

FY 2011 Total Changes (+$21.5 million): Resources will fund the new two-tier strategy initiated in FY 2010. Tier one will provide a longer and continuous base level of prevention communications targeting teens 14-16 (those moving from middle school into high school) at the national level. This effort will continue to evolve the broad "Above the Influence" platform, allowing it to address the general behavior of drug abuse as well as other emerging drug threats for teens. This layer of the campaign would be delivered via a mix of digital and traditional media, opening the Campaign up to greater youth participation and engaging media partners and marketing communications companies.

The second tier involves a wider implementation of targeted initiatives focusing on communities or populations at risk, recognizing that susceptibility to substance abuse is *not* evenly distributed across the youth population, and that different at-risk populations—whether defined demographically, regionally or in some other fashion—are best reached and influenced in different ways with active participation of their communities. Based on the learnings from the pilot projects, resources will be used to implement localized efforts to more communities and/or populations. In addition, this tier includes the required ten percent to focus on methamphetamine demand reduction advertising in geographic areas with the highest level of meth abuse. Resources will also be used to develop and implement a public communications and advertising effort targeting adult influencers of teens, including parents, to help reinforce the localized efforts.

Drug Free Communities

FY 2011 Request: $85.5 Million
(Reflects $9.5 Million Decrease from FY 2010)

The FY 2010 resources of $95.0 million will support the development of community drug-free coalitions throughout the United States. The program provides up to $125,000 per year in grant funding to local drug-free community coalitions which must be matched at a minimum 1:1 ratio by local communities. These grants are awarded through peer-reviewed annual competitions. Community coalitions strive to increase community involvement and effectiveness in carrying out a wide array of drug prevention strategies, initiatives, and activities.

FY 2011 Total Changes (-$9.5 million): Reduced funding will be provided to DFC coalitions in FY 2011.

National Drug Court Institute

FY 2011 Request: $0.9 Million
(Reflects $0.1 Million Decrease from FY 2010)

The FY 2010 resources of $1.0 million will support NDCI's efforts to improve and expand drug courts through its research, training, and technical assistance programs. NDCI will conduct research and produce reports on successful methods of financing and sustaining drug courts. The program will also provide technical assistance to court systems wishing to adopt these methods. NDCI will use resources to continue to develop and encourage standard drug court data collection practices, which allow for comparisons across drug court systems.

FY 2011 Total Changes (–$0.1 million): A reduced amount of funding is requested for the grantee in FY 2011.

Anti-Doping Activities

FY 2011 Request: $9.0 Million
(Reflects $1.0 Million Decrease from FY 2010)

The FY 2010 resources of $10.0 million will continue anti-doping efforts to educate athletes on the dangers of drug use and eliminate doping in amateur athletic competitions recognized by the United States Olympic Committee. Specifically, these funds support athlete drug testing programs, research initiatives, educational programs, and efforts to inform athletes of the newly adopted rules governing the use of prohibited substances outlined in the recently updated World Anti-Doping Code (the Code). In addition, funds will support legal efforts to enforce compliance with the Code and adjudicate athlete appeals involving doping violations.

FY 2010 Total Changes (–$1.0 million): The Budget proposes to reduce funding by $1.0 million reflecting decrease in funding.

Performance Measures Development

FY 2011 Request: $0.2 Million
(Reflects $0.1 Million Decrease from FY 2010)

The FY 2010 resources of $0.3 million will continue to assist in research and evaluation efforts that develop means for continually assessing the performance and effectiveness of drug reduction programs. These funds will be used to obtain critical drug indicator data, and apply those data to studies that permit program managers to respond to changes in drug market conditions, as well as gauge the effectiveness of their efforts.

FY 2011 Total Changes (-$0.1 million): A reduced amount of funding will be provided for the performance research.

National Alliance of Model State Drug Laws

FY 2011 Request: $1.2 Million
(Reflects $0.1 Million Decrease from FY 2010)

The FY 2010 resources of $1.3 million will support the National Alliance for Model State Drug Laws to prepare and conduct state model law summits and assist state officials in the promotion and adoption of summit-based laws. In addition, resources will support the development and distribution of updated model laws, as well as analyses of state laws and bills involving drug issues.

FY 2011 Total Changes (-$0.1 million): A reduced amount of funding is requested for the grantee in FY 2011.

World Anti-Doping Agency Dues

FY 2011 Request: $1.9 Million (Reflects No Change from FY 2010)

The FY 2010 resources of $1.9 million will support WADA's mission to address performance enhancing and illicit drug use in Olympic sports. The organization is jointly funded by national governments and the international sporting movement. The United States continues to play a leadership role in WADA's development by serving on the agency's governing Executive Committee and Foundation Board. Funds will support drug testing operations, athlete drug education and prevention efforts, and research.

FY 2011 Total Changes (no change): There is no program change.

PERFORMANCE

National Youth Anti-Drug Media Campaign

This section on the FY 2009 performance of the Media Campaign program is based on GPRA documents. The table includes performance measures, targets and achievements. In accordance with the 2006 Reauthorization, ONDCP will provide the required annual report on the Media Campaign's effectiveness based on data from Monitoring the Future, National Survey on Drug Use and Health, a special analysis of the Partnership for Drug Free America's PATS survey conducted by GfK North America (Roper) and other relevant studies, including tracking and evaluation data collected according to marketing and advertising standards.

Media Campaign		
Selected Measures of Performance	FY 2009 Target	FY 2009 Achieved
»Percentage of youth ages 12-18 who believe there is great risk of harm from regular marijuana use	50%	53%
»Percentage of teens, 14-16, who think they definitely will not smoke marijuana at any time during the next year	35%	44%
»Percentage of teens, 14-16, who think they definitely will not smoke marijuana if offered by a close friend	35%	47%

DISCUSSION

During FY 2009, Campaign's strategic goals were to: (1) increase awareness of the risk of drug use, (2) change attitudes about drug use among youth and about the value of parental monitoring among parents, and (3) change intentions regarding drug use among youth and parental monitoring among parents.

The multiple and varied highlights of the FY 2009 accomplishments are briefly outlined below according to the three platforms of the Campaign – youth, parents, and meth/other emerging drugs.

FY 2009 Youth-focused Accomplishments

The Campaign successfully maintained 52 weeks of media presence to engage teens with drug prevention messages. For FY 2009, the Campaign reached 97% of teens (ages 12.17) approximately 72 times.

Youth Ad Tracking Study Results

- In FY 2009, Campaign research indicated an average of 76% of the Campaign's target audience were aware of ATI advertising. This figure places ATI at the top of the list along with other teen targeted national brands such as Coca Cola, Burger King and Nike.
- In addition, an average of 82% of teens recognized the ATI brand logo. This logo awareness figure continued to be significantly higher than other national social

marketing campaigns including the American Legacy Foundation's (an anti-tobacco group funded through the Master Settlement Agreement with the tobacco industry) teentargeted antitobacco Truth Campaign, which had an awareness of 63%.

- In addition, there was a positive association between increased awareness levels of Campaign advertising and an increase among antidrug beliefs in the teen target. Specifically, teens that were aware of the Campaign held stronger anti-drug beliefs than teens that were unaware of the Campaign.

Online and Web (AbovetheInfluence.com) Results

- The Campaign extended the ATI message by buying key search terms on search engine sites such as *Google.com* and *Yahoo.com,* so Campaign-related content would appear in search results (e.g., "marijuana," "alcohol," "meth," and "why take drugs").
- Paid search generated 1.1 million clicks to *AbovetheInfluence.com*.
- Search ads outperformed industry standards by a factor of four.
- In addition to buying paid search terms, the Campaign reconfigured pages within the "Drugs Facts" section on *AbovetheInfluence.com* to increase the likelihood that the Campaign Web site would appear on "organic" search results (those results that were not paid advertising), from sites such as *Google.com*, *Yahoo.com* and *Bing.com*. The Web site now appears on the first page of search results for 75 new search terms and 42 new keywords.
- In FY 2009, the Campaign created viral, sharable assets to leverage the social nature of how teens use the Web today while allowing the ATI message to be endorsed by, advocated, and spread through environments where teens spend most of their time online.
- Sharable assets (i.e. widgets, badges) were downloaded or sent to friends nearly 600,000 times in FY 2009.
- Online media delivered 1.5 billion media impressions (the potential number of people who would see, read or hear a message) on 20 teen-targeted sites such as *MySpace*, *Hulu.com*, and *MTV.com.*
- ATI online advertising surpassed industry averages for click-through rates (people who went from a banner ad to click through to go on the Web site), with Campaign banner ads outperforming industry standards by 2.5 times.

FY 2009 Parent-focused Accomplishments

Starting in 2008 and continuing in 2009, the Parents campaign focused on the key emerging drug threat among teens as indicated by the National Survey on Drug Use and Health (NSDUH), prescription medications. Research showed that parents had not been discussing the dangers of prescription abuse with their teens. Using the Campaign's brand for parents, *Parents: The Anti-Drug,* new advertising and outreach communicated to parents the nature of this growing threat and the simple actions they could take to help prevent youth prescription drug abuse. Research continued to show that parents' actions played a crucial role in protecting adolescents from drug use and a wide variety of other risky behaviors.

Parents Campaign Results

- Reached 90% of the parent target audience an average of 10 times from April – June 2009, through paid advertising.

- The Parents Ad Tracking Study showed an increase in parent awareness of the advertising and signs of a positive impact on their beliefs. both important precursors to changing behaviors:
- Parents' belief that prescription drug abuse was prevalent among teens reached its all time high of 87%, from a pre launch average of 77%.
- There had been significant growth in parents' stated intention to properly conceal or dispose of old or unneeded medicines (67% to 75%) and to ask friends and family to safeguard their drugs (42% to 49%).
- The Campaign's advertising effort was bolstered by outreach to news media outlets to get stories about prescription drugs featured in newspaper articles, TV news shows and online sites. The Campaign had initially set a goal of 50 million news media impressions (the potential number of people who would see, read or hear the message) for this initiative. To date, the Campaign has received more than 120 million news media impressions on the initiative, spreading the initiative deeper into local markets.
- The results of a news media content analysis (where a vendor actually reviewed the content of a news story to see if the prescription drug issue was mentioned and also referred to ONDCP/Media Campaign) showed that the Campaign was the most cited source of news stories about prescription drugs. The Campaign was referenced as a resource in news stories more than any other organization, including National Institute on Drug Abuse (NIDA), Substance Abuse and Mental Health Services Administration (SAMHSA), Partnership for a Drug Free America, and the over the counter medicine industry organization, Consumer Healthcare Products Association (CHPA).

Online and Web (TheAntiDrug.com) Results

- During FY 2009, the Campaign's parent Web site (*TheAntiDrug.com*) received 2,267,461 visits, a rate of approximately 190,000 visits per month.
  - Online media delivered 278.3 million media impressions (the potential number of people who will see, read or hear a message) on 15 parent targeted sites, such as *Parents.com*, *iVillage.com*, and *CNN.*
  - Online advertising for the parent campaign surpassed industry averages for click through rates (people who will go from a banner ad to click through to go on the Web site), with campaign banner ads surpassing industry standards by two times.
- The Campaign sought to be in the top places when people searched for drug related terms on the most widely used search engines – thereby providing them with immediate access to accurate drug information.
  - Clicks on paid keyword search terms generated 101,000 clicks to the Web site.
  - Search ads outperformed industry standards by two times.

FY 2009 Anti-Meth Campaign Accomplishments

The Campaign's Anti-Meth efforts were directed to young adults as national drug prevalence data show substantially higher use rates for 18 25 year olds. The most recent NSDUH showed past year usage for young adults aged 18 25 remained over two times higher than past year use rate for teens, ages 12 17. Further, average age of first use remained consistent at 19.2 years.

The 2009 Anti-Meth Campaign launched in September and ran through November 2009. The Campaign delivered most of its advertising weight to specific states with high methamphetamine usage rates based on the NSDUH 20042007 data and/or high levels of meth lab seizures. The Anti-Meth Campaign aimed to prevent methamphetamine use, dispel myths that treatment for meth addiction was ineffective, and encourage people who need help to get into treatment. The FY 2009 Anti-Meth Campaign performed the following:

- The full suite of anti-meth advertising, including television, print, out-of-home (e.g., roadside billboards, convenience store posters and gas pump signs), radio and Internet advertising, was delivered across 16 states.
- Launched a redesigned methresources.gov website to better provide information and materials to individuals and organizations.
- Reached 87% of the target audience an average of 13 times during the campaign. Provided a mechanism for local organizations and community coalitions to receive free anti-meth resources, including customizable versions of the ads (e.g. TV, print, radio, out-of-home billboards, and posters) for use as public-service announcements.

The Campaign's Media Match program has generated approximately $1.28 billion in incremental media value for the Campaign since its inception (1998 through 2009). The Campaign accomplishments are significant and contribute meaningfully to the demand reduction component of the *Strategy*. It is a fact that fewer than 20 percent of American youth receive an evidence-based drug education program in school, and only 25 percent live in a community served by a Drug-Free Community grant. The great majority of American youth are exposed to a rising tide of pro-drug content in their media and social networking environments. The ATI campaign is often-times the only substantive counter to messages normalizing drug use and trivializing the consequences. Youth response to ATI demonstrates that it is reaching youth with clear, consistent, credible messages that strengthen adolescents' ability to resist negative social influences and avoid drug use.

DRUG FREE COMMUNITIES PROGRAM

This section on the FY 2009 performance of the Drug Free Communities Program (DFC) program is based on agency GPRA documents, OMB program reviews, and other agency documents. The table includes performance measures, targets, and achievements for the latest year for which data are available.

Drug Free Communities Program		
Selected Measures of Performance	FY 2009 Target	FY 2009 Achieved
» Percent coalitions that report decreased risk factors in community	60%	63%
» Percent coalitions that report increased protective factors	72%	76%
» Percent coalitions that report improvement in past 30-day youth use of alcohol, tobacco, or marijuana	88%	90%

(Continued).

Drug Free Communities Program		
Selected Measures of Performance	FY 2009 Target	FY 2009 Achieved
» Percent coalitions that report positive change in the age of initiation of tobacco, alcohol, or marijuana	91%	96%
» Percent coalitions that report positive change in youth perception of risk from tobacco, alcohol or marijuana	95%	93%
» Percent coalitions that report positive change in youth perception of parental disapproval of the use of alcohol, tobacco, or marijuana	95%	91%

DISCUSSION

In 2009, the DFC program met or exceeded all but two of their performance goals ("positive change in youth perception of risk from tobacco, alcohol or marijuana" and "positive change in youth perception of parental disapproval of the use of alcohol, tobacco or marijuana"). These measures have historically shown "ceiling" effects: most youth understand that drugs are risky and most parents disapprove of use. As the program has matured, the targets for these measures have risen each year. With the targets approaching 100%, it is increasingly difficult for coalitions to detect and document incremental change.

DFC-funded coalitions are making strides to reduce youth substance use and bolster their communities' response to emerging drug threats. The two coalitions discussed below are examples of resulting reductions in youth substance use.

In rural southeast Iowa, at least 53% of 11th graders reported having had at least one drink in the past 30 days (2005). The Van Buren County SAFE Coalition in Keosauqua, Iowa, brought community organizations and individuals together to address this critical issue. Using DFC funding, the coalition executed a comprehensive environmental strategy, including alcohol compliance checks and merchant education. In addition, the coalition worked with local law enforcement to produce policy change to institutionalize uniform compliance checks: also, incentives for merchants who had all employees trained on the proper and legal sale of alcohol. This coordinated effort led by the Coalition reduced youth alcohol use rates among 11th graders to 34% in 2008.

Tobacco addiction affects both the young and old alike. The Troy Community Coalition in Troy, Michigan, implemented a multi-faceted approach to prevent tobacco use and reduce the number of its residents addicted to the drug. The coalition engaged youth through a variety of activities, such as presentations at all Troy middle schools.

The coalition also educated adults through Smoking Cessation classes. In addition, the coalition partnered with local professional associations, such as the University of Detroit Mercy Dental School and the Arab American Chaldean Association and provided education on the use of hookahs, a type of tobacco pipe. Through coalition efforts, tobacco use among 10th graders dropped from 55% in 1988 to 20% in 2008.

OFFICE OF NATIONAL DRUG CONTROL POLICY

Salaries and Expenses

Resource Summary

	Budget Authority (in Millions)		
	FY 2009 Final	FY 2010 Enacted	FY 2011 Request
Drug Resources by Function			
Interdiction	$5.363	$5.855	$5.169
International	5.363	5.854	5.168
Investigations	3.270	3.570	3.152
Prevention	4.317	4.713	4.160
Research & Development	1.300	1.300	1.235
State and Local Assistance	3.270	3.570	3.152
Treatment	4.317	4.713	4.160
Total Drug Resources by Function	**$27.200**	**$29.575**	**$26.196**
Drug Resources by Decision Unit			
Operations	$25.900	$28.275	$24.961
Policy Research	1.300	1.300	1.235
Total Drug Resources by Decision Unit	**$27.200**	**$29.575**	**$26.196**
Drug Resources Personnel Summary Total FTEs (direct	108	118	98
Drug Resources as a Percent of Budget Total Agency	$0.027	$0.030	$0.026
Drug Resources Percentage	100%	100%	100%

PROGRAM SUMMARY

Mission

The Office of National Drug Control Policy (ONDCP), established by the Anti-Drug Abuse Act of 1988, and reauthorized by the ONDCP Reauthorization Act of 2006, is charged with developing policies, objectives and priorities for the National Drug Control Program. ONDCP seeks to foster healthy individuals and safe communities by effectively leading the nation's effort to reduce drug use and its consequences. ONDCP's responsibilities include developing a *National Drug Control Strategy* and a consolidated National Drug Control Budget. ONDCP also provides oversight on major programs such as the National Youth Anti-Drug Media Campaign, Drug-Free Communities, and High Intensity Drug Trafficking Areas (HIDTA). In addition, ONDCP conducts policy analysis and research to determine the effectiveness of drug programs and policies in accomplishing the *Strategy's* goals.

Budget

In FY 2011, ONDCP requests $26.2 million, which is a decrease of $3.4 million from the FY 2010 enacted level. ONDCP has two major decision units: Operations and Policy Research.

Operations

Total FY 2011 Request: $24.9 Million
(Reflects $3.3 Million Decrease from FY 2010)

The FY 2010 resources of $28.2 million will enable ONDCP to carry out its responsibilities of advising the President on national and international drug control policies and strategies, and to ensure the effective coordination of anti-drug programs among National Drug Control Program agencies. In addition, ONDCP will provide oversight on major programs, such as the National Youth Anti-Drug Media Campaign, Drug-Free Communities, and HIDTA.

FY 2011 Total Changes ($3.3 million): A reduced amount of funding is requested for this program in FY 2011.

Policy Research

Total FY 2011 Request: $1.2 Million
(Reflects $0.1 Million Decrease from FY 2010)

The FY 2010 resources of $1.3 million support policy research to inform the policy making process. ONDCP conducts research to inform drug policy by identifying strategic trends in the supply of and demand for illegal drugs. Because drug trafficking and use is a covert activity, data must be drawn from a variety of sources to understand trends and the reasons behind the trends.

FY 2011 Total Changes (-$0.1 million): The Budget reflects a slight reduction to policy research efforts.

PERFORMANCE

ONDCP supports four key programs: National Youth Anti-Drug Media Campaign, Drug Free Communities Program, Counterdrug Technology Assessment Center, and the High Intensity Drug Trafficking Areas Program. Performance information for these programs is provided in the respective sections of this document.

SMALL BUSINESS ADMINISTRATION

Budget Authority (in Millions)			
	FY 2009 Final	FY 2010 Enacted	FY 2011 Request
Drug Resources by Function			
Prevention	1.000	1.000	1.000

Budget Authority (in Millions)			
	FY 2009 Final	FY 2010 Enacted	FY 2011 Request
Total Drug Resources by Function	1.000	1.000	1.000
Drug Resources by Decision Unit			
Drug-Free Workplace Grants	1.000	1.000	$1.000
Total Drug Resources by Decision Unit	1.000	1.000	$1.000
Drug Resources Personnel Summary			
Total FTEs (direct only)	0	0	0
Drug Resources as a Percent of Budget			
Total Agency Budget (in Billions)*	$0.6	$0.8	$1.0
Drug Resources Percentage	0.17%	0.13%	0.10%

PROGRAM SUMMARY

Mission

The Small Business Administration's (SBA) Drug Free Workplace Demonstrations Program (DFWP) awards grants to Small Business Development Centers (SBDCs) to provide information and assistance to small businesses with respect to establishing drugfree work environments.

Budget

The total FY 2011 drug control request for the Small Business Administration is $1.0 million, reflecting no increase over the FY 2010 enacted level.

Drug Free Workplace Grants

Total FY 2011 Request: $1.0 Million (Reflects No Change from FY 2010)

SBA's Drug-Free Workplace Demonstration Program was established by the Drug Free Workplace Act of 1998 and renamed the Paul D. Coverdell Drug-Free Workplace Program 2000.

The FY 2011 resources of $1.0 million will provide grants to eligible intermediaries to assist small businesses financially and technically in establishing Drug-Free Workplace Programs. Financial assistance may include free and/or reduced costs for training sessions, management/supervisor consultants, employee assistance program services, and drug testing. Technical assistance may include performing needs assessments, writing/reviewing policies and procedures, providing consultation to management on program development, and providing consultation to supervisors on enforcing the DFWP policy and making referrals to drug testing or employee assistance program services.

FY 2011 Total Changes (no change): SBA will continue to support grantees at the same level as in FY 2010.

Performance

This section on the FY 2009 performance of SBA's Drug Free Workplace Program is based on agency GPRA documents. The table includes performance measures, targets, and achievements for the latest year for which data are available.

Small Business Administration		
Selected Measures of Performance	FY 2009 Target	FY 2009 Actual
»Number of small businesses educated	1,450	1,564
» Number of Drug Free Workplace Programs	165	356

Discussion

The Small Business Administration has made great strides to improve performance measurement. By collecting information from program recipients, SBA intends to track changes in employee performance after the implementation of a Drug Free Workplace Program. The collected information reflects on improvements in: (1) absenteeism, (2) tardiness, (3) workplace accidents, (4) employee turnover, (5) insurance premiums, (6) damaged/stolen property costs, and (7) productivity.

For FY 2009, 30 of the responding small businesses reported an improvement in productivity; 36 reported a decrease in damaged or stolen property; 35 reported a decrease in absenteeism; and 34 reported a decrease in employee turnover. It is anticipated that as the small businesses continue to report over the next few years, the data reported will be more accurate and complete.

Department of State

Bureau of International Narcotics and Law Enforcement Affairs

Resource Summary

Budget Authority (in Millions)			
	FY 2009 Final	FY 2010 Enacted	FY 2011 Request
Drug Resources by Function			
Interdiction	$448.365	$191.921	$249.520
International	702.029	678.799	642.482
Total Drug Resources by Function	$1,150.394	$870.720	$892.002
Drug Resources by Decision Unit			

Budget Authority (in Millions)			
	FY 2009 Final	FY 2010 Enacted	FY 2011 Request
Andean Counterdrug Programs	$315.000	$0.000	$0.000
INCLE	547.394	845.720	892.002
INCLE Supplemental	288.000	25.000	0.000
Total Drug Resources by Decision Unit	$1,150.394	$870.720	$892.002
Drug Resources Personnel Summary			
Total FTEs (direct only)	259	259	259
Drug Resources as a Percent of Budget			
Total Agency Budget (in Billions)	$1.9	$1.6	$2.1
Drug Resources Percentage	61.3%	54.5%	41.8%

Funding allocations for Department of State programs are subject to change as more and better information becomes available. The Department of State routinely adjusts its program allocations.

PROGRAM SUMMARY

Mission

The Bureau for International Narcotics and Law Enforcement Affairs (INL) is dedicated to strengthening criminal justice systems, countering the flow of illegal narcotics, and minimizing transnational crime.

Functioning democratic criminal justice systems strengthen international law enforcement and judicial effectiveness, bolster cooperation in legal affairs, and support the rule of law and respect for human rights. Strong criminal justice systems are also essential to counternarcotics efforts and minimizing transnational crime. In addition to traditional counternarcotics activities, such as disrupting the overseas production and trafficking of illicit drugs, INL supports the development of capable police and competent judicial officials. In order for counternarcotics efforts to be sustainable, strong criminal justice systems must be developed. Similarly, minimizing transnational crime requires both specialized assistance and the overall development of criminal justice systems.

Budget

In FY 2011, the Department of State, Bureau for International Narcotics and Law Enforcement Affairs requests $892.0 million for drug control programs, which is a increase of $21.3 million from the FY 2010 level of $870.7 million, which is comprised of $845.7 million FY 2010 enacted funding and $25.0 million in requested FY 2010 supplemental funding. All FY 2011 funding is requested under the International Narcotics Control and Law Enforcement (INCLE) account.

International Narcotics Control and Law Enforcement

FY2011 Request: $892.0 Million
(Reflects $21.3 Million Increase from FY2009)

The FY 2011 request will be used for initiatives designed to minimize the impact of international crime and drugs on the United States and its international partners. To support this, INL develops, implements, and monitors U.S. Government international counternarcotics control strategies and foreign assistance programs that support the President's National Drug Control Strategy. INL programs are designed to advance international cooperation in order to reduce the foreign production and trafficking of illicit coca, opium poppy, marijuana and other illegal drugs. INL commodity, technical assistance, and capacity building programs improve foreign government institutional capabilities to implement their own comprehensive national drug control plans that will reduce trafficking in illicit drugs and money laundering activities. Training and assistance also supports prevention and treatment programs and projects designed to increase public awareness of the drug threat to strengthen the international coalition against drug trafficking. An interregional aviation program supports drug-crop eradication, surveillance and counterdrug enforcement operations.

Projects funded by INL are also directed at improving foreign law enforcement and intelligence gathering capabilities and enhancing the effectiveness of criminal justice sectors to allow foreign governments to increase drug shipment interdictions, effectively investigate, prosecute and convict major narcotics criminals, and break up major drug trafficking organizations. INL also provides technical assistance to U.S. federal law enforcement authorities working overseas in order to enhance their programs. INL is responsible for foreign policy formulation and coordination and for advancing diplomatic initiatives in counternarcotics in the international arena. Specific INCLE programs are described below:

Mexico

FY 2011 Request: $177.0 Million
(Reflects $1.8 Million Decrease from FY 2010)

The FY 2011 drug control request will support continued counternarcotics, law enforcement, and demand reduction programs to advance the shorter-term goal of dismantling drug trafficking and other criminal organizations, and the longer-term goal of strengthening Mexico's law enforcement institutions and expanding their capacity to attack and deter crime affecting the United States. Funds will continue to enhance Mexico's forensics, surveillance, and data collection and analysis capabilities; continue to help develop a secure communications network for national security agencies; provide technical assistance and non-intrusive inspection equipment for land and maritime interdiction; and support the creation of a national network for demand reduction programs.

FY 2011 Total Changes (-$1.8 million): In FY 2011, the focus of counternarcotics programs shifts from procuring high-cost equipment to providing technical assistance on implementing and institutionalizing the changes brought about through the Mérida Initiative.

Colombia

FY 2011 Request: $178.6 Million
(Reflects $26.6 Million Decrease from FY 2010)

The FY 2011 drug control request will continue support for the Government of Colombia's (GOC) implementation of its National Consolidation Plan, which consolidates progress achieved under Plan Colombia while synchronizing security, counternarcotics, and development through a coordinated government approach. Counternarcotics support will also continue to build the GOC's capacity to take over additional counternarcotics responsibilities. Assistance will support aviation programs that focus on interdiction, eradication, humanitarian and high-value target operations, allowing the Colombian military and police the ability to operate in remote regions. Funding will also go towards enhancing the GOC's ability to interdict drugs, particularly along the Pacific coast.

The multi-year Critical Flight Safety Program (CFSP) will continue to ensure aircrew and aircraft safety while maximizing the cost effectiveness of INL's aging Air Wing fleet. By upgrading these aircraft the Department will avoid future costly maintenance and ensure safe aircraft.

FY 2011 Total Changes (-$26.6 million): The decrease continues a glide path in transferring financial and management responsibility for several counternarcotics and security activities to the Government of Colombia. Decreases will be taken from INCLEfunded eradication and interdiction, counternarcotics, and stabilization operations.

Bolivia

FY 2011 Request: $26.0 Million
(Reflects $6.0 Million Increase from FY2010)

The FY 2011 drug control request will support Bolivian efforts to eliminate excess coca cultivation in and around the Chapare and Yungas regions and to eradicate illegal coca in national parks. Funds will also support efforts to interdict cocaine, cocaine derivatives, other drugs, and precursor chemicals. Support is intended to enable the Government of Bolivia (GOB) to improve efficiencies in the prosecution of narcoticsrelated cases, address official corruption, and increase transparency and accessibility in the criminal justice system. Funds will also support drug prevention efforts. A portion of the funds will enhance the capacity of the National Police through training programs.

FY 2011 Total Changes (+$6.0 million): INL will continue to work with the Government of Bolivia to improve efficiencies in the prosecution of narcoticsrelated cases, address official corruption, and increase transparency and accessibility in the criminal justice system.

Peru

FY 2011 Request: $39.5 Million
(Reflects $0.2 Million Decrease from FY 2010)

The FY 2011 drug control request will address narcotics trafficking threats and will assist the Government of Peru (GOP) with security and state presence east of the Andes by supporting secure basing and training for counternarcotics police. Funding will enable GOP capacity to carry out counternarcotics eradication and interdiction operations on multiple fronts, particularly in entrenched coca growing areas and areas of coca expansion.

FY 2011 Total Changes ($0.2 million): INL will continue FY 2010 counternarcotics eradication and interdiction operations.

Ecuador

FY 2011 Request: $7.5 Million
(Reflects $3.5 Million Increase from FY 2010)

The FY 2011 drug control request will support enhanced presence of Ecuadorian security forces at land and sea ports and on the northern and southern borders to deter narcotics trafficking through Ecuador from Colombia and Peru. Interdiction will be improved with support for stationing counternarcotics police along frequently used or emergent trafficking routes.

Funding provides assistance for canine and law enforcement skills training, operational support for recently established money laundering and chemical control units, along with strengthening of administration of justice programs.

FY 2011 Total Changes (+$3.5 million): The increase will continue police operations and incorporate the need for modernization, such as acquisition of sophisticated scanning equipment.

Military operations are anticipated at an increased pace near the porous border region with Colombia, which will require assistance through FY 2011.

Western Hemisphere Regional Security Initiative

FY 2011 Request: $37.5 Million
(Reflects $31.3 Million Increase from FY 2010)

The FY 2011 drug control request for Central America supports programs in Belize, Nicaragua, Guatemala, Panama, El Salvador, Costa Rica, and Honduras. Funds will provide equipment, training and operational support for counternarcotics vetted units including those under the Drug Enforcement Administration (DEA) and U.S. Immigration and Customs Enforcement (ICE) as well as national police units historically supported by INL.

FY 2011 Total Changes (+$31.3 million): The additional drug control funds will support eradication efforts and aviation support in Guatemala, continue and strengthen the DEA and ICE vetted units, expand demand reduction efforts, and enhance support for national police and regional interdiction.

Caribbean Basin Security Initiative

FY 2011 Request: $31.2 Million
(Reflects $31.2 Million Increase from FY 2010)

The FY 2011 drug control request will be used to stem the flow of illegal drugs into the region by strengthening the region's capacity to detect and interdict drug shipments, bring traffickers and other criminals to trial, and attack money laundering and associated corruption.

FY 2011 Total Changes (+$31.2 million): In FY 2011, drug control funding will support both bilateral and regional counternarcotics initiatives, including support for Sovereign Skies, interdiction, eradication, law enforcement reform and development, and demand reduction.

Brazil

FY 2011 Request: $1.0 million (Reflects no change from FY 2010)

The FY 2011 drug control request will be used to support narcotics interdiction programs and to enhance the Government of Brazil's law enforcement efforts.

FY 2011 Total Changes (no change): INL will sustain ongoing programs.

Haití

FY 2011 Request: $3.8 Million
(Reflects $0.5 Million Increase from FY 2010)

The FY 2011 drug control request will provide support for development of Haiti's drug law enforcement infrastructure and expertise, specifically the Haitian National Police (HNP) anti-drugs unit (BLTS, French acronym). Assistance will continue support for the Haitian Coast Guard to strengthen its maritime interdiction capabilities and enhance information sharing and collaboration with the HNP. Funds will also support efforts to restructure the Haitian Financial Investigative Unit to improve its capacity to successfully investigate money laundering and official corruption.

FY 2011 Total Changes (+$0.5 million): Funds in FY 2011 will sustain FY 2010 projects.

West Africa

FY 2011 Request: $13.2 Million
(Reflects $10.0 Million Increase from FY 2010)

The FY 2011 drug control request will be used for counternarcotics projects in West Africa, including Nigeria, Benin, Cape Verde, Ghana, Guinea, GuineaBissau, Sierra Leone, Senegal, Togo, and The Gambia. Programs will develop strong law enforcement investigative abilities and justice sectors capable of prosecuting and convicting narcotraffickers.

FY 2011 Total Changes (+$10.0 million): The majority of the cocaine transiting West Africa flows to Europe, not the United States. The primary concern is the destabilizing effect this trafficking will have on the region and the potential it represents for corroding good governance. The increase will expand support to other West African countries including Benin, Guinea, Sierra Leone, Senegal, Togo, and The Gambia.

East Asia and the Pacific

FY 2011 Request: $1.7 Million
(Reflects $0.1 Million Decrease from FY 2010)

The FY 2011 drug control request will support programs in Laos and Vietnam. In Laos, funds will support counternarcotics law enforcement assistance; alternative livelihood assistance for villages in opium regions of northern Laos, which formerly grew opium and have not yet received prior or sufficient assistance; and drug demand reduction programs. In Vietnam, funds will support drug interdiction programs.

FY 2011 Total Changes ($0.1 million): Funds will sustain drug control program activities in Laos. Vietnam is a new counternarcotics program.

Turkey

FY 2011 Request: $0.5 Million
(Reflects $0.5 Million Increase from FY 2010)

The FY 2011 drug control request of $0.5 million will support antidrug/anti-organized crime training and technical assistance as well as implementation of drug abuse prevention and education and treatment projects.

FY 2011 Total Changes (+$0.5 million): The request will enable support to Turkey.

Iraq

FY 2011 Request: $2.5 Million
(Reflects $1.5 Million Increase from FY 2010)

The FY 2011 drug control request will leverage FY 2010 funding that is providing training and technical assistance to establish a Center of Excellence on Substance Abuse Treatment. In FY 2011, the Center of Excellence will focus on coordinating the efforts of physicians and public health practitioners by developing a comprehensive nationwide demand reduction strategy.

FY 2011 Total Changes (+$1.5 million): The increase of $1.5 million over FY 2010 levels will support more expansive technical assistance as the Government of Iraq forms its nationwide demand reduction strategy in support of the newly established Center.

Morocco

FY 2011 Request: $0.8 Million
(Reflects $0.8 Million Increase from FY 2010)

The FY 2011 drug control request will support training directed at Moroccan customs and border law enforcement agencies and necessary equipment, such as: inspection tool kits, computers, surveillance equipment, and cargo inspection systems.

FY 2011 Total Changes (+$0.8 million): Funds will be utilized for training programs and equipment.

Afghanistan

FY 2011 Request: $250.6 Million
(Reflects $32.0 Million Decrease from FY 2010)

Afghanistan continues to face an environment of continued insecurity; increased insurgent violence; a weak - and in places - corrupt government; and ongoing challenges to democratic stability. Key continuing priorities will be increasing capacity in Afghan government institutions and strengthening the delivery of services at the sub-national level.

In the counternarcotics arena, FY 2011 funds will enhance programs to disrupt drug trafficking and associated criminal activity throughout the country; continue an incentive-based supply reduction program; and change public attitudes towards drug use and cultivation through comprehensive expansion of support to drug prevention and treatment activity. While poppy reduction efforts in Afghanistan have been and will continue to be led by the Afghan government, funding will support Afghan Governor-led efforts in limited areas where on a specific case-bycase basis support may be required. Specifically, funds for counternarcotics in FY 2011 will support programs in the areas of supply reduction, interdiction, public information, and drug demand reduction.

FY 2011 Total Changes (-$32.0 million): Funds in FY 2011 will emphasize the Good Performers Initiative and Counternarcotics Advisory Teams (CNAT) programs continuing these initiatives for the reduction of poppy cultivation, and increasing the focus on province-based dissuasion against planting. INL will provide support for the Counter Narcotics Police of Afghanistan (CNPA) for the expansion of counternarcotics law enforcement into the provinces, as well as for the operation and maintenance of existing and new facilities to support the Afghan Ministry of Interior's interdiction forces. Funds will also strengthen demand reduction efforts through a nationwide treatment delivery system in which the number of residential, outpatient, and mobile treatment centers will be increased to provide counseling and rehabilitation services to Afghans with drug addictions.

Pakistan

FY 2011 Request: $11.2 Million
(Reflects $4.0 Million Increase from FY 2010)

The FY 2011 drug control request will continue to support INL's counternarcotics program in Pakistan. The counternarcotics program is designed to inhibit poppy cultivation; prevent a spillover effect from the poppy growing and opium processing areas in neighboring Afghanistan; reverse poppy expansion into non traditional growing areas; return Pakistan to its zero poppy status; prevent criminal syndicates from taking hold of local economies; and control drug abuse often seen in drug transit countries. INL will continue training and equipping law enforcement agencies focused on counternarcotics and border area drug demand reduction programs– specifically focusing on both treatment and rehabilitation of existing addicts and drug awareness prevention. These funds will continue provision of training, operational support and small scale commodities to a range of law enforcement agencies that share counternarcotics responsibilities, and support aggressive opium poppy monitoring efforts as security allows.

FY 2011 Total Changes (+$4.0 million): The increase of $4 million will support additional demand reduction efforts and increased support to law enforcement agencies.

Interregional Aviation Support

FY 2011 Request: $60.0 Million
(Reflects $0.3 Million Increase from FY 2010)

The FY 2011 drug control request will provide core level services necessary to operate, sustain, and maintain a fleet of over 140 fixed and rotary wing aircraft of eight types. This support includes central system management, contract administration, and oversight of technical functional areas, such as: operations, training, flight standardization, safety, maintenance, and logistics. Additionally, this funding provides for a centralized system for acquiring, storing and shipping parts and commodities in support of all of the overseas locations. The aircraft support counternarcotics aviation programs in Colombia, Bolivia, Guatemala, Peru, Afghanistan, and drug control programs in other temporary deployment locations as required.

FY 2011 Total Changes (+$0.3 million): The increase of $0.3 million will allow for continuation of existing services.

Critical Flight Safety Program

FY 2011 Request: $11.8 Million
(Reflects $3.6 Million Decrease from FY 2010)

FY 2010 was the first year that the Critical Flight Safety Program (CFSP) funds were requested under the Centrally managed account. CFSP is centrally managed funding for drug control programs that address requirements pertaining to Bolivia, Peru, and Afghanistan. The FY 2011 request will continue to modernize the INL air fleet that put in place a fleet management process for INL air assets (life cycle analysis, safety upgrades, and programmed depot level maintenance) like that which is used by DoD and commercial airlines. It allows INL to ensure the safety of and to extend the life of its aviation assets in order to continue to provide requisite aviation support for counternarcotics programs. Funds will address depot level engine requirements, attrition replacements, wiring/avionics upgrades, and programmed depot level maintenance for Huey II helicopters as well as Aircraft/Aircrew Safety items. CFSP activities for Colombia will continue to be requested under the Colombia bilateral program budget line.

FY 2011 Total Changes ($3.6 million): Funds will support CFSP projects associated with the FY 2011 workload. Work not accomplished in FY 2011 will be carried over in this multi year program.

Drug Awareness and Demand Reduction

FY 2011 Request: $12.5 Million
(Reflects $1.5 Million Decrease from FY 2010)

The FY 2011 drug control request supports the U.S. foreign policy priority of reducing drug use, crime and related violence that threatens our national security and hinders the economic development, political stability, and security in emerging democracies and developing countries. INL demand reduction programs are designed to assist the international community in reducing drug consumption in an effort to deprive illegal drug traffickers of their largest source of revenue – the addicted, frequent, high volume drug user thereby reducing the income that criminal and terrorist organizations derive from narcotics trafficking and reducing threats to the health and welfare of fragile states.

FY 2011 Total Changes ($1.5 million): Funds will continue drug demand reduction project activities from FY 2010.

International Organizations

FY 2011 Request: $3.9 Million (Reflects No Change from FY 2010)

The FY 2011 drug control request will support the United Nations Office on Drugs and Crime (UNODC) and the Organization of American States/Inter-American Drug Abuse Control Commission (OAS/CICAD). These programs strengthen foreign government judicial and law enforcement capacity so they can attack drug trafficking and transnational crime groups directly by disrupting their organizations, arresting their leaders, and seizing their assets. Programs also enhance international cooperation among states and help close off safe havens to traffickers and other criminal groups.

FY 2011 Total Changes (no change): Funds will sustain FY 2010 UNODC and OAS/CICAD projects.

Program Development and Support

FY 2011 Request: $20.0 Million
(Reflects $2.7 Million Increase from FY 2010)

The FY 2011 drug control request will be used for domestic salaries, administrative costs, and other Washington based support services costs.

FY 2011 Total Changes (+$2.7 million): The increase of $2.7 million will be used for additional personnel, cover adjustments for inflation, and support other administrative support cost increases.

PERFORMANCE

Introduction

This section on the FY 2009 performance of the State INL programs is based on data reported in their 2008 Performance Plan and Reports (PPR), as available through FACTS Info which represents information provided by country missions.

It is important to note that in FACTS Info, data may not be consistently reported and also, composite data combines drug seizures, both of which lead to a somewhat inaccurate picture. For example, seizing one metric ton of cocaine should be perceived as a greater achievement than one metric ton of marijuana, but is not included in FACTS Info. The 2009 INCSR reports, to be released in March 2010, while based on host nation reports, will provide a more accurate picture of actual seizures, eradication, and coca cultivation in the Western Hemisphere and around the world.

The tables include performance measures, targets and achievements for the latest year for which data are available. This report includes selected program measures from the Western Hemisphere, Asia (Laos), and Afghanistan.

Bureau for International Narcotics and Law Enforcement Affairs		
Selected Measures of Performance	FY 2009 Target	FY2009Achieved
Andean Counterdrug Initiative		

(Continued).

Bureau for International Narcotics and Law Enforcement Affairs		
Selected Measures of Performance	FY 2009 Target	FY2009Achieved
» Number of Hectares (Ha) of coca eradicated in Bolivia, Colombia and Peru in Calendar Year 2009	214,000	188,951
INCLE		
» Number of Hectares (Ha) of illicit opium poppy cultivated in Laos for Calendar Year 2009	<1000	1,800
» Kilos of illicit narcotics seized by host governments in USG-assisted areas in the Western Hemisphere[2]	409,000	1,518,195
Assistance to Rebuilding Countries		
» Reduce cultivation of opium poppy in Afghanistan with the long-term goal of achieving a poppy-free North between 2005 and 2010 (21 out of 34 provinces)	7 poppy-free provinces (PFP) and 7 provinces reducing cultivation (PRC)	18 PFP and 12 PRC

[1] The "FY 2009 Achieved" data is as of December 9, 2009 from host-nation reports since partner countries report eradication on a calendar year basis. The FY 09 actuals reflect considerable under-reporting.

[2] The "FY 2009 Target" and "FY 2009 Achieved" figures are from FACTS-Info and combine all drugs seized.

Discussion

The long-term goal of the Andean Counterdrug Program (ACP) and International Narcotics and Law Enforcement (INCLE) appropriation is to reduce the flow of drugs to the United States, addressing instability in the Andean region and strengthening the ability of both source and transit countries to investigate and prosecute major drug trafficking organizations and their leaders and to block and seize their assets. Among other efforts, INL accomplishes this through aerial eradication, forced and voluntary manual eradication, increasing capabilities for drug interdiction, reducing demand and strengthening rule of law and alternative livelihood efforts.

Eradication is a critical component of the U.S. government's counternarcotics strategy in the Andean region but is not the only metric used in determining success. Eradication data are aggregated by calendar year rather than by fiscal year. Thus, eradication results available are as of December 9, 2009. The 2009 target was for eradication of 214,000 hectares in Bolivia, Colombia, and Peru. In 2009, the Department supported efforts that eradicated over 188,951 hectares (as of December 1) through aerial and manual eradication techniques.

Colombia is assuming greater responsibility for several U.S.-funded programs, enabling the USG to target critical areas through a more coordinated approach with security and alternative development programs. As of December 2009, Colombia eradicated 153,000 hectares of illicit crops – over 100,000 hectares through aerial eradication and over 53,000 hectares by manual eradication efforts. The number of hectares eradicated declined in 2009 because of Colombian budget constraints affecting manual eradication. The Colombian Government's capability to conduct interdiction, however, continues to increase; unofficial estimates for calendar year 2009 show that the 2008 figure will be surpassed by several tons.

Peru exceeded its coca eradication goal of 8,000 hectares for the second year in a row, eradicating over 10,000 hectares in 2009. As of October 2009, Peru seized approximately 17 metric tons of cocaine and destroyed 2,333 cocaine labs.

Also in 2009, Bolivia eradicated over 6,200 hectares of coca nationwide, about 95 percent of which took place in the Cochabamba tropics (Chapare) and Yapacani region. As of October 2009, Bolivia seized 23 metric tons of cocaine. Without a DEA presence in-country, Bolivia interdicted 3 fewer metric tons than the year before, largely due to a lack of enhanced international intelligence and operational support for interdiction forces.

Other efforts in the Western Hemisphere include the Mérida Initiative in Mexico and Central America and the Caribbean Basin Security Initiative, which is under development, as well as other programs in the Southern Cone. USG programs target the criminal organizations that profit from narcotics trafficking. These organizations pose a security threat to the region and the United States with their network of transnational crimes.

Throughout 2009, the Calderon Administration in Mexico continued the unprecedented efforts begun in December 2006 to curb the flow of drugs and curtail the power of drug cartels. In FY 2009, Mérida Mexico programs ramped up assistance to this effort. Despite violent reprisals, Mexican law enforcement arrested over 27,000 persons on drug-related offenses, and extradited over 100 persons from Mexico to the U.S.

As of November 2009, Mexican law enforcement seized 20 metric tons (MT) of cocaine, 788 MT of marijuana, 446 kilograms (kg) of opium gum, 261 kg of heroin, and 3,350 kg of methamphetamine. At the same time U.S. and Mexican law enforcement agencies caution that continued improvements in enforcement will force traffickers to seek alternate routes or alternative enterprises. Central American countries, especially Panama, Guatemala and Honduras, have already seen the violent results of increased criminal activity.

The long-term goal of the International Narcotics Control and Law Enforcement (INCLE) program in Southeast Asia is to remove all countries receiving U.S. assistance from the List of Major Drug Producing and Drug Transit Nations. Thailand was removed in 2004, with the goal of removing Laos prior to 2010. When opium poppy cultivation in Laos is estimated by the U.S. government as less than 1,000 hectares, the country will be removed from the President's list of major illicit drug producing countries. Laos made progress in reducing the number of hectares of opium poppy cultivation in 2007 (USG estimate: 1100 hectares, down from 1700 in 2006) but flat lined in 2008 and increased slightly in 2009. The situation remains precarious and the Department continues to focus on alternative development programs, law enforcement development, and demand reduction programs to support Lao efforts to reduce opium cultivation.

The purpose of the INCLE counternarcotics program in Afghanistan is to reduce opium poppy cultivation in order to create stability in Afghanistan and prevent it from becoming a narco-state controlled by insurgents. The goal of the program is to have 21 of Afghanistan's 34 provinces designated as poppy-free provinces (PFP) or provinces reducing cultivation (PRC) by 2010. The target for CY 2009 was to have 7 poppy free provinces and 7 provinces reducing cultivation. In CY 2009, Afghanistan exceeded its targets, achieving 18 poppy free provinces and 7 provinces reducing cultivation to less than 1000 hectares.

Budget Authority (in Millions)			
	FY 2009 Final	FY 2010 Enacted	FY 2011 Request
Drug Resources by Function			
International	$418.600	$365.132	$365.132
Total Drug Resources by Function	$418.600	$365.132	$365.132
Drug Resources by Decision Unit			
Developmental Assistance Account	$ 48.840	$ 45.271	$ 45.271
Economic Support Fund	276.760	319.861	319.861
Economic Support Fund Supplementals	93.000	-	-
Total Drug Resources by Decision Unit	$418.600	$365.132	$365.132
Drug Resources Personnel Summary			
Total FTEs (direct only)	27	27	27

Funding allocations for Department of State programs are subject to change as more and better information becomes available. The Department of State routinely adjusts its program allocations.

PROGRAM SUMMARY

Mission

The United States Agency for International Development (USAID) is the U.S. government organization responsible for most economic and development foreign aid. It receives overall foreign policy guidance from the US Secretary of the Department of State. USAID advances US foreign policy objectives by supporting economic growth, agriculture and trade, health, democracy, conflict prevention, and humanitarian assistance. USAID's Alternative Development programs support U.S. counternarcotics objectives by helping countries develop economic alternatives to narcotics production. Specifically, to stop the illegal drug trade, USAID offers incentives to farmers to discontinue planting poppy and other illicit crops, and USAID provides training; demonstration centers and farm related business training to help farmers in drug producing countries increase their income from legitimate crops. USAID also supports programs that create off farm employment, improve productive and social infrastructure in drug production areas, strengthen institutions, promote human rights, strengthen small and medium enterprises, improve access to credit, and expand state presence.

Budget

In FY 2011, the Department of State requests $365.1 million in the Economic Support Fund and Development Assistance accounts for Alternative Development (AD) programs in the Andean region and in Afghanistan.

Economic Support Funds and Development Assistance Funds - Andean Region

FY 2011 Request: $180.1 Million (Reflects No Change from FY 2010)

As the source of more than 90 percent of cocaine and about half of the heroin entering the U.S., Colombia and the Andean Region remain the focus of State's efforts to disrupt the market for illegal drugs. USAID administers the Economic Support Fund in Colombia and the Development Assistance (DA) Fund in Bolivia, Ecuador and Peru as sources of funding for alternative development projects and aid in the Andean Region. These resources support projects to advance the development of legitimate crops, legal enterprises and licit employment opportunities in lieu of illicit activities. Alternative Development (AD) funds also strengthen state institutions, support construction of productive and social infrastructure, expand state presence and strengthen community resolve to resist drug trafficking activities.

FY 2011 Total Changes (no change): The Budget will continue to support AD programs that are in alignment with the U.S. counternarcotics strategy in the region.

Economic Support Funds Afghanistan

FY 2011 Request: $185.0 Million (Reflects No Change from FY 2010)

Agriculture is a way of life for seventy percent of Afghanistan's people. However, instability, coupled with the region's four year drought has devastated the country's farms. In fact, eighty percent of the rural population lives in poverty. With its economic support, USAID is renovating irrigation systems, providing farmers with fertilizer and seeds, and is building roads to market centers. Over the past few years, licit agricultural production has nearly doubled, increasing farmers' incomes and encouraging them to produce legitimate crops. However, opium cultivation still occurs. To stop the illegal drug farming and trade, USAID provides alternative economic opportunities to farmers to incentives them to discontinue planting narcotic crops. USAID provides training, demonstration centers and farm related business training to farmers to help them increase their income from legitimate crops.

FY 2011 Total Changes (no change): USAID plans to continue support to a greater number of potential poppy producing provinces, continuing to support activities, such as: cash-for-work projects, availability of agricultural credit, and training and marketing assistance to help farmers increase their income from legitimate crops.

PERFORMANCE

Introduction

This section on the FY 2009 performance of the USAID program is based on agency GPRA documents and the OMB review. The table includes performance measures, targets and achievements for the latest year for which data are available.

USAID		
Selected Measures of Performance	FY 2009 Target	FY 2009 Achieved
»Number of community, producer groups, or associations that signed agreements to become and/or remain "coca-free"	1,554	2,495
» Number of USAID-assisted families that have signed or are included under "coca-free" agreements (cumulative)	242,000	248,764
» Hectares of opium poppies eradicated manually or voluntarily by Alternative Development partners in USAID target areas	n/a	n/a
» Hectares of licit agricultural crops developed or expanded in areas receiving USAID assistance (cumulative)	108,585	58,010
Number of new direct jobs created (agric.& non-agric.) in USAID-assisted areas (annual) »	21,179	46,875
»Increase in sales of licit farm and non-farm products in USAID-target areas of Afghanistan over previous year	23,000,000	169,183,934
»Number of rural households benefiting directly from USAID interventions in Afghanistan	130,000	888,094

Note: The targets for these measures are preliminary. the methodology for developing them is being refined for use in identifying future year targets.

Discussion

USAID/Afghanistan's AD Programs provided assistance to 13 provinces in FY 2009. The AD Program-South provided assistance in Helmand and Kandahar Provinces; the AD Program-North provided assistance in Badakhshan and Takhar provinces; the AD Program–East provided assistance in Kunar, Laghman, Nangarhar, and Nuristan provinces; and the AD Program – Northwest provided assistance in Farah Province. Substantial results have been achieved in FY 2009. An additional 58,010 hectares of alternative crops have been put under cultivation in FY 2009. More than 161,159 individuals have received agricultural, farm management, and business training benefiting over 888,094 families, including over 2,500 women and 47 women's organizations. This assistance has resulted in almost $169 million of increased sales of licit, higher-quality, farm products, much of which are exported to regional markets.

Assistance is helping these farmers to meet improved quantity, quality, and on-time delivery standards.

In the East, the number of families benefiting from alternative livelihoods rose by 12% (from 423,896 to 473,625), and sales of licit products increased by 47% (from $43.6 million to $65.3 million), while ADP programs in the North rehabilitated 95 km of roads and 31 km of irrigation canals, 2,558 families benefited from 63,338 days of labor, and an additional 7% above the target of 3,800 women received short term training in agricultural productivity. Cashfor-work constructed 134 km of roads, providing 88,760 labor days of work, 35, 638 farmers were trained in nursery and orchard management, 954 orchard families benefited from 28,000 paid labor days, sales increased $187,200 over the previous year, 31 veterinary clinics were built and staffed with a para-vet, and four feedlots were built that successfully fattened 720 ruminants on enriched silage.

The Alternative Development (AD) program in Colombia has helped rural families produce nearly 280,000 hectares of agricultural crops and has improved sustainable management practices on almost 260,000 hectares of forest land since 2001. This means that nearly 540,000 hectares of land are being used today for licit activities and are no longer available for production of drug crops.

The AD program in Peru has developed or expanded more than 120,000 hectares of licit crops (particularly cacao, palm oil, and coffee) since 2002, thus generating licit and sustainable livelihoods for over 78,000 families. AD-assisted crops generated over $10 million in sales at farm gate prices in FY 2009.

Bolivia's AD program helped exports of key crops grow by over 250% since 2001. Since 2005, the program has benefited over 42,000 families, and contributed to a significant reduction in poverty in the Yungas region (from 64% in 2004 to 52% in 2009).

The AD program in Ecuador has supported more than 37,000 hectares of legal agricultural crops since 2000 and provided assistance to more than 68 small, medium or large enterprises that created more than 2,700 licit jobs.

DEPARTMENT OF TRANSPORTATION

National Highway Traffic Safety Administration

Resource Summary

Budget Authority (in Millions)			
	FY 2009 Final	FY 2010 Enacted	FY 2011 Request
Drug Resources by Function			
Prevention	2.681	2.688	2.709
Total Drug Resources by Function	$2.681	$2.688	$2.709
Drug Resources by Decision Unit			
Drug Impaired Driving/1	2.681	2.688	$2.709
Total Drug Resources by Decision Unit	$2.681	$2.688	$2.709
Drug Resources Personnel Summary			
Total FTEs (direct only)	2	2	2
Drug Resources as a Percent of Budget			
Total Agency Budget (in Billions)	$0.9	$0.9	$0.9
Drug Resources Percentage	0.32%	0.31%	0.30%

[1] Includes $1.2 million of drug-related resources associated with SAFETEA-LU.

PROGRAM SUMMARY

Mission

The National Highway Traffic Safety Administration's (NHTSA) mission is to save lives, prevent injuries and reduce economic costs due to road traffic crashes, through education, research, safety standards and enforcement activity. The Drug Impaired Driving program contributes to this mission by supporting a range of initiatives intended to reduce impaired driving.

Budget

In FY 2011, NHTSA's budget request reflects $2.7 million for its drug impaired driving activities. Included in this request is $1.5 million for the Drug Impaired Driving program, as well as $1.2 million for drug impaired driving research, as included in Section 2013 of the Safe, Accountable, Flexible, Efficient, Transportation Equity Act: A Legacy for Users (SAFETEA.LU).

Drug Impaired Driving

Total FY 2011 Request: $2.7 Million (Reflects No Change from FY 2010)

The Drug Impaired Driving program, part of the agency's Impaired Driving program, supports infrastructure and sponsors research on the nature and incidence of the drug impaired driving problem. The program maintains and refines the Drug Evaluation and Classification infrastructure to enable accurate detection of drug impairment by trained law enforcement officers. Further, the program provides leadership, guidance and resources to assist states and communities to implement effective programs to reduce drug impaired driving. The program also provides technical assistance and training programs on drug impaired driving for prosecutors, judges and law enforcement officials.

Training

FY 2011 Request: $0.8 Million (Reflects No Change from FY 2010)

In FY 2010, the agency will use $0.8 million to complete the improvement of law enforcement training in the area of drug impaired driving. NHTSA is promoting and facilitating the adoption of the Advanced Roadside Impaired Driving Enforcement curriculum as an intermediate level of training to improve enforcement efforts by officers that are not Drug Recognition Experts (DREs). NHTSA will continue efforts to increase the use of Standardized Field Sobriety Test (SFST) training and application within States, as well as continue to train prosecutors, judges, and other appropriate criminal justice officials regarding drug impairment, detection, sanctions, and treatment options. Training of law enforcement, prosecutors and judges is essential to the success of this program, and as such, the agency will continue these efforts in FY 2011.

Data Collection

FY 2011 Request: $0.5 Million (Reflects No Change from FY 2010)

The $0.5 million in FY 2011 will support data collection efforts to determine the extent of the drug impaired driving problem and to better develop programs and potential countermeasures to address this problem. These objectives will be accomplished through uniform and timely data collection by Drug Recognition Expert (DRE) officers nationwide. This system will provide the data needed to identify trends in drug impaired driving incidents, evaluate the DEC program, and provide information to support federal and state drug impaired driving programs. The system will be internetbased and accessible to law enforcement, toxicologists, prosecutors, NHTSA, and Highway Safety Offices to enter, review, collate and access data relating to drug impaired driving arrests.

Public Information and Outreach

FY 2011 Request: $0.2 Million (Reflects No Change from FY 2010)

The $0.2 million in FY 2011 will support public information and outreach efforts. NHTSA will continue to partner with the International Association of Chiefs of Police (IACP) to support the *Drunk Driving, Over the Limit, Under Arrest* message. NHTSA will accomplish this by offering effective strategies to increase the number of arrests, decrease DWI incidents, increase deterrence, and track and coordinate impaired driving training programs (SFST, ARIDE, and DEC).

In further support of public information and outreach efforts, NHTSA will work with the Community Anti-Drug Coalitions of America to incorporate traffic safety messages into the existing network of community coalitions, with particular focus on alcohol and substance abuse prevention, treatment, and recovery. With this partnership, the agency seeks to provide technical support to coordinate impaired driving messaging through the State and Regional Highway Safety Offices, gain wider distribution of the agency's drug fact sheets for specific audiences (i.e., parents, youth, older drivers, coalitions), and increase support for the national impaired driving crackdowns.

Furthermore, the agency will continue efforts to develop a model statute for States relating to drug-impaired driving, and to coordinate with other Federal agencies. NHTSA will continue to work with IACP and CADCA in FY 2011 to provide technical assistance, training, and effective deterrence strategies.

SAFETEA-LU

FY 2011 Request: $1.2 Million
(Reflects No Change from FY 2010)

Section 2013 of SAFETEA-LU authorizes groundbreaking research on the incidence of drug use among drivers – an area where data is currently extremely limited. In FY 2011 NHTSA will conduct a case-control study to determine the crash risk associated with driving under the influence of drugs other than alcohol.

PERFORMANCE

Introduction

This section on the FY 2009 performance of the Drug Impaired Driving Program is based on agency GPRA documents, the Budget Request, and other agency information. No OMB Assessment has been undertaken of this program.

The program contributes to the Department's long-term goal of reducing the highway fatality rate to no more than 1.0 per 100 million vehicle miles traveled by the end of 2011.

Drug Impaired Driving Program		
Selected Measures of Performance	FY2009 Target	FY2009 Achieved
» Develop and recommend methods for detecting major illegal drugs in drivers.	Detection of at least 5 drugs	No technologies currently exist for detecting drugs

Discussion

NHTSA is undertaking several projects to assess the problem of drug impaired driving. Current NHTSA projects focus on: Methods for detecting illegal drugs, the Roadside Survey of Drug and Alcohol Use By Drivers, and developing procedures for a Case Control Study of the Crash Risk of Drug-Impaired Drivers.

The agency recently completed analysis of the Roadside Survey of Alcohol and Drug Use by Drivers - this survey provides the first nationally representative estimate of drug use among driver populations. These findings will be used to guide future program development and will lead to critical further research regarding the role of drugs in crash causation.

In FY 2009, NHTSA convened an expert group to identify and recommend methods for detecting the presence of major illegal drugs in drivers. The expert group concluded that such technology was not feasible for roadside use in the near future. Therefore, the agency redirected research efforts toward the development of methods to identify drugs that impair driving. The FY 2009 target was not achieved because of this change in research strategy.

In FY 2010, NHTSA will complete a study design and procedures for a Case Control Study of the Crash Risk of Drug-Impaired Drivers. In conjunction with the recently completed Roadside Survey of Drug and Alcohol Use by Drivers, this study will provide key information on drug impairment as a causal factor in crashes. In FY 2011, NHTSA will collect data from 1250 crashes for the Case Control Study, which will mark the halfway point of this study.

Together, these achievements reflect the agency's progress in obtaining essential information for the development of effective countermeasures to drug impaired driving.

Department of the Treasury

Internal Revenue Service

Resource Summary

Budget Authority (in Millions)			
	FY 2009 Final	FY 2010 Enacted	FY 2011 Request
Drug Resources by Function			
Investigations	$60.627	$59.157	$60.349
Total Drug Resources by Function	$60.627	$59.157	$60.349
Drug Resources by Decision Unit			

Budget Authority (in Millions)			
	FY 2009 Final	FY 2010 Enacted	FY 2011 Request
Criminal Investigations	$60.627	$59.157	$60.349
Total Drug Resources by Decision Unit	$60.627	$59.157	$60.349
Drug Resources Personnel Summary			
Total FTEs (direct only)	329	329	329
Drug Resources as a Percent of Budget			
Total Agency Budget (in Billions)	$11.5	$12.1	$12.6
Drug Resources Percentage	0.527%	0.489%	0.479%

Program Summary

Mission

The mission of the IRS Criminal Investigation (CI) Division in federal law enforcement's anti-drug efforts is to reduce or eliminate the financial gains (profits) of major narcotics trafficking and money laundering organizations through the use of unique financial investigative expertise and statutory jurisdiction. These efforts support the goals of the *National Drug Control Strategy* and the *National Money Laundering Strategy*.

CI supports the overall IRS mission by the investigation of criminal violations under its jurisdiction through three program areas: the Legal Income Source Program, the Illegal Income Source Program, and the Narcotics Program. The Narcotics Program supports the National Drug Control Strategy and the National Money Laundering Strategy through continued support of multiagency task forces including Organized Crime Drug Enforcement Task Force (OCDETF), OCDETF Fusion Center (OFC), High Intensity Drug Trafficking Area (HIDTA), and the High Risk Money Laundering and Financial Crimes Areas (HIFCA).

Budget

The total drug control request for the IRS for FY 2011 is $60.4 million, a net increase of $1.2 million over the FY 2010 enacted.

Criminal Investigations

Total FY 2011 Request: $60.4 Million (Reflects $1.2 Million Increase from FY 2010)

The criminal provisions of the Internal Revenue Code (Title 26), the Bank Secrecy Act (Title 31) and the Money Laundering Control Act are particularly useful in the financial investigation (and prosecution) of major narcotics traffickers and money launderers, and the seizure and forfeiture of their profits. CI plays an important role in reducing and disrupting the supply of illegal drugs as a participating member of the OCDETF Program. CI utilizes unique financial skills in the investigation of major drug trafficking and money laundering organizations. By primarily focusing on those sophisticated cases which meet OCDETF designation standards, CI makes a significant contribution to many important investigations, while maximizing the use of its resources. With the globalization of the U.S. economy and the increasing use of electronic funds transfers, investigations have become more international in scope. CI's international strategy places special agents in strategic foreign posts to facilitate the development and use of information obtained in host nations in support of its investigations.

FY 2011 Total Changes (+$1.2 million): The resources of $60.4 million reflects a price growth increase, allow the agency to continue as a member of the OCDETF program.

Performance

Introduction

This section on the FY 2009 performance of the drug control mission of IRS - Criminal Investigation (CI) division's portion of the OCDETF program - is based on agency GPRA documents, an OMB assessment, and other agency information.

The FY 2009 performance information for the IRS CI OCDETF program is shown below.

IRS Criminal Investigation		
Selected Measures of Performance	FY2009 Target	FY2009 Achieved
» Number of investigations completed for OCDETF cases	710	652
» Numberof Convictions	460	462
» Conviction Rate	85%	85%

Discussion

The Internal Revenue Service's Criminal Investigation Division (CI) supports the President's National Drug Control Strategy by dedicating 11% to 13% of total Direct Investigative Time (DIT) to investigation of narcotics related crimes. CI's goal is to use 90% of this DIT through participation in the OCDETF Program. The number of OCDETF Investigations Completed are slightly lower at 652 from the target range of 710, reflecting an 11.6% drop in the OCDETF pipeline inventory from 873 in FY08 to 772 in FY09.

Significant accomplishments during FY 2009 include the successful investigation and indictment of a key defendant on a variety of drug, money laundering, and tax evasion charges. The defendant was convicted of being the leader of a Continuing Criminal Enterprise; conspiracy to possess with the intent to distribute marijuana; conspiracy to commit money laundering; and possession with the intent to distribute marijuana. The sentence includes 20 years in Federal Prison and a $10 million judgment. These drug trafficking offenses were part of a 70-count superseding indictment related to his leadership of a 12-year conspiracy involving the distribution of over 30,000 kilograms of marijuana worth more than $33 million.

Other successes included the sentencing of two Internet pharmacy owners to a five year sentence with an order to pay over $11 million for illegal sales of 10 million worth of hydrocodone pills. The two defendants were illegally selling 9,936,075 pills or dosage units of hydrocodone over the Internet, conspiracy to launder money, engaging in monetary transactions using the proceeds of the illegal drug sales, and filing false tax returns. Additionally, each defendant was ordered to pay $11,870,119 in restitution, which according to court documents, amounted to the gross proceeds derived from the illegal sale of the hydrocodone.

On April 27, 2009, in Columbia, S.C., fourteen defendants were sentenced to prison for their roles in an interstate drug smuggling and money laundering enterprise. The drug organization used several residences to store and sell narcotics, and used vehicles with hidden compartments to transport drugs and money between Columbia and Atlanta. In addition to the prison sentences listed above, the defendants were ordered to forfeit $650,000 in cash, cars, firearms, and other assets used in the conspiracy or purchased with drug money. Some of the defendants, who were in the United States illegally, will be deported following the service of their sentence. The investigation was a joint effort under the OCDETF.

In addition, IRS CI supports the Southwest Border Strategy through OCDETF by providing resources to investigate Mexican Drug Trafficking Organizations (DTOs). A significant number of investigations in the Southwest Region are linked to major Mexican DTOs. CI focuses on identifying and dismantling the financial systems that support the drug trade, and seizing the assets and profits of major criminal organizations. CI dedicates significantly higher resources to field offices along the Southwest border than to non-border field offices. Field offices located along the Southwest Border completed 271, or 41.7%, of the 650 OCDETF investigations completed in FY 2009. The Southwest Border field offices had 192 of the 462 convictions, with an average conviction rate of 78%.

Department of Veterans Affairs

Veterans Health Administration

Resource Summary

Budget Authority (in Millions)			
	FY 2009 Final	FY 2010 Enacted	FY 2011 Request[1]
Drug Resources by Function			
Treatment	$377.751	$389.839	$402.704
Research and Development	15.034	15.184	15.336
Total Drug Resources by Function	$392.785	$405.023	$418.040
Drug Resources by Decision Unit			
Medical Care	$377.751	$389.839	$402.704
Research and Development	$15.034	$15.184	$15.336
Total Drug Resources by Decision Unit	$392.785	$405.023	$418.040
Drug Resources Personnel Summary			
Total FTEs (direct only)	2,764	2,764	2,764
Drug Resources as a Percent of Budget			
Total Agency Budget (in Billions)	$ 99.793	$ 114.035	$ 125.004
Drug Resources Percentage	0.39%	0.36%	0.33%

[1] FY 2011 amounts are enacted levels, provided t hrough advance appropriations by Public Law. 111-118.

Program Summary

Mission

The Veterans Health Administration's (VHA) mission statement is "Honor America's Veterans by providing exceptional care that improves their health and well being." Care for Veterans with mental illnesses and substance use disorders is an important part of overall health care. The goal of VHA's Office of Mental Health Services is to provide effective, safe, efficient, recovery oriented, and compassionate care for those with substance use disorders and mental illness, for those who are vulnerable to substance use disorders, and for those who are in continuing care to sustain recovery.

Consistent with ONDCP guidance, programs and costs described herein will be limited to those services provided in SUD Specialty Treatment.

Methodology

Specialized Treatment Costs

VA's drug budget includes all costs generated for the treatment of patients with drug use disorders treated in specialized substance abuse treatment programs. This budget accounts for drug related costs for VHA Medical Care and Research. The costs do not include those for treatment of substance disorders in general mental health care settings or in other non specialty SUD programs. It does not encompass all of drug related costs for the agency. VA incurs costs related to accounting and security of narcotics and other controlled substances and costs of law enforcement related to illegal drug activity; however, these costs are assumed to be relatively small and would not have a material effect on the aggregate VA costs reported.

As of this submission, Sustained Treatment & Rehabilitation (STAR) program costs have been removed from medical care and treatment actual and estimates for all years. This category has been deleted because these programs serve a broad category of Veterans with significant mental health problems. Although STAR programs, no doubt, include some Veterans with chronic drug abuse or dependence problems, they are not specific to this type of care. As a result, the resource summary reflects this change to the inpatient costs.

Decision Support System

The funding levels are based on costs using the Decision Support System (DSS) which is the official Managerial Cost Accounting System for VA. DSS maps cost to departments, which are then assigned to one of 56,000 intermediate products using Relative Value Units (RVU). Relative Value Units are defined as the determining factor of how much resources it takes to produce an intermediate product. Each Cost Category, for example Fixed Direct Labor or Variable Labor, has an RVU for each intermediate product. All intermediate products are assigned to an actual patient encounter, either inpatient or outpatient, using the patient care data bases. In DSS, the costs are not averaged; rather they are reported by the total of the encounters and can be drilled down to a specific patient.

Also, DSS includes all overhead costs assigned to a facility to include Headquarters, National programs and Network Costs. DSS does not include the costs of capital expenditures; however, it does account for depreciation costs.

Budget

For FY 2011, VHA estimates $418.0 million, which is an increase of $13.0 million from the FY 2010 enacted level.

Medical Care

Total FY 2011 Request: $402.7 Million
(Reflects $12.8 Million Increase from FY 2010)

The Veterans Health Administration, in keeping with modern medical practice, continues to improve service delivery and to provide clinically appropriate care by expanding delivery of substance use disorder services in primary care and shifting delivery of substance use disorder services to ambulatory settings when this is medically appropriate. Within services for Veterans with substance use disorders, this has involved a substantial shift over the past 20 years or so from inpatient to outpatient and residential care settings.

Efforts are continuing to integrate care. Increasingly, mental health and substance use services are being provided in primary care and in non-substance use disorder specialty mental health treatment settings. As a result of this integration of substance use services with other components of care, it is increasingly difficult to disaggregate the costs of care for substance related conditions from costs for other components of care. Accordingly, it must be recognized that the above figure represents solely the cost for care in substance use disorder specialty settings.

Reaching Special Populations

The Uniform Mental Health Services Handbook, approved by the Under Secretary of the Veterans Health Administration on September 11, 2009, specifies substance use disorder services that must be made available to all Veterans in need of them. Secondary prevention services are highlighted among these and include diagnosis and assessment of possible drug abuse problems in patients who receive care in VA mental health clinics or whose presenting medical problem suggests risk of substance abuse (e.g. treatment for Hepatitis C or HIV or care provided in an emergency department for trauma).

Three special populations are targets of particular VA substance use disorder prevention and treatment efforts: service members returned from Iraq and Afghanistan and eligible for VHA services; patients receiving care in Mental Health Residential Rehabilitation Treatment Programs (MH-RRTPs); and patients having Post Traumatic Stress Disorder.

Returning Veterans from OEF/OIF

Interagency efforts with the Department of Defense are underway to assure that newly redeployed Veterans who are referred to VA based on results of their Post Deployment Health Reassessment (PDHRA) are seen quickly by VHA and that results of the PDHRAs are available to mental health care providers in VA.

Patients in Residential Rehabilitation Treatment Programs

VHA offers care in Mental Health Residential Rehabilitation Treatment Programs (MH-RRTPs) to Veterans suffering a range of mental health concerns. Many of these programs are designated as "Substance Abuse RRTPs" and focus on substance use disorder services. Patients receiving care in other types of MH-RRTPs also typically have substance use disorder diagnoses and are at risk for relapse. VHA is now providing each of its "non Substance Abuse" MH RRTPs (that average a census of at least 40 patients) a full time substance use disorder specialist to provide a range of substance use disorder clinical services. These services include substance abuse specific treatment while in the MH RRTP, relapse prevention services, and arrangement of substance abuse treatment follow up services after MH RRTP discharge.

Patients with Post Traumatic Stress Disorder

In light of the frequent co occurrence of substance use disorder problems with Post Traumatic Stress Disorder, VHA is also assigning a full time substance use disorder specialist to each of its hospital level PTSD services or teams. The staff person is an integral member of the PTSD clinical services team and works to integrate substance use disorder care with all other aspects of PTSD related care. Among the position's responsibilities are identification of Veterans in the early stages of a substance use disorder or who are at risk for developing a problem and provision of services to prevent substance abuse.

Increased Treatment Capacity in Targeted Areas

Access to care is also emphasized by the Uniform Mental Health Services Handbook and, as noted, the Handbook commits the VA to providing substance use disorder treatment services to every eligible Veteran regardless of where he or she lives. Additionally, the Handbook specifies that a contact be made by the substance use disorder program within 24 hours of the time care is sought and that a comprehensive assessment be made within 14 days of the initial contact. To further enhance access to substance use disorder treatment, clinics offering these services must offer evening or weekend hours.

Treatment Across the Criminal Justice System – Guiding the Effectiveness of Drug Courts

Interaction with Veterans served by Drug Courts will occur through the Veterans Justice Outreach (VJO) initiative. The Uniform Mental Health Services Handbook affirmed that "Police encounters and pretrial court proceedings are often missed opportunities to connect Veterans with VA mental health services as a negotiated alternative to incarceration or other criminal sanctions." On April 30, 2009, the Under Secretary for Health released "Information and Recommendations for Services Provided by VHA Facilities to Veterans in the Criminal Justice System" (IL 10 2009 005), stating that justice involved Veterans (who are not incarcerated) are as eligible for VA services as those without justice involvement. On May 27, 2009, the Deputy Under Secretary for Health for Operations and Management issued a memorandum requiring VA medical centers to provide outreach to justice involved Veterans in the communities they serve.

In communities where justice programs relevant to Veterans exist (Veterans Courts, Drug Courts, Mental Health Courts, and police Crisis Intervention Teams), VA will take the initiative in building working relationships to assure that eligible justice involved Veterans get needed care. In communities where no such programs exist, VA will reach out to potential justice system partners (judges, prosecutors, police and jail administrators) to connect eligible justice involved Veterans with VA services.

Currently, the VA participates in eight Veterans Court programs located in Santa Ana, CA, Buffalo, NY, Anchorage, AK, San Bernardino, CA, Santa Clara, CA, Chicago, IL,

Rochester, NY, and Tulsa, OK. Elsewhere, VA medical centers have established relationships with a range of justice system and community partners, including police and sheriffs' departments, local jail administrators, judges, prosecutors, public defenders, probation officers, and community mental health providers.

FY 2011 Total Changes (+$13.0 million): The changes are the result of anticipated cost for pay raises and inflation. The majority of VHA's funding goes to support outpatient and residential rehabilitation and treatment services. The Department of Veterans Affairs, through its Veterans Health Administration, operates a national network of substance abuse treatment programs located in the Department's medical centers, residential rehabilitation facilities, and outpatient clinics.

Research and Development

Total FY 2011 Request: $15.3 Million (Reflects $0.2 Increase from FY 2011)

VHA research supports generation of new knowledge to improve prevention, diagnosis, and treatment of substance use disorders as well as to heighten effectiveness, efficiency, accessibility, and quality of Veterans' health care.

Research & Development currently has ongoing projects on drug and alcohol abuse. Topics of investigation range from alcoholism, aging, and brain functions to cognitive factors and relapse in chronic alcoholism to donepezil effects on cocaine craving and pharmacokinetics to neurobehavioral effects of cocaine.

FY 2011 Total Changes (+$0.2 million): The changes are the result of anticipated pay raises and inflation.

PERFORMANCE

This section on the FY 2009 performance is based on agency Government Performance and Results Act (GPRA) documents, an OMB assessment, and other agency information. The table includes performance measures, target and achievement for the latest year for which data are available. VHA reports performance for two separate drug-related initiatives: (1) health care and (2) research and development.

VHA has in place a national system of performance monitoring that uses social, professional, and financial incentives to encourage facilities to provide the highest quality health care. This system has begun to incorporate performance measures related to substance use disorder treatment.

The dollars expended in VHA research help to acquire new knowledge to improve the prevention, diagnosis, and treatment of disease. These funds also generate new knowledge to improve the effectiveness, efficiency, accessibility, and quality of veterans' health care.

Veterans Health Administration		
Selected Measures of Performance	FY 2009 Target	FY 2009 Achieved
Medical Care		
» Percent of clients receiving appropriate continuity of care	47%	52%

(Continued).

Veterans Health Administration		
Selected Measures of Performance	FY 2009 Target	FY 2009 Achieved
Research and Development		
» Number of research studies related to substance use disorder	5	20
» Number of research studies related to alcohol abuse	5	45
» Number of research studies related to both substance use disorder and alcohol abuse	NA	10

Discussion

VA provides three types of 24-hour-a-day care to patients having particularly severe substance use disorders. Two inpatient programs offer acute care, detoxification, and initial stabilization services. Such specialized inpatient treatment for substance use disorders has become rare in VA, just as it has in other parts of the healthcare system, and the remaining substance use disorder inpatient programs in the VA are currently in the process of transitioning into residential rehabilitation programs. These join the large set of 24- hour care settings already classified as residential rehabilitation treatment programs. Finally, 24-hour care is provided for detoxification in numerous inpatient medical and general mental health units throughout the VA system.

Most veterans with substance use disorders are treated in outpatient programs. Intensive substance use disorder outpatient programs provide more than three hours of service per day to each patient, and patients attend them three or more days per week. Standard outpatient programs typically treat patients for an hour or two per treatment day, and patients attend one or two days a week.

In FY 2009, VHA provided services to 114,457 patients with a drug diagnosis, of whom 38 percent used cocaine, 19 percent used opioids, 23 percent used cannabis, and 75 percent had coexisting psychiatric diagnoses. (These categories are not mutually exclusive.)

VHA is steadily expanding the availability of opioid agonist treatment for opioid-dependent veterans. A total of 189 points of care offer buprenorphine treatment, which reflects an increase of 41 new sites in the past year.

VA has implemented a major initiative to create primary care-oriented buprenorphine clinics to increase access to care for opiate-dependent veterans. VA is in the process of implementing initiatives to expand access to intensive outpatient services and to include substance use disorder specialists in large community-based outpatient clinics, mental health residential rehabilitation programs, and services for homeless veterans.

Data collected using the 2008 *Drug and Alcohol Program Survey* (DAPS) was made available in FY 2009 and showed that VA expanded the scope, intensity, and accessibility of substance use disorder treatment services since the comparable 2006 DAPS survey. At the end of Fiscal Year 2008, the Department of Veterans Affairs operated a national network of 260 substance use disorder treatment programs located in the Department's medical centers, mental health residential rehabilitation treatment programs and outpatient clinics.

Current programs consist of 2 medical inpatient programs, 73 residential rehabilitation programs, 112 intensive outpatient programs, and 73 standard outpatient programs. (It should be noted that identification of these programs involves a "roll up" procedure. Lower intensity programs are not counted separately from a higher intensity level program if the lower level intensity program functions as an integrated component of the higher intensity program.)

Based on on-going assessment activities, as of the end of 2009, 12 additional intensive outpatient substance use disorder programs have been added since the 2008 DAPS.

VA is currently conducting a one-year demonstration study at 41 intensive outpatient substance use disorder treatment programs to anticipate and resolve issues that would surround systemwide utilization of the Brief Addiction Monitor (BAM). Efforts involved in the study include monthly conference calls with staff of the demonstration sites, ongoing consultation between them and the VA Center of Excellence for Substance Abuse Treatment and Education in Philadelphia, development of tool kits and responses to "Frequently Asked Questions." An electronic reminder in the medical record has been developed to alert substance use disorder treatment providers to administer the BAM.

IV. Appendices

Other Related Drug Control Funding by Agency

FY2009 –FY2011
(Budget Authority in Millions)

	FY2009 Final	FY2010 Enacted	FY2011 Request
Department of Agriculture			
U.S. Forest Service	15.4	15.4	15.9
Food and Nutrition Service	27.4	29.0	30.4
Total Department of Agriculture	$42.8	$44.4	$46.3
Corporation for National and Community Service	7.2	9.0	11.3
Court Services and Offender Supervision Agency	43.3	43.8	44.0
Department of Health and Human Services			
Administration for Children and Families	30.0	20.0	20.0
Centers for Disease Control and Prevention	10.1	10.1	9.9
National Institute on Alcohol Abuse and Alcoholism	45.5	46.7	42.7
Total Department of Health and Human Services	$85.6	$76.8	$72.6
Department of Homeland Security			
U.S. Secret Service	16.5	17.3	18.1
Federal Law Enforcement Training Center	50.0	48.6	48.7
Total Department of Homeland Security	$66.5	$65.9	$66.8
Department of the Interior			
Bureau of Land Management	7.2	7.2	7.2
National Park Service	7.3	7.3	7.3

(Continued).

	FY2009 Final	FY2010 Enacted	FY2011 Request
Department of Agriculture			
Indian Police Academy	0.5	0.5	0.5
Total Department of the Interior	$15.0	$15.0	$15.0
The Federal Judiciary			
Administrative Office of the U.S. Courts	1,110.5	1,186.9	1,262.4
Department of Justice			
Assets Forfeiture Fund	194.9	186.6	186.6
Alcohol, Tobacco, and Firearms	175.1	185.1	193.1
U.S. Attorneys	679.3	706.5	733.4
Bureau of Prisons	3,200.0	3,204.0	3,449.0
Community Oriented Policing Services	536.9	284.6	217.3
Criminal Division	38.2	41.0	43.0
Federal Bureau of Investigations	140.6	143.4	158.4
Office of Federal Detention Trustee	497.4	565.4	599.7
INTERPOL	0.2	0.2	0.2
U.S. Marshals Service	229.5	273.9	287.6
Total Department of Justice	$5,707.1	$5,590.7	$5,868.3
Department of Labor			
Internal Drug□Free Workplace	0.1	0.1	0.1
Job Corps	6.1	6.2	6.2
Working Partners	0.4	0.0	0.0
Total Department of Labor	$6.6	$6.3	$6.3
Department of State			
Emergencies in the Diplomatic and Consular Service	1.0	0.0	0.0
Department of Transportation			
Federal Aviation Administration	26.4	27.7	28.9
Total	$7,097.0	$7,066.5	$7,421.6

Acknowledgments

Department of Defense
Dario Izquierdo
MAJ Anne-Marie Garcia
Sandra Lawson
Silvia Serban
CDR Tedd Shellenbarger

Department of Education
Larry Cohen
Thomas M. Corwin
William Modzeleski
Deborah Rudy
Thomas P. Skelly

Department of Health and Human Services
Peter Bernardy
Jillian Curtis

Department of Homeland Security
Nichole Brown
Jonathan Evans
Otis France
Aaron Hauer
Barbara Kelly
Wallace Lloyd
Mitchel Martin
Ryan Mitchell
Jessica Reyes
Tracey Wade
Marsha Williams

Office of Counternarcotics Enforcement
Paul Cheshire
Scott Chronister
Bruce Lichtman

Customs and Border Protection
Jules Andersen
Thierry Curtis
Rod Field
Patty Howell
Lisa Kuzma
John Meckley

National Drug Intelligence Center
David J. Mrozowski
Cheryl A. Leleck
Tracy L. Hall

Organized Crime Drug Enforcement Task Force
Simshindo Msola
Jill Aronica
Gene Hausler

Peter Maxey

Office of Justice Programs
Kashan Alamin
Mark Kline

Small Business Administration
Rachel Newman Karton
David Lippold

Department of State
Anthony Gresko
Angela Jeffries
T. David Johnston
Aimee Martin
Anthony Mazzoccoli
Melissa Patsalides
Robinson Ramirez
Laiza Reidenbach
Angelic Young

Department of Transportation
Jeffrey Michael
Melanie O'Donnell

Department of the Treasury
Ronald Pyszczynski

Department of Veterans Affairs
Calvin Seay
John Paul Allen
Mark Yow

Office of Management and Budget
Lisa August
Peter Babb
James Boden
Robert Bullock
Shawn Choy
David Connelly
Michael Crowley
Neil Danberg
Dinee Eriksen
Edna Falk-Curtin
David Harmon
Max Ann Kendrall

Adrian Mathura
Laurie Mignone
Jeptha Nafziger
Kim Newman
John Quinlan
Maria Raphael
Shannon Richter
Narahari Sastry
Tricia Schmitt
Gretchen Trygstad

Office of National Drug Control Policy
Genevieve Beaman
Andree Clark
Meredith DeFraites
Phuong DeSear
Carlos Dublin
VerLyn Francisco
Dan Grayson
Thomas Johnson
Alan Levitt
Mike Lowther
Annie Millar
Richelle Perazich
Michael Reles
Jon Rice
Jane Sanville
June Sivilli
Jack Stein

GLOSSARY

Actuals - A common term used to refer to data on actual performance compared to goals.

Baselines - The starting point from which change is measured and targets are set.

Budget Authority - Authority provided by law to incur financial obligations that will result in outlays.

Demand Reduction - Activities conducted by a National Drug Control Program agency, other than law enforcement, intended to reduce the willingness of individuals to use illicit drugs. Demand reduction activities include drug use education; drug abuse prevention; drug abuse treatment; drug abuse research; drug abuse rehabilitation; drug-free workplace programs; and, drug-testing.

Domestic Law Enforcement - A Drug Control Budget category that combines resources for the following functional units: investigations, intelligence, state and local assistance, and law enforcement research.

Drug Budget Decision Unit - Drug budget decision units correspond to discrete program categories that are identifiable components of budget accounts enumerated in the Budget of the President.

Drug Control Functions - Drug control functions correspond to the nine specific program areas that encompass all possible drug control activities: (1) Prevention; (2) Treatment; (3) Interdiction; (4) International; (5) Investigations; (6) Intelligence; (7) State and Local Assistance; (8) Research and Development; and, (9) Prosecution.

Drug Methodology - The process by which drug-related financial statistics identified for certain agencies or bureaus are calculated. The following bureaus utilize a drug methodology for calculating their aggregate portion of the National Drug Control Budget: Customs and Border Protection; Immigration and Customs Enforcement; U.S. Coast Guard; Centers for Medicare & Medicaid Services; Indian Health Service; Bureau of Indian Affairs; and Veterans Health Administration. All bureaus utilize a drug methodology for presenting their drug budget by drug control function.

Efficiency Measures - Metrics that indicate what outcomes or outputs are realized for a given level of resource use.

Enacted - The drug-related budget authority approved by Congress for the current fiscal year.

Final - The drug-related budget authority approved by Congress, net of rescissions and transfers, for the fiscal year most recently closed.

Fiscal Year - The fiscal year is the Federal Government's accounting period. It begins on October 1st and ends on September 30th. For example, fiscal year 2010 begins on October 1, 2009, and ends on September 30, 2010.

Full-time Equivalents (FTEs) - Civilian employment in the Executive Branch is measured on the basis of full-time equivalents. One FTE is equal to one fiscal work year. Thus, one full-time employee counts as one FTE, and two half-time employees also count as one FTE.

Intelligence - Activities or programs with a primary focus to provide guarded information for use by national policy makers, strategic planners, or operational/tactical elements, principally in the areas of national security and law enforcement. Activities include collecting, processing, analyzing, and disseminating information related to drug production and trafficking organizations and their activities (including transportation, distribution, and finance/money laundering). Additional activities include assessing the willingness and ability of foreign governments to carry out effective drug control programs.

Interdiction - Activities designed to interrupt the trafficking of illicit drugs into the United States by targeting the transportation link. Specifically, interdiction involves intercepting and ultimately disrupting shipments of illegal drugs, their precursors, and the profits of drug distribution.

International - Activities primarily focused on areas outside of the United States, including a wide range of drug control programs to eradicate crops, seize drugs (except air and marine interdiction seizures), arrest and prosecute major traffickers, destroy processing capabilities, develop and promote alternative crops to replace drug crops, reduce the demand for drugs, investigate money laundering and financial crime activities, and promote the involvement of other nations in efforts to control the supply of and demand for illicit drugs.

Investigations - Federal domestic law enforcement activities engaged in preparing drug cases for the arrest and prosecution of leaders and traffickers of illegal drug organizations, seizing drugs and assets, and ensuring that federal laws and regulations governing the legitimate handling, manufacturing, and distribution of controlled substances are properly followed.

National Drug Control Program Agency - An agency that is responsible for implementing any aspect of the *National Drug Control Strategy*, including any agency that receives Federal funds to implement any aspect of the *National Drug Control Strategy,* but does not include any agency that receives funds for a drug control activity solely under the National Foreign Intelligence Program, the Joint Military Intelligence Program, or Tactical Intelligence and Related Activities, unless such agency has been designated – (A) by the President; or (B) jointly by the Director [of ONDCP] and the head of the agency.

Outcome Measures - The intended result or impact of carrying out a program or activity. Outcomes may relate to society as a whole or to the specific beneficiaries of programs, depending on the size and reach of the program.

Output Measures - Metrics that indicate the goods and services produced by a program or organization and provided to the public or others.

Performance Measures - Indicators or metrics that are used to gauge program performance. Performance measures can be either outcome or output measures.

Prevention - Activities focused on discouraging the first-time use of controlled substances and outreach efforts to encourage those who have begun to use illicit drugs to cease their use.

Prosecution - Federal activities related to the conduct of criminal proceedings against drug trafficking and money laundering organizations, with the aim of bringing a civil or criminal judgment against their members, forfeiting their assets, divesting leaders of their power, and, as appropriate, extraditing, deporting, and excluding their members.

Request - The budget authority proposed in the budget of the President, which is submitted to Congress for consideration on the first Monday in February of every year.

Research and Development - Activities intended to improve the capacity, efficiency, or quality of drug control activities.

State and Local Assistance - Federal drug control assistance to help state and local law enforcement entities reduce drug-related violent crime and the availability of illegal drugs.

Supply Reduction - Any activity or program conducted by a National Dug Control Program agency intended to reduce the availability of drugs in the United States and abroad. Supply reduction activities include international drug control; foreign and domestic drug intelligence; interdiction; and, domestic law enforcement.

Targets - Quantifiable or otherwise measurable characteristics that tell how well a program must accomplish a specific performance measure.

Treatment - Activities focused on assisting regular users of controlled substances to become drug-free through such means as counseling services, in-patient and out-patient care, and the demonstration and provision of effective treatment modalities.

INDEX

A

B

C

F

G

H

I

J

L

M

N

O

P

T

U

V

W

X

Y